Stress, Catecholamines, and Cardiovascular Disease

Stress, Catecholamines, and Cardiovascular Disease

DAVID S. GOLDSTEIN

New York   Oxford   OXFORD UNIVERSITY PRESS   1995

Oxford University Press

Oxford   New York   Toronto
Delhi   Bombay   Calcutta   Madras   Karachi
Kuala Lumpur   Singapore   Hong Kong   Tokyo
Nairobi   Dar es Salaam   Cape Town
Melbourne   Auckland   Madrid

and associated companies in
Berlin   Ibadan

Copyright © 1995 by Oxford University Press, Inc.

Published by Oxford University Press, Inc.,
200 Madison Avenue, New York, New York 10016

Oxford is a registered trademark of Oxford University Press

Library of Congress Cataloging-in-Publication Data
Goldstein, David S., 1948–
Stress, catecholamines, and cardiovascular disease / David S. Goldstein.
p. cm.
ISBN 0-19-506538-7
1. Stress (Physiology)
2. Stress (Psychology)
3. Catecholamines—Physiological effect.
4. Cardiovascular system—Diseases—Etiology.
I. Title.
[DNLM: 1. Stress, Psychological—complications.
2. Catecholamines—physiology.
3. Cardiovascular Diseases—etiology.
WM 172 G623s   1994]
QP82.2.S8G65   1994   616.9'8—dc
DNLM/DLC   for Library of Congress   94-19852

9 8 7 6 5 4 3 2 1

Printed in the United States of America
on acid-free paper

Foreword

It is generally accepted that difficult life situations may have adverse effects on health. Almost daily we encounter references to stress: stress at home, in the workplace, at school, and in government; with loss, bereavement, or threat of serious or prolonged illness; after trauma or natural disasters, and so on. There are a plethora of courses, books, lectures, articles, and video tapes on stress reduction and how to deal with stress. It is a subject for comic strip humor, as well as for serious discussion. Textbooks of medicine list ''stress'' among factors that affect asthma, alopecia, atherosclerosis, diabetes, gastritis, hypertension, irritable bowel, and a host of other conditions, as well as a variety of mental disorders. As a topic for scientific investigation, however, ''stress'' has proven to be an elusive concept with almost as many definitions of the term as there are scientists working in the field.

The problems are complex because of the multiple systems involved. Scientific approaches to studies of stress require a detailed knowledge of neuroanatomy, physiology, biochemistry and other fundamental sciences, as well as expertise in behavioral research and clinical medicine. Experimental models inadequately control for all possible factors, and it is extremely difficult to quantify the stressors being studied. We have limited knowledge about mechanisms linking mental and other biological functions. We do not understand the complex interactions of previous experience and genetic constitution in determining response patterns. Yet there is a vast literature on stress, with multiple symposia, governmental reports, thousands of scientific communications, and even entire journals devoted to research on stress. Perhaps the strongest evidence for a role of stress in the pathogenesis of somatic disorders has been with regard to cardiovascular diseases. This field is certainly ripe for further productive investigations seeking new knowledge to yield better therapies.

In writing *Stress, Catecholamines, and Cardiovascular Disease,* Dr. David Goldstein has produced a remarkable book. Certainly, it is unusual for a single author to attempt to assess as complex and multidisciplinary a topic as represented by this field. For Dr. Goldstein, however, this monumental task was a labor of love for which he was well prepared. He graduated Yale University Cum Laude with Honors with Exceptional Distinction in Psychology. Then he went on to receive an M.D. degree from the Johns Hopkins University, combined with a Ph.D. in Behavioral Sciences for his work on cardiovascular conditioning. After completing an internship and residency in Internal Medicine at the University of Washington in Seattle, he served as a Clinical Associate, Medical Staff Fellow, and Senior Investigator in the National Heart, Lung, and Blood Institute. At present, Dr. Goldstein is Chief, Clinical Neurochemistry Section in the Clinical Neuroscience Branch of the National Institute of Neurological Disorders and Stroke. He is Board Certified in Internal Medicine, is a Fellow of the American College of Physicians, was elected to the American Society of Clinical Investigation, and holds an appointment as Clinical Associate Professor of Medicine (Cardiology) at George-town University. Over the last 20 years, Dr. Goldstein has published more than 200 articles and three dozen chapters in various books and symposia describing his original research in cardiovascular physiology, catecholamines, and various aspects of stress. He has lectured throughout the world on stress and its implications for health and disease and is a well recognized expert in this field.

In this volume, Dr. Goldstein has attempted to discuss candidly the major issues concerning stress as a subject for scientific study. Well-informed discussions of the studies by Cannon on homeostasis and on sympathoadrenal "fight or flight" responses, and of the controversial views of stress that were popularized by Selye provide useful and interesting historical perspectives. There follows a series of well-balanced, detailed, state-of-the art presentations of current investigations as well as Dr. Goldstein's view-points about mechanisms of peripheral sympathetic and central adrenergic function, their responses to different stressors, and the cardiovascular consequences of these responses. The text is clearly and interestingly written, with an unusual depth of under-standing and span of interest. I know of no other source that provides such a vast store of well-referenced information about this unique interdisciplinary subject. The publi-cation of this book should spur the development of a new field: Neurocardiology.

IRWIN J. KOPIN, M.D.

another angel who, obviously enraged, was running in circles, sweating, his mouth contorted in a fierce grimace with teeth and fists clenched. The caption was: "He really should slow down! It was stress that brought him here in the first place!" Placemats of the Roy Rogers™ fast food chain have proclaimed: "Roy's Hot & Delicious Chicken. Stress relief in a bucket or a box." A villain in the Batman™ comic book dated June 1, 1993, screams as he attacks his victim with a knife: "I'm really the man who needs your freshly *harvested heart* . . . its *noradrenaline* and *adrenaline* . . . its deliciously bubbling *stress hormones* . . . all the natural ingredients for a stew of *organic fear* . . ." The Joker, mastermind of the plan to kill by fear, watching through binoculars, says to himself, "No you *moron!* You were supposed to *kidnap*—not *kill* him!"

As might be predicted, the number of claims of cardiovascular disability and death allegedly due to job-related stress has increased markedly. A 1988 *Newsweek* report estimated that the cost of stress, including stress-related absenteeism and compensation claims, was $150 billion per year (*Newsweek on Health,* Winter 1988, p. 8). The Chief of the Behavioral Medicine Branch of the National Heart, Lung, and Blood Institute, stated that between $50 billion and $75 billion are spent per year in the United States for stress-linked diseases (Eliot, 1988). According to DeCarlo and Gruenfeld (1989), in California stress now accounts for 22% of occupational disease cases, having increased five-fold between 1980 and 1986; and according to the syndicated columnists, Jack Anderson and Michael Binstein, stress-related claims in California increased 7-fold in the last decade (*Washington Post,* December 27, 1992, p. C7). In Wisconsin, work-related stress cases increased 15-fold between 1978 and 1985 (DeCarlo and Gruenfeld, 1989).

As might also be predicted, entrepreneurs in the nascent stress management business have contracted with large companies to develop programs to alleviate stress and thereby improve the productivity, morale, and health of workers:

> Vendors of stress relief say that although their industry is in its infancy, it has the potential for rivaling those twin titans of self-help, diet and exercise. "In the next 10 years, stress can be a $15 billion industry," said Ted Barish, an executive who developed marketing programs for Weight Watchers and Pritikin. (*New York Times,* March 19, 1988, p. 34)

The burgeoning of popular interest and media attention about stress, which seem to be increasingly affecting health policy, medicolegal decisions, and the economy, contrasts with a wilting of academic interest and research attention. These considerations incited the present attempt to re-evaluate stress as a medical scientific entity.

The acceptability of ideas about the health consequences of stress depends on the validity of stress as a scientific construct. This book views stress not as an inescapable burden of life, an intuitive notion, a legal term, or a justification for business schemes, but as the subject of a *scientific theory;* and the measure of the worth of a theory of stress, as that of any theory, is not intrinsic truthfulness but the ability to generate hypotheses that observation or experiment can test.

The physicist, Stephen Hawking, has written:

Preface

When asked "What is stress?" a few years ago, a friend of mine, paraphrasing the late Supreme Court Justice, Potter Stewart, replied: "Stress is like obscenity. I can't define it, but I know it when I see it!"

Analogously, most researchers have not defined stress before delving into its endocrinological, physiological, and psychological effects. Some have skirted the issue by defining stress empirically—but actually circularly—by those effects.

This approach, while conducive to production of literature, has retarded scientific acceptance of the field as a whole and has left the impression that stress can be virtually anything that does anything to anyone and that it can cause or contribute to virtually any disease. One researcher put it this way: "Stress, in addition to being itself, and the result of itself, is also the cause of itself" (*Time,* June 6, 1983, p. 49).

Because of this circularity and vagueness, one might long ago have dismissed stress as a scientific idea. By now, however, stress is ingrained in American vernacular, and folk wisdom presumes that the stress of modern life threatens our mental and physical well-being. Reports about the health consequences and treatment of stress abound in the popular media. In the July 22, 1990 edition of *Parade,* the highest circulation periodical on earth (MacWhirter, 1988, p. 210), the header for the article, "Stressbusters," claimed: "'Stress is taking a terrible toll on the nation's health and economy,' says one of the experts who are teaching people how to control it." The painting on the cover of *Time* June 6, 1983, depicted a shrieking man's head exploding out of a concrete cube, under the headline: "Stress! Seeking Cures for Modern Anxieties." On May 4, 1993, the cover story of the supermarket check-out tabloid, *The National Examiner,* carried the banner: "10 Ways to Beat Stress—Before It Beats You—and Makes You Sick." A "Grin and Bear It" cartoon showed two angels commenting about a theory is just a model of the universe, or a restricted part of it, and a set of rules that relate quantities in the model to observations that we make. It exists only in our minds and does not have any other reality (whatever that means). A theory is a good theory if it satisfies two requirements: It must accurately describe a large class of observations on the basis of a model that contains only a few arbitrary elements, and it must make definite predictions about the results of future observations . . . Any . . . theory is always provisional, in the sense that it is only a hypothesis: you can never prove it . . . As philosopher of science Karl Popper has emphasized, a good theory is characterized by the fact that it makes a number of predictions that could in principle be disproved or falsified by observation. (Hawking, 1988, p. 10)

Stress seems weak as a scientific medical concept for three reasons. First is the lack of a widely accepted, non-circular definition of stress from which testable hypotheses can be derived. Second is a lack of suitably designed, ethical experiments to test patho-physiologic hypotheses—especially about chronic effects that only longitudinal studies can address. Instead, overgeneralization from inappropriately designed or inadequately conducted studies has often incited acrimonious debate. And third is the difficulty of conducting research about integrative aspects of neurocirculatory regulation. Studying one system or one substance is always easier than studying more than one simultaneously, and studying effects of a drug or a non-physiologic amount of an endogenous substance is always easier than studying a homeostatic system. Moreover, full comprehension of the factors determining the activities of homeostatic systems requires *in vivo* studies, and neither *in vivo* studies nor integrative physiology currently seem in vogue. Nevertheless examining the potentially important role of stress in the development and expression of cardiovascular disease depends vitally on understanding the principles of operation of homeostatic systems.

The first chapter of this book therefore concentrates on stress as a scientific concept. The discussion includes historical and theoretical analyses, definitions of stress and distress, the role of the sympathetic nervous system in the constellation of circulatory homeostatic effectors, and stress in evolutionary perspective. Finally, a new homeostatic theory of stress is proposed.

The presentation pays particular attention to Selye's theory, the most prominent current theory of stress. Central to his view is the doctrine of non-specificity which holds that stress is the non-specific response of the body to any demand. Results of many neuroendocrine studies, involving simultaneous measurements of activities of several effectors, have indicated instead that stress responses do have a degree of specificity; however, no stress theory seems to have incorporated the patterning of stress responses in any comprehensive way. Such a theory is developed and presented here.

Specifically, stress is defined as a condition where expectations—whether genetically programmed, established by prior learning, or deduced from circumstances—do not match current or anticipated sensations about the internal or external environment, and this discrepancy between what is expected and what is sensed elicits patterned, compensatory responses. The patterned responses result from the operations of ''homeo-stats,'' physiological comparators that regulate activities of multiple effectors in parallel and therefore influence cardiovascular function complexly. Some stress effectors include the sympathetic nervous system, the adrenomedullary system, the pituitary-adrenocortical system, the parasympathetic nervous system, the renin-angiotensin-aldosterone system, vasopressin, and endogenous opioids.

Different forms of stress have different experiential, behavioral, neuroendocrine, and physiological facets. In particular, distress is viewed as a form of stress characterized by a conscious, aversive experience motivating avoidance or escape behavior, largely instinctive behavioral and autonomic signs, and homeostatic resetting that produces increased pituitary-adrenocortical and adrenomedullary outflows. The theory does not assume that distress causes or contributes to any cardiovascular disease, rendering this issue amenable to experimental testing.

The homeostat theory borrows heavily from Cannon, Darwin, and ethologists such as Lorenz and Dawkins in emphasizing the evolutionary significance of stress responses. Regulation of homeostatic systems seems so important to survival one may hypothesize that as effectors evolved, so did mechanisms integrating them, resulting in the expression of primitively specific neuroendocrine patterns supporting the behaviors elicited by different stressors.

Homeostatic physiological systems operate according to several principles, such as inhibitory feedback regulation, which explains the increased variability in effector activity and levels of monitored variables after disruption of homeostats; multiple effectors, which provides the bases for compensatory activation and patterning of effector responses; effector sharing by different homeostats, which results in weak or absent relationships between measures of effector activity and levels of any single monitored variable; and resetting, which is especially apparent during distress and may have both acute and long-term pathophysiologic consequences.

The second chapter describes several of the most powerful and extensively researched stress effectors and emphasizes the remarkable array of their interactions. The mechanoreceptor reflexes, or baroreflexes, have been a major topic of neurocirculatory research, and since they exemplify all the principles by which stress systems operate, the second chapter considers baroreflex regulation of the circulation in some detail.

Most research about mind-body interactions has dealt with skeletal muscle responses to exteroceptor input, independently of visceral responses to interoceptor input. Catecholaminergic systems span this unnatural conceptual chasm; for instance, catecholamines probably delay skeletal muscle fatigue during distress and mediate baroreflex regulation of the circulation. Many hypotheses relating stress to cardiovascular disease have included a catecholaminergic link between stressful experiences and circulatory dysfunction. The third chapter describes the peripheral catecholaminergic systems—the well-known neuronal sympathetic and hormonal adrenomedullary systems and the less well-known autocrine/paracrine dopaminergic system. Steps in catecholamine synthesis, storage, release, uptake, and metabolism are summarized, and adrenoceptors and the physiological effects of circulating catecholamines are then considered. The chapter introduces the idea of separate regulation of activities of these systems, a theme developed further in the chapter about stress response patterns.

Widely cited findings about other peripheral systems or substances that influence cardiovascular performance have for several years overshadowed the catecholaminergic systems. The third chapter reemphasizes the crucial role of catecholaminergic systems, not only in adaptive circulatory responses during emergency reactions, but also in the regulation of tonic levels of cardiovascular performance.

The fourth chapter deals with the central neuroanatomy of sympathoneural outflow to the cardiovascular system and with the roles of catecholamines in the brain. This is a long, difficult chapter because the abundance of research literature about connections among cardiovascular regulatory "centers" and about catecholaminergic chemical neuroanatomy contrasts with a lack of organizing concepts about the relationship between activities of catecholaminergic neurons in the brain and sympathetically-mediated release of catecholamines in the periphery. Complexly (but not randomly) organized periodic discharges of clusters of relatively few brainstem neurons, particularly in the rostral ventrolateral medulla (RVLM), generate sympathetic outflow, with modulation by other clusters at several sites in the neuraxis. Although the RVLM contains catecholamine-synthesizing cells, the role of the catecholamines in regulating the neuronal outflows to sympathetic preganglionic neurons remains poorly understood. Almost nothing is known about patterned alterations in the activity of those centers in stress and cardiovascular disease, or about how their functions reset during distress. Appropriate laboratory techniques have only recently been introduced for examining the release of norepinephrine in the brain *in vivo* and relating this to sympathetically-mediated release of norepinephrine in the periphery. The discovery of a large number of neuropeptides and other putative co-transmitters has introduced the possibility of complex chemical "coding" of central neurotransmission; if there is such a code, it has not yet been broken.

Understanding the role of stress in clinical cardiovascular disease requires means to examine aspects of catecholaminergic—especially cardiac sympathoneural—function in people. The fifth chapter updates clinical approaches for assessing catecholaminergic function. These approaches include biochemical techniques, such as measurements of levels of catechols and their metabolites in body fluids, direct sympathetic nerve recording, and imaging techniques to visualize regional sympathetic innervation.

Plasma levels of different catechols reflect different aspects of sympathoneural function. Simultaneous estimates of regional spillover rates of DOPA, norepinephrine, and its metabolites into the bloodstream provide a comprehensive picture of local synthesis, release, uptake, and metabolism of norepinephrine in sympathetic nerve terminals. Approaches combining measurements of norepinephrine spillover with direct microneurographic recordings of skeletal muscle sympathetic activity can shed light on the function of receptors on sympathetic nerve terminals and of cellular uptake processes that crucially influence the relationship between sympathetic outflow and the occupation of receptors on cardiovascular smooth muscle cells. The principles underlying the use of positron-emitting analogs of catecholamines or sympathomimetic amines for positron emission tomographic (PET) scanning of cardiac sympathetic innervation and function are presented, along with initial clinical findings from the use of this new technology in humans.

The sixth chapter describes the involvement of the sympathoneural, adrenomedullary, dopaminergic, and other effector systems in the expression of stress response patterns. A major thesis of this book is that the activities of these systems are coordinated with other systems to produce patterned behavioral, neuroendocrine, and cardiovascular adjustments that preserve the internal environment during stress. Several lines of evidence reinforce the view introduced in the first chapter that stress responses have a degree of specificity. The multiple interactions of neuronal and hormonal systems support their separate regulation to produce distinctive and adaptive response patterns to different stressors. Distress-induced adrenomedullary activation seems linked more closely to that of another major stress system, the pituitary-adrenocortical system, than to the sympathoneural system.

These six chapters constitute a long but necessary introduction to the seventh, main chapter of the book. This is about catecholaminergic systems in cardiovascular disorders. A failed attempt at homeostasis can explain much of the pathogenic role of the sympathoneural and adrenomedullary systems in heart disease. For instance, effective treatments for congestive heart failure work by countering cardiopulmonary overfilling, vasoconstriction, and retention of salt and water, all of which result at least partly from increased sympathoneural and adrenomedullary activity. In teleologic terms, these systems were not designed to ameliorate congestive heart failure but to regulate the delivery of life-sustaining fuels to vital organs, by maintaining effective arterial blood volume and appropriate blood concentrations of glucose and oxygen. These parameters take precedence over peripheral resistance to blood flow, blood pressure, or extracellular fluid volume. Decreased ability of the heart to deliver blood into the arterial tree therefore activates these homeostatic systems to maintain effective arterial blood volume. This is why, when a patient in heart failure undergoes treatment with an arterial vasodilator, ''unloading'' the heart, the improved arterial filling decreases the recruitment of sympathetic activity, even though the same vasodilator administered to a healthy person increases sympathetic activity reflexively. Sympathoneural activation in ''compensated'' heart failure generally is homeostatic, since the administration of sympatholytic agents to patients at this stage can rapidly usher in circulatory collapse and shock. Cardiac sympathetic stimulation and expansion of intra-cardiac volume, however, increase myocardial contractility, increase myocardial oxygen requirements due to increased cardiac filling, afterload, rate, and contractility, and can decrease myocardial oxygenation due to pulmonary edema; all these effects may produce net worsening rather than improvement in the overall clinical situation. Thus, in heart failure, while sympathoneural activation is homeostatic in purpose, the activation can be pathologic in effect because of exacerbation of a largely independent pathologic state.

The approach in the chapter about cardiovascular diseases therefore considers the role of catecholaminergic systems first as homeostatic in purpose and effect, second to be homeostatic in purpose but pathologic in effect, and third, only after the first two roles are excluded, to be etiologic. Perhaps the most persuasive evidence for the latter is in pheochromocytomas, tumors that release catecholamines into the bloodstream, and in neurogenic orthostatic hypotension due to pure autonomic failure. Increased sympathoneural activity and release of norepinephrine attend the development of hyperten-

sion in spontaneously hypertensive rats (SHR's) of the Okamoto strain; still unresolved, however, are the locus of the abnormality in the sympathetic neuraxis and whether the increased sympathetic activity specifically causes the hypertension or merely accompanies behavioral hyperactivity that also characterizes this strain. The multiplicity of neurochemical and neurophysiological abnormalities described in SHR's and in relatively young patients with hypertension leads to the suggestion that an altered genetic ''algorithm,'' rather than any single genetic defect, favors the development of high blood pressure. The chapter also analyzes the sometimes contentious research literature about stress and catecholamines in coronary heart disease, cardiomyopathy, sudden cardiac death, and functional cardiorespiratory syndromes.

Because of the pervasiveness of the stress concept in modern parlance, one must attempt continually to separate facts from opinions about the role of stress in cardiovascular disease. The eighth and final chapter analyzes critically several topics in this area, including stress as a unitary phenomenon, ''life change'' inventories, job stress, and the reactivity hypothesis. Issues considered in analyzing available research literature on these topics include selection biases, reproducibility, experimental design (controls, retrospective vs prospective, longitudinal vs cross-sectional), clinical importance as distinguished from statistical significance, and extrapolation from acute to chronic stress effects.

One can categorize research literature about medical aspects of stress in terms of physiological and psychological stressors and in terms of physiological and psychological stress responses, yielding four categories: physical-physical, mental-physical, physical-mental, and mental-mental. Viewed in this light, gaps in information and concepts become apparent; much of the literature about psychopathological responses to psychological stressors seems unacceptably speculative, relying often on analogy to physical-physical concepts or on intuitive speculation. Studies of mental-physical and physical-mental aspects of stress often appear scientific in purpose but flawed in design or practice, due to insurmountable ethical and pragmatic limitations.

The last chapter also predicts trends in the area of stress, catecholaminergic systems, and cardiovascular disease. To emphasize gaps in current knowledge, the last chapter asks many questions. Comprehensive presentation of any scientific subject requires not only accurate description and interpretation of what is known but also recognition of what is not known. We remain largely ignorant about the molecular basis of homeostasis; the mechanisms of homeostat resetting during distress; the central neural mechanisms integrating and regulating sympathoneural and adrenomedullary outflows with activities of other homeostatic neuroendocrine systems during stress, and the roles of central catecholamines in that regulation; the identity and functioning of psychological homeostats; the genetic determinants of patterns of neuroendocrine stress responses; and the pathophysiologic significance of chronic distress and of increased sympathetic cardiovascular tone.

The state of science may now be adequate, both in terms of the ability to generate testable hypotheses and in terms of technical advances allowing appropriate experiments, for the emergence of ''neurocardiology'' as a new discipline in clinical medicine. The last chapter also outlines the subject matter and some techniques of this discipline.

This book was written with several audiences in mind. Psychologists and psychological researchers, as well as investigators already immersed in the stress field, may wish to consider the homeostatic stress theory presented here. Medical students and academic clinicians should benefit from overviews of stress systems, including catecholaminergic systems, in the body economy during different conditions. Cardiologists and cardiovascular researchers can acquaint themselves with the regulation of hemodynamic factors that depends on nerves outside the heart and organs above the neck, just as neurologists and neurological researchers can acquaint themselves with neural inflows other than those from external sense organs and neural outflows other than those to skeletal muscle. Finally, clinicians who diagnose, treat, and manage patients with cardiovascular disease will receive an update about what is known, and what is not yet known, about how catecholamines mediate effects of stress on the cardiovascular system.

The effort of writing this book will have been worthwhile if the ideas presented here arouse sufficient interest that they are assimilated by students, considered by clinical practitioners, and tested by researchers.

I have greatly appreciated discussions with Dr. Irwin Kopin, who has served as a mentor for much of my research, and with many colleagues at the NIH, whose friendship and stimulation I have valued, including (in alphabetical order) Drs. Ines Armando, Peter Chang, Anna Deka-Starosta, Graeme Eisenhofer, Giora Feuerstein, Ehud Grossman, Moshe Garty, Harry Keiser, Richard Kvetnansky, Jacques Lenders, Paul Levinson, Karel Pacak, Katalin Szemeredi, Efrat Wolfovitz, Gal Yadid, Reuven Zimlichman, and Zofia Zukowska-Grojec. The expertise and dedication of Courtney Holmes, Robin Stull, and Rod Turner enabled the development, validation, and application of assay techniques upon which most of my research has been based. Finally, I thank my wife, Minka, and our family for their support and encouragement and for allowing me the time to develop and reduce to writing my thoughts on the topic of stress, catecholamines, and cardiovascular disease.

Potomac, Md.   D.S.G.

Contents

Abbreviations

Compounds

ACTH	corticotropin
ANP	atrial natriuretic peptide (also called atriopeptin, atrial natriuretic factor)
ATP	adenosine triphosphate
AVP	arginine vasopressin (also called antidiuretic hormone, ADH)
cAMP	cyclic 3'-5'-adenosine monophosphate
β-CCE	β-carboline-3-carboxylic acid ethyl ester
cGMP	cyclic 3'-5'-guanosine monophosphate
CRH	corticotropin-releasing hormone
DA	dopamine
DARPP-32	dopamine- and cAMP-regulated phosphoprotein of M_r 32,000
DAGO	D-Ala^2, MePhe^4, Gly-ol^5-enkephalin
DG	diacylglycerol
DHPG	dihydroxphenylglycol (also called DOPEG)
DHPR	dihydropteridine reductase
DOCA	deoxycorticosterone
DOPA	dihydroxphenylalanine
DOPS	dihydroxyphenylserine

DOPAC   dihydroxphenylacetic acid (also called DHPAA)

DPDPE   D-Pen^2, D-Pen^5-enkephalin

EDRF   endothelium-derived relaxing factor

EPI   epinephrine (also called adrenaline)

GABA   γ-aminobutyric acid

GDP   guanosine diphosphate

GH   growth hormone

GRH   growth hormone releasing factor

GTP   guanosine triphosphate

5-HT   serotonin

HDL   high-density lipoprotein

HEAT   2-[β-(4-hydroxyphenyl)-ethylaminomethyl]tetralone

HVA   homovanillic acid

IP$_3$ inositol triphosphate

LDL   low-density lipoprotein

β-LPH   β-lipotropin

MHPG   methoxyhydroxyphenylglycol (also called MOPEG)

MIBG   meta-iodo-benzylguanidine

MN   metanephrine

γ-MSH   γ-melanocyte-stimulating hormone

α-MT   (α-methyl-*p*-tyrosine)

NE   norepinephrine (also called noradrenaline)

NGF   nerve growth factor

NMDA   *N*-methyl-D-aspartic acid

NMN   normetanephrine

NO   nitric oxide (also called endothelium-derived relaxing factor, EDRF)

NPY   neuropeptide Y

6-OHDA   6-hydroxydopamine

OMeDOPA   *O*-methyldihydroxyphenylalanine (also called 3-methoxytyrosine)

PK   protein kinase

POMC   pro-opiomelanocortin

SAM   *S*-adenosylmethionine

TYR   tyrosine

VMA   vanillylmandelic acid

VIP   vasoactive intestinal peptide

Enzymes

ACE	angiotensin-converting enzyme
βARK	β-adrenergic receptor kinase
COMT	catechol-*O*-methyltransferase
CPK	creatine phosphokinase
DBH	dopamine-β-hydroxylase
DDC DOPA	decarboxylase (L-aromatic amino acid decarboxylase, L-AAADC)
DHPR	dihydropteridine reductase
LCAT	lecithin-cholesterol acyltransferase
LDH	lactate dehydrogenase
MAO	monoamine oxidase
PKA	cyclic AMP-dependent protein kinase, protein kinase A
PKC	protein kinase C
PNMT	phenylethanolamine-*N*-methyltransferase
PST	phenolsulfotransferase
TH	tyrosine hydroxylase

Systems

AHS	adrenomedullary hormonal system
HPA	hypothalamo-pituitary-adrenocortical
PNS	parasympathetic nervous system
RAS	renin–angiotensin–aldosterone system
SNS	sympathetic nervous system (sympathoneural system)

Neuroanatomic Locations

ACE	central nucleus of the amygdala
AP	area postrema
AV3V	anteroventral third ventricle region of the hypothalamus
BNST	bed nucleus of the stria terminalis
CT	central tegmental tract
CVLM	caudal ventrolateral medulla
DNB	dorsal noradrenergic bundle (also called dorsal bundle, DB)
HACER	hypothalamic area controlling emotional responses
LC	locus ceruleus (also spelled locus coeruleus)
MFB	medial forebrain bundle

NA   nucleus ambiguus
nCVL   nucleus reticularis caudoventrolateralis
NTS   nucleus of the solitary tract
OVLT   organum vasculosum of the lamina terminalis
PGi   nucleus paragigantocellularis lateralis
PrH   nucleus prepositus hypoglossi
PVN   paraventricular nucleus
RVLM   rostral ventrolateral medulla
RVMM   rostral ventromedial medulla
SFO   subfornical organ
SN   substantia nigra
SON   supraoptic nucleus
VLM   ventrolateral medulla
VNB   ventral noradrenergic bundle (also called ventral medullary catechol-amine bundle)

Other

APUD   amino precursor uptake and decarboxylation
CSF   cerebrospinal fluid
CVP   central venous pressure
HPLC   high-pressure liquid chromatography (also called high-performance liquid chromatography)
LCED   liquid chromatography with electrochemical detection
icv   intracerebroventricularly (or intracerebroventricular)
LBNP   lower body negative pressure
MRFIT Multiple Risk Factor Intervention Trial
MSA   multiple system atrophy (also called Shy–Drager syndrome)
PAF   pure autonomic failure
PET   positron emission tomography
RSD   reflexive sympathetic dystrophy
SHR   spontaneously hypertensive rat
SIF   small intensely fluorescent
SMSA   skeletal muscle sympathoneural activity
SPN   sympathetic preganglionic neuron
TAC   time–activity curve
WCGS   Western Collaborative Group Study
WKY   Wistar-Kyoto

Stress, Catecholamines, and Cardiovascular Disease

Stress and Science

Scientific medicine attempts to explain diseases by a continuing process of formulating and testing theories. Consideration of stress, catecholamines, and cardiovascular disease must begin with a theory about what stress is.

This chapter develops such a theory. The chapter begins with two fundamental concepts—Bernard's *milieu intérieur* and Cannon's "homeostasis"—analyzes the stress theory of Selye, proposes new definitions of stress and distress, and views stress from the perspective of evolution.

Bernard and the *Milieu Intérieur*

About 150 years ago Claude Bernard concentrated on the fundamental physiological issue of the time: How does the living body work? Do living beings share a vital essence beyond understanding by physical or chemical laws? Or can principles based on observation and experimentation explain bodily processes? These were the opposing views of the vitalist and determinist schools. Bernard was the foremost proponent of the determinist view.

His creed was that by scientific observation one could grasp the laws governing and so predict the activities of body systems. The foundation of what he called "scientific determinism" was the criterion of deduction from experiment. If the experimental conditions were identical, then the experimental results would be the same; that is, the results would be determined.

This belief is so basic to modern biology, it seems intuitively obvious. For most of medical history, however, from Galen's second-century writings until the publication of William Harvey's description of the circulation of the blood in 1628, the opposing vitalist doctrine dominated medical thought.

Vitalism

Vitalism holds that life processes are uniquely different from physicochemical phenomena and so are beyond understanding by physicochemical laws. Vitalist explanations always have offered a pleasing sense of order and purpose. For instance, according to Galen, the veins distributed "natural spirits" formed in the liver, the arteries distributed "vital spirits" formed in the heart, and the nerves distributed "animal spirits," associated with sensation and emotion, formed in the brain. Blood entering the right side of the heart would contact air flowing from the lungs via the pulmonary veins to the heart, the mixture imbuing the blood with the "vital spirit" and igniting a biological flame that would literally heat the blood and so the body. This explained simply why during life the blood always is warm. Thus, for 1,500 years, the heart was viewed not as a pump but as a furnace (Miller, 1978).

The existence of the spirits could not be proven or disproven; however, Galen proposed specific physiological and anatomical mechanisms for the instillation of the spirits in the blood. According to Galen, the blood in the veins and arteries was confined in separate pools. Galen recognized that the possibility of rapid and complete exsanguination by arteriotomy required some communication between the two pools, and he hypothesized that blood warmed by the "vital spirit" passes through pores in the septum between the right and left ventricles—the "septal pore hypothesis."

The notion that warmed blood traverses the septum was a testable—and in this sense scientific—idea, although many centuries passed before William Harvey disproved this tenet of Galenic physiology. The refutation led to the abandonment of the theory of natural and vital spirits. The vitalist element nevertheless persisted in physiological thought, eventually inciting the disputations of Claude Bernard.

Mechanism

The opposite of the vitalist view, the purely mechanistic view, holds that physical and chemical laws can explain all physiological processes, with no need to posit intervening influences such as "goals" or "purposes" for those processes.

Mechanistic theories have also received criticism, for two reasons. First, considered cursorily, mechanism does not appear to account for organization, a characteristic of all living things:

> A metaphysical concept prevalent among medical scientists is that the properties of a whole system can be fully derived from information about the behavior of its isolated parts . . . This . . . assumption neglects the fact of organization—the first fact, indeed, that strikes one about organisms. (Strauss, 1960, p. 805)

Mechanistic theories, however, do not have to ignore the "fact of organization." In particular, Charles Darwin proposed his theory of evolution, a type of mechanistic theory, to explain the complexity of the structure and the apparent purposefulness of the behavior of organisms. Modern-day Darwinians emphasize that genetic variation and natural selection, operating over the eons, can explain organized complexity, without imputing an overall goal or design. Indeed, Dawkins (1987) has argued that the theory of evolution is the *only* theory in principle capable of doing so.

Second, mechanistic theories often seem insufficient in that they depend on temporal relationships to yield inferences about cause and effect. If phenomenon A can cause phenomenon B only if A precedes B, then how can one apply a mechanistic theory to explain goal-directed behaviors, which precede their effects?

A mechanistic theory need not require responses only to past events. For instance, a chess computer can *simulate* consequences of alternative actions and, according to programed algorithms, choose the move most likely to produce checkmate. The analogous ability of higher organisms to simulate, as discussed below, provides a ready mechanistic explanation for anticipatory stress responses.

Thus, neither the organized complexity of living things nor temporal limitations preclude a mechanistic theory of stress.

Regarding the apparent purposiveness of stress responses, Walter B. Cannon, the most influential of early twentieth-century American physiologists, wrote:

> Since a response in the organism has certain definite consequences, however, we should frankly regard them as being integrated with what has immediately preceded them. The various stages in the response that lead to the consequences may then be looked upon as *purposive*. If a crumb lodges in the larynx, for example, nerve impulses pass to the lower brain stem and, reflexly, impulses are discharged to abdominal muscles so that a cough results and the crumb is expelled. The sensory and neuromuscular sequences of the reflex action are all meaningless unless the aim is considered, unless attention is paid to the end effect toward which the complicated act is directed. (Cannon, 1945, pp. 108–109)

One can extend Cannon's example to note that stroking the tracheal lining evokes a coordinated, effective cough reflex, even in unconscious individuals; indeed, intensivists depend on this reflex for pulmonary toilette in intubated, comatose patients. The goal-directedness and coordination—the apparent purposiveness—of this reflex does not imply that the patient senses the suctioning catheter consciously or coughs voluntarily, just as the apparent purposiveness of a thermostat does not imply that the thermostat is either conscious of or "wants" to maintain the temperature of a room. The argument about protective reflexes, which can be viewed as primitive stress responses, may extend to all stress responses.

Teleology

Any biological theory depending on the notion of purposiveness is to some extent teleological. Teleology is the doctrine that an overall design or purpose determines natural phenomena. Bernard's theory of the *milieu intérieur,* presented below, contains an element of teleology, not by asserting the application of a Creator's supernatural will, but by imputing an overall purpose for the operations of body systems. Continuing this tradition, Cannon wrote: "My first article of belief is based on the observation, almost universally confirmed in present knowledge, that what happens in our bodies is directed toward a useful end" (Cannon, 1945, p. 108).

The themes of compensatoriness, adaptiveness, and purposiveness of stress responses, which will resurface repeatedly in this book, correspond roughly to mechanistic, Darwinian, and teleological views. Purposiveness, while helpful in deriving testable hypotheses, cannot constitute the essence of a rigorously scientific stress theory, since all the elements of such a theory should be both necessary and testable, and how does one prove the necessity and existence of purposiveness? Compensatoriness alone, while possibly adequate for a parsimonious definition of stress, seems inadequate to explain why and how stress responses evolved, as evidence discussed below suggests they did. A scientific theory of stress therefore should avoid including the notion of purposiveness and should transcend the notion of compensatoriness to include the survival advantage of adaptiveness. The theory presented later in this chapter attempts to do this.

In order to posit a scientific stress theory, to comprehend the immense "stress" literature, and to enable acceptance of the field of stress research by medical researchers, one must deal continually with the ideas of compensatoriness, purposiveness, and adaptiveness, and with their distinction—a thorny semantic if not philosophical problem. For now the key point is that the ability to test derivative ideas—hypotheses—by observation and experiment strongly favored the theory of Bernard, even with its hint of teleology, over vitalist theories. By this criterion, all vitalist theories proposed to date have either been refuted (e.g., Galen's hypothesis about septal pores) or discarded.

Modern-day notions about stress and disease derive from Bernard's simple but crucially important concept about the existence and maintenance of the internal environment—the *milieu intérieur.*

The Theory of the *Milieu Intérieur*

Why do body systems function as they do? Bernard's theory answered the question simply: They function as they do in order to maintain a stable internal environment.

Bernard's conception of the *milieu intérieur* evolved over several years and was presented in distilled form in a series of lectures in 1876. Before this Bernard had emphasized that the nearly constant composition and temperature of fluids bathing living cells of higher organisms protected and nourished them. Now he suggested something more profound: that the body maintains this constant internal environment by myriad, continual, compensatory reactions, tending to restore a state of equilibrium, and thereby allowing independence from the external environment. He wrote: "It is the fixity of the *'milieu intérieur'* which is the condition of free and independent life. All the vital mechanisms, varied as they are, have only one object, that of preserving constant the conditions of life in the internal environment" (Bernard, 1878).

Figure 1–1 illustrates the two main means by which body processes maintain the internal environment in the face of alterations in the external environment: internal

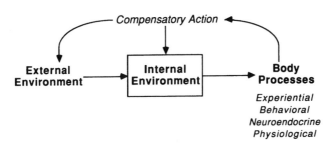

Figure 1–1. Bernard's *milieu intérieur*. Claude Bernard's simple but profound explanation for the purpose of body processes was to maintain a stable internal environment, or *milieu intérieur*. According to the theory, myriad, continual compensatory responses, both internal (e.g., hormonal) and external (e.g., behavioral), enable freedom from changes in the external environment.

adjustments, such as produced by changes in levels of hormones; and behaviors, such as avoidance or escape, which decrease or eliminate the environmental perturbation.

The idea that body systems maintain a constant internal environment engendered many fundamental concepts in medicine. For instance, it led directly to the cybernetic concept of feedback regulation:

> Walter Cannon, going back to Claude Bernard, emphasized that the health and even the very existence of the body depends on what are called homeostatic processes . . . the apparent equilibrium of life is an active equilibrium, in which each deviation from the norm brings on a reaction in the opposite direction, which is of the nature of what we call negative feedback . . . Our inner economy must contain an assembly of thermostats, automatic hydrogen-ion concentration controls, governors and the like, which would be adequate for a great chemical plant. (Weiner, cited in Virtanen, 1960, p. 88)

The same concept has also led to major hypotheses in psychosomatic medicine. One of these, to which we shall return several times in this book, is that emotional responses that throughout evolution have been advantageous in natural selection, facilitating fighting or fleeing behaviors, have by now become "maladaptive," causing organic disease when those emotions are repeated and unfulfilled.

Bernard's views tended to conflict with those of Pasteur, the father of microbiology and of the germ theory of disease. The two argued over the cause of alcoholic fermentation, Pasteur claiming that fermentation requires the presence of living organisms, germs, and Bernard claiming that fermentation is a strictly chemical intrinsic decomposition. Analogous debates among their students dealt with the cause of diseases: Are diseases due to external threats to the well-being of the organism or to inappropriate or inadequate responses of the body to those threats? To paraphrase Osler, is disease due to the "seed" or to the "soil"?

During the era of ascendance of the germ theory of disease at the end of the 1800s, the importance of the equilibrium of the organism was relatively ignored. Now, in the era of immunology and molecular genetics, which view disease as the result of deleterious interactions between heredity and environment, or from genetic flaws outright, Bernard seems vindicated.

On his deathbed Pasteur is said to have conceded, "Bernard was right. The microbe is nothing: the soil is everything" (Selye, 1956).

Bernard's idea of the *milieu intérieur* is the first and main guiding principle for the present theory of stress: All life forms possess means to preserve their integrity, by activation of compensatory systems to maintain the constancy of the internal environment.

Cannon and Homeostasis

According to Bernard's theory of the *milieu intérieur,* most of our cells are not in direct contact with the external environment. Instead, a continuously maintained internal environment bathes and nurtures them. Walter B. Cannon extended Bernard's concept by showing that the maintenance of a stable internal environment depends on the sympathetic nervous system.

Recall that Galen taught that there were three types of spirits—natural, vital, and animal. The nerves distributed the "animal spirits" in the body. This fostered consent, or "sympathy," among the body parts. The idea of the sympathetic nervous system, which we now know to be essential for appropriate cardiovascular adjustments during stress, was Galen's; it antedated the concept of the circulation itself by about fourteen centuries. Galen's view that the nerves coordinate activities of body organs was essentially, ironically, correct.

One can trace the existence of the sympathetic system to primordial challenges all higher organisms have faced as a consequence of complex structure. Whereas single-celled organisms normally are surrounded by the nutrient medium they need, higher organisms must use internal systems—especially the cardiovascular system—to maintain cellular temperature, take in and distribute oxygen, ingest and deliver fuel and water, and rid themselves of metabolic waste. The evolution of increasingly complex (and increasingly energy-requiring) systems to deliver fuel and remove waste has paralleled the evolution of the organized complexity that has afforded resistance to the vicissitudes of the external environment. The cost of the maintenance of internal systems to deliver fuel, remove waste, provide water of the correct tonicity, and optimize temperature for cellular processes, is the price of independence from the external environment.

Efficient functioning of the cardiovascular system requires continuous monitoring and coordination of blood flows to the various organs, allowing appropriate redistribution of the cardiac output to meet internal and external demands, yet maintaining blood flow to the vital organs—the heart, lungs, and especially the brain. The monitoring depends on perceptions of the outside world and sensations from the inside, and the coordination depends mainly on the sympathetic nervous system.

Adjustments in sympathetic activity accompany virtually every human action and reaction and are the main means for acute regulation of cardiovascular function—from the subtle, unconscious shifts of the distribution of blood volume that occur each time we stand, to the desperate distress syndrome of shock.

Homeostasis

Cannon coined the term ''homeostasis'' to describe the ''coordinated physiological processes which maintain most of the steady states in the organism'' (Cannon, 1929a, 1929b, 1939a). Many of his experiments were so beautifully designed, conclusive, and relevant to current understanding of the role of catecholaminergic systems in stress responses, they are cited in several places in this book. This chapter highlights Cannon's conceptual framework more than his experimental findings.

According to Cannon, the most important process determining the phylogenetic development of physiological and even psychological patterns of response has been essentially the same process determining the development of anatomic patterns—natural selection:

> The perfection of the process of holding a stable state in spite of extensive shifts of outer circumstance is not a special gift bestowed upon the highest organisms but is the consequence of a gradual evolution. (Cannon, 1939a, p. 23)

Cannon suggested that rapid activation of homeostatic systems preserves the internal environment by producing compensatory and anticipatory adjustments that enhance the likelihood of survival of the organism. He explained the emotional responses of rage and fear—which he called ''fight or flight'' responses—in these terms (Cannon, 1939a, p. 228).

One would predict from this view that in cardiovascular disorders, alterations in sympathetic activity would reflect an attempt at compensation to maintain homeostasis, rather than reflect a primary etiologic abnormality. As discussed later, this is the essence of the problem in elucidating the role of the sympathetic system in cardiovascular disorders.

A glance at the large constellation of effects of sympathetic stimulation in the schema in Figure 1–2 raises two questions. Depending on the specific threat, would not one or more of these effects be irrelevant to homeostasis? Cannon recognized this potential limitation, and his explanation is discussed later in this chapter. Second, during emergency situations such as ''fight-or-flight'' encounters, what is homeostasis? Values for all the variables depicted in the schema should be regulated at new levels, in essence redefining homeostasis, at least temporarily. This Cannon did not recognize.

From the work and ideas of Cannon we glean the following principles: Homeostatic systems maintain most of the steady states in the organism; and the sympathetic system regulates cardiovascular performance to maintain homeostasis, especially during emergency reactions.

The theories of Bernard and Cannon did not incorporate stress per se as a scientific concept, or the relationship between stress and disease. Hans Selye concentrated on these issues.

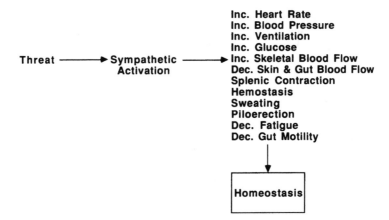

Figure 1–2. Cannon's concept of homeostasis. Compensatory or anticipatory activation of the sympathoadrenal system stimulates the cardiorespiratory system, accelerates hemostasis, shunts blood to skeletal muscle, decreases fatigue, inhibits vegetative functions, and increases blood glucose levels, enabling the organism to meet threats to homeostasis during emergencies.

Selye and the General Adaptation Syndrome

Hans Selye popularized stress as a scientific and medical idea. Having observed as a medical student that all sick patients seemed to share a "syndrome of just being sick," he eventually elaborated a theory of stress as a condition shared by all organisms in their interaction with the environment: "Stress is the nonspecific response of the body to any demand upon it" (Selye, 1974, p. 14).

The Doctrine of Nonspecificity

Selye emphasized that stress and stress responses are nonspecific; that is, they can be brought on regardless of the stimulus. His first publication about this idea, "A Syndrome Produced by Diverse Nocuous Agents," published as a letter to *Nature* in 1936 (Selye, 1936), was based on the similarity of responses in animals receiving injections of any of a variety of chemicals; and in one of his last papers, Selye maintained his stand: "Stress is the sum of the nonspecific biologic phenomena (including damage and defense), and consequently, a stressor agent is by definition nonspecific since it produces stress" (Selye, 1982, p. 4).

According to Selye's theory, after specific responses were removed from consideration, a nonspecific syndrome would remain. Although nonspecific with respect to the inciting agents, the stress response itself was viewed to consist of a stereotyped pattern, with three components: enlargement of the adrenal glands, involution of the thymus gland (associated with atrophy of lymph nodes and inhibition of inflammatory responses), and peptic ulceration of the stomach (Figure 1–3). A decrease in the circulating number of eosinophils was added later to this triad. All these responses are inducible by exogenous administration of glucocorticoids.

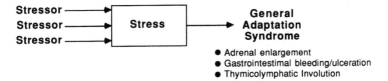

Figure 1–3. Selye's concept of stress. All stressors elicit a stereotyped general adaptation syndrome, characterized by adrenal enlargement, gastrointestinal bleeding or ulceration, and decreased function of immune system organs such as the thymus and lymph nodes.

The General Adaptation Syndrome

The stress response was also thought to have characteristic stages, in a triphasic "General Adaptation Syndrome" (Figure 1–4). The first phase was a rapid "alarm" reaction, including hypothermia, hypotension, neural depression, decreased muscle tone, hemoconcentration, altered capillary and red blood cell permeability, catabolism, hyperkalemia, acidosis, leucopenia followed by leucocytosis, hyperglycemia followed by hypoglycemia, and gastric erosions (Selye, 1950). The alarm stage was thought to consist of two periods: "shock" and "counter-shock," the latter due to responses of the adrenal cortex, releasing "corticoids," and of the adrenal medulla, releasing "adrenalines." The counter-shock responses were thought to reverse many of the above abnormalities and to induce hypertension, hyperglycemia, increased blood volume, alkalosis, diuresis, and often hyperthermia (Selye, 1950). Morphologically there would be enlargement of the adrenal cortex and acute "involution of the thymico-lymphatic apparatus" due to the release of anti-inflammatory corticoids (Selye, 1950).

After an undefined length of time, a longer-lasting stage of "resistance" would ensue, with increased resistance to the particular stressor but decreased resistance to other stimuli (Selye, 1950). During this stage, most of the above morphological and biochemical changes would disappear. The stage of resistance was dominated by a balanced effect of "syntoxic" and "catatoxic" hormones of the adrenal cortex. The adrenal corticosteroids (cortisol in humans, corticosterone in rats) were thought to be syntoxic in that they would help the body to put up with aggressors by acting as "tissue tranquilizers," inhibiting defensive reactions such as immune and inflammatory responses. Catatoxic agents were thought to be proinflammatory, destroying aggressors by destructive enzymatic attack. The catatoxic hormones of the body were never identified conclusively.

The stage of resistance would end with the depletion of stores of "adaptation energy," ushering in the third stage, "exhaustion." There would be a resurgence of pituitary–adrenocortical hyperactivity, with attendant gastrointestinal ulcers, immunologic failure, and eventual death of the organism.

Eustress, Distress, and Diseases of Adaptation

According to Selye's theory, stress is not necessarily deleterious. He coined the term "eustress" to refer to stress that is not harmful and possibly is helpful to the body

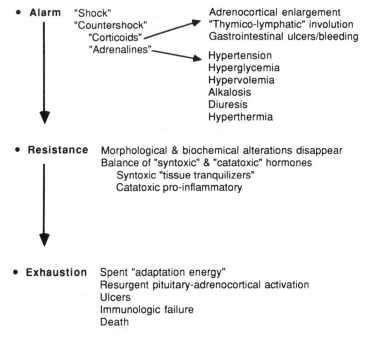

Figure 1–4. Stages of Selye's General Adaptation Syndrome. The G.A.S. consists of three phases: alarm, resistance, and exhaustion. During the alarm stage, the adrenal cortex secretes adrenocortical steroids and the adrenal medulla secretes "adrenalines." During the resistance stage, the signs of stress regress, due to a balance of syntoxic anti-inflammatory and catatoxic pro-inflammatory hormones. During the exhaustion stage, the signs of stress recur, and the organism dies when adaptation energy is spent.

(Figure 1–5). "Distress" referred to damaging or unpleasant stress (Selye, 1974, p. 18). Excessive, repeated, or inappropriate stress responses were viewed as maladaptive, and Selye coined the phrase "diseases of adaptation" to refer to situations where the General Adaptation Syndrome is "derailed" (Selye, 1956, p. 47). The contributions of stress to the diseases of adaptation were suggested mainly from effects of large doses of glucocorticoids or mineralocorticoids. If abnormal (hyper-, hypo-, or dys-adaptive) responses did not directly cause these diseases, then they were thought to predispose the individual to develop these diseases, based on tendencies called "conditioning factors."

Selye proposed an immense list diseases of adaptation. Hyperfunctional and dysfunctional conditions included Cushing's disease, adrenal tumors, chromaffinomas, renal artery stenosis, hypertension, periarteritis nodosa, nephrosclerosis, nephritis, rheumatic and inflammatory diseases, gouty arthritis, peptic ulceration, eclampsia, diabetes, allergic and hypersensitivity disorders, and psychosomatic disorders. Hypofunctional conditions included Addison's disease, Waterhouse–Fredrichsen syndrome, cancer, and

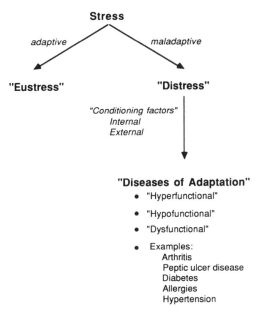

Figure 1–5. Selye's concepts of distress, eustress, and diseases of adaptation. Distress is noxious and eustress beneficial. Organisms develop diseases of adaptation based on conditioning factors in the setting of distress.

diseases of resistance in general (Selye, 1950, 1974). The most severely affected targets were thought to be the cardiovascular system, the joints, and metabolism.

Critique of Selye's Stress Theory

Selye's stress theory became and remains popular. Among other things, the theory provides a ready explanation for how any distressing experience can lead to virtually any disease state. By 1982, Selye's International Institute of Stress had catalogued over 200,000 publications about various aspects of the stress concept (Selye, 1982).

The theory also aroused intense controversy. Bombastic publicity amplified the theory's controversiality. For instance, the book jacket of Selye's *The Stress of Life* carried the following:

> Here is a revolutionary new concept of mental and physical illness, explained by its discoverer. This startling new theory of disease may be the most important and far-reaching idea in the history of medicine. It has often been compared with the contributions of Pasteur, Ehrlich, and Freud . . .
>
> Hans Selye has been acclaimed throughout the world by scientists, physicians, and psychologists for his brilliant exposition of the stress theory. Here, in language easily understandable by the general reader, the man who has been called ''the Einstein of medicine'' explains his modern stress concept.

Although Selye's stress theory has certainly provoked much thought and research, the theory has proven deficient in several crucial respects.

Circularities

Four circularities vitiate Selye's theory. The first is based on the assumption that stress is a nonobservable condition that leads invariably to the General Adaptation Syndrome. Stress was the condition producing the syndrome; however, the occurrence of the syndrome was the only means by which the existence of the condition could be deduced.

In order to explain how different patients could evince different diseases of adaptation, Selye hypothesized that "conditioning factors" selectively enhance or inhibit particular stress effects. The conditioning factors could be internal (e.g., hereditary predispositions, aging, and sex) or external (e.g., drugs and nutritional factors). Conditioning could explain any deviation from the predicted pattern of stress-induced lesions; however, the presence of conditioning could be detected only by this deviation.

"Distress" was defined as stress that was unpleasant or harmful to the body (Selye, 1974, p. 18). The only means to determine whether a particular stress was a distress or "eustress" was the occurrence of observable tissue damage or shortened survival.

"Adaptation energy" was defined as that which was consumed during adaptive work. Depletion of this energy would usher in the state of exhaustion leading to death. The measure of the success of the adaptive response to a particular stressor was not the ability to mitigate the intensity or noxiousness of the stressor but its effects on pathology and survival. If these were adverse then the response was viewed as maladaptive. If there were no pathologic consequences to a stress response, then the active and passive defenses were viewed as in balance, but if there were pathologic consequences, then they were viewed as due to an imbalance. The only way to determine whether such an imbalance had occurred was by the pathologic effects.

Selye claimed that all he knew about adaptation energy was that constant exposure to any stressor would exhaust the adaptation energy (Selye, 1956, p. 209). He considered the human life-span to be determined primarily by the amount of available adaptation energy. Indeed, Selye suggested that there was a fundamental, specific element of life, a unit of reactivity to biologic stimuli, that could be used to define life. He called this functional unit of life a "reacton" (Selye, 1956, p. 233). The idea of adaptation energy not only constitutes a circularity in Selye's theory, it also smacks of vitalism.

Inconsistencies

As noted above, Selye defined stress as the nonspecific *response* of the body to any demand. Elsewhere, he claimed that this was an operational definition and that stress was the "sum of all the wear and tear in the body caused by life at any one time" (Selye, 1956, p. 222), or that stress was a non-observable *condition* (Selye, 1956, p. 41) leading invariably to and therefore detectable and measurable by the General Adaptation Syndrome.

The stage of resistance was thought to be characterized by decreased responsiveness to the stressor to which the organism had been exposed repeatedly, but also increased responsiveness to other stressors. Although several studies have confirmed this observation (e.g., Nisenbaum and Abercrombie, 1992; Nisenbaum et al., 1991), the phenomenon of "stress-switch hyper-responsiveness" argues against the doctrine of nonspecificity.

The Doctrine of Nonspecificity

Cannon, to whom Selye referred as the "Great Old Man" (Selye, 1956, p. 191), was one of the first critics of Selye's stress theory. Cannon's critique centered on the doctrine of nonspecificity and the implicit assumption that a stereotyped response pattern can be adaptive, regardless of the character of the stressor. The General Adaptation Syndrome could be viewed as adaptive in the sense of preserving the internal environment effectively in the face of widely differing challenges. Since a nonspecific stress response would not have provided an advantage in natural selection, a stereotyped stress response would not have evolved.

As research has uncovered more and more systems that participate in stress responses and serve distinct homeostatic needs, it becomes less and less clear whether, after removing these specific reactions from consideration, any truly nonspecific reactions would remain.

Mason (Mason, 1971, 1975a) also disputed Selye's doctrine of nonspecificity, noting that in response to different stressors, activity of the pituitary–adrenocortical system can increase, decrease, or remain unaffected (Mason, 1971). This means that the triad of the General Adaptation Syndrome could not infallibly indicate the occurrence of stress. Mason suggested that the basis for similarities in neuroendocrine responses to different physical stressors was not the nonspecificity of responses of the body to any demand but that all the stressors used in Selye's research produced the experience of emotional distress, resulting in similar neuroendocrine consequences. A central nervous system source of distress responses would also help to explain one of the main admitted failures of stress research testing Selye's theory: the inability to identify carriers of the "alarm signals" from peripheral sites (Selye, 1982).

Emphasis on Inflammation and the Pituitary–Adrenocortical Axis

Selye overemphasized analogies to inflammation and the role of the pituitary–adrenocortical system in the stress response. By dwelling on only one effector system, Selye virtually defined the presence or absence of stress by the presence or absence of pituitary–adrenocortical activation; however, many other neuroendocrine systems participate in different stress responses, as discussed in the chapter about stress response patterns. Because Selye never incorporated these other systems adequately into his theory, he did not consider possible adaptive patterning of responses of these systems.

Selye overgeneralized from the effects of pharmacologic doses of adrenocortical steroids to the occurrence of "diseases of adaptation," thought to result from maladaptive stimulation of endogenous release of those steroids. For instance, although Selye was correct that deoxycorticosterone combined with high salt intake produces hypertension in uninephrectomized rats, and that clinical diseases such as hyperaldosteronism produce salt-sensitive hypertension, he erred in implying that excessive release of mineralocorticoids into the bloodstream characterizes, causes, or even contributes to more common forms of hypertension. His suggestion that adrenalectomy or hypophysectomy could be beneficial in hypertensive patients in general (Selye, 1956, p. 143) has been discarded.

Had Selye obtained data about activities other stress effector systems besides the pituitary–adrenocortical system, he probably would not have proposed the stages of the General Adaptation Syndrome. For instance, repetition of immobilization stress does not result in habituation of plasma catecholamine responses, and no stage of exhaustion occurs (Kvetnansky and Mikulaj, 1970; R. Kvetnansky, personal communication).

As discussed in the chapter about stress response patterns, neuroendocrine evidence has suggested that stimuli perceived as novel may selectively activate the pituitary–adrenocortical system (Frankenhaeuser, 1975; Herd, 1986). This leads to the hypothesis that the stage of resistance in Selye's General Adaptation Syndrome may actually reflect habituation of central neural processes regulating pituitary–adrenocortical outflow during repetitive exposure to noxious but no longer novel stimuli. Thus, for instance, chronically repeated exposure of rats to cold attenuates corticosterone responses to acute exposure to cold (Burchfield et al., 1980). Since hypercortisolemia characterizes a proportion of patients with depression (Gold et al., 1988), the occurrence of pituitary–adrenocortical activation during clinical "giving up" (Henry et al., 1986) may indicate a phenomenon corresponding roughly to the stage of exhaustion.

Two conclusions from Selye's theory and experiments do seem justified, and the present theory incorporates them: Stress is an unobservable condition that leads to adaptive responses; and adrenal release of glucocorticoids often accompanies stress responses.

Current Definitions of Stress

Cannon rarely used the term "stress" and never defined it:

> Perhaps a comparative study would show that every complex organization must have more or less effective self-right adjustments in order to prevent a check on its functions or a rapid disintegration of its parts when it is subjected to stress . . . (Cannon, 1939a, pp. 23–25)

One may infer that he viewed stress as a stimulus, such as decreased external temperature or hypoglycemia, arousing increased activity of the sympathetic system as a compensatory process. Some modern theorists continue to define stress the same way: "In psychological and biological terms, stress may be defined as any stimulus or interference with the organism that results in a change in bodily functions" (Beamish et al., 1991, p. 232).

By considering stress to reflect the imposition of an external influence on the organism, this approach tends to ignore the contribution to the responses by the organism's perception and interpretation of events in the external and internal environment. Both

Cannon and Selye imposed such overwhelming threats—such as asphyxia, hemorrhage, sepsis, and injections of large doses of toxic substances—that their theories could ignore these perceptions. Current stress theories presume that in the absence of a perception or sensation of a threat to homeostasis, stress responses do not and cannot occur.

Conversely, the perceptions of the individual probably are the main determinant of the occurrence and character of stress responses, even if those perceptions are erroneous or are elicited by conditioned or symbolic stimuli that actually pose no direct challenge to homeostasis. In modern society, direct agonistic confrontation evokes distress relatively rarely, compared with the frequent experience of distress in response to subtle psychosocial cues at home or work.

This interpretive process affects not only the occurrence but also the character of cardiovascular and neuroendocrine stress responses. For instance, in response to contrived laboratory psychological stressors in humans, cognitions influence importantly the quality and intensity of emotional experiences (Johnson and Leventhal, 1974; Schachter and Singer, 1962). Field observations of nonhuman primates have supported this view (Sapolsky, 1990a, 1990b).

The interpretation of environmental and internal stimuli in the elaboration of stress responses is a key element of several stress theories. Skinner (1985) has suggested that stress is a cerebral reaction of a particular individual to a stimulus event, rather than being an inherent feature of the stressor itself. Pickering (1990) has suggested that three types of factors mediate the relationship between stress and cardiovascular disorders: the nature of the environmental stressor, personality or individual factors, and the individual's physiological susceptibility (the latter apparently not very different from Selye's "conditioning" factors). Krantz and Lazar (1987) have proposed that psychological stress should be defined not solely in terms of environmental conditions or response variables but in terms of a "transaction" between the organism and the environment. Weiner (1991a) has argued that although physiological responses to several stressors are similar, species differ in the interpretation of the stressors. Lazarus (1991) has stated that a definition of psychological stress requires references to the individual's motivation and how the individual defines and evaluates relationships with the environment—a process of appraisal. And Levine and Ursin (1991) have viewed stress as part of an adaptive biological system, where a state is created when a central processor registers an informational discrepancy.

Most modern stress theories therefore discard Selye's notions about the non-specificity and stereotyped nature of the stress response, in favor of adaptive, compensatory response patterns elicited by challenges to homeostasis as the organism perceives those challenges.

According to Weiner (1991a, 1991b), stressors are selective pressures from the physical and social environment that threaten or challenge the organism, and they elicit compensatory response patterns. Weiner also asserts that the concept of homeostasis has by now lost its usefulness because there are no truly steady states in living organisms, and that the body's "fundamental operating modes" are oscillatory. Weiner argues that illness or disease occurs when the stability of a system's usual operating mode is lost.

The circular definition proposed by Eliot (1988) also emphasizes the importance of perceptions in the elicitation of stress responses:

> We now know the consequences of "stress" more precisely than we know the definition of it. Stress may be viewed as the body's response to any real or imagined events perceived as requiring some adaptive response and/or producing strain. (Eliot, 1988, p. 1)

As noted above, a major weakness of the doctrine of nonspecificity in Selye's theory is the characterization of stress in terms of a nonspecific, stereotyped response pattern, since this ignores the operation of selective pressures favoring the evolution of truly adaptive responses. Weiner (1989, 1991a) has applied Darwin's theory of natural selection to derive a concept about the adaptiveness (and therefore specificity) of responses to stress. The present theory agrees with this; however, Weiner (1989) does not distinguish carefully stress as a stimulus external to the organism from stress as an experience within the organism: "The term *'stress'* covers a wide variety of phenomena and experiences occurring external to the organism" (Weiner, 1989, p. 405).

Eliot and Buell (1985) and Eliot (1989) have proposed a chronological dimension of stress, analogous to that of Selye, with the hypothesis that sympathetic activation predominates during short-term stress, exemplified by fight-or-flight responses; and that pituitary–adrenocortical activation predominates during long-term stress ("vigilance"), when the individual struggles continually to maintain control and self-esteem. They offer no experimental support for this distinction, nor for their view that both forms of stress contribute to cardiovascular morbidity and mortality. On the contrary, current evidence indicates that chronic emotional distress is associated with long-term activation of catecholaminergic as well as pituitary–adrenocortical systems (Henry, 1992), as discussed in the chapter about stress response patterns.

Chrousos and Gold (1992) defined stress as a state of disharmony or of threatened homeostasis, evoking adaptive responses that can be specific to the stressor or generalized and nonspecific and that usually occur stereotypically when the threat to homeostasis exceeds a threshold. The theory seems to dwell on homeostasis as a psychological sense of well-being. The authors have postulated that increased or decreased activity of "the stress system," consisting mainly of corticotropin-releasing hormone (CRH) and the "locus ceruleus-norepinephrine/sympathetic system," produces abnormal levels of glucocorticoids, norepinephrine, and epinephrine in the periphery and contributes to several disorders, ranging from psychiatric (e.g., melancholic depression, anorexia nervosa, and obsessive-compulsive disorder), to medical (e.g., hypothyroidism, Cushing's syndrome, and inflammatory disease). These views seem similar to Selye's doctrine of nonspecificity, his listing of numerous "diseases of adaptation," and his emphasis on "adrenalines" and especially on the pituitary-adrenocortical system in stress. Both theories do not recognize stressor-specificity of responses of the adrenomedullary, sympathoneural, and other effector systems; both fail to distinguish well stress from distress; and both explain stress-related disorders circularly in terms of maladaptiveness. Chrousos and Gold (1992) have deleted several of Selye's "diseases of adaptation," most notably peptic ulceration and hypertension, from the list of 21 disorders associated with dysregulation of ''the stress system.''

Hennessy and Levine (1979) elaborated a ''psychoendocrine hypothesis'' of stress and arousal. Their theory and the present one share key elements, including defining stress as a type of intervening variable, with central neural comparator processes determining adrenocortical responses to psychological stimuli. Their theory, however, refers to stress mainly in terms of pathological organ responses to physical, noxious stimuli and to arousal in terms of physiological or behavioral responses to psychological stimuli, and their theory views arousal, drive, and psychological stress as essentially synonymous. Their theory does not deal with distress as a distinct entity and considers only the pituitary–adrenocortical system as a stress effector.

A New Definition of Stress

Selye appeared to be closer to a valid definition when he asserted that stress is a ''condition'' or a ''state'' than when he asserted that stress is a nonspecific, stereotyped response pattern. In the former sense, stress can be thought of as a generic form of what in psychology is called an ''intervening variable.'' This is the starting point for the present definition.

Stress as an Intervening Variable

An intervening variable is a theoretical construct in psychology that links a stimulus and a behavioral response (Figure 1–6).

Motivational states such as hunger are intervening variables. If one were to deprive an individual of food, one would make that individual hungry, but the stimulus, the withdrawal of food, would not itself be the hunger. Observing an individual gorging himself at a buffet table, one would infer that the individual must be hungry, but the behavior, while perhaps indicating the intensity of the hunger, would not be the hunger itself. The hunger is not directly observable. It is experiential.

Emotions such as anger are also are intervening variables. Certain stimulus situations are likely to elicit this emotion, and several behaviors or measurements of hemodynamic or biochemical parameters may measure its intensity, but the anger itself, although experienced by the individual, cannot be observed directly.

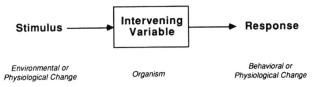

Figure 1–6. An intervening variable. Intervening variables are theoretical constructs linking a stimulus and a response. They represent all the neurological and experiential intervening mechanisms.

The present theory views stress as a type of intervening variable, with several characteristics as described below. The stimulus and response may be physiological or psychological. Indeed, in some cases, such as conditioned avoidance responses attended by autonomic activation, this distinction becomes blurred.

Levine and Ursin (1991) have provided an analogous definition of stress that includes three elements: stimulus input, a central processing system, and response output, with biological and psychological processes viewed as integral parts of a general homeostatic principle. The present theory expands the psychological stress model proposed by Lazarus (1966, 1991) to include physiological stress and neuroendocrine and circulatory responses.

Proponents of different psychological schools have debated the value of emotions and motivational states as scientific constructs. Being experiential, emotions and motivational states are not amenable to direct examination, and given two theories, one with and one without an untestable component, the law of parsimony favors the simpler one. The behaviorist school posits that the study of the rules governing relationships between stimuli and responses is a sufficient and appropriate basis for experimental psychology.

The same argument applies to all intervening variables and therefore to stress. One may question the scientific necessity of stress as an intervening variable. Does adding the word ''stress'' to hypoglycemia or hemorrhage enhance understanding of how these manipulations lead to responses of neuroendocrine effector systems? Nevertheless, one may conceptualize ''hunger'' more easily than ''the collection of central neural and neuroendocrine mechanisms initiated by food deprivation that produce the search for and ingestion of food.'' Much of this book deals with neurophysiological and neurochemical mechanisms, and in explaining them, the term ''stress,'' as the term ''hunger,'' may provide a useful conceptual abbreviation. Moreover, since all people are hungry at some time or other, the experience leads to a sense of shared reality that seems to transcend simple stimulus–response relationships; the same may hold true for stress.

Unlike emotional and motivational intervening variables, the occurrence of stress does not imply a conscious experience. The present theory defines stress as a condition, not an experience:

> *Stress is a condition where expectations, whether genetically programmed, established by prior learning, or deduced from circumstances, do not match the current or anticipated perceptions of the internal or external environment, and this discrepancy between what is observed or sensed and what is expected or programmed elicits patterned, compensatory responses.*

The following discussion elaborates on the main elements of this definition.

Homeostats

Not all intervening variables are stresses. The main determinant of whether an intervening variable is a stress is the effort at a *compensatory* response. Stress depends on the organism's sensing something that leads to a compensatory reaction. It matters little whether the reaction is rational or successful for the reaction to indicate stress. Whether the response is adaptive or maladaptive, however, depends on the success (or perceived success) and effects of the response.

In stress the organism senses a disruption or a threat of disruption of homeostasis. This sensation requires a comparative process, where the brain compares available information with set points for responding. Consider the analogy of a thermostat. Feedback about temperature reaches a thermostat set for a certain temperature. A sufficiently large discrepancy between the measured temperature and the set temperature turns on the furnace, and sufficient reduction of the discrepancy shuts down the furnace, keeping room temperature within a certain range, and with the average temperature corresponding to the thermostat setting.

The body has many such homeostatic comparators; they can be called ''homeostats.'' Each homeostat compares information with a set point for responding, determined by a regulator (Figure 1–7). The homeostat uses one or more effectors to change values for the controlled variable. The loop is closed by monitoring changes in the levels of the controlled variable, via one or more monitored variables.

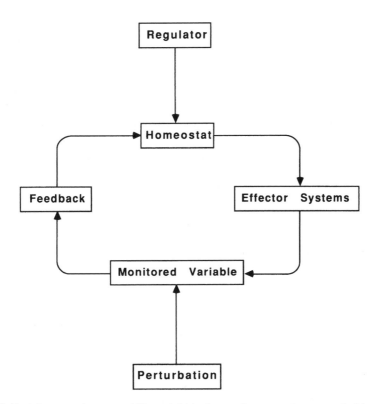

Figure 1–7. A homeostatic system. Afferent information to a homeostat is compared with a set-point for responding. The homeostat uses one or more effectors to change values for the controlled variable. The loop is closed by monitoring changes in the levels of a variable that faithfully indicates the controlled variable. At least one homeostat regulates each stress response.

Several treatments used in modern medicine entail artificial homeostats or effectors to correct or replace deranged stress systems. In patients with diabetes mellitus, the endogenous glucostatic system fails to regulate blood glucose levels adequately. An implanted glucose sensor can measure levels of the monitored variable, glucose, and regulate the rate of insulin injection. Analogously, to treat patients with orthostatic hypotension due to pure autonomic failure, Polinsky et al. (1983) developed a "sympathetic neural prosthesis," consisting of a transducer to monitor arterial blood pressure and an injector to infuse norepinephrine, so that when the patient would stand, the monitor would sense the fall in blood pressure, and the pump would infuse norepinephrine to maintain blood pressure within a set range.

The implantable defibrillator constitutes perhaps the most extreme example of an artificial homeostat (Mirowski et al., 1980). No natural compensatory mechanism has ever evolved against ventricular fibrillation, an invariably and rapidly lethal arrhythmia. Electrical defibrillation can reverse ventricular fibrillation; however, the survivors are prone to develop ventricular fibrillation again. The implanted defibrillator senses the loss of cardiac rhythm, diagnoses ventricular fibrillation, and delivers a defibrillatory shock.

Stress systems require sensors that monitor the controlled variable faithfully. The organism responds not to the perturbation itself, not even to alterations in values of the variable that researchers think the system is "designed" to control, but to changes in values of the variable that the sensor actually monitors. Understanding the function of any stress system requires elucidating the relationship between the "supposed" regulated variable (the controlled variable) and the actually sensed variable (the monitored variable)—a repeated theme in this chapter and book. From the analogy of the thermostat, the "purpose" of the device is to maintain room temperature, the controlled variable. The temperature itself does not determine whether the thermostat turns on the furnace; rather, when the temperature changes, metal ribboned strips in the thermostat expand differentially, bending the ribbon and closing an electrical contact. The extent of bending of the ribbon is the monitored variable. Of course, in this case, the monitored variable reflects the controlled variable with very high fidelity. But suppose one of the metal bands corrodes, so that the ribbon bends less for a given change in temperature; or suppose that the two bands begin to separate. The system would continue to regulate the monitored variable, the extent of bending, but the room temperature could drift to a new level.

As discussed in detail in the next chapter, in the human arterial baroreceptor reflex, stretch receptors in the walls of major arteries such as the carotid arteries sense pulse-related distortion of the vessel wall (Figure 1–8). Cardiovascular researchers have thought that the "purpose" of the system is to regulate arterial pressure (hence the name "baroreceptor"), although pulse pressure and pulse rate also affect baroreceptor afferent activity (Gero and Gerova, 1967). The afferent information to the brain leads to reflexive responses, including sympathetic inhibition, which, among other things, relaxes blood vessels and counters the initial perturbation of blood pressure. Under normal circumstances, the extent of receptor stretching, the monitored variable, faithfully indicates the extent of change in pressure, the presumed controlled variable. In

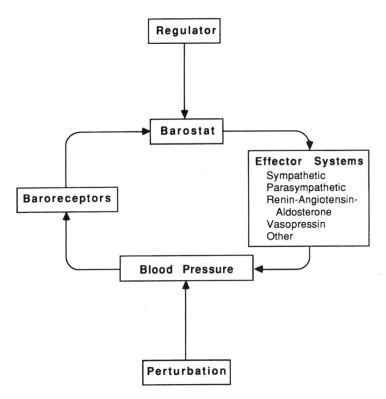

Figure 1–8. A barostatic system. Baroreceptors, stretch receptors in cardiovascular walls, sense distortion related to the pressure pulse and send afferent information to the barostat. The barostat compares this information with its regulated set-point, and if there is a discrepancy, the barostat changes efferent activities from effector systems in order to decrease the discrepancy.

arteriosclerosis, however, when thickening and rigidification of arterial walls decrease the extent of pulse-related distortion, even if the baroreceptors themselves functioned normally, the decreased distortion would attenuate the amount of baroreceptor stimulation. This would decrease the afferent baroreflex information, tending to increase sympathetic outflow and therefore blood pressure. In other words, all other things being the same, arteriosclerosis resets the function of the barostatic system in such a manner that blood pressure and sympathetic outflow increase. In fact, encasing the carotid sinus in a cast does increase blood pressure (Kezdi, 1967). Since in many populations, arterial rigidity increases with normal aging, this phenomenon may help to explain why blood pressure and sympathetic nerve activity tend to increase with age, as discussed in the chapter about cardiovascular diseases.

Another key to understanding the function of homeostatic systems is to identify the homeostats that actually mediate observed biochemical, neurochemical, or physiological responses. The neuroendocrine response to water deprivation illustrates this point. The response pattern in this setting does not result from the deprivation itself but from the deprivation-induced changes in at least *two* monitored variables, serum osmolality and blood volume, each of which a homeostat regulates. Cells in the hypothalamus sense osmolality, and the main known effector used by the "osmostat" is vasopressin (arginine vasopressin, AVP, anti-diuretic hormone, ADH). Effective circulating blood volume is monitored not by volume sensors per se but by "low pressure" stretch receptors (i.e., low pressure baroreceptors) in the cardiac atria and to a lesser extent in the ventricular myocardium and other cardiovascular regions; the "volustat" also uses the AVP effector. AVP therefore serves as an effector for *both* the osmostat and the volustat. Since water deprivation tends to increase osmolality and decrease blood volume, and since in this setting the osmostat and volustat both direct increases in AVP release, AVP levels increase markedly during water deprivation (e.g., Seckl et al., 1986; Shore et al., 1988).

What happens to AVP levels when the perturbation tends to increase *both* osmolality and blood volume concurrently? According to the homeostatic model in Figure 1–9, the osmostat would stimulate AVP release, whereas the volustat would inhibit AVP release. Depending on the gain of the two homeostats, and on the dynamics of the monitored variables, AVP levels could increase, decrease, or not change at all. Thus, in baboons chronically ingesting hypertonic saline (Turkkan and Goldstein, 1991a), and in dogs on a high-salt diet with constant water intake (Krieger et al., 1990), circulating AVP levels do not change, despite the osmolar load. In humans, ingestion of oral hypertonic saline after dehydration transiently decreases plasma AVP levels from the high levels that result from dehydration alone (Seckl et al., 1986). Quillen and Cowley

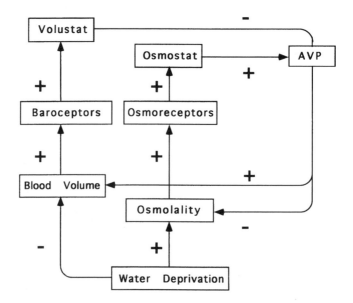

Figure 1–9. Vasopressin and homeostatic responses to water deprivation. Water deprivation decreases effective blood volume, as sensed by low pressure baroreceptors, and increases plasma osmolality. Both the "volustat" and osmostat use vasopressin (AVP) as an effector.

(1983) reported that hypervolemia shifts to the right the curve relating AVP levels to osmolality. In other words, hypervolemia increases the set point of the osmostat. These results demonstrate that in order to predict the response of an effector to a perturbation, one must take into account the effects of the perturbation on all homeostats that use the effector.

A tremendous array of homeostatic systems detect perturbations of monitored variables (Figure 1–10). Arterial baroreceptors, as noted above, monitor distortion of arterial walls and use the sympathetic and parasympathetic effectors to regulate blood pressure acutely. Chemoreceptors in the macula densa of the kidney monitor ionic concentrations in the glomerular filtrate and use renin–angiotensin–aldosterone system (RAS) effector to regulate sodium and potassium balances. Chemoreceptors in the carotid sinus region and in the brainstem monitor arterial concentrations of oxygen, carbon dioxide, and hydrogen ions, and use the phrenic and sympathetic nerves to regulate arterial oxygen, pH, and carbon dioxide levels. Nociceptors in the skin send information about pain via spinothalamic tracts and elicit sympathoneural, adrenomedullary, and pituitary–adrenocortical activation as components of distress responses. Gastrointestinal distention by food stimulates local increases in blood flow, regional sympathoneural inhibition, and vagally mediated parasympathetic activation. Glucose and temperature sensors, probably located in the hypothalamus, elicit different efferent patterns, with hypoglycemia stimulating release of growth hormone and corticotropin (ACTH) from the anterior pituitary gland, cortisol from the adrenal cortex, glucagon from the pancreas, and epinephrine from the adrenal medulla, and inhibiting pancreatic release of insulin. Effectors for temperature regulation include cholinergic and noradrenergic nerve fibers in the skin.

According to the current definition, even a simple homeostatic reflex such as the arterial baroreflex may reflect stress, in that a perceived discrepancy between a set point for a monitored variable and information about the actual level of that variable elicits compensatory responses to decrease the discrepancy. Is stress, defined in this way, too general to be meaningful, since stress responses would encompass virtually all physiological and psychological adjustments? As discussed at the beginning of this chapter, the value of the definition will depend on the ability to generate hypotheses that are testable by observation and experiment. One such prediction, about the homeostatic bases for AVP responses to water deprivation, was discussed above. Homeostatic systems seem to operate according to several principles, presented below; from these principles one can derive testable hypotheses.

Given the multiplicity of homeostatic systems, predictions about patterns of responses to stressors that potentially affect many homeostats, each of which may have particular gains and time constants for several effectors, seem to require sophisticated computer modeling (Bogen, 1989). One would prefer choosing this complexity over regressing to Selye's dubious doctrine of nonspecificity.

An alternative theory distinguishes homeostatic responses from stress responses, with the latter implying maladaptiveness and therefore potential harm. Such a theory cannot define stress as a condition, since a condition should occur independently of the adaptiveness of the response. Defining stress in terms of maladaptiveness also

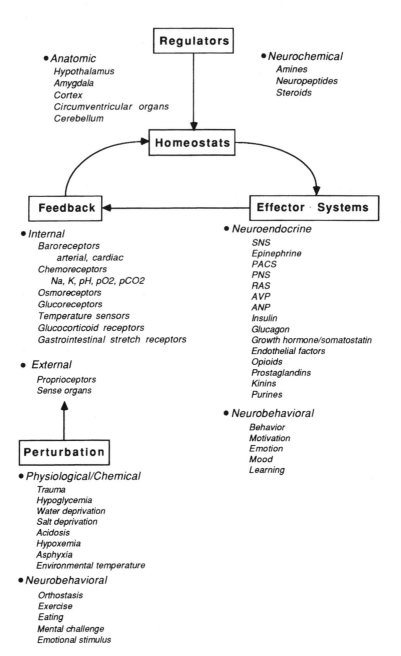

Figure 1–10. Homeostatic systems of the body. The body possesses many homeostatic systems, and this diagram is by no means comprehensive. Receptors sense external and internal perturbations. Internal receptors include chemoreceptors, baroreceptors, glucoreceptors, osmoreceptors, thermal receptors, nociceptors, gastrointestinal stretch receptors, and proprioceptors. Effectors include neuroendocrine and neurobehavioral systems. The neuroendocrine effector systems include nerves (to skeletal muscle, sympathetic (SNS) and parasympathetic nerves (PNS)), hormones (e.g., epinephrine, renin–angiotensin–aldosterone system (RAS), pituitary–adrenocortical system (PACS), vasopressin (AVP), insulin, atriopeptin (ANP), endogenous digitalis-like substances, glucagon, opioids, growth hormone, somatostatin), and paracrine/autocrine substances (e.g., prostaglandins, endothelin, endothelium-derived relaxing factors, dopamine, kinins, purines).

risks the problem of circular reasoning that led to abandonment of Selye's definition of distress.

Principles of Homeostat Operation

Homeostatic systems operate according to a few principles, which, despite their simplicity, can explain complex physiological phenomena and can help to resolve persistently controversial issues in the area of stress and cardiovascular disease.

Monitored vs. Controlled Variables

In the analogy with a thermostat as a homeostatic system, the distinction between the monitored and the controlled variable seemed largely semantic. In real stress systems, the distinction is crucial. The monitored variable is a tangible, measurable entity, such as the extent of cellular stretching or the concentration of hydrogen ions. The body does not directly sense the controlled variable, regulation of which is the "goal" of the homeostatic system. A controlled variable is a theoretical construct that helps us to comprehend and to predict—that is, to "explain"—phenomena. One should feel free to discard a controlled variable (as will be done in Chapter 2), if empirical observations disagree with predictions based on its regulation. In a homeostatic schema, therefore, the controlled variable either does not appear or else appears in the designation of the homeostat itself ("osmostat," "glucostat," etc.). One can much more confidently include the monitored variable.

Substantial progress has been made in identifying the physical location and regulation of brain centers mediating baroreflex regulation of the circulation, as discussed in detail in Chapters 2 and 4. The central nervous pathways have been mapped out, and simple baroreflex arcs have been identified. These results have helped to identify central neural sites and mechanisms of the baroreflex; they cannot identify with surety what and why the barostat *is*.

Negative Feedback

Homeostatic systems always include regulation by negative feedback. Increases in values of the monitored variable result in changes in effector activity that oppose and thereby "buffer" changes in that variable. Thus, hypercortisolemia inhibits pituitary–adrenocortical system activity; stimulation of arterial baroreceptor afferents inhibits sympathoneural activity; increased cardiopulmonary filling inhibits vasopressin release; increases in the filtered load of sodium inhibit renin–angiotensin–aldosterone system activity; and atrial decompression inhibits atriopeptin release. This feedback regulation can be modulated at several levels and therefore can be quite complex.

In homeostatic diagrams such as in Figure 1–9, the symbol "+" denotes a stimulatory relationship and "−" an inhibitory relationship. Each "−" changes the sign of the next relationship in the circuit, whereas each "+" does not affect the sign of the next relationship. In a stable system (i.e., a system where the monitored variables are maintained within a certain "steady-state" range), all the loops must have at least one "+" and one "−." For each perturbation of a monitored variable, the net effect of at least one effector must have a sign opposite to that of the perturbation. For instance, Figure 1–9 depicts two homeostatic loops, one for the sequence of relationships determining AVP responses to decreased blood volume and one for the relationships determining AVP responses to increased serum osmolality. Following the sequences of "+" and "–" signs, both circuits are stable, because decreased blood volume eventually increases AVP levels, tending to increase blood volume, and because increased serum osmolality eventually increases AVP levels, tending to decrease serum osmolality.

If a loop has "+" relationships but no "–" relationships (a positive feedback loop), the system, if otherwise unchecked, will "explode," because activity in the system will increase without restraint. Since positive feedback loops are essentially unstable, an organism cannot tolerate them for long. One must therefore suspect any hypothesis that includes a positive feedback loop.

In the field of stress and cardiovascular disease, a few hypotheses have included positive feedback loops; they have been either wrong or incomplete. One of these is the "epinephrine hypothesis" for the mechanism of essential hypertension (Majewski et al., 1981, 1982; Rand and Majewski, 1984). According to the epinephrine hypothesis, circulating epinephrine is taken up into sympathetic nerves and coreleased with norepinephrine. The coreleased epinephrine binds to presynaptic receptors to augment further release of norepinephrine, and the augmented norepinephrine release increases blood pressure. Since epinephrine would stimulate its own release as well as that of norepinephrine, levels of epinephrine, norepinephrine, and blood pressure all would increase without limit. The chapters about peripheral catecholaminergic systems and about cardiovascular diseases discuss the epinephrine hypothesis in more detail.

Another hypothesis with a suspicious positive feedback loop asserts that epinephrine stimulates pituitary β-adrenoceptors, increasing release of ACTH (Axelrod and Reisine, 1984). According to the hypothesis, in response to a stressor, elevated epinephrine levels augment ACTH release. ACTH, via adrenal corticosteroids, regulates activity of phenylethanolamine-N-methyltransferase, a key enzyme in epinephrine synthesis, and injected ACTH increases circulating epinephrine levels (Valenta et al., 1986). If epinephrine stimulated ACTH release, and ACTH stimulated epinephrine release, then stress levels of both hormones would increase rapidly to infinity.

Positive feedback loops do occur in clinical medicine. When they do, they always signify an unstable situation. For instance, when an insulin-dependent diabetic contracts a bacterial infection, septicemia rapidly can ensue, the patient presenting with both hypotension and diabetic ketoacidosis. The fall in blood pressure disinhibits sympathetic outflow reflexively, and endotoxin increases circulating catecholamine levels (Gullichsen et al., 1989; Murray et al., 1989). Catecholamines counter insulin effects in several ways (Garber et al., 1976; Shah et al., 1984), and this worsens the ketoacidosis.

Mechanisms of cardiac decompensation in heart failure probably involve several positive feedback loops. Ventricular chamber enlargement normally augments contractility and performance, according to Starling's law of the heart (Braunwald et al., 1968; Frye and Braunwald, 1960). In patients with heart failure and cardiomegaly, for a given increment in chamber size, the increment in ventricular performance decreases; that is, the slope of the performance–volume relationship flattens. If the slope were to become negative, then with further enlargement of the ventricular chamber, ventricular performance would decrease rather than increase, resulting rapidly in myocardial depression and fatal pulmonary edema.

Most patients with heart failure die before the descending portion of the Starling curve would apply. A major reason for this is the operation of other positive feedback loops, in which the sympathetic nervous system figures prominently. The maintenance of ventricular performance in compensated heart failure depends not only on the Starling mechanism but also on sympathetic neural outflow (Gaffney and Braunwald, 1963). In patients with heart failure, myocardial sympathetic outflow, as indicated by the spillover rate of norepinephrine into the cardiac venous drainage, increases markedly (Hasking et al., 1986). High myocardial levels of catecholamines such as norepinephrine predispose to the development of arrhythmias. Any arrhythmia in this setting would rapidly decrease cardiac output, reflexively evoking further increases in cardiac sympathetically-mediated release of norepinephrine, which would further increase the likelihood of developing a fatal ventricular arrhythmia.

The concurrence of heart failure and coronary ischemia causes a second type of sympathetic positive feedback loop in heart failure. Heart failure recruits cardiac sympathetic outflow, which increases myocardial oxygen consumption by increasing cardiac rate and contractility. This worsens the imbalance between oxygen supply and demand and can precipitate a lethal myocardial infarction or ventricular arrhythmia. Hypoxic ischemia also can evoke norepinephrine release by local effects at the sympathetic terminals (Schomig et al., 1987).

Simultaneous increases in sympathetic outflow to the heart and to other body regions produce a third type of sympathetic positive feedback loop in heart failure. These changes increase cardiac filling and work, due to direct and indirect sodium-retaining effects of renal sympathetic stimulation (Hasking et al., 1986) and to peripheral vasoconstriction. The increases in cardiac afterload may impair ventricular performance more than the increases in cardiac filling augment ventricular performance, because the heart operates here at a flattened portion of the Starling curve. The net worsening of ventricular performance stimulates sympathetic outflow further. Cardiac overfilling also leads to pulmonary edema, producing hypoxemia, acidosis, and respiratory distress, all of which exaggerate the sympathetic response. The combination of these factors produces cardiac decompensation and death.

Multiple Effectors

Homeostatic systems generally use more than one effector. For instance, activation of the body's glucostats rapidly increases glucagon and growth hormone levels, augments activities of the adrenomedullary and pituitary–adrenocortical systems, and suppresses insulin release; and unloading of cardiopulmonary baroreceptors increases skeletal sympathoneural outflow and renal release of renin, whereas cardiac release of atriopeptin (ANP, atrial natriuretic factor, ANF) declines.

Since multiple effectors enhance the range and refinement of control of regulated variables, natural selection would have favored the evolution of systems including multiple effectors.

This redundancy has several consequences. One is that disabling an effector compensatorily activates the others, assuming no change in homeostat settings (Figure 1–11). This enables partial or even complete maintenance of the monitored variable at the previous setting. The efficiency of the other effectors determines whether the compensatory activation actually normalizes values for the monitored variable.

The chapter about stress response patterns contains several examples of compensatory activation, including augmentation of sympathoneural responsiveness by adrenalectomy or hypophysectomy and augmented adrenomedullary responsiveness by sympathectomy.

Because of compensatory activation, blockade or destruction of a single effector to assess the contribution of the effector to a monitored variable may underestimate that contribution—or even fail to detect it—if the homeostat uses effectors other than the blocked or destroyed one. As discussed in the chapter about cardiovascular diseases, the multiplicity of effectors regulating blood pressure helps to explain inconsistent results of studies using sympatholytic procedures or adrenoceptor blockade to evaluate the sympathetic contribution to high blood pressure. Elucidating such a contribution requires either monitoring or control of the activities of the other effectors.

A second consequence of multiple effectors is the potential for patterning of effector responses. Patterning of neuroendocrine, physiological, and behavioral effectors increases the likelihood of adaptiveness to the particular challenge to homeostasis, providing another basis for natural selection to favor the evolution of systems with multiple effectors.

Experimental evidence supporting this patterning (e.g., de Boer et al., 1989, 1990; Henry, 1992; Rappaport et al., 1982; Young et al., 1984) refutes Selye's doctrine of nonspecificity. This patterning is crucial not only for stress theory but also for elucidating the role of catecholaminergic systems in mediating the relationships between stress and cardiovascular disease; the patterning of stress responses is discussed in its own chapter.

Effector Sharing

Conversely, several homeostats can regulate the activity of a single effector system (Figure 1–12). A previous section of this chapter discussed sharing of the AVP effector by the osmostat and volustat. Other examples of effector sharing abound in physiology. Both arterial hypotension and decreased cardiopulmonary filling stimulate sympathoneural activity; both hypoglycemia and emotional distress stimulate adrenomedullary activity; both exercise and hypoglycemia stimulate growth hormone secretion; and both decreased sodium concentration in the glomerular filtrate and decreased renal perfusion pressure stimulate RAS activity.

Sharing of the activity of an effector by more than one homeostat increases the likelihood of drawing a false negative conclusion (''Type I'' error) about the relationship between the state of activity of the effector and the extent of activation of any homeostat using that effector. For instance, debate has raged for years about whether

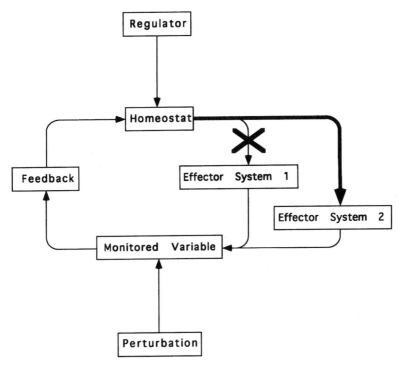

Figure 1–11. Compensatory activation. One consequence of multiple effectors is the ability to continue to regulate a controlled variable by compensatory activation of the effectors that remain functional. Another consequence is patterning of effector responses for a given stressor.

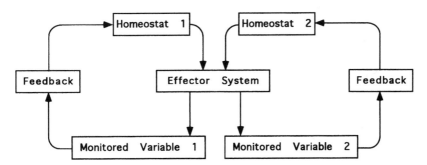

Figure 1–12. Effector sharing. When two or more homeostats share the same effector, then the ability to detect a relationship between the activation of the effector and the activation of any homeostat requires monitoring or controlling the concurrent regulation of the effector's activity by the other homeostats.

borderline hypertensives have increased sympathetic nerve activity. Many homeostats share the sympathoneural effector. When the activity of one of them, the low-pressure barostatic system, is monitored by measurements of central venous pressure, then excessive skeletal muscle sympathetic activity *for a given central venous pressure* becomes obvious (Rea and Hamdan, 1990); in the absence of this monitoring, the frequency distributions of nerve activities in hypertensive and normotensive groups overlap.

Effector sharing alone cannot explain poor correlations between values for activity of the effector and values for a monitored variable, if the effector is the only one determining the level of the monitored variable. For instance, in Figure 1–12, even though two homeostats determine the activity of the same effector, changes in the function of Homeostat 1 do not affect the *relationship* between the activity of the effector and the activity of Monitored Variable 2. If the activity of the effector decreases, the level of Monitored Variable 2 decreases, according to whatever defines the relationship between the two. In general, the presence of a single arrow in a homeostatic schema implies a consistent relationship between the connected variables, regardless of the complex interactions among other variables in the schema.

Virtually every monitored variable, however, is subject to influences by more than one effector, as discussed above. The combination of multiple effectors and effector sharing can easily explain the notoriously poor correlations between values for activity of a single effector and of a single monitored variable—such as the correlations between sympathetic nerve activity and blood pressure in "resting" subjects. Blood pressure is only one of many factors determining sympathetic activity (effector sharing); and many systems besides the sympathetic nerve system contribute to blood pressure regulation (multiple effectors). Inadequate consideration of these two principles of operation of homeostatic systems will produce Type I errors.

Effector systems can also interact directly. Chapter 2 discusses many of these interactions, such as effects of glucocorticoids on sympathoneural outflow epinephrine synthesis and effects of sympathoneural and adrenomedullary outflows on activity of the RAS.

Release from Homeostatic Restraint

Blockade of afferent information to or interference with the function of a homeostat increases the variability of the monitored variable. Thus, baroreceptor deafferentiation increases the variability of blood pressure (Cowley et al., 1973), as does destroying bilaterally the likely brainstem site of the arterial barostat (Nathan and Reis, 1977; Snyder et al., 1978).

A more difficult issue is whether release of a monitored variable from homeostatic restraint causes the variable to drift to a new level—a level that may be pathophysiologic. In particular, as discussed in the chapters about the baroreflex and about cardiovascular diseases, researchers have debated for many years whether baroreceptor "debuffering" increases "resting" blood pressure (i.e., whether debuffering produces a form of neurogenic hypertension).

Part of the problem here lies in the meaning of the term, "resting." Many interacting systems determine blood pressure levels, and activities of these systems never cease in life. Even if one were to avoid use of the term and were rigorously to control environmental conditions, organisms with impaired baroreflexes could have excessive classically conditioned sympathetic responses to seemingly neutral cues (Nathan et al., 1978). Moreover, debuffering may decrease thresholds for arousal, vigilance, or rage (Bartorelli et al., 1960; Lacey, 1967; Lacey and Lacey, 1970), and the accompanying sympathetic activation would then increase blood pressure.

In contrast with clinical hypertension, a largely statistical disease of modern man, hypotension due to traumatic hemorrhage has always posed an immediate and mortal threat. Natural selection must have favored the evolution of systems to support blood pressure during emergencies. As Cannon (1914a, 1929a, 1939a) demonstrated, prominent among these systems is the sympathetic system, activation of which increases blood pressure. If the sympathetic system were an emergency system, then one would expect that release of the sympathoneural effector from baroreceptor restraint would bias blood pressure upwards. Thus, baroreflexes should buffer hypotension more effectively than buffer hypertension (Rea and Eckberg, 1987).

Interference with homeostatic regulation of blood pressure therefore increases the variability of blood pressure, augments hypertensive responses to various stressors, and produces acute hypertension. In rabbits (Berthelot et al., 1982) and baboons (Shade et al., 1990), denervation of the carotid sinus and aortic baroreceptors elicits sustained increases in both variability and mean levels of blood pressure, with increased plasma levels of norepinephrine, the sympathetic neurotransmitter. In humans, baroreceptor debuffering due to surgical denervation (Ahn et al., 1989), or vagal and glossopharyngeal local anesthesia (Fagius et al., 1985; Guz et al., 1966), acutely increases blood pressure and indices of sympathetic nervous activity; however, a patient with irradiation-induced arterial baroreceptor denervation reported by Aksamit et al. (1987) had episodes of paroxysmal hypertension and very high plasma norepinephrine levels without sustained hypertension.

Resetting

Homeostat resetting in essence redefines homeostasis. Selye suggested resetting of the pituitary–adrenocortical system during stress:

> It had been claimed a few years ago that . . . a real increase of corticoids in the blood could never develop during stress . . . But as I found to my surprise in 1940, *during stress this moderator system is largely by-passed.* It turned out that the alarm signals (discharged from the various cells of our tissues during stress) can stimulate ACTH-secretion, even when the concentration of corticoids in the blood reaches the highest attainable levels . . . If the feed-back mechanism were perfect we could never survive a seriously stressful experience. (Selye, 1956, pp. 198–199)

Challenges to homeostasis may or may not require homeostat resetting for the individual to respond appropriately. During orthostasis or performance of the Valsalva maneuver, as cardiac filling and output decrease, sympathetic vasomotor outflows increase reflexively; the resulting vasoconstriction maintains mean arterial pressure at about baseline, without any obvious change in the functioning of the reflex. In contrast, during exercise, homeostatic resetting caused by altered "central command" releases skeletal sympathoneural outflow from baroreceptor restraint, enabling sympathetically mediated vasoconstrictor tone to counter effects of vasodilator substances that if unopposed would decrease blood pressure and flow to the brain.

Short-term changes in homeostatic settings during stress generally enhance the long-term well-being and survival of the organism (responses during exercise provide an obvious example). When superimposed on a substrate of cardiovascular pathology, however, homeostatic resetting can cause harm, because during many stresses (exercise and cold exposure are examples), the hemodynamic effects of homeostat resetting include increased cardiac work or afterload, due to global or patterned increases in sympathetic outflow. As discussed in the chapter about cardiovascular diseases, the resetting may then worsen a largely independent cardiac pathologic state.

Homeostatic resetting in pathologic conditions can therefore produce unexpected clinical consequences. Patients with chronic obstructive pulmonary disease often have decreased chemoreceptor responsiveness to hypercarbia, thus depending upon hypoxic drive to regulate ventilation. Administering pure oxygen eliminates this drive, causing hypoventilation, accumulation of carbon dioxide, and possibly coma or respiratory arrest.

The efficacy of nitroglycerine in angina pectoris may depend on baroreflex resetting due to decreased cardiovascular compliance. In healthy volunteers, nitroglycerine increases pulse rate reflexively as stroke volume falls (Goldstein, 1983a). Since systolic blood pressure declines, whereas heart rate increases, the pressure–rate product, an index of myocardial oxygen consumption, remains largely unchanged. In patients with angina pectoris, nitroglycerine reduces the imbalance between myocardial oxygen demand and coronary arterial oxygen supply, relieving the chest discomfort. An explanation for this beneficial effect is that stiff cardiovascular walls splint baroreceptors, preventing reflexive sympathetic cardiovascular stimulation during nitroglycerine-induced decreases in cardiac filling, thereby decreasing myocardial oxygen consumption.

Distress

Distress is a form of stress with four additional defining features: consciousness, aversiveness, externally observable signs, and pituitary–adrenocortical and adrenomedullary activation.

Consciousness

The occurrence of stress does not require consciousness. Selye would have agreed, since he claimed that stress reactions can occur in anesthetized animals, in lower animals without nervous systems or undergoing mechanical damage to denervated limbs, and even in cells cultured outside the body (Selye, 1956, p. 53). In contrast, *dis*tress does require consciousness, because distress involves not only a challenge to homeostasis but also a perception by the organism that homeostatic mechanisms may not suffice—that is, conscious interpretation of sensory information and simulation of future events.

This is a more generalized statement of the concept of psychological stress as a consequence of a perceived inability to cope (Lazarus, 1966). The sense of an inability to cope or of a lack of controllability is basic to psychological theories about feelings associated with distress (Krantz and Lazar, 1987; Lazarus, 1966, 1991). An organism experiences distress when it perceives the inadequacy of compensatory adjustments to either a psychological or physiological stressor.

One need not separate psychological and physiological models of stress, despite independent development of the two research "traditions" (Krantz and Lazar, 1987). The present stress model shares main elements with the psychological stress model proposed by Lazarus (1966): appraisal processes based on afferent information, perception of threats to homeostasis, elicitation of compensatory response patterns, and continuous reappraisal of the success of the homeostatic effort.

Fundamental questions remain about whether psychological stress can bring on physical disease in otherwise healthy individuals and about whether physiological stress contributes to psychopathology. The existence, location, regulation, and pathology of psychological "homeostats" associated with the experience of distress remain largely unknown.

Aversiveness

Distressed organisms avoid situations that may produce the same distressing experience. Distress can therefore motivate escape and avoidance learning.

The experience of distress would be expected to enhance vigilance behavior and longterm memory of the distressing event. These adaptive neurological adjustments may involve catecholamines in the brain, as discussed in Chapter 4.

Most animals can react instinctively not only to a stressor but also to symbolic substitutes resembling the natural stimulus. Monkeys become visibly upset upon exposure to a snake, without ever having seen one before; rabbits freeze when a hawk-shaped shadow glides by; stickleback fish attack any red object in their territory; and mallards scurry to the water in response to a foxlike piece of red-brown skin dragged along the edge of the pond (Lorenz, 1952).

The plasticity afforded by learning decreases the likelihood of inappropriate instinctive responses to symbolic cues. One definition of learning is modification of behavior based on experience. According to this definition, learning requires memory. Even "primitive" animals have the capacity to learn to withdraw or escape from noxious stimuli (Kandel, 1983), or to habituate after prolonged or repeated exposure to a stimulus. These forms of learning mirror each other, the former reflecting a sensitization and the latter a desensitization. The fact that "primitive" animals have these capabilities indicates the remarkably durable survival advantage of learning.

Classical (or Pavlovian) conditioning represents an important refinement of these responses (Pavlov, 1927; Figure 1–13). Habituation and sensitization exemplify non-associative learning, where the organism learns about single stimuli. In contrast, clas-

● **Classical Conditioning**

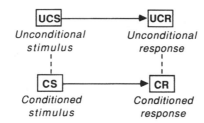

● **Operant (Instrumental) Conditioning**

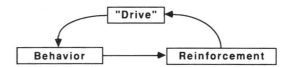

● **Combined Classical and Operant Conditioning**

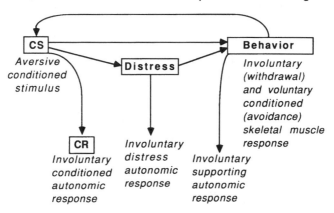

Figure 1–13. Conditioning paradigms. In classical (Pavlovian) conditioning, learning of a conditioned response occurs as a result of the repeated pairing of an unconditioned stimulus (UCS), which evokes an involuntary unconditioned response (UCR), with a previously neutral conditioned stimulus (CS). Learning occurs when the CS evokes all or part of the UCR. The acquired response is the conditioned response (CR). If the UCS is aversive, exposure to it or to the CS can elicit distress. In instrumental (operant) conditioning, the organism learns a behavior because elicitation of the behavior results in reward (positive reinforcement) or punishment (negative reinforcement). Operant conditioning models often include intervening variables—drives—such as motivational or emotional states. In combined aversive classical-operant conditioning, the organism learns to avoid an unpleasant CS, because the CS evokes distress.

sical conditioning (and operant conditioning, to be discussed shortly) involves learning associations among stimuli.

In classical conditioning, repeated pairing of a neutral stimulus (e.g., a bell ringing) with an unconditioned stimulus (UCS) that elicits an instinctive unconditioned response (UCR—e.g., salivation at the presentation of meat powder to a hungry dog; limb withdrawal after a local shock) results eventually in the elicitation of the UCR (or components of it) by the previously neutral conditioned stimulus (CS). The CS elicits a conditioned response (CR). For instance, depending on the UCS with which the ringing is paired, the dog may salivate or withdraw a leg when the bell rings.

Pavlov taught that the acquisition of conditioned reflexes requires cerebral cortices—the "crowning achievement in the nervous development of the animal kingdom" (Pavlov, 1927, p. 1); however, even invertebrates such as the sea snail, *Aplysia,* have the capacity to learn by classical conditioning (Kandel, 1983; Kandel and Tauc, 1965).

Although most classical conditioning experiments have involved an external UCS, such as an electric shock to the skin, this does not imply that the UCS must be external. For instance, rats can acquire hyperglycemia as a CR after repeated pairing of a previously neutral cue with injections of insulin (Siegel, 1972). Pavlov (1927, p. 36) himself demonstrated classically conditioned nausea and vomiting after repeated pairing of a CS (approach of the experimenter) with an internal UCS (injected morphine). Moreover, although classical conditioning experiments often have focused on presumably involuntary alimentary, glandular, or cardiovascular responses mediated by smooth muscle, Pavlov emphasized that conditioned reflexes include both external motor and internal secretory components (Pavlov, 1927, p. 17).

Instrumental, or operant, conditioning, appears to represent a more advanced form of learning, requiring a cerebral cortex (Thornton and Van-Toller, 1973). In instrumental conditioning, the likelihood of a behavior increases when the behavior leads to positive reinforcement (reward) and decreases when the behavior leads to negative reinforcement (punishment). Conversely—but circularly—reinforcement can be defined as an event that strengthens the response it follows (Rubin and McNeil, 1987). The conditioning is "operant" in that the individual's behavior operates on the environment, determining the occurrence of reinforcement; and the conditioning is "instrumental" in that the learning is a means to an end, with the occurrence of reinforcement contingent on the behavior. Operant conditioning therefore differs from Pavlovian conditioning, where delivery of the reinforcement occurs independently of the individual's behavior.

Both forms of conditioning require remembering an association between reinforcement and behavior. In Pavlovian conditioning, behavior (the UCR and CR) depends on the reinforcement (the UCS), whereas in operant conditioning, reinforcement depends on the behavior.

According to Hull's drive-reduction theory (Hull, 1943), an individual acquires a behavior because the behavior reduces a drive. For instance, a hungry rat learns to press a bar in order to receive food pellets, since the reinforcement—food—reduces the drive, hunger. Drive-reduction theory encountered several criticisms, beyond the scope of this presentation. Discarding intervening variables such as "drives" from the mechanism of instrumental learning seems to have necessitated the inclusion of a circular definition of reinforcement.

In avoidance learning, a form of operant conditioning, the individual learns to avoid negative reinforcement by producing behaviors that decrease the likelihood of that reinforcement. According to the drive-reduction theory, the punishment increases the experience of fear or anxiety, and learning the avoidance behavior reduces the drive. This is where the present view of distress enters the picture. If an organism experiences distress consistently in a given situation, subsequent perception of reexposure to the situation elicits distress as a classically conditioned response. Thus, in the morphine experiment described by Pavlov, when the experimenter entered the room, the dog became ''restless,'' not as a CR to morphine injection but as a CR to the experimenter. In anthropomorphic terms, the dog recognized that every time the experimenter entered the room, suffering followed, and this realization elicited a feeling of distress as a CR in response to the CS of the experimenter.

Aversive CR's lead to at least two types of behavioral response. One is a rapid, involuntary, conditioned withdrawal response. The response may be so rapid that the individual may not have time to consider the significance of the CS. The sheer rapidity of withdrawal (or escape) responses helps to explain their endurance in evolution.

A second response is avoidance. The basis for learning avoidance behavior is the reinforcement provided by reducing the distress. Concrete examples may help here: Suppose there are two signal lights in an animal's cage, one red, the other white. When the red light is on, there is a likelihood that an electric shock to the tail will follow. When the white light is on, there is no chance of shock. When the red light is on, pulling a lever in the box decreases the likelihood but does not completely prevent the occurrence of the shock. What does the animal learn to do when the red light turns on, and what would the cardiovascular consequences be?

By classical conditioning, the red light acquires the properties of an aversive CS. The cardiovascular reaction mimics that to the UCS (i.e., shock). Skeletal muscle in the tail contracts as a conditioned withdrawal response. In addition, the animal experiences distress, associated with patterned neuroendocrine changes producing cardiovascular effects. By operant avoidance conditioning, the animal learns to pull the lever, reducing its distress. Patterned neuroendocrine and cardiovascular changes accompany both the operantly and classically conditioned skeletal muscle contractions.

Another example, more relevant to modern human life: What happens when a speeder notices a red flashing light in the rear-view mirror? From prior experience, being caught speeding causes delay, confrontation, and humiliation, all delivered by a UCS in uniform. The light therefore is a CS, signifying an approaching car containing an aversive UCS. What does the speeder do? Virtually instantaneously, the right foot lifts from the accelerator—a skeletal muscle CR. Second, the speeder's heart rate increases—a visceral CR. This occurs because the red light has been paired in the past with confrontation and humiliation, and these constitute a UCS, increasing sympathetic outflow to the heart. Third, the speeder experiences distress, due to anxiety about whether the police car actually is going to signal the speeder to pull over and deliver the UCS, or is going to pass by. The distress also increases cardiac sympathetic outflow. Fourth, the speeder may flip down the rear-view mirror, rendering the red light less glaring, or turn on the cruise control, rapidly adjusting the car speed to a rate within the legal limit. The speeder may even search for a raffle ticket from a recent fund-raising campaign of the police benevolent association! These avoidance behaviors decrease the distress. Since they consist of skeletal muscle movements, sympathetic neural changes support the circulation during the skeletal muscle contractions.

These examples highlight sharing of the sympathoneural effector by several homeostats, including those related to skeletal muscle contraction and to the experience of distress. They also suggest that situations evoking distress typically involve a complex interplay of classically and operantly conditioned behaviors.

Communication

A third characteristic of distress, in addition to consciousness and aversiveness, is evocation of signs that other members of the species can interpret as indicating the emotional state and intent of the organism.

Darwin (1965) emphasized that the various outward manifestations of emotion provide important means of intraspecific communication with survival value for the species; and that physiological arousal, by intensifying emotions, amplifies further the physiological stress responses that accompany those emotions.

The latter constitutes a psychological positive feedback loop. From the previous discussion, such a loop is unstable. This can explain why fear, if not checked by some interposed negative feedback, degenerates into self-destructive panic.

Perceptions of signs of distress by other members of the species elicit involuntary, instinctive responses. Lorenz (1952) described the behavior of two fighting wolves after one submitted and extended its neck to the victor:

> A dog or wolf that offers its neck to its adversary . . . will never be bitten seriously . . . Since the fight is stopped so suddenly by this action, the victor frequently finds himself straddling his vanquished foe in anything but a comfortable position. So to remain, with his muzzle applied to the neck of the ''under-dog'' soon becomes tedious for the champion and, seeing that he cannot bite anyway, he soon withdraws . . .
>
> Why has the dog the inhibition against biting his fellow's neck? Why has the raven an inhibition against pecking the eye of his friend? . . . Should the raven peck, without compunction, at the eye of his nest-mate, his wife or his young, in the same way as he pecks at any other moving and glittering object, there would, by now, be no more ravens in the world. Should a dog or wolf unrestrainedly and unaccountably bite the neck of his packmates and actually execute the movement of shaking them to death, then his species also would certainly be exterminated within a short space of time. (Lorenz, 1952, pp. 188–191)

This principle applies analogously in humans, where the fiercest combat usually ends abruptly when one side shows universally understood signs of surrender and submission.

The communication value of external signs of distress helps to explain the continued elaboration of observable components of distress responses, despite the relative rarity of true "fight-or-flight" reactions in humans. Even in the wild, all social animals continually elicit and instinctively comprehend psychosocial cues (Sapolsky, 1990).

Alterations in sympathoneural activity often produce these external signs. For instance, sympathetic nerves to cutaneous blood vessels mediate facial blushing (Drummond and Lance, 1987; Metz et al., 1978), indicating embarrassment or humiliation. In a confrontation between two people, if one turns pale, quivers, averts his eyes, mumbles, and exposes his palms, and the other flushes, stands erect, glowers, shouts, and clenches his fists, the former evinces signs of submission and capitulation, and the latter signs of dominance and triumph. In evolution, these signs may have been by-products of genetically determined neurocirculatory adjustments supporting fleeing and fighting. In modern society, they serve signal functions of their own.

Crying in human newborns exemplifies the communication value of distress responses. Studies of expression of common emotions in primitive cultures and in blind infants (Eibl-Eibesfeldt, 1970) suggest that newborns cry not because of an emotional experience but as part of an instinctive pattern (Izard, 1977; Izard et al., 1980). One may surmise the "goal" of the behavior from what stops the crying—warmth, nursing, and being held protectively. Birth removes the fetus from an environment that has maintained its temperature, supplied metabolic fuels, and sheltered it from physical trauma. For these the newborn now depends entirely on its interaction with its mother. This being a matter of survival, natural selection must have favored the development of expressions fostering this interaction.

The mother's response to the cry may also include substantial genetic "loading." Thus, both the infant's expressions and temperamental characteristics and the mother's emotional experiences, expressive behaviors, and personality traits predict the infant–mother attachment during the first year of life (Izard et al., 1991).

In psychology, the issue of the relationship between emotional expression and emotional experience remains controversial (Izard, 1990). Eventually, the infant experiences distress when it cries. Distress, as all emotional experiences (Izard, 1978), can in turn motivate learning. Any parent can confirm that, at some point in an infant's development, the infant cries not only from distress but also as a learned behavior. Crying leads to positive reinforcement, in the form of parental provision of comfort and food.

Neuroendocrine Activation due to Homeostat Resetting

A fourth characteristic of distress is neuroendocrine activation—in particular, enhanced adrenomedullary release of catecholamines and adrenocortical release of steroids. As discussed in the chapter about stress response patterns, increased adrenomedullary release of epinephrine constitutes perhaps the most sensitive neurochemical index of this activation.

Neurochemical activation alone does not itself produce distress (Cameron et al., 1990). The experience of distress requires both physiological arousal and appropriate cognitions by the organism (Schachter and Singer, 1962). Although several emotions include distressing elements (e.g., fear, anxiety, panic, guilt), other emotions do not (e.g., libido, joy), yet adrenomedullary activation accompanies even positive emotional experiences (Frankenhaeuser, 1975). According to the present concept, adrenomedullary activation does not imply the experience of distress, because such an experience requires appropriate cognitions and because sympathetic activation can accompany even nondistressing emotions; however, in organisms with a functional adrenomedullary system, the absence of adrenomedullary activation excludes the experience of distress.

Cannon viewed the neuronal and hormonal components of the sympathetic system to act as a unit in preserving homeostasis. Describing the pattern of neuroendocrine activation attending distress requires a distinction between the sympathetic neuronal and adrenomedullary systems, because according to the present conception, specifically the adrenomedullary hormonal component characterizes distress. Subsequent chapters of this book will return to the theme of dissociated sympathetic neural and adrenomedullary hormonal responses during different forms of stress.

Distress always resets homeostats. For instance, as discussed in Chapter 2, stimulation of the "defense area" of the hypothalamus or elicitation of the "defense reaction" decreases the sensitivity of the cardiac limb of the arterial baroreflex (Koizumi and Kollai, 1981; Lundin et al., 1983, 1984; Sleight et al., 1978). Reversible resetting of homeostats during distress produces the associated neurocirculatory and neuroendocrine activation, including activation of the hypothalamic–pituitary–adrenocortical and adrenomedullary systems. The prominence of changes in pituitary–adrenocortical and adrenomedullary outflows during distress results from sharing of these effectors by so many homeostats that reset during distress.

Stress-associated resetting provides at least a theoretical basis for virtually all psychosomatic concomitants of cardiovascular disease. For instance, resetting of arterial baroreflex function due to repeated "defense reactions" remains a viable mechanistic hypothesis for the pathogenesis of hypertension (Folkow, 1982, 1987, 1988).

If distress invariably resets homeostats, why does it do so? The present conception views the many physiological, neurochemical, and psychological adjustments attending distress as products of preprogramed strategies that include alterations in learning and memory which, in turn, enable simulations of future events. The evolution of means to make these adjustments even *in anticipation* of distress-evoking situations implies that the survival advantage of anticipatory changes outweighed the potentially deleterious effects of redefining homeostasis temporarily.

What are these adjustments, the products of these resettings, during distress? Hemodynamically, blood flow is diverted to skeletal muscle, in order to meet the markedly increased demand for glucose and oxygen and to remove metabolic waste during strenuous exercise, without compromising blood flow to the brain and heart. Platelet aggregability increases, enhancing the ability to plug vascular holes. Biochemically, blood glucose levels rise, owing to decreased insulin-mediated cellular uptake of glucose, glycogenolysis, and accelerated gluconeogenesis, increasing availability of this vital fuel. Sweating increases, with evaporative heat loss to avoid increases in body temperature resulting from accelerated metabolism. Behaviorally, hyperventilation maximizes oxygenation, removes carbon dioxide, increases pH, and decreases serum potassium, the latter perhaps to counter acidosis and hyperkalemia produced by tissue trauma. Alertness, strength, and resistance to fatigue increase. Memory processes change to facilitate long-term recall of the distressing event and escape and avoidance learning.

The appearance and actions of the individual instinctively communicate information about the internal state.

Levine and Ursin (1991) and Weiner (1991a) have used the terms "distress" and "stress" largely interchangeably. The present conception considers the distinction to be more than semantic, viewing distress as a form of stress with additional, defining features—a conscious, aversive experience related to the perception of a failure of homeostatic mechanisms, autonomic and behavioral communicated signs that are largely instinctive, and adrenomedullary and pituitary–adrenocortical activation due to homeostat resetting.

A second distinction of the present view from others about stress and distress is the emphasis on homeostat resetting that always accompanies distress. According to the present conception, higher brain centers determine this resetting as part of the elaboration of coordinated behavioral, endocrine, and physiological patterns. Thus, homeostasis is not static at all and, instead, is continually redefined. There are no "steady states," not only because some effector systems are inherently oscillatory, but because homeostatic settings are continually readjusted. The above theories do not emphasize such resetting. A major task for future research is to identify central neural processes underlying these "homeodynamic" readjustments and their results—stress response patterns.

With repetition of exposure to a situation evoking distress, the organism habituates, in the sense that effector components whose expression depends on novelty or unpredictability recede; concurrently, however, the organism becomes hyperreactive to other potential stressors (Abercrombie et al., 1992; Kvetnansky et al., 1984; McCarty et al., 1992; Nisenbaum et al., 1991), a phenomenon called stressor-switch hyperresponsiveness, or dishabituation (McCarty et al., 1992).

Habituation to a stressor recalls the stage of resistance, the second phase of Selye's General Adaptation Syndrome; however, in the stage of resistance, all the components of the unitary stress response would diminish, not only those components dependent on novelty or unpredictability. As noted above, the occurrence of dishabituation refutes Selye's doctrine of nonspecificity, since the stress response in this setting would depend on the type of stressor.

Distress vs. the General Adaptation Syndrome

How does the present view of distress differ from Selye's General Adaptation Syndrome?

First, as noted above, Selye's theory emphasized the non-specificity of the General Adaptation Syndrome. According to the present conception, the elicitation of distress responses depends importantly on the character, intensity, and meaning of the stressor as perceived by the organism and on the organism's perceived ability to cope with it.

Second, distress responses—as all stress responses—are viewed here as compensatory in origin and purpose, attempting in some way to mitigate the effects of a stressor. This applies not only to neuroendocrine aspects of those responses (such as the glucose counterregulatory actions of pituitary–adrenocortical and adrenomedullary stimulation during insulin-induced hypoglycemia) but also to psychological aspects (such as conditioned aversive and instrumental avoidance learning). In this sense the present conception agrees with that of Gray (1991):

> Fear or anxiety that is associated with real or perceived threat constitutes psychological stress. This "stress" or so-called defense response is composed of a set of relatively well-defined biological changes . . . These changes help to promote the readiness and execution of behaviors that will ultimately increase the probability of survival of the organism. (Gray, 1991b, p. 39)

Gray, however, does not distinguish stress as an experiential entity from stress as a stereotyped biological pattern, just as Selye sometimes defined stress as a condition and sometimes as a response pattern.

Third, according to Selye, the General Adaptation Syndrome consisted of a series of well-defined stages: alarm, resistance, and exhaustion; however, experimental results have not consistently confirmed either the habituation or exhaustion of adrenomedullary responses after chronically repeated episodes of distress (Kvetnansky and Mikulaj, 1970; McCarty et al., 1992). The present theory does not depend on these stages.

Fourth, the present theory views distress as a consciously experienced condition. Neither adrenomedullary nor pituitary–adrenocortical activation implies the experience of distress. Since Selye never developed a clear distinction between stress (which could be conscious or unconscious) and distress, his theory did not state whether the experiential requirement would distinguish them.

Fifth, and most relevant to the subject matter of this book, the present theory does not assume that distress causes disease. Distress, while unpleasant, is not by definition pathologic. Selye characterized distress as unpleasant or harmful (Selye, 1974, p. 18), without separating these two very different characteristics. He never incorporated the relationship between distress and disease explicitly in his theory; he appears to have added distress as a concept long after he proposed maladaptation from excessive or inappropriate stress responses or the operation of "conditioning factors." Thus, the index to his treatise about stress and diseases of adaptation (Selye, 1950) does not include an entry under "distress"; and in his book for laypeople, *Stress Without Distress,* he did not elaborate on the relationship between distress and disease.

Perhaps Selye recognized the paradox of stress as simultaneously homeostatic and pathologic. Rather than concluding that the relationship between stress and disease was a matter for research, he simply defined a new term, distress, to denote stress that causes disease. As suggested above, he seems to have developed this idea rather late in his career. Writers about stress have also generally not recognized this paradox of Selye's theory and have either assumed the linkage between stress and psychiatric and physical disease or else adopted the term, distress, without explaining its meaning specifically (Asterita, 1985; Beamish et al., 1985; Eliot, 1974).

Stress theorists have also argued that because of modern societal constraints on emotional expression, people repeatedly suppress behavioral responses during emotional distress without the ability to suppress the physiological and biochemical concomitants, resulting in psychological or physical pathology: "[D]istress or end-organ dysfunction can occur as a result of the accumulation of many unresolved 'fight or flight' responses" (Asterita, 1985, pp. 170–171).

Folkow (1987, 1988) similarly has suggested that chronic, frequent repetition of even mild "defense reactions" can produce high blood pressure. More generally:

> [L]imbic–hypothalamic patterns are basically designed to protect the individual and species from adverse environmental influences in primitive life . . . Thanks to our more advanced neocortex, man differs here from animals mainly in two ways. First, we learn to cope with some environmental stimuli and thus delimit undue emotional engagements; second, when once elicited we can often suppress the behavioural link . . . As we cannot suppress the autonomic-hormonal links, however, they then occur more or less "in vain," and such socially enforced dissociations of per se normal response patterns may not in the long run be healthy. (Folkow, 1988, p. 61)

This notion is a founding—and largely unproven—tenet of psychosomatic medicine.

Weiner (1991b) seems to have adopted Selye's circular argument that stress is harmful when it causes disease:

> [T]he linear relation between stressful experience and disease, which Selye described, occurs when the experience is injurious, unavoidable, or incontrollable. In most other instances, however, when it is not, little or no organ damage occurs. (Weiner, 1991b, p. II-2).

The assertion that stressful experience probably leads to disease only in predisposed individuals (Weiner, 1991b, p. II-2) seems to add another layer of circularity.

The present conception implies no necessary link between stress or distress and the long-term development of physical disease. This does not mean that acute stress, by evoking neuroendocrine activation, cannot evoke severe and even fatal cardiovascular events. For instance, a large plasma epinephrine response during exercise in a patient with coronary heart disease can augment myocardial oxygen consumption, platelet aggregability, and ventricular irritability, resulting in angina pectoris, myocardial infarction, or sudden death. Nor does this suggest a lack of reasonableness for the assertion that chronic emotional distress has pathological consequences. Rather, the present conception views the pathologic effects of stress and distress as a matter for experimental testing, especially using longitudinal controlled studies.

Stress in Evolutionary Perspective

Darwin and Ethology

Charles Darwin introduced the notion that emotional expressions and their autonomic accompaniments evolved. Based on numerous interviews, readings, and observations, Darwin suggested the inheritance not only of physical characteristics but also of emotional behaviors. In fact, he used the latter to support his theory of the descent of man:

I have endeavored to show in considerable detail that all the chief expressions exhibited by man are the same throughout the world. This fact is interesting, as it affords a new argument in favor of the several races being descended from a single parent-stock, which must have been almost completely human in structure, and to a large extent in mind, before the period at which the races diverged from each other. (Darwin, 1965, p. 359)

The naturalistic studies of the ethologists, Lorenz and Tinbergen, largely confirmed Darwin's views about the evolution of instinctive behaviors. Indeed, Darwin provided much of the conceptual foundation for the field of ethology, the branch of zoology that deals with instinctive animal behaviors. In the preface to an edition of Darwin's classic, *The Expression of the Emotions in Man and Animals* (originally published in 1872, a century before Lorenz received the Nobel Prize in Physiology and Medicine), Lorenz wrote:

[T]he adaptation of the behavior patterns of an organism to its environment is achieved in exactly the same manner as that of its organs, that is to say on the basis of information which the species has gained in the course of its evolution by the age-old method of mutation and selection. This is true not only for relatively rigid patterns of form or behavior, but also for the complicated mechanisms of adaptive modification, among which are those generally subsumed under the conception of learning (Darwin, 1965, p. xii)

Darwin himself wrote:

My object is to show that certain movements were originally performed for a definite end, and that, under nearly the same circumstances, they are still pertinaciously performed through habit when not of the least use. That the tendency in most of the following cases is inherited, we may infer from such actions being performed in the same manner by all the individuals, young and old, of the same species. (Darwin, 1965, p. 42)

As far as we can judge, only a few expressive movements . . . are learnt by each individual . . . The far greater number of the movements of expression, and all the more important ones, are, as we have seen, innate or inherited; and such cannot be said to depend on the will of the individual. (Darwin, 1965, p. 351–352)

Geographically diverse societies appear to have essentially the same forms of emotional expression. For instance, members of the Minangkabau culture in Bukittingi, western Sumatra, express fear, anger, sadness, and disgust similarly to Americans, and production of facial expressions of fear or anger produce immediate increases in heart rate in both cultures (Levenson et al., cited in ''Science Notebook,'' *The Washington Post,* January 23, 1989, p. A10).

Darwin recognized that the autonomic concomitants of emotion have proved advantageous not only in preparing the organism for emergency responses, but also for providing the basis for visible signs that serve important, universally understood communication functions within the species:

The movements of expression in the face and body, whatever their origin may have been, are in themselves of much importance for our welfare. They serve as the first means of communication between the mother and her infant; she smiles approval, and thus encourages her child on the right path, or frowns disapproval. We readily perceive sympathy in others by their expression; our sufferings are thus mitigated and our pleasures increased; and mutual good feeling is thus strengthened. The movements of expression give vividness and energy to our spoken words. They reveal the thoughts and intentions of others more truly than do words, which may be falsified. (Darwin, 1965, p. 364)

Research on primates in the wild (Sapolsky, 1990a, 1990b) has suggested that in everyday life, most ''stress'' system activation accompanies instinctive social behaviors—e.g., dominance displays, sexual pursuit, and submissive escape—rather than mitigating threats to physiological or metabolic homeostasis.

Darwin was acquainted with the work of Claude Bernard but had only a vague understanding of the role of the sympathoadrenal system in producing the observable signs of emotional distress. Darwin did recognize, however, the origin of these signs in the nervous system:

[C]ertain actions which we recognize as expressive of certain states of mind, are the direct results of the constitution of the nervous system, and have been from the first independent of the will, and, to a large extent, of habit. When the sensorium is strongly excited nerve-force is generated in excess, and is transmitted in certain directions, dependent on the connection of the nerve-cells, and, as far as the muscular system is concerned, on the nature of the movements which have been habitually practiced . . . Claude Bernard also repeatedly insists, and this deserves especial notice, that when the heart is affected it reacts on the brain; and the state of the brain again reacts through the pneumogastric nerve on the heart; so that under any excitement there will be much mutual action and reaction between these, the two most important organs of the body.

. . . any sensation or emotion, as great pain or rage, which has habitually led to much muscular action, will immediately influence the flow of nerve-force to the heart, although there may not be at the time any muscular exertion. (Darwin, 1965, pp. 66–75).

The current theory of stress and distress therefore relies on concepts Darwin introduced: Autonomic changes that accompany emotional experiences and their behavioral manifestations evolved, because the autonomic changes were advantageous in natural selection; one advantage of autonomic arousal was provision of rapid or anticipatory adjustments in cardiovascular function, and another was provision of universally understood means of intraspecific communication.

Behavioral evolution requires a genetic substrate. Several strains of laboratory animals have genetic differences in activities of major stress systems. For instance, spontaneously hypertensive and borderline hypertensive rats of the Okamoto strain have excessive responses of renal sympathetic nerve activity or plasma catecholamine levels during various forms of psychological stress (Lundin and Thoren, 1982; McCarty and Kopin, 1978). ''Lewis'' rats have a genetic deficiency of ACTH responses after injection of substances evoking inflammation (Sternberg, Young et al., 1989) and have low plasma levels of epinephrine at rest (Goldstein, Garty et al., 1993). Plasma catechol-amine levels differ in rats inbred for differences in response to stress (Blizard et al., 1980). "Brattleboro" rats lack hypothalamic production of AVP.

Studies of identical twins have indicated relatively high heritability of levels of various neurochemicals, including catecholamines, in humans (Luft et al., 1987; Miller et al., 1980; Williams et al., 1993). Monozygotic twins tend to have similar rates of directly recorded skeletal muscle sympathetic nerve traffic (Wallin et al., 1993) and twins tend also to have similar cardiovascular stress responses (Carmelli et al., 1985). Lacey and Lacey (1958) elaborated a principle of autonomic response-stereotypy, in which individuals respond with a consistent physiological activation pattern across stressors. Consistent with their concept, rates of directly recorded skeletal muscle sympathetic traffic have remarkable intraindividual reproducibility even after a decade between measurements, despite substantial interindividual variability (Fagius and Wallin, 1993).

Considering the genetic component of stress responses, the same selective pressures that determined the evolution of physical characteristics should have determined the evolution of stress responses. More generally, the ethologist Richard Dawkins has presented a comprehensive theory about the evolution of behavior (Dawkins, 1989). The following propositions summarize his "selfish gene" theory:

1. The fundamental unit of selection is either the species nor, strictly speaking, the individual but rather, the gene, the unit of heredity. A gene is any portion of chromosomal material that potentially lasts for enough generations to serve as a unit of natural selection. A gene is not a single physical piece of DNA in a chromosome but all replicas of that piece, distributed throughout the world. Groups of genes can be selected as units.
2. "Survival of the fittest" means survival of the stable. Selection has favored genes that cooperate within a body, so that it is usually convenient to consider the body as an integral agent for preserving and propagating genes—a "survival machine."
3. In animals, behavior, mediated by muscles, evolved because it enabled rapid movement. Generating complex, timed movements requires coordination by a computer, the brain, the unit of which is the neuron. The genes control behavior indirectly, like a computer programmer. They set up the machine but cannot control it, because of time-lag problems. Genes work by controlling protein synthesis, which is powerful but slow. They provide strategies, preprogramed behavioral policies. An evolutionarily stable strategy is one which, if most members of a population adopt it, cannot be bettered by an alternative strategy.
4. Genes predict behavioral strategies by incorporating a capacity for learning, which requires memory and feedback. Learning can occur by trial and error. Simulations represent vicarious trial-and-error predictions of future events. The evolution of the capacity to simulate has culminated in subjective consciousness.

From the selfish gene theory one may hypothesize that natural selection favored the evolution of stress responses, the body's means for preserving a stable internal environment. The continual adjustments in activities of homeostatic systems reflect genetically determined algorithms, learning by combinations of classical and operant conditioning, and conscious simulations of likely future events. The mystery, and the challenge for stress research, is not to explain why stress responses evolved, but how they work. Although research has begun to elucidate the molecular events underlying classical conditioning, such as in *Aplysia* (Kandel, 1983), the genetic instructions dictating these events, and therefore the bases for evolution of stress responses, remain unknown.

Ascending the phylogenetic scale, organisms have depended increasingly on complex, energy-requiring systems and on close coordination of behavioral, neuroendocrine, and physiological responses. For instance, reef corals—relatively simple animals—live a fragile existence, surviving only in unusual, suitable niches within a small range of salinity, turbulence, and temperature. Although they benefit from the lack of energy expenditure to maintain cellular temperature, they cannot live in water colder than 18°C. More versatile cold-blooded reptiles and other lower vertebrates survive a larger range of external temperature by instinctively using both sun and shade (Brattstrom, 1965; Swanson, 1987) and probably by adjusting cardiovascular system performance, but this mechanism requires more organization and more energy.

The big-eye tuna, which has muscles adapted to warm water, possesses a circulatory heat exchanger, where a network of vessels containing blood warmed by exercising muscles wraps around vessels containing blood chilled as a result of their closeness to the fish's outer surface. The heat exchangers regulate the temperature of the blood before the blood enters the heart. When the tuna ascends to warm water, the exchanger shuts off, accelerating the ability of the fish to warm the blood before the fish descends again to the cool depths (Holland et al., 1992). The rapidity of the shutdown in the heat exchanger suggests a form of neurocirculatory regulation.

Warm-blooded mammals require and use much more fuel than do reptiles or fish, simply to maintain body temperature. As in reptiles, mammals possess not only physiological but also instinctive behavioral means to regulate temperature. Ecological niches determine the adaptive value of this inheritance. For instance, llamas, having evolved in a cold, mountainous, treeless climate, do not instinctively seek shade from the sun. Transported to and kept on a Caribbean island, many of these animals, with coats that prevented evaporative heat loss, succumbed to heat stroke (*New York Times,* April 21, 1989, p. 1). Humans spend most of their lives wrapped in protective clothing or in environments where the external temperature itself is regulated.

Other stress responses are also phylogenetically very old. Even relatively simple organisms such as *Aplysia* have withdrawal or escape responses to physical or chemical manipulation (Kandel, 1983; Kandel and Tauc, 1965).

Mechanisms for preserving body water, ionic composition, and essential nutrients—oxygen and glucose—must also have developed early in evolution. The classic paper by Macallum (1926) postulated a "paleochemistry" of body fluids: ". . . the blood plasma of Vertebrates and Invertebrates with a closed circulatory system is, in its inorganic salts, but a reproduction of the sea water of the remote geological period in which the prototypic representatives of such animal forms first made their appearance." (Macallum, 1926, p. 322)

The remarkably large repertoire of glucose "counterregulatory" systems indicates the importance of appropriate adjustments in blood glucose levels in different situations, including exercise, emotion, and the postprandial state. Many behaviors increase glucose utilization in different organs, and therefore a variety of means to maintain glucose levels evolved with those behaviors. Since all cells require glucose, these situations often call for generalized metabolic responses, elicited by hormones reaching all tissues of the body. Conversely, cellular glucoprivation poses a generalized threat, where no patterned neural response or readjustment of blood volume distribution can suffice. Glucopenia therefore evokes marked hormonal responses, including large, rapid increases in adrenomedullary secretion of epinephrine. Generalized threats such as glucopenia often elicit emotional distress. In insulin-induced hypoglycemia, the patient's anxious, pale, and sweaty appearance constitutes an important clinical sign. Drugs that block effects of epinephrine mask this protective response and can render the patient and those caring for him or her unaware of the life threat.

Agonistic behavior, such as attack and dominance displays, also includes strong genetically determined components and evolved. Aggression facilitates predation, reproduction, social organization, and the division of ecological space (Lorenz, 1963). Since unchecked aggression would also threaten gene propagation, instinctive means to limit intraspecific aggression have also evolved, as discussed above.

The assumption of an upright posture—orthostasis—has posed a relatively recent challenge in evolution. The ability of snakes to maintain blood pressure during orthostasis illustrates the interplay between ecology and physical, physiological, and behavioral characteristics of a species (Lillywhite, 1988). In climbing snakes, the heart is located relatively close to the head, and the thin tail minimizes pooling of blood during climbing. In contrast, in sea snakes, the heart is located in the center of the body. Exposure of sea snakes to orthostatic stress in a tilting tube causes their blood pressure to fall, whereas climbing snakes in the same situation maintain their blood pressure, both because of the above physical features and because of active muscle pumping behavior.

In mammals, internal sensations and perceptions of changes in the body's orientation in space during orthostasis lead to patterned neural discharges that result in constriction of arterioles in the legs and gut, increased pulse rate, and increased total peripheral resistance to blood flow, all tending to redistribute blood volume toward the heart and brain. Skeletal muscle pumping contributes to this redistribution. Ordinarily, these rapid and effective concerted neural responses, mediated mainly by the sympathetic nervous system, counter the stressor unconsciously.

The importance of these mechanisms for human well-being is illustrated by several clinical autonomic disorders, discussed in the chapter about cardiovascular diseases, and the effects of weightlessness in space flight. Weightlessness is, of course, a novel stressor in human evolution. Several manifestations of "space sickness" result from the lack of evolution of physiological and neuroendocrine mechanisms to counter the absence of gravitational force. During exposure to zero-gravity, the absence of orthostatic blood pooling increases venous return to the heart, in turn altering activities of several systems that maintain cardiac filling. Excretion of water and salt increases, probably due to decreased renal sympathetic activity, decreased activity of the renin-angiotensin-aldosterone system, increased atrial natriuretic factor release by the heart, and decreased vasopressin release by the pituitary gland. Blood volume falls and becomes dissociated from cardiac filling. A new state of equilibrium occurs, and sympathoneural activity, as indicated by plasma norepinephrine levels, is about normal during prolonged space flight (Davydova et al., 1989; Kvetnansky et al., 1988), despite hypovolemia. When the astronauts return to earth, orthostatic pooling of blood combines with the relatively low blood volume and possibly with resetting of cardiopulmonary baroreflexes to evoke symptomatic orthostatic hypotension.

Catecholaminergic systems, major stress effectors, seem to have evolved in sequence, with dopamine the most primitive catecholamine. For instance, sea anemones contain the catecholamine precursor dihydroxyphenylalanine (DOPA) but do not contain catecholamines or the enzyme catalyzing the conversion of DOPA to catecholamines (Carlberg, 1983). In most invertebrates, dopamine is the dominant catecholamine; concentrations of norepinephrine, when detected, are less than those of dopamine; and epinephrine is absent (Welsh, 1972). In organs or plasma of amphibia, epinephrine is the dominant catecholamine; in reptiles, either norepinephrine or epinephrine may predominate; and in mammals norepinephrine predominates (Holzbauer and Sharman, 1972). Hart et al. (1989) reported that of 31 animal groups, the lamprey had the highest basal circulating concentrations of dopamine and epinephrine; sharks and domestic animals had high concentrations of norepinephrine; and the eel and lumpfish had low concentrations of norepinephrine.

Autocrine/paracrine systems can theoretically meet the needs of simple organisms that lack mechanisms of neurocirculatory regulation, whereas more sophisticated organisms use hormones to coordinate organ functions, and in the most complicated organisms, including humans, autonomic nerve networks enable complex central neural regulation of regional resistances to blood flow and of glandular secretion. The regulation of nerve networks by the brain also fosters a close association between learned skeletal muscle movements and autonomic outflows to smooth muscle that support those movements. These principles may help to comprehend the evolution of catecholaminergic systems.

The autocrine/paracrine catecholaminergic systems still appear to operate, at least in the kidneys, adrenal glands, and gut. In the kidneys, locally formed dopamine contributes to regulation of sodium balance (Carey et al., 1990; Siragy et al., 1989). In the adrenal cortex, locally formed dopamine inhibits aldosterone secretion. In both organs, however, more powerful hormonal and neuronal systems now seem to predominate. In the gastrointestinal tract, dopamine, which can be formed locally from DOPA (Vieira-Coelho and Soares-da-Silva, 1993), stimulates bicarbonate secretion (Flemstrom et al., 1993; Knutson et al., 1993) and may constitute a catecholaminergic effector for the "brain-gut axis" (Glavin, 1991). In rabbit myocardium, nests of chromaffin cells have been observed at all ages studied, even in the fetus (Friedman et al., 1968). Ruminants have very high pulmonary concentrations of dopamine (Juorio and Chedreses, 1990), for unknown reasons. The source and significance of these cells, and other scattered cells—APUD (amino precursor uptake and decarboxylation) and enterochromaffin cells of the gut, SIF (small intensely fluorescent) cells in sympathetic ganglia, and mast cells in the lungs—remain mysterious. Perhaps they constitute remnants of a primordial autocrine/paracrine aminergic system.

Dopamine concentrations in plasma are remarkably low, and concentrations of the inactive conjugate dopamine sulfate exceed those of unconjugated dopamine by about 50 fold. The source and physiological meaning of conjugated dopamine are unknown. Since the conjugation causes circulating concentrations of free dopamine to be far lower than required to produce physiological effects, and since dopamine injection in humans rapidly increases plasma levels of dopamine sulfate (Ratge et al., 1991), one may speculate that conjugation inactivates dopamine escaping from organs into the bloodstream, localizing changes in tissue function due to alterations in release of dopamine as an autocrine/paracrine agent. In the gut, sulfation may provide a "gut–blood barrier" for ingested catecholamines (Cuche et al., 1990).

Selective factors favoring the evolution of coordination of activities of hormonal stress systems may explain the architectural arrangement of the adrenal cortex and medulla. In mammals, the adrenal cortex envelops the medulla. The two components of the adrenal gland have entirely different embryological sources (Langman, 1969). Adrenal medullary cells arise from ectodermal sympathetic neuroblasts that migrate anteriorly to penetrate the fetal adrenal, of mesodermal origin. Since adrenal blood flows in a corticomedullary direction, this arrangement produces very high local concentrations of adrenocortical compounds in blood passing through the adrenal medulla. As noted in the chapter about peripheral catecholaminergic systems, glucocorticoids contribute importantly to regulation of adrenomedullary epinephrine synthesis. Since angiotensin II is formed in the adrenal cortex, and since angiotensin II stimulates catecholamine secretion in cultured adrenomedullary cells (Zimlichman, Goldstein, Zimlichman et al., 1987), high local concentrations of angiotensin II may contribute to adrenomedullary secretion.

The sympathetic nervous system is immature at birth (Friedman et al., 1968). From the concept that ontogeny recapitulates phylogeny, this immaturity may indicate relatively late development of the sympathetic nerve network in evolution. Maturation of the sympathetic nervous system after birth allows a degree of plasticity of symphatoneural development based on experiences of the individual early in life. In contrast, as noted above, the adrenal medulla forms during fetal development in mammals, and low and unchanging basal tissue concentrations of epinephrine persist in sympathetically innervated organs throughout the life-span (Friedman et al., 1968).

Primitive Specificity

A major thesis of this book is that activities of stress effector systems are coordinated in relatively specific patterns, including neuroendocrine patterns. These patterns, produced by the actions of different homeostats, serve different homeostatic needs.

For each stress, neuroendocrine and physiological changes are coupled with behavioral changes. For instance, the regulation of total body water in humans depends on an interplay between behavior (the search for water and drinking), an internal experience or feeling (thirst), and the elicitation of a neurohormonal response pattern (in this case dominated by AVP, the antidiuretic hormone; and to a lesser extent angiotensin, a potent dipsogen, or stimulator of drinking). Evoked changes in homeostat function often produce not only neuroendocrine and physiological effects but also behavioral responses; however, because of traditional boundaries among physiology, endocrinology, and psychology, interactions producing integrated patterns of response remain incompletely understood. For instance, studies about vasopressin and activity of the renin–angiotensin–aldosterone system during blood volume depletion rarely have included controls for or monitoring of thirst and salt hunger.

This situation developed partly because of the long-held view that acts of skeletal muscle—the province of neurology and psychology—mediate the voluntary, conscious responses of the organism to the external environment, whereas autonomic and endocrine changes—the province of physiology and endocrinology—mediate the involuntary, unconscious responses of smooth muscle and glands to maintain the internal environment. Findings in neuroendocrinology refute this distinction. Conclusive evidence has accrued that the external environment, via the central nervous system—in particular the hypothalamus—affects autonomic and endocrine activity. Biofeedback and conditioning studies suggested learned modifications of some autonomic functions (Goldstein et al., 1977; Miller, 1969; Siegel, 1972). The state of physiological arousal affects behavior by, among other things, intensifying emotions (Schachter and Singer, 1962) and communicating external signs of internal states. Finally, recent findings involving circumventricular organs, sites in the brain that are devoid of a blood–brain barrier, have introduced the possibility that hormones can reach central neural sites, eliciting various behaviors and altering autonomic and neuroendocrine activity.

Folkow (1988) has argued that limbic–hypothalamic patterns, protecting the individual during exposure to adverse environmental conditions, are always expressed as a triad of closely linked, situation-specific, somatomotor behavioral, visceromotor autonomic, and hormonal changes. One may speculate that patterns of behavioral, experiential, neuroendocrine, and autonomic activities during stress intertwined so tightly in evolution that they are now expressed as units, since, as noted above in the discussion of Dawkins's "selfish gene" theory, groups of genes can be selected as a unit.

The notion of stressor-specific response patterns disagrees with the theories of both Cannon and Selye. Cannon, largely ignoring other systems, asserted that sympathoadrenal activation meets most or all important threats to the internal environment.

> The amazing feature of the role played by the sympathico-adrenal system is its applicability to the widespread range of possible disturbances that we have just noted. As stated earlier, the system commonly works as a unit. It is very remarkable indeed that such unified action can be useful in circumstances so diverse as low blood sugar, low blood pressure, and low temperature . . . The appearance of inappropriate features in the total complex of sympathicoadrenal function is made reasonable, as I pointed out in 1928, if we consider, first, that it is, on the whole, a unitary system; second, that it is capable of producing effects in many different organs; and third, that among these effects are different combinations which are of the utmost utility in correspondingly different conditions of need. (Cannon, 1939a, pp. 298–299)

According to Cannon, the neuronal and hormonal components of the sympathoad-renal system function as a unit. This book emphasizes the separate regulation of sympathoneural and adrenomedullary responses, with a close association between adrenomedullary responses and responses of the pituitary–adrenocortical system. Differential regulation of the sympathoneural and adrenomedullary systems during different forms of stress supports the concept of primitive specificity.

This differential regulation therefore also argues against Selye's doctrine of nonspecificity. Selye, like Cannon, overemphasized responses of a single system—in Selye's case, the pituitary–adrenocortical system. This activation produces thymicolymphatic degeneration and adrenal hypertrophy but only provides a glimpse at the spectrum of systemic responses to stress. Deriving a concept based on heterogeneous neuroendocrine responses during stress has required simultaneous measures of several endogenous substances indicating activities of different stress systems, and descriptions of assays for these measurements appeared only long after Cannon and Selye had published their unitary theories.

Different emotional behaviors can have also different cardiovascular concomitants, reflecting differential regulation of sympathoneural outflows. For instance, in baboons, attack toward the observer and orienting behavior are associated with a pattern of markedly decreased renal flow, increased heart rate and iliac flow, and decreased arterial pressure (Smith et al., 1988). Exposure to a conspecific of the opposite sex decreases renal flow, increases iliac flow, increases heart rate, and increases arterial pressure; whereas exposure of a monitored male baboon to a male conspecific produces profound, prolonged decreases in renal flow and increases in heart rate, with small and variable increases in blood pressure and iliac flow. In anticipation of overt attack by a dominant male, renal and mesenteric flow decrease, and heart rate and blood pressure increase (Astley et al., 1991).

Because of the importance of dominance in the daily life of male baboons, determining access to food, territory, attention, and sexual partners, one would expect that challenges to dominance would produce especially large stress responses in these animals. Smith and co-workers (1988) concluded that "each definable behavior seems to carry its own cardiovascular signature. It also seems to be the case that rather simple behaviors may include dramatic cardiovascular responses." By analyses of relevant environmental changes, video recordings of behavior, and telemetered cardiovascular changes, these investigators hope to develop a code relating behavioral with cardiovascular dynamics (Astley et al., 1991). One would hope further that the code will incorporate the neuroendocrine responses that link these dynamics, and the homeostats that determine them all.

Summary and Conclusions

Claude Bernard suggested that the body maintains a constant internal environment by myriad, continual compensatory reactions, tending to restore a state of equilibrium, thereby allowing independence from the external environment. Cannon extended Bernard's concept by showing that the maintenance of a stable internal environment depends importantly on circulatory regulation by the sympathoadrenal system. Cannon coined the term "homeostasis" to describe the "coordinated physiological processes which maintain most of the steady states in the organism."

Homeostatic systems maintain most of the steady states in the organism. Adjustments in sympathetic activity accompany virtually every human action and reaction and are the main means for acute regulation of cardiovascular function.

Hans Selye popularized stress as a scientific and medical concept. His theory was founded on the doctrine of nonspecificity, that various stimuli elicit the same stress response, consisting of enlargement of the adrenal glands, thymicolymphatic involution, and peptic ulceration. High circulating levels of adrenal corticosteroids produce all these effects. The General Adaptation Syndrome had characteristic stages: alarm, resistance, and exhaustion. Several major problems with Selye's stress theory, including circularities, inconsistencies, and the doctrine of nonspecificity, have led to its abandonment by many researchers.

According to the present conception, stress is a type of intervening variable. It is a condition where expectations—whether genetically programed, established by prior learning, or deduced from circumstances—do not match the current or anticipated perceptions of the internal or external environment, and this discrepancy between what is observed or sensed and what is expected or programed elicits patterned compensatory responses.

Distress is a consciously experienced form of stress, characterized by specific behavioral and autonomic communicated signs, pituitary–adrenocortical and adrenomedullary activation, and a negative feeling that motivates escape behavior or avoidance learning.

The body has homeostatic comparators, which can be generically called "homeostats." All share several characteristics. Homeostatic systems are subject to negative feedback regulation. They usually include more than one effector, extending the range of control, allowing for a degree of compensatory activation of effectors to achieve homeostatic goals, and enabling elaboration of relatively specific patterns of effector responses. Homeostats can share an effector system, obscuring relationships between effector system activity and values for any single physiological parameter. These features explain why, in the absence of rigorous controls, plasma levels of norepinephrine, the sympathetic neurotransmitter, rarely correlate positively with mean arterial pressure across subjects, despite the importance of the sympathoneural system as a pressure-regulating effector system.

Disruption of a homeostatic system increases the variability of the monitored variable and tends to result in drifting of the absolute value to a new level. Dysfunction of circulatory homeostatic reflexes therefore would be expected to contribute to cardiovascular instability and possibly to stress-related pathology.

Homeostatic settings can reset when the challenge to homeostasis reaches consciousness. These mechanisms enable homeostasis to be redefined continually in life. Distress resets homeostats.

Charles Darwin introduced the notion that emotional expressions and their autonomic accompaniments evolved. The process determining the phylogenetic development of physiological and even psychological patterns of response has been essentially the same as the process that has determined the development of anatomic patterns—that is, natural selection. As homeostatic systems evolved, so did mechanisms regulating them.

Activities of the body's stress systems are regulated in primitively specific patterns. Many of these patterns, which are at least partly inherited, can be understood teleologically on the basis of preservation of the internal environment and natural selection in evolution. The physiological, biochemical, experiential, and behavioral components usually are closely linked.

The scientific worth of the homeostat theory and its applications in elucidating relationships between stress and cardiovascular disease will depend on the ability to generate hypotheses that observation and experiment can test. The rest of this book presents and analyzes some of the relevant research.

2

The Fact of Organization

This chapter develops two themes introduced in Chapter 1. The first is that the body possesses many stress effector systems, including the sympathetic nervous system (SNS), the adrenomedullary hormonal system (AHS), the hypothalamic–pituitary–adrenocortical (HPA) system, the parasympathetic nervous system (PNS), the renin–angiotensin–aldosterone system (RAS), and systems involving vasopressin (AVP) and endogenous opioids. These systems act both indirectly, by altering levels of monitored variables, with consequent reflexive adjustments determined by homeostats, and directly, by altering the release or effects of chemical messengers.

All stress effector systems have central neural as well as peripheral facets, with the chemical messengers used by those systems acting in or released in the brain as well as in other organs. Remarkably little is known about what, if anything, the release of a messenger in the brain has to do with release of that messenger in the periphery.

The second theme of this chapter is that cardiovascular functioning depends on many homeostatic systems, with different set-points, gains, and time constants (Guyton, 1991). Two of these systems, which predominate in cardiovascular regulation acutely, receive afferent information from arterial high-pressure and cardiac (or great venous) low-pressure baroreceptors, stretch or distortion receptors in the walls of arteries (especially the carotid sinus region at the bifurcation of the common carotid artery) and walls of the cardiac chambers.

Several points justify dwelling on these barostatic systems here: First, baroreflexes play key roles in cardiovascular regulation and dysregulation; second, an enormous body of experimental research has focused on the functioning and regulation of these reflexes, providing a large database; third, the baroreflexes use catecholaminergic effectors—especially the SNS; and fourth, and most relevant to the theme of this book, baroreflexes illustrate all the principles of operation that homeostatic systems obey, including regulation by negative feedback, effector sharing, compensatory activation, increased variability evoked by homeostat disruption, and resetting. The latter process explains many of the acute effects of distress on the cardiovascular system.

Traditional concepts have viewed the arterial high-pressure baroreceptors as monitoring stretching of arterial walls, eliciting reflexive adjustments that maintain arterial pressure; and have viewed the cardiac low-pressure baroreceptors as monitoring stretching of cardiac or pulmonary arterials walls, eliciting reflexive adjustments that maintain central blood volume. Applying these concepts, one may designate the homeostat subserved by the arterial high-pressure baroreceptors as the "barostat" and that subserved by the cardiopulmonary low-pressure baroreceptors as the "volustat." Discussion to follow deals with the "goals" of these homeostats.

Barostatic set-points change continually in life. Programmed patterns of central neural activation, elicited instinctively (i.e., under fairly direct genetic control), by conditioning, and by simulation (in the sense defined in Dawkins's "selfish gene" theory in Chapter 1) dictate this resetting.

Stress Effector Systems

The body's effector systems determine the physiological and chemical responses attending stress. From the distinctive actions of these effectors, one may speculate as to the natural selective forces that fostered their evolution.

The Sympathoneural System

The sympathoneural system (SNS), the neuronal component of what Cannon considered the sympathoadrenal system, consists of nerve networks. The axons derive from cells in ganglia (from the Latin and Greek words for swellings or tumors), accumulations of nervous tissue strung along each side the spinal column, rather than deriving directly from the spinal cord or brainstem. Sympathetic nerves therefore consist mainly of postganglionic neurons. Sympathetic nerves and nerve terminals enmesh the adventitial (from the Latin for "coming from abroad") and adventitial–medial layer of arterioles, the smallest and most numerous nutrient blood vessels; and form lattices in the myocardium and glands such as the salivary and sweat glands.

In primates, the main sympathetic ganglia with nerves projecting to the heart are the superior and middle cervical ganglia and the stellate ganglion (Armour and Hopkins, 1984). Peripheral nerves contain sympathetic fibers that supply the vasculature of the skeletal muscle and skin, innervate sweat glands, and carry afferent traffic from nociceptors.

Sympathetic nerve stimulation almost instantaneously constricts arterioles, increasing regional resistance to blood flow. The increased vascular resistance shifts the blood to other regions with less resistance. Sympathoneural activation in the kidneys, splanchnic region, and skeletal muscle therefore elicits rapid changes in the distribution of blood volume. Diffuse sympathetic stimulation increases total arteriolar resistance to blood flow, and since sympathetic activation in the heart increases the force and rate of cardiac contraction, blood pressure increases from both increased peripheral resistance and increased cardiac output.

Stimulation of nerves to the salivary glands increases salivation, to the eye dilates the pupil, to sweat glands increases sweating, to hair follicles causes goosebumps (piloerection), to the kidneys inhibits excretion of sodium, and to skeletal muscle causes trembling.

The chemical transmitter at sympathetic nerve endings is norepinephrine, or noradrenaline. Sympathetic stimulation releases norepinephrine, and noradrenergic binding to adrenoceptors (specific receptors for catecholamines) on cardiovascular smooth muscle cells causes the cells to contract. Sympathoneural norepinephrine therefore satisfies the main criteria defining a neurotransmitter: It is a chemical, released from nerve terminals by electrical action potentials, that interacts with specific receptors on nearby structures to produce specific physiological responses.

Structurally, norepinephrine is a catecholamine, a chemical consisting of an organic (i.e., benzene) ring, two adjacent hydroxyl groups on the ring (the combination defining a catechol), and a short organic tail containing an amine group (Figure 2–1).

Sympathoneural release of norepinephrine, with occupation of the adrenoceptors on smooth muscle or secretory cells, therefore affects blood flow distribution, cardiac function, and glandular activity (Figure 2–2). The adjustments usually are not noticed consciously. Because of the network architecture of the SNS, different stressors can elicit different patterns of sympathoneural outflows to the various vascular beds, redistributing blood flow.

Examples of situations associated with prominent changes in sympathoneural outflows include orthostasis, mild exercise, postprandial hemodynamic changes, mild changes in environmental temperature, and performance of nondistressing locomotor tasks.

The Adrenomedullary Hormonal System (AHS)

The AHS consists of chromaffin cells in the inner portion, or medulla, of the adrenal gland (Figure 2–3). The word ''chromaffin'' is a histologic classification based on staining by chromium salts. The cells receive mainly preganglionic input from cell bodies of the intermediolateral columns of the spinal cord. The adrenomedullary cells secrete catecholamines—in humans mainly epinephrine, or adrenaline—directly into the bloodstream. The adrenomedullary system therefore is hormonal.

Epinephrine affects the function of most body organs. Exogenously administered epinephrine rapidly increases the rate and force of cardiac contraction; increases myocardial cell automaticity; dilates bronchioles and increases the rate of breathing; redistributes blood volume toward the heart, brain, and skeletal muscle and away from the skin, kidneys, and gut; enhances the aggregability of platelets; relaxes smooth muscle of the uterus and gut; increases blood glucose by a variety of means including glycogenolysis and antagonizing insulin; dilates pupils; increases activity of the RAS; decreases serum potassium concentrations; increases the metabolic rate; and produces

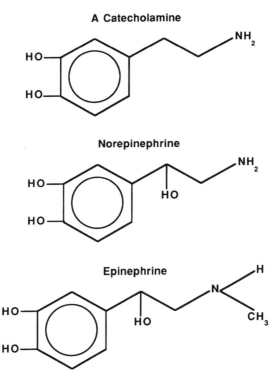

Figure 2–1. Catecholamine structures. A catecholamine consists of a catechol nucleus connected to a amine-containing tail. A catechol nucleus is an aromatic ring with two adjacent hydroxyl groups. Norepinephrine (noradrenaline) and epinephrine (adrenaline) are catecholamines. Their structures differ only in that epinephrine has a methyl group attached to the nitrogen moiety. The amine groups on catecholamines are positively charged at physiological pH.

psychological effects such as increased alertness, decreased fatigue, and intensification of emotions.

All these effects usually enhance survival during emergencies such as traumatic hemorrhage, hypoglycemia, asphyxiation, cardiac collapse, and emotional distress, when the individual senses an overall threat to well-being or survival.

The Hypothalamic–Pituitary–Adrenocortical (HPA) System

HPA system activation releases hormones such as cortisol from the cortex of the adrenal glands into the bloodstream.

Cortisol is a ''glucocorticoid'' (Figure 2–4). Exogenously administered cortisol increases blood levels of glucose; conversely, patients with adrenocortical failure due to Addison's disease tend to have hypoglycemia.

Cortisol also inhibits delayed inflammatory responses. The anti-inflammatory effects of glucocorticoids figure prominently in the stress theory of Selye, discussed in Chapter

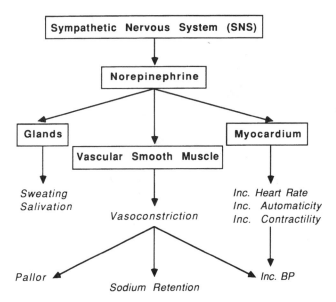

Figure 2–2. Overview of the sympathetic neural effector. Because the sympathetic nervous system is a neural network, sympathetic nerves to different regions can be activated differentially during stress, producing redistributions of blood flow to body organs. Norepinephrine released from sympathetic nerves generally contracts smooth muscle cells, eliciting glandular secretion, vasoconstriction, and myocardial contraction. Renal vasoconstriction produces an anti-natriuretic effect. Cutaneous vasoconstriction produces pallor. The net effect of systemic vasoconstriction is to increase the total peripheral resistance to blood flow in the body. This, combined with myocardial stimulation, increases blood pressure.

1. Glucocorticoids at high doses can improve the condition of patients with inflammatory diseases or shock. Conversely, adrenocortical failure, as in Addison's disease, markedly increases susceptibility during exposure to a variety of stressors.

The bases for the requirement of normal adrenocortical function in order to weather acute stress remain obscure. Deficiency of circulating glucocorticoids increases capillary permeability, attenuates cardiac and vascular responses to catecholamines, and reduces blood volume, decreasing the threshold for circulatory collapse. Adrenalectomized animals fail to maintain hepatic glycogen stores after brief starvation, rendering them hypersensitive to insulin.

As with catecholamines, glucocorticoids when exogenously administered affect virtually all body organs; however, these effects are much slower than those of catecholamines. Chronically elevated glucocorticoid levels can produce a form of diabetes mellitus. The anti-inflammatory effects increase susceptibility to some infections, such as tuberculosis. Other effects include redistribution of body fat, leading to central, or truncal, obesity and a moon-faced appearance; retention of sodium and excretion of potassium by the kidney, leading to increased extracellular fluid volume, hypertension, and hypokalemia; catabolism of proteins, leading to muscle wasting; gastrointestinal

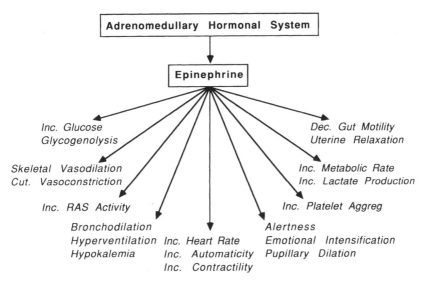

Figure 2–3. Overview of the adrenomedullary hormonal effector. In humans, the main hormone released by the adrenal medulla is epinephrine (adrenaline). Epinephrine affects the function of most organs and produces generalized effects such as increased metabolic rate, increased blood glucose levels, hypokalemia, increased lactate production, increased alertness, increased platelet aggregability, and intensification of emotions.

bleeding, (one of the defining components of the stress response of Selye); decreased sympathoneural and adrenomedullary outflows and increased cardiovascular sensitivity to catecholamines (Szemeredi et al., 1989); and several forms of psychiatric disturbance.

Corticotropin, or ACTH (an abbreviation for adrenocorticotropic hormone), regulates release of adrenocortical glucocorticoids. The anterior lobe of the pituitary gland releases ACTH, a polypeptide consisting of 39 amino acids. The pituitary, a pea-sized gland, sits in a bony cavity called the sella turcica (from its shape resembling a Turkish saddle) at the end of a thin stalk (infundibulum) extending from the base of the brain. The pituitary gland is also known as the hypophysis, from the Greek words for a growth beneath the brain.

Corticotropin-releasing hormone (CRH, Vale et al., 1981; Figure 2–5) importantly influences pituitary ACTH secretion. CRH release in the hypothalamus, the region of the brainstem giving rise to the pituitary gland, responds to several stressors. Other central neuropeptides (such as AVP, Al-Damluji, Thomas et al., 1990), catecholamines in the brain (Al-Damluji, 1988), and feedback inhibition from circulating glucocorticoids interact complexly with CRH in determining ACTH release.

Intracerebroventricular administration of CRH increases not only plasma levels of ACTH but also levels of epinephrine and norepinephrine (e.g., Brown and Fisher, 1984, 1985). Simultaneous CRH-induced activation of the body's three main stress systems—HPA, sympathoneural, and adrenomedullary—has led to speculation about CRH being

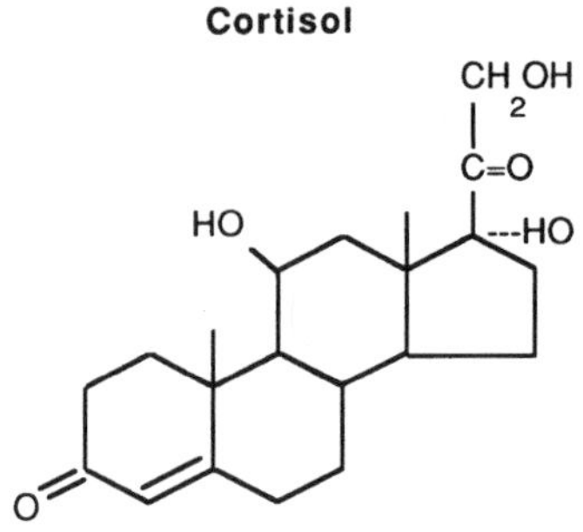

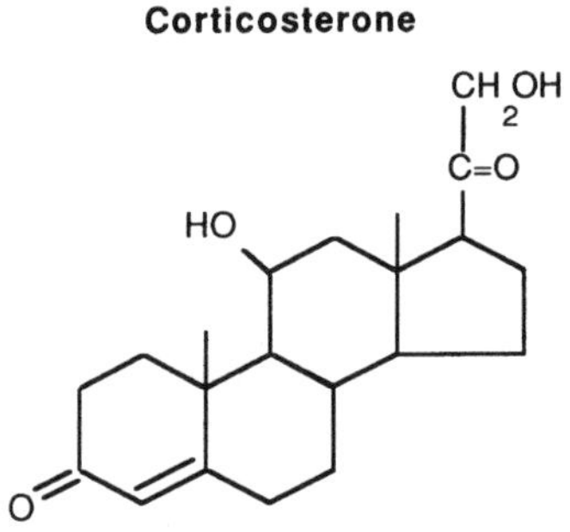

Cortisol

Corticosterone

Figure 2–4. Cortisol and corticosterone. Cortisol and corticosterone are glucocorticoids. Cortisol is the main glucocorticoid in humans, and corticosterone is the main glucocorticoid in rats. The two glucocorticoids differ structurally by the presence of a hydroxyl group.

a "master stress hormone," which would support Selye's unitary theory of stress. This issue receives more attention below in the section about interactions among stress systems.

The Vasopressin (AVP) System

Water deprivation poses a distinct homeostatic challenge. Another stress system, the AVP system, seems to have evolved as the main effector for maintaining total body water content.

AVP (Figure 2–6), a peptide consisting of nine amino acids and a disulfide bond, is synthesized as part of a larger precursor molecule in magnocellular cells of the paraventricular and supraoptic nuclei of the hypothalamus. Neurosecretory granules flow in the axoplasm to nerve terminals in the posterior pituitary; during the transport, AVP detaches from the precursor molecule. In the posterior pituitary, granules store AVP until AVP is released by neurosecretion from the nerve terminals into the bloodstream. AVP therefore is a prototypical neurohormone.

Increased serum osmolality, reflecting relatively inadequate serum water, potently

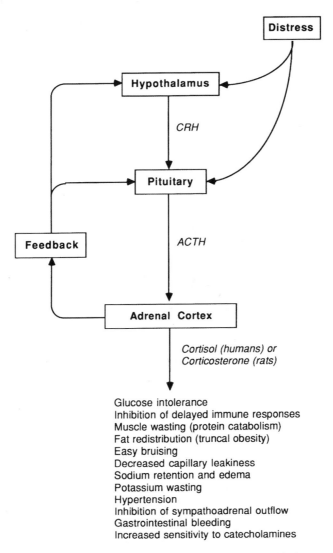

Figure 2–5. The hypothalamic–pituitary–adrenocortical (HPA) system. This hormonal system controls release of the glucocorticoids corticosterone (in rats) and cortisol (in humans). The HPA system is a classic example of a homeostatic system regulated by negative feedback. Corticotropin (ACTH) stimulates adrenocortical release of glucocorticoids. ACTH release from the pituitary is complexly regulated. One prominent determinant of ACTH release is corticotropin-releasing hormone (CRH), synthesized in the hypothalamus. Many other endogenous substances, including vasopressin and catecholamines, alter ACTH release, either directly or via effects on CRH.

Vasopressin

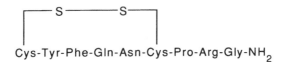

$$\text{Cys-Tyr-Phe-Gln-Asn-Cys-Pro-Arg-Gly-NH}_2$$

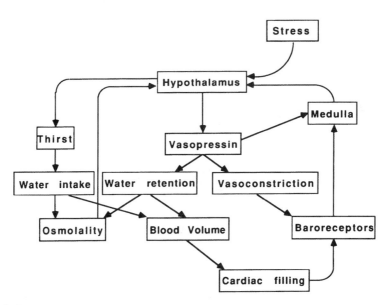

Figure 2–6. The vasopressin system. Vasopressin (arginine vasopressin, AVP, antidiuretic hormone, ADH) is a peptide containing nine amino acids and a disulfide bond. It is transported from the hypothalamus to the posterior pituitary, from which it is released as a neurohormone. The main systemic effects of AVP are retention of free water (explaining the name, antidiuretic hormone) and vasoconstriction (explaining the name, vasopressin). Vasopressin also potentiates arterial baroreflex sensitivity. Vasopressin figures prominently in regulation of water balance.

stimulates AVP secretion (Shore et al., 1988). Decreased cardiac filling pressure, such as occurs during hemorrhagic hypotension, also stimulates AVP release.

As noted in Chapter 1, the osmostat and volustat interact in regulating AVP levels. Hypervolemia shifts to the right the curve for the relationship between AVP levels and osmolality (Quillen and Cowley, 1983); that is, hypervolemia increases the set point of the osmostat.

AVP exerts an antidiuretic effect (hence its other name, antidiuretic hormone, or ADH) by stimulating specific AVP receptors, V_2 receptors, on the abluminal membrane of renal tubular cells in the ascending loop of Henle and the collecting duct. Occupation of the V_2 receptors increases generation of the intracellular second messenger, cyclic AMP (cAMP), which increases the permeability of the luminal membrane to water and promotes the fusion of water-trapping endosomes with the luminal membrane. The endosomes take up water via protein–water channels, resulting in concentration of the urine. Consequently, AVP inhibition, such as produced by alcohol, evokes a diuresis, with the urine hypotonic with respect to plasma.

By promoting excretion of concentrated urine, the renal actions of AVP increase retention of "free water" when water is available to drink. Free water retention, in concert with decreased delivery of water to diluting segments of the nephron due to decreased glomerular filtration, explains hyponatremia in edematous states such as heart failure. Excessive ADH release in clinical pathologic states (syndromes of inappropriate ADH secretion, SIADH) decreases serum osmolality and causes hyponatremia.

As its other name, "vasopressin," implies, exogenously administered AVP increases blood pressure, via peripheral vasoconstriction elicited by occupation of V_1 receptors on vascular smooth muscle cells. Endogenous AVP probably does not participate in tonic blood pressure regulation in healthy humans; however, after sympathoneural ablation in laboratory animals, endogenous AVP does contribute to maintaining blood pressure (Hatzinikolaou et al., 1982). Intravenously administered AVP has been used clinically to ameliorate upper gastrointestinal hemorrhage due to variceal bleeding, by producing vasoconstriction and decreasing portal venous pressure.

AVP also augments arterial baroreflex inhibition of sympathetic nerve activity, as discussed below in the section about AVP–catecholamine interactions, and augments baroreflex stimulation of cardiac parasympathetic activity.

The Renin–Angiotensin–Aldosterone System (RAS)

The body possesses impressively efficient means to preserve sodium, with the RAS (Figure 2–7) the most prominent effector. Dietary salt restriction stimulates RAS activity; salt loading virtually shuts it down.

Renin is a glycoprotein synthesized in and released from modified vascular smooth muscle cells, juxtaglomerular cells, in the afferent arterioles to the renal glomeruli. The main stimuli for release of renin are decreased renal perfusion pressure, sensed by the juxtaglomerular cells; decreased renal tubular concentrations of sodium, sensed by cells of the macula densa in the distal nephron near the juxtaglomerular apparatus; decreased cardiac filling pressures, sensed by low-pressure baroreceptors in the heart; and occupation of β-adrenoceptors by norepinephrine released from sympathetic nerves terminating at the juxtaglomerular cells and by epinephrine reaching those receptors via the circulation. Angiotensin II, discussed below, inhibits renin secretion.

Renin has no known activity of its own, but it catalyzes the conversion of a large α-2 globulin, angiotensinogen, to a decapeptide, angiotensin I. Angiotensin I also has no known physiological action; however, angiotensin-converting enzyme (ACE) catalyzes conversion of angiotensin I to the physiologically active octapeptide, angiotensin II (AII, previously called hypertensin or angiotonin). ACE inhibitors are widely used clinically to treat hypertension.

AII potently constricts blood vessels in all vascular beds, and exogenous AII increases blood pressure. On a weight basis, AII is a more potent vasoconstrictor

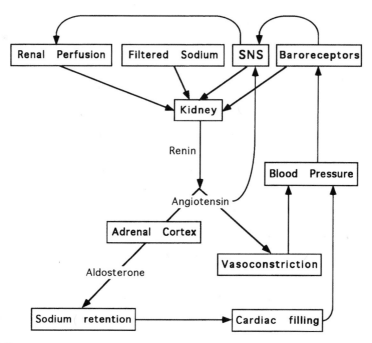

Figure 2–7. The renin–angiotensin–aldosterone system (RAS). Angiotensin and aldosterone both are active hormones. Angiotensin produces vascular smooth muscle contraction, stimulates adrenocortical secretion of aldosterone, and may stimulate sympathoneural and adrenomedullary secretion. Aldosterone is a mineralocorticoid that causes sodium retention and potassium depletion.

than is norepinephrine in healthy individuals. AII exerts little direct effect on the heart, and after bolus injection of AII, heart rate decreases reflexively. This provided the basis for the first means to test the gain of the arterial barocardiac reflex in humans (Smyth et al., 1969).

AII also stimulates the adrenal cortex to release aldosterone, the main mineralocorticoid in humans. Aldosterone augments renal sodium retention (hence its designation as a mineralocorticoid) by stimulating exchange of sodium for potassium, so that hyperaldosteronism tends to produce sodium retention, expansion of extracellular fluid volume, hypertension, and potassium wasting.

Angiotensinases rapidly destroy circulating AII. One of these, aminopeptidase, cleaves an Asp residue from the N-terminal end of the molecule (Figure 2–8). The metabolite angiotensin III has about 40% the pressor activity of AII and is equally potent with AII in stimulating aldosterone secretion.

RAS activation therefore increases blood pressure both by angiotensin-induced vasoconstriction and by aldosterone-induced sodium retention and expansion of extracellular fluid volume.

In the brain, exogenously administered AII elicits thirst (AII is one of the most potent known dipsogens), salt hunger, and secretion of AVP and ACTH. Catecholaminergic

Angiotensinogen

Asp-Arg-Val-Tyr-Ile-His-Pro-Phe-His-Leu-Val-Ile-His-R

Angiotensin I

Asp-Arg-Val-Tyr-Ile-His-Pro-Phe-His-Leu

Angiotensin II

Asp-Arg-Val-Tyr-Ile-His-Pro-Phe

Angiotensin III

Arg-Val-Tyr-Ile-His-Pro-Phe

Aldosterone

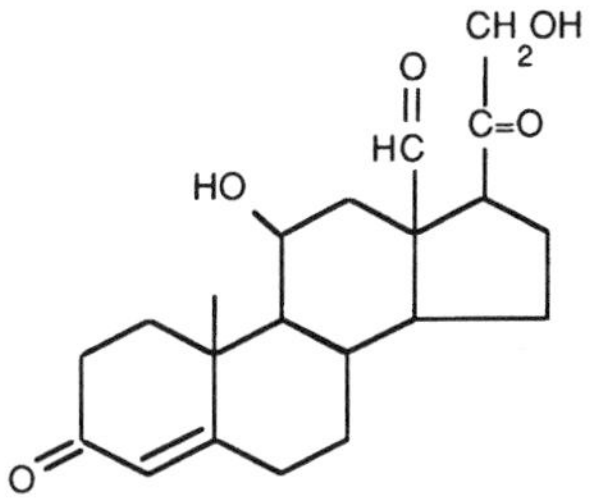

Figure 2–8. Angiotensin and aldosterone. Angiotensin II is a peptide consisting of eight amino acids, whereas aldosterone is a steroid produced from corticosterone. Cleavage of the N-terminal Asp residue of angiotensin II produces angiotensin III, which is also physiologically active.

effects of AII in the brain and periphery are discussed below in the section about renin–catecholamine interactions.

Selye held the now abandoned view of aldosterone as a ''proinflammatory'' hormone.

The Parasympathetic Nervous System (PNS)

The PNS consists of two sets of nerves (Figure 2–9), one derived from the brainstem, constituting the cranial parasympathetic outflow, and the other derived from the intermediolateral columns of the sacral spinal cord, constituting the sacral parasympathetic outflow. These sites of origin contrast with those of sympathetic nerves, which emanate from the the thoracic and lumbar spinal cord. The SNS and PNS are called the autonomic nervous system.

Parasympathetic nerves subserve mainly vegetative, conservative processes; parasympathetic activity decreases during many but by no means all stresses. As would be predicted from this teleological view, parasympathetic stimulation activates digestive

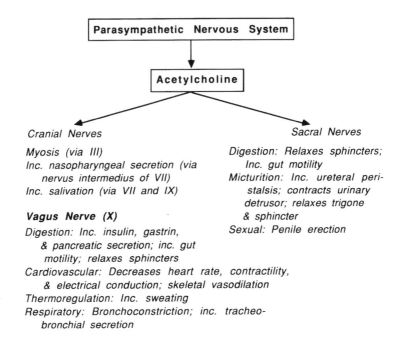

Figure 2–9. The parasympathetic nervous system (PNS). The PNS consists of cranial and sacral nerves that release acetycholine. Activation of the PNS generally supports vegetative activities such as digestion. The PNS and sympathetic nervous system are the two components of the autonomic nervous system. Their activities generally oppose each other. The vagus nerve, the tenth cranial nerve, is the medium for parasympathetic regulation of the heart and blood vessels.

processes, including release of gastrin and insulin (Kaneto et al., 1967; Steffens et al., 1986), and increases gut motility; cardiac parasympathetic stimulation decreases the force and rate of myocardial contraction. When sympathoneural activity increases, parasympathetic activity usually decreases. Whereas increased SNS and AHS activity expends metabolic energy during emergency conditions, increased PNS activity tends to replenish energy stores during periods of quiescence.

The main parasympathetic nerve, the vagus nerve (so named because of its wandering course in the body), emanates from the medulla of the brainstem, where it is the tenth cranial nerve, and innervates the heart, bronchioles, stomach, skin, and gut. Unlike sympathetic ganglia, which lie in chains on either side of the spinal column, parasympathetic ganglia are located very close to or inside the innervated organs. The postganglionic nerves therefore are short or nonexistent, and the vagus contains preganglionic fibers. The vagal preganglionic fibers originate from the dorsal motor nucleus of the vagus, an intermediate zone, the nucleus ambiguus, and the ventrolateral nucleus ambiguus of the medulla (Armour and Hopkins, 1984).

Stimulation of the right vagus nerve slows the discharge rate of the sinus node, whereas stimulation of the left vagus induces less slowing in the sinus rate but a larger amount of blockade of atrioventricular conduction (Randall, 1984).

In the 1920s, Otto Loewi proposed that a chemical messenger substance, acetylcholine, produced the physiological effects of vagal stimulation. Loewi's experiment was a milestone because it identified a new type of endogenous substance—a neurotransmitter; for this work he shared the Nobel Prize in Physiology or Medicine in 1936. Loewi stimulated the vagus nerve of the perfused heart of a donor frog. During the stimulation, the perfusate was applied to the heart of a recipient frog. Stimulation of the vagus nerve of the donor frog decreased the rate of cardiac contraction, as expected; application of the perfusate to the recipient's heart decreased the rate of contraction of the recipient's heart as well. Loewi called the substance that was released in the first heart and slowed the rate of the second, "Vagusstoff," or the substance of the vagus. Using other bioassay preparations, where the substance produced responses identical to those produced by acetylcholine, in 1926 Loewi and Navratil identified the Vagusstoff as acetylcholine.

Loewi used virtually the same bioassay preparation to demonstrate that in the frog heart, epinephrine is the sympathetic neurotransmitter (Loewi, 1921); and Cannon used bioassay preparations to measure the release of epinephrine from the adrenal glands (Cannon and De la Paz, 1911; Cannon and Rapport, 1921).

All parasympathetic nerves release acetylcholine as the neurotransmitter. Parasympathetic neurons therefore are cholinergic. Other cholinergic nerves mediate neuromuscular transmission, adrenomedullary and sweat gland secretion, and, in some species, sympathetic vasodilation (Ellison and Zanchetti, 1971; Sanders et al., 1989a; Takeuchi and Manning, 1971).

Acetylcholine is synthesized from the choline acetyltransferase-catalyzed transfer of acetylcoenzyme A to choline (Figure 2–10) and is inactivated by acetylcholinesterase almost immediately after release of the transmitter from nerve endings.

Specific receptors mediate the effects of acetylcholine. Classically they have been divided into nicotinic and muscarinic (Dale, 1914). Atropine blocks muscarinic but not nicotinic receptors, and hexamethonium and related drugs block nicotinic receptors but not muscarinic receptors. Nicotinic receptors mediate cholinergic transmission from pre- to postganglionic sympathetic neurons in the sympathetic ganglia and cholinergic stimulation of adrenomedullary secretion. Muscarinic receptors, named for the toxin in toadstools, stimulate gut smooth muscle contraction and glandular secretion. Muscarinic receptors on sympathetic nerve terminals inhibit norepinephrine release, as discussed below. At skeletal neuromuscular junctions, acetylcholine binds to nicotinic receptors that are pharmacologically distinct from those in the autonomic nervous system.

Acetylcholine itself is not used as a drug in clinical medicine, because of the diverse toxic effects and susceptibility to rapid degradation. Exogenously administered cholinergic agonists (e.g., bethanecol) are used to treat nonobstructive urinary retention and gastric atony. These drugs stimulate digestive processes and intestinal motility, increase salivation, and increase sweating, with relatively little change in heart rate. Drugs that inhibit acetylcholinesterase (e.g., neostigmine, physostigmine, edrophonium) reverse central nervous depression due to overdose of anticholinergics. Edrophonium rapidly stimulates cardiac cholinergic receptors and is used to treat paroxysmal supraventricular tachycardia. Anticholinergics are used clinically in several conditions, including

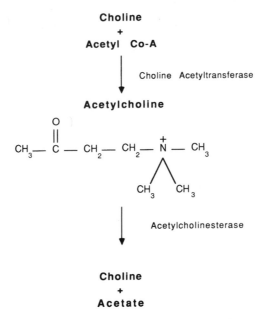

Figure 2-10. Synthesis and degradation of acetylcholine. Acetylcholine is responsible for sympathetic ganglionic, parasympathetic, and neuromuscular neurotransmission and for neuronal stimulation of adrenomedullary secretion. Acetylcholine is degraded metabolically extracellularly soon after its release, in contrast with catecholamines, which are removed by cellular uptake and intracellular metabolism.

asthma, insomnia, peptic ulcer disease, symptomatic bradycardia or heart block, diarrhea, hyperhidrosis, Parkinson's disease, and mushroom poisoning.

Release of acetylcholine from parasympathetic terminals (and release of acetylcholine from sympathetic terminals in skeletal muscle) usually produces local vasodilation. The vasodilator effect of acetylcholine depends on intact endothelium (Furchgott, 1983). Denudation of endothelium unmasks a vasoconstrictor effect of exogenous acetylcholine and potentiates responses to neuronally released norepinephrine (Urabe et al., 1991). Acetylcholine increases the local generation of endothelium-derived relaxing factors (EDRF), one of which is nitric oxide (NO). Thus, *N*-methylarginine-induced blockade of NO production prevents vasodilation produced by acetylcholine. Nonadrenergic, noncholinergic mechanisms mediating penile erection may also depend on local generation of NO (Rajfer et al., 1992).

The Endogenous Opioid System

The endogenous opioid system contributes to the experience of pain and to stress-related analgesia. Activity of this system is linked with those of the HPA and adrenomedullary systems (Hargreaves et al., 1986; Troullos et al., 1989).

Martin first hypothesized the existence of different receptors for opiates (Martin,

1967). Three types of receptors were suggested, based on in vivo observations: "mu" (for morphine); "kappa" (for ketocyclazocine); and "sigma" (for the investigational drug SKF-10,047). In vitro bioassay evidence identified a fourth type of receptor, "delta" (for mouse vas deferens). The anesthetic, fentanyl, stimulates mu receptors; whereas morphine stimulates mu and delta receptors.

Pert and Snyder (1973) demonstrated the existence of opiate receptors in brian tissue and hypothesized that endogenous morphinelike neurochemicals—opioids—could determine the experience of pain. The first identified class of endogenous opioids were the enkephalins—methionine–enkephalin and leucine–enkephalin—small peptides (5 amino acids each) with either methionine or leucine at the end of a chain, and with the first 4 amino acids being Tyr-Gly-Gly-Phe (Figure 2–11). Enkephalins are packaged together with catecholamines and released with them during adrenomedullary stimulation (Gaumann et al., 1988). Every known endogenous opioid peptide, collectively termed endorphins, contains the Tyr-Gly-Gly-Phe sequence of amino acids. Narcotic activity appears to depend on the Tyr residue.

A pituitary hormone of unknown function, β-lipotropin, or β-LPH, contains met-enkephalin but was found not to be its source. The opioid fragment of β-lipotropin is not the 5-residue but a 31-residue peptide, β-endorphin. β-endorphin is in turn a portion of a precursor peptide, pro-opiomelanocortin (POMC), which is also the precursor of ACTH, melanocyte-stimulating hormone (γ-MSH), and β-LPH. In the anterior pituitary, POMC gives rise to ACTH, as well as β-LPH, which is cleaved to form α-LPH and β-endorphin. As suggested by the name, β-endorphin is an endogenous opioid that acts as a central neurotransmitter. The highest concentrations of β-endorphin in the body are in the pituitary gland. CRH increases plasma levels of both ACTH and β-endorphin.

Since β-LPH was found not to be the source of the enkephalins, the source of the enkephalins was unknown until the early 1980s. By now it is known that there are three precursor molecules for the endogenous opioids: POMC, as noted above; a second precursor, giving rise to leu- and met-enkephalin; and a third precursor, giving rise to dynorphin, a powerful peptide that begins with the leu-enkephalin sequence.

Many types of stress increase circulating levels of β-endorphin, and increases in plasma β-endorphin and epinephrine levels during real-life stress are highly correlated in humans (Troullos et al., 1989). The role or roles of endogenous opioids in the regulation of SNS and AHS outflows and circulatory parameters remain incompletely understood. Most reports have suggested indirect inhibitory effects on sympathetic outflow or neurotransmission.

Studies about physiological roles of endogenous opioids have relied heavily on use of naloxone, which blocks the effects of all endogenous opioids. Naloxone is short-acting but very effective in the treatment of opiate overdose. Opioid antagonism by naloxone can reverse septic, hemorrhagic, or endotoxic shock (Faden and Holaday, 1979), consistent with the view that endogenous opioids participate in the apparently paradoxical sympathoinhibition that occurs in these conditions. Opioids attenuate norepinephrine release from the locus ceruleus in the brainstem, and fentanyl produces a central vagotonic and sympatholytic effect, helping to explain the benefit of morphine

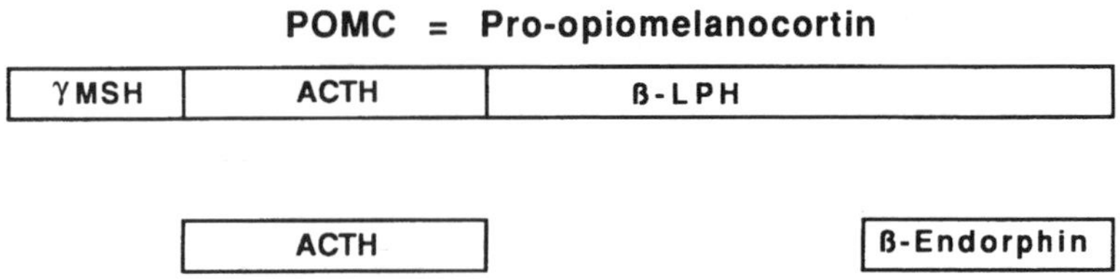

POMC = Pro-opiomelanocortin

γMSH	ACTH	β-LPH

ACTH		β-Endorphin

β-Endorphin

Gly-Gly-Lys-Lys-His-Ala-Asn-Lys-Val-Ile-Ala-Asn-Lys
                                                   |
                                                  Phe
                                                   |
Tyr-Gly-Gly-Phe-Met-Thr-Ser-Glu-Lys-Ser-Gln-Thr-Pro-Leu-Val-Thr-Leu

Leu-Enkephalin

Tyr-Gly-Gly-Phe-Leu

Met-Enkephalin

Tyr-Gly-Gly-Phe-Met

Dynorphin

Tyr-Gly-Gly-Phe-Leu-Arg-Arg-Ile-Arg-Pro-Lys-Leu-Lys-Trp-Asp-Asn-Gln

Figure 2–11. The pro-opiomelanocortin (POMC) family. ACTH, β-endorphin, and melanocyte-stimulating hormone are components of the same parent peptide, POMC. The structurally related endogenous opioids, the enkephalins, are not derived from POMC.

in the prevention of sudden death due to ventricular fibrillation in heart attack patients (DeSilva et al., 1978). Farsang and Kunos (1979) reported that naloxone administration reversed the hypotensive effect of the sympatholytic α_2-adrenoceptor agonist clonidine, perhaps by interfering with a system whereby stimulation of α_2-adrenoceptors in the nucleus of the solitary tract (NTS) of the medulla leads to release of an endogenous opioid; however, the relationship between endogenous opioids and the function of central adrenoceptors remains unclear. Pressor stimuli can induce analgesia (Dworkin et al., 1979), suggesting that input from arterial baroreceptors can release endorphins in the brain.

Endogenous opioids interact differentially with the receptor types, with enkephalins more effective at δ-receptors, dynorphins at κ-receptors, and endorphins at δ- and μ-receptors (Bennett, 1990).

High enkephalin concentrations in the dorsal columns of the spinal cord suggest involvement in the transmission of sensory information to the brain. Enkephalins in the spinal cord inhibit transmission of pain impulses ascending in the lateral spinothalamic tract to the thalamus. Injection of β-endorphin or fentanyl into the cerebrospinal fluid space produces analgesia, and both have been used to treat pain in patients with terminal cancer. Release of β-endorphin in the brain may be the basis for analgesia produced by acupuncture and placebos.

Other Stress Effector Systems

As with digestive processes, sexual activity declines during periods of distress. This is reflected by decreased circulating levels of gonadotropins and of sex steroids such as testosterone (e.g., Kreuz et al., 1972).

Growth hormone (GH) is required for normal linear growth. Serum factors called somatomedins mediate effects of GH on growth. As an anabolic hormone, growth hormone stimulates amino acid uptake in some systems, and amino acids such as arginine stimulate GH release. Growth hormone acts synergistically with insulin in stimulating amino acid uptake into cells. Pituitary release of growth hormone is regulated by both a hypothalamic growth hormone-releasing factor (GRH) and a growth hormone release-inhibitory factor (somatostatin). Hypoglycemia is a potent stimulus for growth hormone release; conversely, GH is a minor glucose counter-regulatory hormone.

Interactions Among Stress Effector Systems

Neuroendocrine response patterns during stress reflect different contributions of many effector systems. For instance, manipulations of glucose availability produce responses of insulin secretion, the AHS, the HPA system, and levels of other glucostatic hormones (glucagon, GH); orthostasis elicits SNS and RAS activation; fainting is associated with PNS and AHS activation; manipulations of dietary salt intake markedly affect RAS activity; and manipulations of water intake importantly influence AVP levels.

In addition to the coordinated participation of effector systems in most stress responses, these systems exert many direct effects on each other, by influencing the release or actions of the chemical messengers. Because of this multitude, the following discussion must be incomplete; moreover, the relevance of many of these interactions to physiology and pathophysiology remains to be established.

Cholinergic–Catecholamine Interactions

Alterations in SNS activity are usually associated with opposite changes in PNS activity. For instance, increases in arterial baroreceptor afferent activity reflexively inhibit sympathoneural outflow and stimulate vagal outflow. Stimulation of the anterior hypothalamus usually produces vagally mediated bradycardia and hypotension, whereas stimulation of the posterior hypothalamus produces sympathetically mediated tachycardia and hypertension (Hess, 1949). Nevertheless, stimulating selected hypothalamic sites can alter differentially the central neural processes mediating parasympathetic and sympathetic outflows (Koizumi and Kollai, 1981).

Several other antagonistic interactions parallel the opposite changes in sympathetic and parasympathetic activities resulting from central neural determinants (Table 2–1). Vagal stimulation can abolish tachycardic responses to right stellate ganglion stimulation in anesthetized dogs (Levy, 1988). Stimulation of cholinergic receptors in the heart inhibits norepinephrine release during sympathetic stimulation (Levy, 1971; Levy and Blattberg, 1976; Levy and Martin, 1984). The inhibition results from stimulation of muscarinic receptors, presumably located on the sympathetic terminals (Hollenberg et al. 1965; Lindmar et al., 1968; Loffesholz and Muscholl, 1969). Conversely, during sympathetic stimulation, neurally released neuropeptide Y may inhibit vagally mediated effects (Warner et al., 1991).

"Accentuated antagonism" (Rosenblueth and Simeone, 1934) refers to the augmented bradycardic effect of cholinergic stimulation in the presence of increased cardiac sympathetic tone. A given amount of vagal stimulation decreases heart rate more in the presence of concurrent sympathetic stimulation than in the absence of sympathetic stimulation. Sympathetic–vagal interactions appear to be more important in influencing cardiac automaticity than conduction velocity (Levy and Martin, 1984; Levy and Zieske, 1969; Wallick et al., 1982). A vagal–sympathetic interaction also influences regulation of left ventricular myocardial contraction, since in anesthetized dogs, sympathetic neural stimulation or norepinephrine infusion augments the depressant effect of vagal stimulation or intracoronary injection of acetylcholine on myocardial contractility (Hollenberg et al.,1965).

Vagal activity helps to maintain myocardial electrical stability in the setting of increased cardiac sympathetic activity during emotional stress or myocardial infarction (Lown and Verrier, 1976; Verrier and Lown, 1981). In anesthetized dogs, stellate ganglion stimulation decreases the ventricular fibrillation threshold by about 60%, infusion of norepinephrine decreases the threshold by about 40%, and increased vagal activity can prevent this augmentation of ventricular susceptibility (Kolman et al., 1975). Pretreatment with physostigmine, which inhibits acetylcholinesterase, decreases the frequency of ventricular fibrillation after ligation of the left anterior descending coronary artery and attenuates the arrhythmogenic effect of subepicardial injections of epinephrine (Das, 1984).

Different effects on cyclic nucleotides, both prejunctionally and postjunctionally, at the cellular level may explain the antagonism between the two divisions of the autonomic nervous system. Prejunctionally, acetylcholine appears to bind to muscarinic

Table 2–1. Acetylcholine–Catecholamine Interactions

Brain: Cholinergic agonists stimulate adrenomedullary and sympathoneural outflows

SNS: Acetylcholine inhibits NE release

    Acetylcholine is responsible for sympathetic ganglionic neurotransmission

    "Accentuated antagonism" in the heart

    Acetylcholine mediates sympathetic active vasodilation in some regions (e.g., skeletal muscle)

Adrenals: Nicotine stimulates adrenomedullary secretion

Reflexes: Atropine augments BP responses to pressor amines

receptors to inhibit release of norepinephrine during sympathetic stimulation. The intracellular mechanism is unknown. Postjunctionally, vagal stimulation increases intracellular cGMP levels, whereas β-adrenoceptor stimulation increases cAMP levels. Muscarinic stimulation increases activity of an inhibitory protein, G_i, which both inhibits adenyl cyclase and catalyzes the hydrolysis of GTP to GDP. The latter may decrease the availability of GTP for activation of the stimulatory G protein for adenylate cyclase, G_s. Thus, the net postjunctional effect of muscarinic stimulation is to block β-adrenoceptor-mediated stimulation of adenyl cyclase and therefore to inhibit formation of cAMP. Brown (AM Brown, 1990) has proposed a molecular basis for accentuated antagonism based on interactions of G-proteins regulating ion channels.

Stimulation of central cholinergic receptors increases efferent sympathetic nerve traffic, adrenomedullary catecholamine release, and blood pressure (Brezenoff and Giuliano, 1982; RM Robertson et al., 1993). In humans, central cholinergic stimulation increases plasma epinephrine levels more than it does plasma norepinephrine levels (Janowsky et al., 1985; Kennedy et al., 1985). Combined peripheral and central cholinergic blockade with atropine decreases arterial plasma levels of norepinephrine (Goldstein and Keiser, 1984).

During vasovagal depressor reactions, AHS activity increases, whereas SNS activity decreases (Goldstein, Spanarkel et al., 1982; Wallin and Sundlof, 1982; Ziegler et al., 1986). The antagonism between the PNS and SNS therefore does not apply to the AHS.

Glucocorticoid–Catecholamine Interactions

Activities of the HPA and catecholaminergic systems interact at several levels (Table 2–2). These interactions suggest sharing of the HPA, adrenomedullary, and sympathoneural effectors by many homeostats.

Physiological or metabolic stimuli that increase adrenomedullary secretion (e.g., hypoglycemia, hemorrhage, and surgery) often increase HPA system activity concurrently (Udelsman et al., 1987a, 1987b). Emotional distress also elicits combined adre-

Table 2–2. HPA-Catecholamine Interactions

Brain: ICV CRH stimulates sympathoadrenal outflows
 Central NE stimulates ACTH release
 Cortisol inhibits sympathoadrenal outflows and α_2-adrenoceptor-mediated NE release
 β-Endorphin exerts α_2-adrenoceptor agonist-like actions
Pituitary: β-Agonists inhibit ACTH release
 Hypophysectomy increases sympathoadrenal activity and reactivity
SNS: Steroids inhibit Uptake-2
 Hypercortisolemia augments β-adrenoceptor-mediated responses
 Chromaffin tissue contains functional CRH receptors
Adrenals: Steroids increase adrenal PNMT
 Adrenalectomy augments sympathoneural responses
Reflexes: Steroids increase BP, reflexively inhibiting sympathetic outflows.

nomedullary and HPA activation. For instance, viewing Disney nature films decreases, and viewing stressful (mainly anxiety-provoking) films increases urinary 17-hydroxy-corticosteroid and epinephrine excretion (Levi, 1965). During the mental challenge of playing a video game, responses of arterial plasma levels of ACTH and epinephrine correlate strongly positively across individual subjects (Goldstein, Eisenhofer et al., 1987), even when mean ACTH levels remain unchanged.

In the absence of a functioning AHS, disruption of the HPA compensatorily activates the SNS. Thus, adrenalectomized monkeys have exaggerated responses of plasma norepinephrine levels during surgical stress several months later, and the magnitude of this augmentation varies inversely with the amount of glucocorticoid pretreatment (Udelsman et al., 1987a). Adrenalectomized rats have high plasma levels of norepinephrine under resting conditions and have especially high norepinephrine levels in response to immobilization (Kvetnansky et al., 1993) or ether inhalation (Brown and Fisher, 1986). Knife-cut lesions interrupting CRH and AVPergic innervation of the median eminence attenuate ACTH responses to immobilization stress but exaggerate the responses of plasma norepinephrine levels (Makara et al., 1986). Adrenalectomized humans tend to have increased urinary excretion of norepinephrine (von Euler et al., 1954). Finally, hypophysectomy produces large increases in plasma levels of norepinephrine and epinephrine in rats (Goldstein, Garty et al., 1993).

Exogenous administration of agonists at glucocorticoid receptors inhibits sympathoneural and adrenomedullary activity, and exogenous administration of adrenoceptor agonists tends to inhibit HPA activity. Thus, administration of cortisol or dexamethasone to rats decreases basal plasma levels of norepinephrine and especially of epinephrine (Brown and Fisher, 1986; Szemeredi et al., 1988). Dexamethasone can blunt acute plasma catecholamine responses during exposure to different stressors (Brown and Fisher, 1986; Komesaroff and Funder, 1994), and hypercortisolemia abolishes α_2-adrenoceptor blockade-induced increases in plasma norepinephrine levels (Szemeredi et al., 1990). Hypercortisolemia also inhibits α_2-adrenoceptor blockade-induced norepinephrine release in the brain (Pacak et al., 1992a). In humans, exogenously administered glucocorticoid decreases directly recorded sympathetic nerve traffic and plasma norepinephrine levels (Golczynska et al., unpublished observations). In rats, fetal dexamethasone exposure retards the development of cardiac noradrenergic innervation (Bian et al., 1993).

Intracerebroventricular administration of CRH evokes large increases in plasma levels of ACTH and catecholamines (Brown and Fisher, 1984, 1985; Lenz et al., 1987) and in directly recorded adrenal nerve activity (Kurosawa et al., 1986). High doses of CRH administered into the fourth ventricle of monkeys increase plasma epinephrine but not norepinephrine levels (Insel et al., 1984), and children with hypocorticotropic hypopituitarism have normal plasma levels of norepinephrine at rest and during exercise but markedly reduced levels of epinephrine (Rudman et al., 1981).

Intracerebroventricular administration of the CRH receptor antagonist α-helical CRH$_{9-41}$ does not affect basal plasma levels of catecholamines but attenuates plasma epinephrine responses to hemorrhage and to insulin-induced hypoglycemia (Brown et al., 1986), consistent with a role of endogenous CRH in mediating the adrenomedullary responses to these stressors. A recent study failed to replicate the latter effect (Goldstein, Garty et al., 1993).

Lewis rats have deficient corticotropin responses during inflammatory stresses, apparently due to deficient hypothalamic CRH secretion (Sternberg, Young et al., 1989). These rats also have low baseline plasma levels of epinephrine, compared with levels in histocompatible Fischer rats (Goldstein, Garty et al., 1993).

Conversely, central noradrenergic receptors participate in regulation by hypothalamic CRH secretion and pituitary ACTH release. Activation of central α_1-adrenoceptors stimulates release of AVP, which in turn facilitates ACTH responses to CRH (Al-Damluji, 1988; Al-Damluji and White, 1992; Al-Damluji and Francis, 1993; Al-Damluji, Perry et al., 1987; Al-Damluji, Thomas et al., 1990; Al-Damluji, White et al., 1990).

Sympathetic ganglia and adrenomedullary cells possess functional CRH receptors (Udelsman et al., 1986). ACTH (probably via adrenal corticosteroids) increases activities of dopamine-β-hydroxylase and phenylethanolamine-N-methyltransferase (Wurtman and Axelrod, 1966), enhancing the capacity to synthesize norepinephrine and convert norepinephrine to epinephrine. ACTH administered at pharmacological doses can stimulate catecholamine release (Valenta et al., 1986), and glucocorticoids augment catecholamine synthesis and increase catecholamine stores in PC12 pheochromocytoma cells (Tischler et al., 1983). Thus, whereas steroids act in the brain to decrease sympathoneural outflows, steroids act in the periphery to enhance catecholamine synthesis.

Although it had been proposed that epinephrine stimulates pituitary release of ACTH (Axelrod and Reisine, 1984), administration of the β-adrenoceptor agonist, isoproterenol, if anything decreases circulating ACTH and epinephrine levels in humans (Eisenhofer et al., 1987; Goldstein, Zimlichman et al., 1986a; Ludwig et al., 1989).

Hypercortisolemia augments β-adrenoceptor-mediated heart rate responses in rats (Szemeredi et al., 1989), and glucocorticoids stimulate the transcription of genes coding for β_2-adrenoceptors in hamster smooth muscle cells (Collins et al., 1988).

As noted in the chapter about peripheral catecholaminergic systems, steroids inhibit the extraneuronal uptake of catecholamines (Salt, 1972).

Renin–Catecholamine Interactions

Major stimuli for release of renin include decreased renal perfusion pressure and decreased cardiac filling. In these situations, associations between reflexive alterations in sympathoneural and RAS activities result from sharing of the effector systems by both the high-pressure barostat and low-pressure volustat. Consistent with this view, many studies have reported positive correlations between plasma levels of norepinephrine and renin activity across individuals, the relationship being especially apparent among groups of patients with essential hypertension (Agabiti-Rosei et al., 1983, 1984; Chobanian et al., 1978; DeQuattro et al., 1976; Esler et al., 1977; Miura and DeQuattro, 1975).

These systems also interact more directly (Table 2–3). Stimulation of juxtaglomerular cell β-adrenoceptors, by neuronal norepinephrine or circulating epinephrine, evokes renin release (Osborn et al., 1983; Saynavalammi et al., 1982; Weber et al., 1983).

Table 2–3. Renin–Catecholamine Interactions

Brain: Angiotensin II stimulates sympathetic outflow

SNS: Angiotensin II augments NE release

Adrenals: Angiotensin II stimulates adrenomedullary secretion, and dopamine inhibits aldosterone secretion

Kidneys: Epinephrine and renal nerve stimulation evokes renin release

Reflexes: Angiotensin II decreases baroreflex–sympathoneural gain; after chemical sympathectomy, the RAS maintains flood pressure

Conversely, exogenous AII augments release of norepinephrine during sympathetic stimulation (Hughes and Roth, 1971; Zimmerman, 1978, 1981), and application of AII to primary cultures of adrenomedullary cells stimulates rapid release of catecholamines into the medium (Zimlichman, Goldstein, Zimlichman et al., 1987). Whether endogenous AII augments sympathoneural release of norepinephrine or adrenomedullary release of epinephrine in humans is unknown.

The brain contains all the elements of the RAS (Ganten et al., 1983). AII-like immunoreactivity has been identified in several brain regions, including the NTS, paraventricular nucleus of the hypothalamus, the subfornical organ, and the supraoptic nuclei and hippocampus; and AII receptors in the NTS, paraventricular nucleus of the hypothalamus, subfornical organ, and area postrema. In quietly resting, conscious animals, centrally administered AII increases sympathetic outflow, especially when unmasked by disruption of baroreflexes (Aars and Akre, 1968; Keim and Sigg, 1971). Endogenous AII, however, does not appear to exert a tonic influence on sympathetic outflow, since blockade of angiotensin receptors or ACE fails to alter renal sympathetic activity (Dorward and Rudd, 1991). Animals that have received chronic systemic AII infusion develop a neurogenic form of hypertension (Cox and Bishop, 1991).

The location of AII receptors in circumventricular organs suggests that both circulating and central AII can reach the receptors. Centrally administered AII elicits thirst, sodium hunger, pituitary secretion of ACTH and AVP, and sympathetic activation, and AII appears to act in the NTS to decrease baroreflex sensitivity (Casto and Phillips, 1985). All these effects are consistent with a homeostatic system to maintain extracellular fluid or blood volume. AII-containing neurons project from the paraventricular nucleus of the hypothalamus to the NTS, where AII release may inhibit baroreflex function to increase sympathetic outflow and blood pressure.

Destruction of sympathetic nerve terminals by the neurotoxin 6-hydroxydopamine increases plasma renin activity (PRA) by about 145% in conscious, unrestrained rats (Micalizzi and Pals, 1979). Whereas administration of the ACE inhibitor perindopril produces little effect on blood pressure in intact, conscious rats, administration of the drug to rats with guanethidine-induced destruction of peripheral sympathetic fibers produces immediate, marked hypotension (Julien et al., 1990). Thus, sympathetic destruction activates the RAS compensatorily, masking the role of the SNS in maintaining blood pressure.

Dopamine attenuates adrenocortical secretion of aldosterone in response to sodium depletion (Lombardi et al., 1988, 1989) or exogenous AII (Missale et al., 1988), via occupation of local DA_2 receptors. Adrenocortical dopamine production depends importantly on uptake and decarboxylation of circulating DOPA (Buu and Lussier, 1990).

AVP–Catecholamine Interactions

Studies about interactions between catecholamines and AVP have focused mainly on the effects of catecholamines in the brain on AVP release, on the relative roles of the sympathoneural and AVP systems in mediating hypertensive responses to brainstem lesions, and on the effects of AVP on baroreflex regulation of sympathoneural outflow (Table 2–4).

Stimulation of α-adrenergic receptors by injected norepinephrine suppresses circulating AVP levels (Berl et al., 1974), probably owing to the use of the AVP effector by the high-pressure barostat, discussed below.

In the brain, catecholaminergic pathways contribute to regulation of AVP release. Central administration of 6-hydroxydopamine causes adipsia and an inability to conserve administered fluids. Animals treated with 6-hydroxydopamine do not have increased serum AVP levels, despite the dehydration (Davis et al., 1987), although further hypovolemia resulting from intraperitoneal polyethylene glycol does evoke large increases in AVP secretion.

Bilateral lesions of the NTS markedly increase AVP levels. Ganglionic blockade alone does not attenuate the hypertension, whereas combined ganglion blockade and administration of an AVP antagonist abolishes the hypertension (Sved et al., 1985). Intravenous administration of clonidine can ameliorate both the hypertension and the elevated levels of AVP resulting from bilateral lesions of the NTS in rats (Sved, 1985), consistent with a role of central neural α_2-adrenoceptors in determining the AVP response.

Lesions of the A1 noradrenergic cells of the ventrolateral medulla elicit fulminant hypertension, also due to sympathetic stimulation and AVP release (Blessing et al., 1982; Imaizumi et al., 1985). Ganglionic or α-adrenoceptor blockade abolishes and administration of a AVP antagonist attenuates A1 hypertension (Sved and Reis, 1985). Since systemic administration of 6-hydroxydopamine also ameliorates A1 hypertension, and since AVP-deficient Brattleboro rats can develop A1 hypertension, sympathoneural activation determines this form of hypertension, despite 100-fold increases in plasma AVP levels (Minson et al., 1986).

The localization of parvocellular neurons projecting to medullary and spinal cord centers involved with sympathetic outflow and of magnocellular neurons contributing to AVP release suggests that the paraventricular nucleus (PVN) of the hypothalamus

Table 2–4. Vasopressin–Catecholamine Interactions

Brain: Destruction of A1 or A2 noradrenergic neurons evokes vasopressin release

Reflexes: Vasopressin increases baroreflex–sympathoneural gain; after chemical sympathectomy, vasopressin maintains blood pressure provides a site for interaction between AVP and peripheral catecholaminergic systems. Stimulation of the PVN increases blood pressure, the pressor effect apparently independent of AVP release, since PVN stimulation increases pressure even in Brattleboro rats (Porter and Brody, 1985, 1986a). Acute sinoaortic denervation unmasks a stimulatory effect of parvocellular cells on blood pressure and on splanchnic, renal, and skeletal muscle vasoconstriction, whereas magnocellular stimulation in this setting exerts little effect on blood pressure but causes marked hindquarters vasodilation (Porter and Brody, 1986b). Electrical stimulation of the circumventricular subfornical organ increases blood pressure by causing diffuse vasoconstriction, especially of the mesenteric bed, and ganglion blockade abolishes and AVP blockade attenuates the responses (Mangiapane and Brody, 1986).

Surgical disruption of CRH and AVP pathways to the median eminence attenuate plasma ACTH responses but augment plasma catecholamine levels during immobilization stress (Makara et al., 1986). Conversely, chemical sympathectomy increases plasma AVP levels (Hatzinikolaou et al., 1982).

In laboratory animals, circulating AVP inhibits renal sympathetic nerve activity indirectly via a pathway from the area postrema to the NTS (Suzuki et al., 1989), suggesting effects of AVP on baroreflex function, as discussed below. Stimulation by AVP of medullary centers regulating baroreflexes attenuates reflexive increments in regional sympathoneural outflows (Guo, Sharabi et al., 1982; Hasser et al., 1987, 1988; Imaizumi and Thames, 1986). In humans, AVP administration inhibits directly recorded skeletal muscle sympathetic activity (Floras et al., 1987) and augments baroreflex inhibition of sympathoneural outflow (Aylward et al., 1986). Concurrent sensitization of baroreceptor–sympathoneural reflexes may mask the pressor action of pharmacologic doses of AVP (Floras et al., 1987).

Chemical sympathectomy markedly increases plasma AVP levels (Hatzinikolaou et al., 1982) and decreases blood pressure. Vasopressinergic inhibition after chemical sympathectomy produces profound, persistent hypotension. As noted above for the RAS, this finding illustrates how compensatory activation of alternative effectors can lead to underestimation of the role of a single effector system (in this case, the SNS) in determining "basal" levels of a monitored variable (in this case, blood pressure).

Opioid–Catecholamine Interactions

Studies about opioid–catecholamine interactions have concentrated mainly on central neural mechanisms, discussed in the chapter about central functional neuroanatomy. In general, stimulation of mu-opioid receptors on noradrenergic terminals inhibits norepinephrine release, both in the brain (Hertting et al., 1990) and in the periphery (Bucher et al., 1992). This inhibitory modulation seems related complexly to α_2-adrenoceptors (Al-Damluji, Bouloux et al., 1990; Bucher et al., 1992), which exert similar actions in the brain and periphery (Budai and Duckles, 1989). This interaction may depend on shared linkage to an intracellular transduction pathway (Hertting et al., 1990).

In humans, endogenous opioids limit sympathoneural responses to isometric handgrip exercise, since administration of naloxone augments skeletal muscle sympathetic nerve responses in this setting (Farrell et al., 1991). Naloxone does not augment sympathoneural responses during nitroprusside infusion or the cold pressor test, which elicit similar increases in skeletal sympathetic outflow. These results suggest stressor specificity in opiate modulation of central mechanisms determining skeletal sympathoneural responses.

Baroreflex Regulation of the Circulation

Two general types of homeostat regulate the circulation reflexively: the arterial high-pressure barostat and the low-pressure system barostat.

Since monitored and controlled variables differ, one must hypothesize the ''goals'' of these systems. Most researchers have accepted the ''goal'' of the high-pressure baroreflex to be to regulate mean arterial pressure and of the low-pressure baroreflex to regulate central venous pressure, cardiac filling, cardiac output, extracellular fluid volume, or ''effective'' blood volume.

Schrier (1990) argued instead for a single ''goal'' for both the low- and high-pressure baroreflexes: maintenance of ''effective arterial blood volume.'' According to this conception, arterial vasodilation decreases arterial baroreceptor afferent activity to the brain, resulting in activation of the AVP system, SNS, and RAS, leading to water retention, increased vasoconstrictor outflow, and sodium retention. These processes, coupled with the increased cardiac output resulting directly from the vasodilator, would maintain effective arterial blood volume. A different perturbation, hypovolemia, would decrease cardiac filling, decreasing cardiac baroreceptor afferent activity and thereby eliciting the same neuroendocrine activation, again maintaining effective arterial blood volume.

Schrier's theory assumes that decreases in cardiac filling and in arterial resistance produce the same neurohumoral ''profile.'' Decreases in cardiac filling, however, elicit especially large increases in PRA (Egan et al., 1987); atrial stretching increases cardiac sympathetic outflow (Karim et al., 1972), whereas vasoconstriction decreases cardiac sympathetic outflow (Ninomiya et al., 1971); and inhibition of cardiac baroreceptor afferent activity by application of lower body negative pressure (LBNP) increases skeletal sympathoneural activity and regional vascular resistance more than does inhibition of carotid arterial baroreceptor afferent activity by application of negative pressure at the neck (Abboud et al., 1976; Baily et al., 1990).

In Schrier's model, a single homeostat maintains levels of a controlled variable (effective arterial blood volume) based on afferent information from two monitored variables (cardiac filling and arterial pressure), using a single effector (the neurohumoral profile). The structure of this system resembles that of a hypothetical homeostatic system to regulate ''effective total body water'' by monitoring cardiac filling and serum osmolality and using the AVP effector. Since neither monitored variable is the controlled variable, values for both monitored variables would tend to fluctuate. In the ''effective total body water'' model, values for both serum osmolality and cardiac filling would vary, as long as this variability did not affect the value for effective total body water. In fact, however, organisms cannot tolerate the osmotic shock resulting from a precipitous fall in osmolality, cellular dehydration produced by a hyperosmolar state, or severe cardiac over- or underfilling, which would precipitate pulmonary edema or cerebral ischemia. The body keeps both osmolality and cardiac filling within a narrow range (i.e., both variables seem to be controlled variables). If so, then two homeostats must regulate them, even if the two homeostats share the AVP effector. The "effective total body water" model must therefore be abandoned.

Schrier's model analogously assumes maintenance of effective arterial blood volume to be the "goal" of a single circulatory homeostat. If effective arterial blood volume were the controlled variable, then the monitored variables, cardiac filling and arterial pressure (more precisely, intracardiac end-diastolic pressure and arterial pulsatile stretching) would be allowed to vary. In healthy people, however, both variables seem controlled.

The arterial baroreceptors unquestionably do restrict the range of arterial pressure, since all relevant studies have agreed that disruption of the arterial baroreflex markedly and permanently increases pressure variability. It is reasonable therefore to presume that maintaining arterial pressure is a "goal" of the arterial baroreflex homeostatic system. One may question, however, whether it is *the* goal, since not only mean arterial pressure but also pulse pressure and heart rate influence the afferent input from the arterial baroreceptors to the brain (Gero and Gerova, 1967; Schmidt et al., 1972). One may alternatively hypothesize the "goal" of the arterial baroreflex to be the maintenance of delivery of blood to the brain, which is not necessarily the same as the maintenance of arterial blood pressure. This would explain nicely the positioning of the carotid sinus baroreceptors at the arterial gateway to the brain.

In contrast, evidence has not accrued about the effect of disruption of low-pressure baroreflexes on variability of cardiac filling. The "goal" of the low-pressure baroreflex homeostatic system therefore remains obscure. From the above discussion of Schrier's model, more than one homeostat probably mediates baroreflex circulatory regulation. The low-pressure barostat may or may not be the "volustat"; however, for the rest of this chapter and book, the two terms are used largely interchangeably, referring to the parameter controlled by the homeostat that receives low-pressure baroreceptor information.

The Arterial Baroreflex

In the arterial baroreflex, nerves from distortion receptors in the walls of major arteries, including the carotid sinus region, transmit afferent information about at least one monitored variable, arterial blood pressure, to the brain; the medulla oblongata of the brainstem contains the homeostat, which directs the reflexive compensatory responses of several effectors. The hypothalamus contains regulatory centers that adjust arterial barostat settings. The sympathoneural and parasympathetic vagal systems are the two most prominent effectors in this reflex (Figure 2–12).

As noted above, the arterial baroreceptors sense systemic blood pressure indirectly, by the extent of stretching of baroreceptor nerve endings in the walls of the aorta and carotid arteries. Injection of a vasoconstrictor drug into a healthy subject increases blood

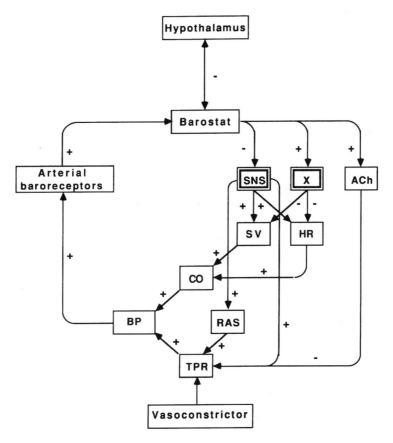

Figure 2-12. Overview of the arterial high-pressure baroreflex homeostatic system. High-pressure baroreceptors in the walls of the aorta and carotid sinus send afferents via the vagus (aortic depressor) and glossopharyngeal (carotid sinus) nerves to the nucleus of the solitary tract, eliciting reflexive compensatory changes in heart rate (HR), stroke volume (SV), cardiac output (CO), and total peripheral resistance (TPR) to blood flow. Several effectors, including nervous [parasympathetic (PNS), sympathetic noradrenergic (SNS), sympathetic cholinergic (ACh)] outflows, and changes in levels of hormones [vasopressin (AVP), renin–angiotensin–aldosterone (RAS)] mediate these changes. The "goal" of the high-pressure baroreflex may be maintenance of arterial pressure, since disruption of the reflex always increases blood pressure variability. The homeostat regulating this system is therefore called a "barostat." The doubly outlined effectors seem most prominent in the reflex.

pressure acutely, and stretching of the arterial walls containing the baroreceptors increases afferent nerve traffic to the NTS in the medulla of the brainstem. This leads to reflexively decreased SNS and increased PNS outflows, tending to normalize blood pressure by relaxing blood vessels and the heart and by decreasing heart rate.

The arterial baroreflex is so efficient at buffering changes in blood pressure, injection of vasoconstrictor into healthy young people may produce surprisingly small increases in pressure (Goldstein, 1983a); conversely, interference with baroreflex buffering markedly enhances the pressor response for the same dose of the drug (Goldstein and Keiser, 1984; Page and McCubbin, 1963).

Most relatively simple physiological homeostatic systems such as the arterial baroreflex system function rapidly and silently. When a person stands up, the person usually senses nothing unusual, despite almost immediate reflexive adjustments in heart rate and in the caliber of blood vessels. Nevertheless, orthostasis constitutes a threat to homeostasis, as demonstrated by the consequences of any of several types of neurological degeneration that cause failure to release norepinephrine adequately reflexively from sympathetic nerve terminals. Blood then pools in the legs and splanchnic bed during orthostasis, venous return to the heart decreases, and hypotension ensues. If cerebral blood flow decreases enough, the patient loses consciousness. The adjustments in sympathetic and parasympathetic outflows evoked by orthostasis therefore constitute relatively simple but unequivocal stress responses.

Arterial baroreceptor stimulation reflexively inhibits sympathetic nervous outflows to the heart and blood vessels, decreasing the force and rate of cardiac contraction, increasing venous compliance, and dilating arterioles. The arterial dilation results not only from sympathetic noradrenergic inhibition (Ninomiya et al., 1971; Spickler et al., 1967) but also, to a variable extent, from sympathetic cholinergic stimulation (Folkow and Uvnas, 1948; Rengo et al., 1976; Takeuchi and Manning, 1971). Stimulation of the carotid sinus nerve in humans therefore decreases cardiac output and total peripheral resistance (Carlsten et al., 1958; Epstein et al., 1969).

The reflexive sympathetic inhibitory effects of arterial baroreceptor activation are diffuse among several vascular beds (Ninomiya et al., 1971); however, cutaneous sympathoneural activity, which is quite sensitive to psychological stress, seems relatively insensitive to alterations in input from hemodynamic interoceptors (Delius et al., 1972a, 1972b).

Carotid Sinus Baroreflex

The baroreceptors in the carotid sinus region, at the bifurcation of the common carotid artery, have long served as an object of neurocirculatory research. Hering described the reflexive role of the carotid sinus nerve—also known as Hering's nerve— in the 1920s; however, the discovery of where in the brain this nerve leads took about another half century. Afferent impulses from the carotid sinus mechanoreceptors travel via the glossopharyngeal nerve to synapse in the NTS (Calaresu et al., 1984; Seller and Illert, 1969). The chapter about central functional neuroanatomy discusses this nucleus and its neural and neurochemical connections.

In humans, carotid arterial reflex affecting muscle sympathetic activity responds more to decreases in blood pressure than to increases in pressure (Rea and Eckberg, 1987). This suggests a curvilinear relationship between the extent of carotid sinus distention and the extent of inhibition of sympathetic outflow, with a steeper slope when blood pressure falls than when blood pressure rises.

During neck suction to stimulate carotid arterial baroreceptors, reduced total peripheral resistance causes most of the reflexive decrease in blood pressure, although heart rate also decreases. Since atropinization attenuates the depressor response in this setting

(Goldstein and Keiser, 1984), cholinergic vasodilator systems (either sympathetic or parasympathetic) may participate in the reflexive vasodilation produced by stimulation of carotid baroreceptors in humans. Consistent with this view, atropine augments pressor responses to norepinephrine in intact cats (Page and McCubbin, 1963) and to phenylephrine in humans (Goldstein and Keiser, 1984).

Aortic Baroreflex

Because of technical convenience, research about the arterial baroreflex in rats and humans mainly has involved either the carotid sinus baroreceptors or reflexive responses to diffuse alterations in systemic blood pressures. In rabbits, the carotid sinus and aortic arch baroreceptors are amenable to separate study, because the aortic depressor nerve can be distinguished from the vagus, which itself appears to carry no arterial baroreceptor afferents in this species (Alexander and De Cuir, 1963). By tightening a snare around the aortic depressor nerve, one can assess the effects of acute section of the nerve in conscious rabbits.

Neither carotid nor aortic denervation impairs baroreflex control of renal nerve activity in anesthetized rabbits (Thames and Ballon, 1984), suggesting that aortic and carotid baroreflexes interact by occlusive or mutually inhibitory summation in influencing renal nerve activity. Unlike the case for renal nerve activity, denervation of carotid or aortic baroreceptors in anesthetized rabbits does impair reflexive heart rate responses, and combined denervation virtually abolishes most cardiac and vascular baroreceptor-mediated responses (Guo et al., 1982). Each arterial baroreceptor system therefore compensates fully in terms of the ability to inhibit sympathetic outflow when the other system is destroyed, but neither system compensates fully in terms of activation of vagal neurons.

In humans, one can examine separately the aortic and carotid sinus arterial baroreflexes, by manipulating arterial pressure and controlling carotid sinus distending pressure, using a neck cuff (Sanders et al., 1989b). Systemic infusion of nitroprusside decreases blood pressure and reflexively increases skeletal muscle sympathetic activity. Stimulating carotid baroreceptors by applying neck suction augments the depressor response, suggesting that unloading carotid arterial baroreceptors contributes to blood pressure maintenance during vasodilation. Neck suction in this setting fails to decrease skeletal muscle sympathetic activity from the increased levels, in contrast with a bradycardic effect, consistent with a contribution of aortic baroreceptors to reflexive skeletal sympathoneural responses in humans.

Other Arterial Baroreflexes

Regions other than the aortic arch and carotid sinus can give rise to mechanoreceptor afferents. These include mesenteric vessel walls, the liver, spleen, and kidneys (Kampine and Kostreva, 1986). Recent attention has focused on ''reno-renal'' reflexes (Stella and Zanchetti, 1991). Renal afferent nerve traffic from mechanosensitive or chemosensitive receptors reaches the spinal cord and brainstem—in particular, the NTS (Simon and Schramm, 1984). Efferents may then travel along established sympathoneural pathways.

These other mechanoreceptor regions appear to contribute little to baroreflex-mediated bradycardia, because section of the aortic depressor and carotid sinus nerves in rabbits abolishes reflexive bradycardia during systemic hypertension in rabbits with intact vagus nerves (Alexander and De Cuir, 1963). Genovesi et al. (1993) have suggested that renal pelvic pressure and urine flow rate—diuretic activity—is a major influence on renal afferent nerve traffic.

The contributions of renal afferents to blood pressure and efferent sympathoneural activity therefore remain unclear. Webb and Brody (1987) reported that stimulation of renal afferent nerves decreases arterial pressure and produces mesenteric vasoconstriction and hindquarters vasodilation, with the mesenteric vasoconstriction depending on an intact periventricular preoptic region of the hypothalamus and the hindquarters vasodilation depending on an intact NTS or parabrachial nucleus. Stella et al. (1987), however, reported that electrical stimulation of afferent renal nerves increases blood pressure and heart rate, by diffuse sympathetically mediated vasoconstriction. Several other studies have used unilateral renal denervation or blockade to establish the existence of tonically active, inhibitory reno-renal reflexes (Stella and Zanchetti, 1991). The role of the reno-renal reflexes in hypertension and other cardiovascular disorders is unknown.

Central Pathways

The [^{3}H]-2-deoxyglucose autoradiographic technique can map central neural pathways involved in the arterial baroreflex (Ciriello et al., 1983). In this technique, metabolically active brain regions take up and retain the tracer-labeled analog of glucose more avidly than do metabolically inactive regions. As expected, baroreceptor stimulation increases metabolic activity in the NTS. Metabolic activity also increases in the dorsal motor nucleus of the vagus, the nucleus ambiguus, the parabrachial nucleus, the inferior olivary nucleus, and the ventrolateral reticular formation; in the hypothalamus, increased glucose utilization occurs only in the paraventricular and supraoptic nuclei. The paraventricular and supraoptic nuclei are the main sites of origin of AVP synthesis in the brain, the nucleus ambiguus is the main site of origin of vagal outflow mediating bradycardia, and the ventrolateral reticular formation contains the probable main site of origin of pathways descending in the spinal cord to the sympathetic preganglionic neurons. The chapter about central functional neuroanatomy discusses these centers.

Whether and how central pathways mediating the arterial baroreflex–cardiac vagal reflex differ from those mediating the arterial baroreflex–sympathoneural reflex remain unclear. In 1924, Hering (cited in Heymans and Neil, 1958) found that atropine abolished the heart rate changes during mechanical stimulation of the carotid sinus but did not affect the blood pressure responses. Analogously, stimulating the hypothalamic "defense area" suppresses baroreflex–cardiac inhibition, usually without affecting baroreflex-mediated depressor responses (Djojosugito et al., 1970; Gebber and Snyder, 1969). Destruction of the medial reticular formation eliminates the blood pressure response but not the bradycardic response to carotid sinus nerve stimulation (Humphrey,

1967), and destruction of the ventral medulla eliminates the heart rate response but not the blood pressure response to dorsal medullary stimulation (Peiss, 1960).

In rabbits, section of the aortic depressor nerve produces tachycardia without hypertension, whereas section of the carotid sinus nerve evokes hypertension (Alexander and De Cuir, 1963); and baroreflex control of heart rate can be impaired even when reflexive control of vascular resistance remains unaffected (Guo, Thames et al., 1982). Bilateral destruction of the rostral ventrolateral medulla, however, abolishes both the reflexive hypotension and bradycardia elicited by carotid sinus stretch or afferent stimulation of the vagus nerve (Granata, Ruggiero et al., 1985). In humans, anesthesia of the carotid sinus increases mean arterial pressure with only small increases in heart rate (Tuckman et al., 1967), and electrical stimulation of the carotid sinus nerve decreases blood pressure with only small decreases in heart rate (Epstein et al., 1969).

Clinical investigations of arterial baroreflex function have often failed to appreciate the likely differences in central pathways responsible for baroreflex-induced bradycardia and for baroreflex-induced depressor or sympathoinhibitory responses. No studies have addressed directly whether pathways mediating adrenomedullary reflexive responses differ from those mediating sympathoneural responses.

Arterial Baroreflex "Sensitivity"

The prominent, rapid, mainly vagal bradycardia produced by acute increases in blood pressure has provided the basis for the most commonly used clinical technique to assess arterial baroreflex sensitivity. In this approach, introduced by Smyth et al., in 1969, a subject whose blood pressure and heart rate are monitored continuously after injection of a vasoconstrictor, such as angiotensin (Smyth et al, 1969) or phenylephrine (Bristow et al., 1969), as an intravenous bolus. Blood pressure increases, evoking reflexive bradycardia. The slope of the relationship between the electrocardiographic R–R interval and the blood pressure is referred to as the gain, or sensitivity, of the reflex. (The clinical literature has used baroreflex "gain" and "sensitivity" interchangeably, whereas in other contexts, sensitivity is defined as the set point for responding.)

Analogous clinical methods to assess baroreflex–cardiac sensitivity include the decrease in the R-R interval as blood pressure falls after intravenous bolus injection of a vasodilator such as nitroglycerine; the change in the R-R interval during external application of pressure or suction at the neck to decrease or increase carotid transmural pressure; and the changes in R-R intervals during the hypotension and hypertension of phases II and IV of the Valsalva maneuver (Goldstein, Horwitz et al., 1982).

Recent clinical approaches have examined the arterial baroreflex–sympathoneural reflex, using responses of directly recorded skeletal muscle sympathetic activity after systemic administration of a vasoconstrictor or vasodilator (Matsukawa et al., 1991a) or during stimulation or unloading of carotid sinus or cardiac baroreceptors (Rea and Eckberg, 1987; Rea and Wallin, 1989), or using the changes in plasma norepinephrine levels and blood pressure after administration of vasoactive substances (Floras et al., 1988b; Grossman et al., 1982). Studies have not yet determined whether baroreceptor–sympathoneural reflex gain correlates with baroreceptor-vascular gain.

Cardiac "Low Pressure" Baroreceptors

Mechanoreceptors in the cardiac atria and ventricles respond to changes in cardiopulmonary filling and evoke complex reflexive effects on sympathoneural outflows, with the apparent dual purposes of preserving effective circulating blood volume and preventing cardiac overfilling. Little is known about the central pathways mediating cardiac reflexes (Hainsworth, 1991).

Increased cardiac filling usually inhibits sympathetic outflows reflexively (Figure 2–13). Thus, in humans, water immersion to the neck, which increases cardiac filling, decreases plasma levels and urinary excretion of norepinephrine, the sympathetic neurotransmitter (Grossman, Goldstein et al., 1992). During ganglion blockade, which prevents reflexive sympathoneural responses, even a minor increase in blood volume, such as induced by transfusion in humans, increases central blood volume, cardiac output, and left ventricular stroke work (Frye and Braunwald, 1960), indicating that during acute hypervolemia, autonomically mediated reflexive vasodilation and decreased myocardial contractility buffer the acute changes in circulatory dynamics.

Conversely, orthostasis, tilting, and application of LBNP decrease cardiac filling, and the "unloading" of cardiac mechanoreceptors contributes to reflexive increases in sympathoneural outflows, especially in skeletal muscles (Baily et al., 1990).

Cardiac reflexes involve both myelinated and unmyelinated afferent fibers, traveling in vagal and sympathetic nerves, from mechanoreceptors and chemoreceptors, in the atrial and ventricular myocardium. Not surprisingly, patterns of sympathoneural reflexive responses to alterations in traffic along these afferent pathways can be quite heterogeneous. Stimulation of sympathetic afferents may increase, rather than inhibit, efferent sympathoneural traffic, and circulatory models including this positive feedback loop have attracted increasing attention. The diversity of responses to stimulation of discrete reflexogenic areas in the heart leads one to doubt the validity of subsuming all cardiopulmonary reflexes under the heading "low pressure baroreflexes" or "volume reflexes" (Hainsworth, 1991).

Separating reflexive changes due to alterations in cardiac baroreceptor activity from changes due to alterations in arterial baroreceptor activity can be very difficult. Although it is widely accepted that application of small amounts of LBNP selectively unloads cardiac baroreceptors, because there are no changes in heart rate or mean arterial pressure, disruption of arterial baroreflexes unmasks hypotensive responses to even a slight amount of LBNP (Cornish et al., 1988), consistent with the view that arterial baroreceptors can respond to decreases in cardiac filling by sensing associated decreases in pulse pressure.

Atrial Baroreflex

The most frequently studied cardiac mechanoreceptors are the so-called Paintal receptors (Paintal, 1953), unencapsulated receptors in the atrial endocardium—especially near the junctions of the great veins and atria—that lead to myelinated vagal afferent nerves. Type A receptors discharge with the "a" wave of atrial systole, Type B with the "v" wave of atrial filling, and Type AB receptors with either or both. This clas-

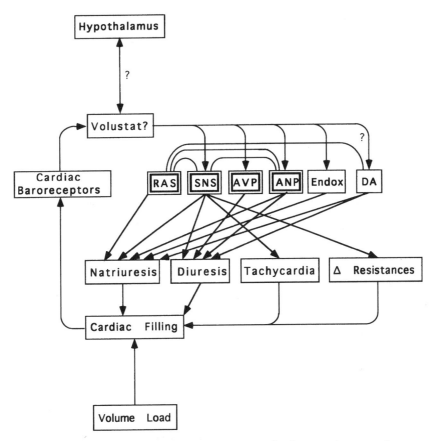

Figure 2–13. Overview of the cardiac low-pressure baroreflex homeostatic system. Low-pressure baroreceptors in the walls of atria, venoatrial junctions, and possibly ventricles send afferents via the vagus nerve to the nucleus of the solitary tract, eliciting reflexive compensatory changes in heart rate, retention of free water, sodium excretion, and regional resistances to blood flow. Several effectors, including nervous (parasympathetic, sympathetic noradrenergic) outflows and changes in levels of hormones [vasopressin, renin–angiotensin–aldosterone, atriopeptin (ANP), and probably others such as dopamine (DA), an endogenous digoxin-like glycoside (endoxin), and an endogenous diuretic (not shown)], mediate these changes. These changes predictably affect cardiac filling. The exact "goal" of the low-pressure barostat is unclear but is probably maintenance of cardiovascular blood volume. The homeostat regulating this system is therefore called a "volustat." The doubly outlined effectors seem most prominent in the reflex. The pattern of neuroendocrine changes in the low-pressure baroreflex differs somewhat from that in the high-pressure baroreflex.

sification may actually reflect different locations of the same receptors in the atria (Hainsworth, 1991). All the Paintal receptors are distortion receptors and therefore respond to alterations in atrial volume; and all receptors with the Type A discharge pattern are localized to the venous–atrial junctions (Linden and Kappagoda, 1982).

Ledsome and Linden (1964) used an ingenious technique to stimulate stretch receptors at the pulmonary vein–atrial junctions without affecting atrial pressure or interfering with the systemic circulation. The investigators tied off the left lung root and placed small balloons at the pulmonary vein–atrial junctions. In this preparation, total venous return passes through the right lung, and inflating the balloons stimulates the atrial stretch receptors. This stimulation increases afferent vagal nerve traffic along myelin-ated fibers and reflexively increases heart rate due to increased cardiac sympathetic efferent activity (Linden and Kappagoda, 1982). These findings confirm the persistently controversial report of Bainbridge (1915) that acute increases in cardiac filling increase heart rate.

Distention of the pulmonary venous–atrial junctions decreases renal sympathetic out-flow, with little effect on abdominal or peripheral sympathetic outflows (Karim et al., 1972). Increased vagal afferent activity appears to mediate the reflexive renal sympa-thoinhibition (Morita and Vatner, 1985b). These findings indicate that, in contrast with the diffuse, directionally similar changes in regional sympathoneural outflows elicited by alterations in arterial baroreceptor activity, alterations in atrial baroreceptor activity produce heterogeneous sympathoneural responses.

Atrial distention does not reflexively increase the inotropic state of the ventricle. Atrial mechanoreceptors predominate in the control of the efferent sympathetic nerves to the sinoatrial node (Hainsworth, 1991).

Ligation of the inferior vena cava, which immediately decreases cardiac filling, also stimulates cardiac sympathetic outflow (Honda et al., 1987). This at first would seem inconsistent with the findings of Karim et al. (1972), since increased cardiac sympathetic nerve traffic would result from both decreased and increased stretch of cardiac mech-anoreceptors. Consideration of the threats to homeostasis posed by the two different manipulations can explain this apparent discrepancy. Stretching at the pulmonary venous–atrial junction resembles severe cardiac overfilling; this should recruit cardiac sympathetic outflow selectively to relieve the overfilling by enhancing the ejection of blood. Thus, heart failure in humans produces marked increases in cardiac spillover of norepinephrine (Hasking et al., 1986). Inferior vena caval ligation resembles hypoten-sive hemorrhage in producing marked cardiac underfilling; this should recruit diffuse stimulation of sympathoneural outflow to maintain viable levels of blood pressure and to distribute blood to vital organs. Thus, the cardiac sympathoneural response to alter-ations in cardiac filling is probably U-shaped, with both severe underfilling and over-filling increasing cardiac sympathetic activity, and with mild increases in filling inhib-iting cardiac sympathetic activity.

Stimulation of right (Kappagoda et al., 1973) or left (Linden, 1986) atrial mecha-noreceptors evokes a natriuresis and diuresis. The natriuresis depends at least partly on intact renal innervation and therefore on renal sympathoinhibition (Sreeharan et al., 1981). In contrast, the diuresis does not depend on intact renal nerves. Thus, atrial stretching evokes a diuresis even in isolated, perfused kidneys (Carswell et al., 1970); and when hemodynamic effects of atrial stretching are prevented, and the heart and kidney are denervated pharmacologically, atrial stretching increases urinary volume without changing sodium excretion (Linden and Sreeharan, 1981).

The latter finding implies that atrial distention increases free water clearance. Since AVP is the antidiuretic hormone (ADH), the diuresis would be expected to result at least partly from ADH inhibition. Atrial distention does decrease ADH levels (Bennett et al., 1983; Ledsome et al., 1983; Schultz et al., 1982); however, the AVP inhibitory response to acute expansion of cardiopulmonary blood volume seems unimpressive compared to the marked stimulatory responses to decreased cardipulmonary filling pressure and increased serum osmolality (Robertson and Berl, 1986). Whether ADH inhibition actually causes the diuresis attending atrial distention therefore remains unclear. In Brattleboro rats, which do not secrete ADH, atrial distention still increases urine flow, even in animals with renal denervation (Kaufman and Stelfox, 1987). The identity of the other hormonal diuretic substance, if one exists, is unknown. Since the agent is stable at pH 3.2, is of low molecular weight, is not deactivated by boiling in water, and is weakly acidic (Hainsworth, 1991), an enticing possibility is that the substance is DOPA, which is converted to the natriuretic and diuretic catecholamine dopamine in the kidney. The chapter about peripheral catecholaminergic systems discusses the renal DOPA–dopamine system.

Since vagotomy attenuates both the natriuretic and diuretic responses to blood volume expansion and to atrial distention (Bennett et al., 1984; Morita and Vatner, 1985b; Vatner et al., 1986), vagal afferents at least partly mediate these responses. Other mediators by which atrial stretch may evoke natriuresis include release of atrial natriuretic peptide (Edwards et al., 1988; Goetz et al., 1986; Sagnella et al., 1986), decreased PRA (Schultz et al., 1982), and release of an endogenous digoxin-like substance (''endoxin'').

The activation of atrial cells to release atrial natriuretic peptide (ANP) depends on actual mechanical distortion of the cells, not the pressure to which they are exposed (Edwards et al., 1988). Isolated rat myocytes release ANP in response to osmotic stretch (Greenwald et al., 1989). Although as the name implies, exogenously administered ANP evokes a natriuresis, release of endogenous ANP probably cannot account for the natriuretic response to atrial stretch, because in animals with cardiac denervation, atrial distention increases circulating ANP levels but does not increase urine flow or sodium excretion (Goetz et al., 1986).

Decreases in PRA usually decrease production of AII, in turn decreasing secretion of the sodium-retaining steroid aldosterone and therefore enhancing natriuresis. Potential mechanisms for inhibition of RAS activity during atrial stretch include decreased renal sympathetic nerve activity and inhibitory effects of ANP on adrenocortical secretion of aldosterone. Although distention of the left atrium decreases levels of PRA (Schultz et al., 1982), results about distention of the right atrium have been inconsistent (Kaufman, 1987).

The natriuretic response to cardiac receptor stimulation may also involve actions of dopamine in the kidney (Sowers et al., 1984), since treatment with a dopamine receptor blocker can prevent the natriuretic response to lower body positive pressure in humans (Bennett et al., 1982).

Decreases in cardiopulmonary filling decrease plasma ANP levels and increase plasma norepinephrine levels in humans (Miller et al., 1991). Unloading of cardiac baroreceptors also stimulates renin release (Egan et al., 1987). All these changes would be expected to produce antinatriuretic homeostatic effects, restoring cardiac filling.

Ventricular Baroreflexes

Most ventricular afferent nerves are nonmyelinated (Hainsworth, 1991). It is unclear to what extent ventricular stretching, volume, inotropic state, and chemical factors affect activities along these nerves; and it is also unclear exactly what responses they induce.

In 1927, Daly and Verney described an inhibitory reflex produced by distention of the left ventricle, with decreases in pulse rate and blood pressure mediated by non-myelinated vagal afferent fibers. It has been proposed that during orthostasis in volume-depleted subjects, ventricular walls can snap together at end-systole, and the paradoxical stimulation of mural mechanoreceptors can cause vasovagal syncope (Barcroft and Edholm, 1945; Oberg and Thoren, 1972; Sharpey-Schaefer, 1956). This mechanism, although widely accepted, has never actually been demonstrated as a cause of vasovagal syncope (Hainsworth, 1991). Infusion of a vasodilator can evoke vasodepressor syncope in heart transplant recipients, in whom ventricular baroreceptor afferent activity would be expected to be absent (Scherrer et al., 1990a).

A rapidly expanding literature has supported the existence of sympathetic cardiac afferents; however, their role in clinical cardiology is unclear. It has been proposed that they initiate a positive feedback loop, eliciting reflexive increases in efferent sympathetic nerve traffic and blood pressure (Malliani, 1986). Increased afferent sympathetic activity can occur in myocardial ischemia (Brown, 1967; Felder and Thames, 1981; Minisi and Thames, 1991), aortic or coronary distention (Malliani, 1986), and intra-coronary injection or epicardial application of bradykinin (Baker et al., 1980; Felder and Thames, 1982). Since dorsal root section from C8 to T6 augments reflexive bradycardia during increases in aortic pressure (Malliani et al., 1986), the afferent cardiac sympathetic activity may tonically inhibit baroreflexes. This excitatory input may provide an explanation for increases in plasma and cerebrospinal fluid levels of norepinephrine that occur during dorsal column stimulation in humans (Levin and Hubschmann, 1980). Gross overdistention of the left ventricle, especially when accompanied by weak or absent contraction, potently stimulates cardiac afferent sympathoneural traffic (Hainsworth, 1991). In patients with endstage ischemic cardiomyopathy, a sympathetic cardiac afferent–efferent positive feedback loop could result in spiraling increases in sympathoneural outflow.

Multiple Effectors

The arterial and atrial mechanoreflexes possess many effectors. As discussed above, stimulation of arterial baroreceptors evokes not only diffuse reflexive sympathoinhibition but also prompt, marked, reflexive, vagally-mediated bradycardia, sympathetic cholinergic vasodilation in skeletal muscle, and, to a variable extent, decreased activity of the RAS (Egan et al., 1987) and decreased AVP levels (Thames and Schmid, 1981). Analogously, stimulation of cardiac baroreceptors usually evokes reflexive cardiac sympathetic stimulation, renal sympathoinhibition, decreased AVP and ANP levels, and decreased PRA.

Bilateral carotid occlusion, which decreases inhibitory afferent activity from carotid sinus baroreceptors, produces particularly large increases in renal and cardiac release of norepinephrine into the bloodstream, whereas increments in arterial epinephrine levels seem surprisingly small, considering the rather severe experimental manipulation (Reison et al., 1983). The larger sympathoneural than adrenomedullary stimulation by decreased arterial baroreflex afferent activity is consistent with separate reflexive regulation of these two systems, a repeated theme in this book.

The multiplicity of effector systems regulating cardiopulmonary filling and systemic arterial pressure obscures the important role of the SNS in the maintenance of tonic levels of cardiovascular performance. Thus, as noted above, chemical sympathectomy produces relatively small decreases in blood pressure; however, when a sympathectomized individual receives an AVP antagonist that itself exerts little effect in the intact organism, blood pressure rapidly falls to shock levels (Hatzinikolaou et al., 1982). The reason is that in the absence of a functioning SNS, compensatorily increased plasma AVP levels (as well as epinephrine and AII levels) assume prominent roles in maintaining the blood pressure.

Sharing of the Sympathoneural Effector

Barostats share the sympathoneural effector with other homeostats. For instance, during sustained baroreceptor stimulation, mental stress increases directly recorded muscle sympathetic activity (Anderson et al., 1991). Dietary salt restriction also increases sympathetic activity and plasma norepinephrine levels (Anderson et al., 1989; Kaufman and Vollmer, 1984; Robertson, Shand et al., 1979), even in the absence of changes in systemic blood pressures. Glucoprivation induced by insulin or 2-deoxyglucose increases skeletal muscle sympathetic activity (Fagius and Berne, 1989; Frandsen et al., 1989), although whether this is due to direct stimulation of sympathetic outflow as part of a glucostatic system or is secondary to hemodynamic changes produced by glucopenia has not been established.

Sharing of the same effector system by different homeostats obscures the relationship between activity of the effector and values for a variable regulated by one of the homeostats. This helps to explain why, across individuals, arterial baroreflex–cardiac sensitivity correlates only weakly inversely with plasma norepinephrine concentrations (Goldstein, 1983; Grossman et al., 1982) and helps to explain the inconsistent literature about reflexive regulation of sympathetic neurocirculatory outflow in patients with cardiac transplants, discussed below.

Interaction of Cardiac and Arterial Barostats

In general, interference with arterial baroreceptor function enhances responses to cardiac baroreceptor stimulation or unloading, and interference with cardiac baroreceptor function enhances responses to arterial baroreceptor stimulation or unloading (Hainsworth, 1991). Since both the cardiac and arterial baroreflexes use the sympathoneural effector system, the relationship between mechanoreceptor stimulation and reflexive alterations in sympathoneural activity depends importantly on the interaction of the cardiac and arterial barostats.

Unloading of arterial and cardiac mechanoreceptors produces additive effects on AVP and renin release. Denervation of sinoaortic baroreceptors in normovolemic rats increases glucose utilization (indicating increased metabolic activity) in the median eminence and posterior pituitary gland and increases secretion of AVP (Lekan et al., 1990). Hemorrhage in the denervated rats, unloading cardiac "low pressure" barore-ceptors, further increases the regional glucose utilization and AVP release. More exten-sive hemorrhage (20% of blood volume) increases glucose utilization in the paraven-tricular and supraoptic nuclei, area postrema, and subfornical organ. The latter regions are circumventricular areas where circulating hormones, such as AII and AVP, may act to augment reflexive autonomic responses. Analogously, in humans, maximal responses of PRA occur during simultaneous unloading of cardiopulmonary and carotid barore-ceptors (Egan et al., 1987).

Patterns of reflexive responses elicited by carotid and cardiac baroreceptor unloading appear to have a degree of selectivity. In humans, when external suction at the neck is used to increase carotid transmural pressure and therefore to stimulate carotid sinus baroreceptors, blood pressure and pulse rate decrease, whereas forearm vascular resist-ance remains unchanged (Abboud et al., 1976). When LBNP is used to decrease cardiac filling and to inhibit cardiac baroreceptor afferent activity, forearm vascular resistance and splanchnic resistance increase. When the two manipulations are combined, neck suction inhibits the increases in splanchnic resistance and heart rate during application of LBNP, but neck suction does not alter the increases in forearm vascular resistance during LBNP (Abboud et al., 1979). These results suggest that cardiac and carotid baroreceptors both contribute to reflexive regulation of cardiac and splanchnic neural activity, whereas cardiac baroreceptors predominate in the regulation of responses of forearm vascular resistance. Consistent with this view, unloading cardiac baroreceptors in humans selectively increases sympathoneural activity in skeletal muscle, when the estimated spillover rate of norepinephrine into arterial plasma remains unchanged (Baily et al., 1990). Cardiac baroreceptor unloading seems also to be much more effective than arterial baroreceptor unloading in stimulating release of renin into the circulation (Egan et al., 1987). These results suggest that cardiac baroreceptors figure especially prominently in the reflexive regulation of RAS activity and of sympathetic outflow to skeletal muscle.

Patients with recent heart or heart–lung transplants have denervated hearts. Assess-ments of reflexive sympathetic neurocirculatory in these patients therefore have the potential to determine effects of disruption of low-pressure baroreflex arcs in humans. Clinical results so far have been inconsistent. Mohanty et al. (1987) reported impairment of responses of forearm vascular resistance and of plasma norepinephrine levels during application of LBNP in heart transplant recipients; Banner et al. (1990) reported that heart–lung transplant recipients had blunted responses of PRA but augmented responses of total peripheral resistance and plasma norepinephrine levels during passive head-up tilting.

Local release of norepinephrine from sympathetic terminals in forearm skeletal mus-cle contributes importantly to antecubital venous levels of the transmitter. In the study of Mohanty et al. (1987), denervation of low-pressure baroreceptors could have blunted responses of both norepinephrine levels and forearm vascular resistance, due to decreased responses of skeletal sympathoneural outflow. In the study of Banner et al.

(1990), cardiac baroreceptor denervation could have augmented arterial baroreflex inhibition of overall sympathoneural outflow. Since head-up tilting decreases stroke volume, the resulting decreased pulse pressure could have released sympathetic nerves from the augmented restraint, producing exaggerated responses of total peripheral resistance.

Whereas in the study of Mohanty et al. (1987), heart transplant patients had blunted norepinephrine responses during LBNP, in the study of Banner et al. (1990), heart–lung transplant patients had exaggerated norepinephrine responses during head-up tilting. Consideration of the meaning of the term "response" here may help resolve this apparent discrepancy. In the study of Mohanty et al. (1987), baseline norepinephrine levels in the transplant patients averaged less than 1/2 that in the controls, whereas in the study of Banner et al. (1990), baseline norepinephrine levels in the transplant patients averaged about 50% higher in the patients than in the controls. In both studies, the *proportionate* increases in norepinephrine levels in response to decreased cardiac filling averaged about 50% and were roughly similar in the patients and controls. According to this explanation, heart transplant recipients may actually have normal proportionate increases of antecubital venous norepinephrine levels during exposure to stimuli that decrease cardiac filling, not because the cardiac baroreceptors do not tonically inhibit sympathetic outflow, but because destruction of the cardiac baroreflex compensatorily increases arterial baroreflex restraint of sympathetic outflow.

An alternative explanation arises from the possibility that head-up tilting produces relatively more inhibition of arterial baroreflex afferent activity than does LBNP. If decreased cardiac baroreceptor afferent activity preferentially evoked reflexive increases in skeletal muscle sympathetic outflow, whereas decreased arterial baroreceptor activity evoked more diffuse increases in sympathetic outflow to several vascular beds, then during LBNP, heart transplant patients would have attenuated responses of skeletal sympathetic outflow and antecubital venous norepinephrine levels, and during head-up tilting they would have preserved norepinephrine responses to the arterial baroreceptor unloading. Again, however, for plasma norepinephrine responses to be *augmented* during head-up tilting would require compensatory activation of the arterial baroreflex restraint of sympathetic outflow in heart transplant patients.

Studies of heart transplant recipients involve many potentially confounding factors, including treatment with cyclosporine or steroids. Moreover, neither head-up tilting nor LBNP decreases cardiac baroreceptor afferent activity without decreasing arterial baroreceptor afferent activity concurrently, even at a maintained level of mean arterial pressure, because, as noted above, decreases in cardiac filling decrease pulse pressure, which the arterial baroreceptors sense (Cornish et al., 1988).

Donald and Shepherd (1978) obtained further evidence that cardiac, aortic, and carotid arterial baroreceptor effects interact. In laboratory animals, various combinations of carotid occlusion (to unload carotid sinus baroreceptors) and cooling of the vagus nerves (to inhibit cardiac, aortic, and pulmonary baroreceptor afferents) were applied. Vagal block augmented pressor responses during carotid occlusion, and carotid occlusion augmented pressor responses during vagal block. Thus, depending on arterial and cardiopulmonary pressures, arterial and cardiac baroreceptor effects can reinforce each other.

Since large increases in carotid distending pressure reflexively decrease systemic pressure and plasma AVP levels, even during concomitant vagal cold block (Thames and Schmid, 1981), the interactions between the carotid and cardiopulmonary baroreceptor homeostats influence vasopressinergic responses analogously to sympathoneural responses.

Baroreflex Resetting

The arterial baroreflex is prone to resetting. During sustained hypertension, vagal and sympathoneural activities return toward baseline values, and acute changes in arterial pressure from the newly established level again elicit the reflexive responses (McCubbin et al., 1956; Sleight et al., 1977). These findings indicate resetting of the set point for the reflex. In rabbits, baroreflex-elicited bradycardia in response to hypertension does not last more than 1 hour (Alexander and De Cuir, 1963).

Some of this resetting results directly from effects of hypertension on the receptors themselves, due to changes in the viscoelastic relaxation characteristics, vascular rigidification, and genetic abnormalities in membrane permeability (Shepherd, 1990). In renal hypertensive rabbits, Kezdi (1967) measured carotid sinus nerve impulse frequency as a function of distending pressure. When the pressure in an isolated carotid sinus was prevented from increasing for 6 to 8 months, then resetting did not occur on the side of the protected sinus.

Since the baroreceptors are distortion receptors in the walls of large arteries, processes that increase the stiffness of those walls would be expected to interfere with the ability of the receptors to sense changes in pressure. Atherosclerosis therefore is associated with resetting of arterial baroreflexes, due to splinting of the receptors in the stiffened arterial walls (Munch and Brown, 1985). In hypertensive rabbits, Aars (1968) reported that both changes in characteristics of the arterial wall and fatigue or loss of baroreceptors were responsible for baroreflex resetting.

Structural adaptation of arterioles in hypertension, resulting in an increased wall: lumen ratio (Folkow, 1982), is associated with enhanced vasoconstrictor responses even for a normal amount of shortening of vascular smooth muscle cells. Appropriate baroreflex-mediated changes in sympathetic vasoconstrictor outflow would then lead to exaggerated changes in total peripheral resistance and blood pressure.

The function of the arterial baroreceptors themselves can reset reversibly (Munch et al., 1983; Salgado and Krieger, 1973); however, changes in the receptors or their milieu can account for only part of baroreflex resetting. This sort of explanation cannot account easily for the ability to respond approximately normally to acute perturbations of blood pressure from the new setpoint, for rapidly reversible resetting (Xie et al., 1991), and for simultaneously abnormal arterial baroreflex–cardiac sensitivity and normal baroreflex–vascular sensitivity. For instance, isotonic exercise rapidly resets carotid baroreflex function to a higher operating point, permitting the blood pressure to increase and preventing decreases in pressure due to vasodilation (Melcher and Donald, 1981), and cardiac transplantation can reverse the marked impairment of baroreflex–cardiac sensitivity in patients with congestive heart failure (Ellenbogen et al., 1987). Renal hypertensive rabbits can have normal arterial baroreflex control of lumbar sympathetic nerve activity and of hindlimb vascular resistance at the same time that baroreflex control of heart rate is markedly decreased (Guo et al., 1983).

Most relevant to the present discussion, a large body of experimental evidence indicates that physiological and biochemical manipulations can produce *central* resetting of the baroreflex. In general, controlling influences from the hypothalamus and higher levels impinge on medullary centers to modify characteristics of the reflex. Central resetting appears to be especially prominent for the cardiac vagal—i.e., bradycardic—component of the arterial baroreflex.

When healthy individuals exercise, SNS activity does not decrease reflexively as blood pressure increases. The barostat seems to reset based on changes in "central command," so that the same afferent information from the baroreceptors does not elicit the same reflexive response. Moreover, other homeostatic systems besides the arterial barostat may affect sympathoneural activity during exercise; the combined influences of several neuroendocrine systems and metabolic byproducts affect vascular tone during exercise, so that the same reflexive changes in sympathetic activity do not lead to the same effects on blood pressure; and the transmission of information along baroreceptor pathways to the brain may change. Thus, the relationship between arterial blood pressure and SNS activity during exercise is dynamic and influenced importantly by feedback about the circulatory, metabolic, and even psychological status of the individual.

During exercise, although the set point for the carotid baroreflex probably resets rapidly, alterations in hemodynamics complicate interpretation of the data. In humans with an implanted carotid sinus nerve stimulator, stimulation of the carotid sinus nerve at rest decreases mean arterial pressure by 23% (14 mm Hg), due to both decreases in cardiac output and total peripheral resistance (Epstein et al., 1969); stimulation during supine bicycle exercise decreases mean arterial pressure by 16% (16 mm Hg), without a decrease in cardiac output. Bevegard and Shepherd (1966) similarly reported that during exercise, neck suction to stimulate carotid baroreceptors produced about the same absolute decreases in heart rate and blood pressure as under resting conditions. Thus, exercise does not significantly impair the ability of carotid sinus afferent stimulation to decrease blood pressure or heart rate, although exercise does prevent reflexive decreases in cardiac output. It is possible that carotid arterial baroreflex–vagal responses may reset during exercise, whereas baroreflex–sympathoneural responses may not; alternatively, since exercise increases blood pressure and heart rate, proportionate changes in values for these variables may decrease during exercise. Cardiopulmonary baroreflexes seem unaffected by exercise (Melcher and Donald, 1981).

Studies of stimulation of hypothalamic "defense" or pressor areas have provided further evidence for hypothalamic resetting of arterial baroreflex function. The results lead to the overall view of a mutually inhibitory interaction between hypothalamic and arterial baroreflex influences on sympathetic outflow. Gebber and Snyder (1969) reported that baroreceptor activation induced by pressor doses of exogenous norepi-

nephrine reduced or abolished responses of sympathetic discharges in the inferior cardiac and splanchnic nerves evoked by hypothalamic stimulation; conversely, posterolateral hypothalamic stimulation eliminated the bradycardic response to carotid sinus
stretch. Similarly, Koizumi and Kollai (1981) reported that stimulation of the hypothalamic defense area abolished the increased vagal efferent activity produced by stimulation of the carotid sinus nerve. Carotid sinus nerve stimulation, in turn, was sufficiently
powerful to block the sympathetic excitation resulting from defense area stimulation.
Combined carotid sinus nerve and defense area stimulation produced little change in
blood pressure, although pulse rate increased. After sinoaortic denervation, stimulation
of the posterior hypothalamus augments pressor, vasoconstrictor, and sympathoneural
responses (Barron and Heesch, 1990). Conversely, bilateral lesions of the posterior
hypothalamus augmented both reflexive bradycardia and sympathoinhibition produced
by intravenous phenylephrine in rats (Tanabe and Bunag, 1991). Mifflin and Felder
(1990) summarized direct electrophysiological evidence that descending inputs to the
NTS from the hypothalamic perifornical defense area and the parabrachial nucleus alter
the responsiveness of the neurons to baroreceptor input.

Stimulation of several other central neural sites thought to contribute to autonomic
responses accompanying emotion, including the amygdala (Knuepfer et al., 1991;
Schlor et al., 1984; Stock et al., 1981), the LC (Chan et al., 1992), and the mesencephalic central gray region (Kumada and Sagawa, 1974), also produces baroreflex
resetting.

Central administration of drugs that are vasoactive peripherally often affects baroreflex–cardiac sensitivity. For instance, baroreflex–cardiac sensitivity decreases after
central administration of AII (Cox and Bishop, 1991), yohimbine (Huchet et al., 1982),
or CRH (Fisher, 1988) and increases after central administration ANP (Imaizumi et al.,
1987; Parkes et al., 1990), clonidine (Badoer et al., 1983; Korner et al., 1974), α-
methyldopa (Badoer et al., 1983), guanfacine (Fabris et al., 1986), morphine (Weinstock
et al., 1984), AVP (Aylward et al., 1986; Guo et al., 1986; Imaizumi and Thames,
1986), or the ACE inhibitor, captopril (Clementi et al., 1986). ANP appears also to
augment responses of vagal afferent activity (Thoren et al., 1986).

These drugs produce generally analogous effects on baroreflex–cardiac and on baroreflex–vascular or baroreflex–sympathoneural activity. In conscious rabbits, intracerebroventricular administration of AII augments renal sympathoneural responses to slow
ramp decreases in mean arterial pressure without affecting the response to increases in
mean arterial pressure (Dorward and Rudd, 1991). AVP enhances baroreflex–sympathoneural sensitivity in laboratory animals (Gupta et al., 1987) and in humans (Floras
et al., 1987), probably both by direct actions on baroreceptors (Abboud et al., 1986;
Guo et al, 1986) and by effects in the brain (Imaizumi and Thames, 1986). The antihypertensive action of clonidine depends at least partly on augmentation of baroreflex–
sympathoneural gain (Haeusler, 1973). In patients with implanted carotid sinus nerve
stimulators, clonidine augments depressor responses to ''baropacing'' (Myers, 1977).
Morphine or endogenous opiates increase baroreflex restraint of cardiac (Weinstock et
al., 1984) and renal (Morita et al., 1988) sympathoneural outflows, and ANP increases

baroreflex-mediated inhibition of lumbar and renal sympathetic activity (Imaizumi et al., 1987).

Psychological manipulations evoking distress decrease baroreflex–cardiac and baroreflex–sympathoneural gain (Baccelli et al., 1981; Schlor et al., 1984; Sleight et al., 1978; Stephenson et al., 1981). In baboons trained using operant conditioning to increase diastolic blood pressure, decreases in baroreflex–cardiac sensitivity occur concurrently with the pressor episodes (Goldstein et al., 1977). Defense reactions elicited by hypothalamic stimulation inhibit baroreflex-mediated heart rate responses in animals (Djojosugito et al., 1970; Kumada et al., 1975). In baboons performing a presumably distressing shock avoidance task during concurrent cyclic changes in blood pressure by constriction of the descending aorta, reflexive heart rate responses to the aortic constriction are smaller than those during performance of a presumably nondistressing food reinforcement task (Stephenson et al., 1981). In spontaneously hypertensive rats, "mental" stress (air puffs to the snout) overrides baroreflex-mediated influences on sympathetic neural activity (Lundin et al., 1983, 1984).

Clinical data about possible resetting of arterial baroreflex gain during psychological stress have been inconsistent. Brooks et al. (1978) and Sleight et al. (1978) reported decreased baroreflex–cardiac sensitivity, measured by the phenylephrine injection technique, during performance of mental arithmetic in humans, and Anderson et al. (1991) found that during sustained stimulation of arterial baroreceptors by phenylephrine infusion, mental stress increased directly recorded skeletal muscle sympathetic activity. Conway et al. (1984) suggested that during emotional arousal, decreased baroreflex–cardiac sensitivity can cause pressor hyperresponsiveness. Acute stimulation of the carotid sinus nerve in humans attenuates stress-related increases in blood pressure (Ruddel et al., 1986; von Eiff et al., 1970). Forsman and Lindblad (1983), however, did not observe alterations in carotid baroreceptor control of heart rate or blood pressure during the color–word conflict test.

Goldstein and Keiser (1985) and Kuchel et al. (1987) reported cases of patients with emotion-induced hypertensive paroxysms, high plasma catecholamine levels, flushing of the face, neck, and upper chest, and markedly decreased baroreflex–cardiac sensitivity. In the case reported by Goldstein and Keiser (1986), administration of diazepam, which acts predominantly in supracollicular structures (Antonaccio and Halley, 1975), normalized the baroreflex–cardiac sensitivity.

Indirect clinical evidence has suggested that stimulation of afferent baroreceptor pathways inhibits cortical "arousal." Fagius et al. (1985) reported that arousal stimuli that elicited discharges of skin sympathetic activity did not always produce discharges of skeletal muscle sympathetic activity in humans; however, in subjects with temporary debuffering produced by anesthesia of the vagus and glossopharyngeal nerves, the same arousal stimuli produced parallel discharges in skin and skeletal muscle sympathetic activity. These results suggest that baroreceptor afferent activity may inhibit arousal-induced increases in sympathetic activity in skeletal muscle. Dworkin et al. (1979) reported that baroreceptor stimulation decreased reactivity to noxious stimulation, leading to the provocative suggestion that hypertension may be positively reinforcing.

Disruption of the Arterial Baroreflex Increases Pressure Variability

The reflexive responses to arterial baroreceptor stimulation all tend to counter, or buffer, blood pressure perturbations. Nerves carrying arterial baroreceptor afferent traffic therefore have been termed "buffer" nerves. Upon disruption of a homeostat, values for the monitored variable fluctuate. Consistent with this principle, section of the buffer nerves—"debuffering"—produces marked lability of blood pressure (Thomas, 1944). Bilateral lesions of the NTS in cats produce labile hypertension (Nathan and Reis, 1977). In this setting, exposure to any pressor stimuli—including classically conditioned stimuli—produces exaggerated pressor responses (Nathan et al., 1978).

Whether and to what extent interference with the arterial baroreflex can produce sustained "neurogenic" hypertension has been controversial, as discussed in the chapter about cardiovascular disorders. Interruption of the baroreflex arc by destruction of the NTS produces fulminant hypertension in rats (Doba and Reis, 1973; Snyder et al., 1978) and labile hypertension in cats (Nathan and Reis, 1977). In baboons, carotid sinus denervation increases blood pressure acutely, and sinoaortic denervation produces chronic hypertension (Shade et al., 1990).

In humans, bilateral local anesthesia of the glossopharyngeal and vagus nerves by lidocaine injection produces marked hypertension (Guz et al., 1966), and high blood pressure following carotid sinus nerve section can last from 30 minutes to several weeks (Tuckman et al., 1967). Electrical stimulation of the carotid sinus nerve was used successfully to control severe hypertension in humans (Bilgutay et al., 1967), before the ascendance of pharmacotherapy supplanted the procedure.

Patients with the Shy–Drager syndrome (Shy and Drager, 1960), a rare cause of autonomic failure, appear to have deficient functioning of both the arterial high-pressure barostat and the cardiac low-pressure volustat, resulting in marked and rapid fluctuations of blood pressure. Figures 2–12 and 2–13 help to localize the homeostatic lesion. Patients with the Shy–Drager syndrome have a failure to increase plasma norepinephrine levels normally during standing (Ziegler et al., 1977a; Polinsky et al., 1981); and they have excessive blood pressure responses to pressor drugs, as indicated by an increased slope for the relationship between blood pressure and drug dose (Polinsky, 1992). In contrast, patients with pure autonomic failure have both an increased slope for this relationship and a shift of the relationship to the left, when the drug is an adrenoceptor agonist. These findings are consistent with attenuated arterial baroreflex responsiveness in Shy–Drager patients and with both decreased baroreflex responsiveness and up-regulation of postsynaptic adrenoceptors in patients with pure autonomic failure. Shy–Drager patients have decreased chronotropic responses to atropine (Mathias and Bannister, 1992), suggesting decreased basal PNS outflow and abnormal arterial baroreflex–cardiac function.

Shy–Drager patients also have low levels of PRA (DiBona and Wilcox, 1992). Since both the volustat and arterial barostat use the RAS effector, this abnormality does not distinguish which reflex is dysfunctional, although the above-mentioned prominence of the volustat in regulating RAS activity implicates the volustat. Decreases in cardiac filling evoke increased AVP release, and Puritz et al. (1983) and Kaufmann et al. (1992) reported blunted orthostatic responses of AVP levels in Shy–Drager patients.

The locus ceruleus of the pons, the site of origin of most norepinephrine in the brain, responds sensitively to decreased cardiac filling. Shy–Drager patients have low concentrations of norepinephrine metabolites in cerebrospinal fluid (Polinsky, Jimerson et al., 1984) and low concentrations of norepinephrine in locus ceruleus tissue (Spokes et al., 1979). Degeneration of locus ceruleus neurons in the brain may therefore participate in the central neural pathology that causes defective function of the barostat and volustat in these patients. Since cerebrospinal fluid from Shy–Drager patients can contain immunoreactivity to rat locus ceruleus (Polinsky et al., 1991), an immune mechanism destroying locus ceruleus neurons may contribute to the degeneration.

Robertson and colleagues have described a syndrome of arterial baroreflex failure (D. Robertston et al., 1993). Patients with this syndrome have marked hemodynamic instability, with sympathetically-mediated pressor and tachycardic episodes and a failure of vasoactive drugs to elicit baroreflex-mediated changes in heart rate.

Summary and Conclusions

The body possesses many effector systems for maintaining homeostasis, including the SNS, AHS, HPA system, PNS, RAS, and systems involving AVP and endogenous opioids.

These systems interact both indirectly and directly. Their indirect interactions result from their regulation in common by homeostats. Their direct interactions result mainly from modulatory effects of chemical messengers on release of other messengers by other effectors.

In general, PNS activation inhibits sympathetically mediated release of norepinephrine, the sympathetic neurotransmitter. "Accentuated antagonism" refers to the augmented bradycardic effect of cholinergic stimulation in the presence of increased cardiac sympathetic tone. During vasovagal depressor reactions, AHS activity increases whereas SNS activity decreases.

Glucocorticoids block extraneuronal uptake of catecholamines and are required for normal rates of epinephrine synthesis and normal β-adrenoceptor-mediated responses. The absence of endogenous glucocorticoid effects augments sympathoneural stress responses. SNS and AHS activation increases renin release, and AII tends to augment adrenomedullary and sympathoneural responsiveness and attenuates baroreflex gain. AVP and endogenous opioids enhance baroreflex inhibition of sympathoneural outflow.

Two homeostats that predominate in acute cardiovascular regulation receive afferent information from arterial high-pressure and cardiac low-pressure baroreceptors. Their exact "goals" have not been identified conclusively. Both homeostats use the SNS, RAS, and AVP effectors, demonstrating effector sharing, but the patterns of neuroendocrine response differ. The cardiac low-pressure baroreceptor system ("volustatic" system) also uses ANP and probably other effectors, and the high-pressure baroreceptor system also uses the PNS effector.

The arterial barostatic and cardiac volustatic systems interact complexly and generally compensatorily. Disruption of the arterial barostat always increases blood pressure variability and augments pressor reactivity to stressors. Hypothalamic and other brain centers regulate baroreflex settings. Arterial baroreflex function resets during a variety of stress responses. Distress acutely alters the set point and often the gain of baroreflexes. The body's barostatic systems therefore function in accordance with all the principles of homeostat operation presented in Chapter 1.

The next chapter considers in more detail the body's powerful effector systems that work by way of catecholamines.

3

Peripheral Catecholaminergic Systems

Catecholamines in the heart, blood vessels, and kidneys determine most of the acute circulatory effects of stressors. Hypotheses about pathological cardiovascular effects of stress therefore have virtually always imputed catecholamines.

Concepts about the role of stress in cardiovascular disease should incorporate regulation of not only levels of these compounds at the receptors but also regulation of the receptor numbers and of the intracellular mechanisms affected by receptor occupation. Research testing of these concepts usually has not examined these aspects of regulation simultaneously, thereby disregarding the homeostatic functions that probably actually channeled the evolution of catecholaminergic effector systems.

The organization of this chapter reflects this separation of spheres of research interest. The first section deals with synthesis, release, uptake, and metabolism of catecholamines and the roles of norepinephrine, epinephrine, and dopamine in cardiovascular homeostasis. The second section deals with adrenoceptors and effects mediated by those receptors. This chapter presents peripheral catecholaminergic systems, whereas the next chapter, about functional central neuroanatomy, considers central regulation of sympathetic outflow and catecholaminergic cells and pathways in the brain.

As discussed in the chapter about stress and science, three types of endogenous catecholaminergic systems operate outside the central nervous system: the sympathetic nervous system (SNS), the adrenomedullary hormonal (AHS), and the DOPA–dopamine system (Table 3–1). These systems exemplify the major known means by which chemical messengers act on cells. Norepinephrine (NE) is the neurotransmitter of the SNS; epinephrine (EPI, adrenaline) is the main hormone of the AHS; and dopamine (DA), the natriuretic catecholamine, acts in the kidneys and probably elsewhere as an autocrine/paracrine substance.

Table 3–1. Catecholaminergic Systems

Peripheral
- Sympathoneural
- Adrenomedullary
- Dopa–Dopamine
    Renal
    Adrenal?

Central
- Dopaminergic
- Noradrenergic
- Adrenergic?

As discussed in the chapter about stress, Cannon considered the neuronal and hormonal catecholaminergic systems to function as a unit, the sympathoadrenal system, with the neuronal component (SNS) consisting of nerve networks and the hormonal component (AHS) consisting of the adrenal medulla. The renal DOPA–DA system exemplifies a third, much more recently described, yet possibly more phylogenetically old, peripheral catecholaminergic system. In this system, nonneuronal cells take up DOPA and convert it to DA, which then acts locally by binding to specific receptors within the same organ or even on the same cell.

The SNS and AHS play key roles in the expression of cardiovascular stress responses. The renal DOPA–DA system probably contributes more indirectly, by affecting sodium homeostasis and therefore blood volume regulation.

The Sympathoadrenal System: Historical Overview

Concepts about the organization and functions of catecholaminergic systems developed from neuronal and hormonal investigative traditions that originally were distinct and then merged in the early twentieth century, the fusion persisting until now.

Networks of sympathetic nerves have been recognized from antiquity. The term "sympathetic nerve" originated in the second century ideas of Galen, who taught that the chain of ganglia alongside the spinal column provided the medium for producing consent, or "sympathy," among the body parts.

In the early 1850s, Bernard and Brown-Sequard demonstrated the profound vascular effects of sympathetic nerve section and stimulation (Bernard, 1852; Brown-Sequard, 1852). By the beginning of the twentieth century, after Pavlov's reports about the effects of neural stimulation of the heart, the anatomy and physiology of the sympathetic innervation of the heart had been described in detail (Cyon, 1907; Keng, 1893).

The contribution of the adrenal medulla to circulatory function, however, remained unknown until 1895, when Oliver and Schafer reported the marked cardiovascular effects of injections of adrenal extracts. Soon afterwards, Abel and Crawford (1897) identified the active principle of the adrenal extracts, EPI. Abel's 1902 report about EPI was the first to describe the synthesis of a hormone. About the same time, Takamine (1901) also isolated EPI from the adrenal gland. American medical literature uses Abel's appellation for the adrenomedullary hormone: epinephrine; British medical literature uses Takamine's term: adrenaline. "Adrenalin" is a registered trademark of Parke-Davis.

Until about the turn of the twentieth century, the nervous and endocrine systems were thought to be distinct, with nervous impulses to and from skeletal muscle mediating interactions with the external environment, and with chemical substances (i.e., hormones) transported in the bloodstream, determining the states of activity of internal organs. The work and ideas of Elliott and Loewi melded the neural and endocrine traditions in medicine. Elliott (1904) and his mentor, Langley, noted the similarity between the effects of adrenal extracts and those produced by stimulating sympathetic nerves. In 1904, Elliott proposed a revolutionary idea:

> [A] mechanism developed out of the muscle cell, in response to its union with the synapsing sympathetic fibre, the function of which is to receive and transform the nervous impulse. Adrenalin(e) might then be a chemical stimulant liberated on each occasion when the impulse arrives at the periphery. (Elliott, 1904, p. xxi)

Sir Henry Dale (1960) credited the idea of chemical neurotransmission, a founding principle of neuropharmacology, to Elliott's explanation for the similarity between the effects of adrenaline and those of stimulating sympathetic nerves.

Confirmation of EPI as both the adrenomedullary hormone and the sympathetic neurotransmitter would have led to a complete merger conceptually of the hormonal and neural adrenergic components, to form a single neuroendocrine, sympathoadrenal system. After Loewi (Loewi, 1921; Loewi and Navratil, 1926) demonstrated chemical neurotransmission by both acetylcholine and EPI in the frog heart (where the main catecholamine is EPI), Cannon and Rosenblueth (1933) obtained evidence for either release of a substance other than EPI during stimulation of sympathetic nerves, or else conversion of EPI to a different substance in the effector cells. Cannon erroneously backed the latter view. In anesthetized cats "sensitized" with cocaine and pretreated with ergotoxine, hepatic or lower abdominal sympathetic nerve stimulation increased blood pressure, whereas administration of EPI decreased blood pressure. We now know that blockade of α-adrenoceptors by ergotoxine and the greater affinity for EPI than for NE by vascular β_2-adrenoceptors can explain these results, but the report by Cannon and Rosenblueth (1933) appeared 15 years before the introduction of the idea of adrenergic receptors. Cannon instead proposed two forms of the released transmitter: excitatory "sympathin E" and inhibitory "sympathin I."

Cannon never identified the sympathetic neurotransmitter. In 1939, he and Lissak formally proposed EPI as the sympathetic neurotransmitter, with differences in organ responses to EPI and to "sympathin" due to conversion of the latter to another substance in activated effector cells:

> [S]ympathetic neurones liberate adrenaline at their terminals and . . . this agent, when it escapes into the blood stream, has been modified in such manner that it has the peculiar

actions of sympathin on remote organs in the body. The designation, "adrenergic nerve fibers," would thus be quite exact. (Cannon and Lissak, 1939, p. 774)

After the suggestion of Bacq (1934), von Euler identified the neurotransmitter of the mammalian SNS as NE, the precursor of EPI (von Euler, 1946, 1948). Peart (1949) confirmed von Euler's results. Loewi shared the Nobel Prize with Dale in 1936, and von Euler shared the Nobel Prize with Axelrod in 1970, but Cannon, despite his seminal work and ideas about catecholamines and homeostasis, never received a Nobel Prize. His failure to identify correctly the sympathetic neurotransmitter was probably the reason.

Based on Cannon's influential experiments and writings, the sympathoadrenal system came to be considered to function as a unit, preserving homeostasis during exposure to extreme environmental or physiological stimuli and during "fight or flight" responses (Cannon, 1929a, 1929b). Cannon coined both the terms "homeostasis" and "fight-or-flight." Later, Selye incorporated "adrenalines," a generic term for all the catecholamines released from the adrenal medulla, in his concept of the "alarm" reaction, the first stage of the General Adaptation Syndrome (Selye, 1950).

Numerous findings in neuroendocrinology, indicating complex interactions between nerves and hormones, have by now demonstrated the oversimplification of both Cannon's and Selye's concepts. For instance, neural events in the brain regulate release of many hormones; conversely, the internal state of the organism importantly influences behavior. The same compounds that act as neurotransmitters or neuromodulators in the brain can also act as hormones in the periphery. Hormones can modulate release of transmitters by binding to specific receptors on nerve terminals. Nonendocrine organs and nuclei in the brain can synthesize and release hormones. Some hormones act only within a confined portal circulation in the brain and do not normally attain active concentrations in the systemic circulation, and others in the bloodstream probably influence central neural processes by reaching circumventricular organs lacking a blood–brain barrier. Cytokines released in the periphery can alter release of neurotransmitters in the brain. Finally, hormones released by the brain into the bloodstream can act at functional receptors on peripheral nervous tissues to affect the release of other hormones.

In particular, accumulating evidence supports independent regulation of the sympathoneural and adrenomedullary systems (SNS and AHS), refuting the concept of a unitary sympathoadrenal system. Differential activation of the neuronal and hormonal catecholaminergic systems during stress also constitutes one of the main arguments against Selye's doctrine of nonspecificity. Nevertheless, Selye's theory still dominates present-day concepts about the neuroendocrinology of stress, and Cannon's views about the unitary function of the neural and hormonal components of the sympathoadrenal system still prevail in research about the physiology of emergency reactions.

In response to perceived global, metabolic threats, whether from external or internal stimuli, increased neural outflow to the adrenal medulla elicits catecholamine secretion into the adrenal venous drainage. EPI therefore rapidly reaches all cells of the body (with the exception of most of the brain), producing a wide variety of hormonal effects at low blood concentrations. One can comprehend all the many effects of EPI in terms of countering acute threats to survival that mammals perennially have faced, such as sudden depletion of metabolic fuels, trauma with hemorrhage, intravascular volume depletion and hypotension, and fight-or-flight confrontations. Thus, as discussed in the chapter about stress response patterns, even mild hypoglycemia elicits marked increases in plasma levels of EPI, in contrast with small increases in plasma levels of NE. Distress accompanies all of these situations, the experience undoubtedly fostering the long-term survival of the individual and the species by motivating avoidance learning and producing signs universally understood among other members of the species.

In contrast, the SNS provides a nerve network for regional alterations in vascular tone and glandular secretion. During orthostasis, after eating a meal, or during mild or moderate amounts of exercise, redistributions of blood flow and glandular (sweat, salivary) secretion suffice to maintain the internal environment. In these situations, the organism usually does not feel distressed.

Increases in adrenomedullary activity, as indicated by plasma EPI levels, often correlate more closely with increases in pituitary–adrenocortical activity, as indicated by plasma levels of corticotropin (ACTH), than with increases in sympathoneural activity, as indicated by plasma NE levels. For instance, insulin-induced hypoglycemia produces drastic increases in plasma EPI and ACTH levels, with rather mild NE responses (e.g., Cryer, 1980, 1993; Darlington et al., 1989; Garber et al., 1976; Jezova et al., 1987; Shah et al., 1984). The same pattern occurs in healthy volunteers during glucopenia induced by intravenous administration of 2-deoxy-D-glucose (Fagius and Berne, 1989; Goldstein, Breier et al., 1992). In humans recovering post-operatively from general anesthesia and relatively minor surgery, plasma ACTH and EPI levels increase simultaneously, whereas NE levels remain unchanged; during the surgery, NE levels tend to increase, whereas ACTH and EPI levels remain unchanged (Udelsman et al., 1987b). Playing a video game elicits correlated increases in arterial plasma levels of EPI and ACTH (Goldstein, Eisenhofer et al., 1987).

About the same time that von Euler's identification of NE as the sympathetic neurotransmitter disproved Cannon and Lissak's suggestion about sympathin E and sympathin I, Ahlquist (1948) proposed another basis for different cardiovascular effects of NE and EPI: that these catecholamines differentially stimulate specific receptors, adrenergic receptors, or adrenoceptors. Ahlquist proposed the existence of two types of adrenoceptors, α and β. Numerous pharmacological and molecular biological studies have by now not only confirmed this suggestion but also elucidated the molecular structures of adrenoceptors and provided detailed descriptions of the mechanisms that link occupation of receptors in the cell membrane to processes inside the effector cells.

Sympathetic Innervation of the Heart and Blood Vessels

The sympathetic nerves are distributed widely in the walls of blood vessels and in the parenchyma of most organs—especially the heart, spleen, and salivary glands. Sympathetic nerve endings are so extensively arborized that a single sympathetic postganglionic neuron can have 20,000 varicosities over a total length of 10 cm (Stjarne, 1988).

The neuroeffector junctions in the arteriolar walls and in the heart constitute the main sites for sympathetic nervous control of cardiovascular function.

The development of the sympathetic nervous system depends on nerve growth factor (NGF). Indeed, the discovery of NGF, the first identified neurotrophic substance, arose from the observations of effects of mouse sarcomas on growth of sensory and sympathetic ganglia (Cohen et al., 1954; Levi-Montalcini, 1987). NGF is taken up by sympathetic nerves and transported retrogradely to the perikarya where, by mechanisms still poorly understood, it modulates the phenotypic expression of the cells. Thus, NGF acts not only as a vital trophic factor in development but also as a stimulator of differential nerve growth. Administration of antiserum to NGF to newborn mammals results in the virtual disappearance of sympathetic ganglia—immunosympathectomy.

Cardiac Sympathetic Innervation

Soon after the development of chemical methods to assay catecholamine concentrations in tissues and body fluids, Outschoorn and Vogt (1952) reported that sympathoneural stimulation released NE but not EPI into the venous drainage of the heart, providing in vivo confirmation of NE as the sympathetic neurotransmitter in the mammalian cardiovascular system.

In the heart, sympathetic nerves pervade the myocardial parenchyma, with filamentous fibers coursing alongside myocardial cells of the atria and ventricles (Dahlstrom et al., 1965; Friedman et al., 1968).

Most information about pathways of sympathetic innervation in the heart derive from studies of dogs. Sympathetic nerves to the canine ventricles travel through the ansae subclaviae, branches of the left and right stellate ganglia. The fibers in the ansae subclaviae pass along the dorsal surface of the pulmonary artery into the plexus that supplies the left main coronary artery. Whereas in dogs cardiac sympathetic nerves originate mainly from the middle cervical ganglion, in primates they originate about equally from the superior, middle, and inferior cervical (stellate) ganglia (Armour and Hopkins, 1984).

Individual cardiac nerves supply relatively localized regions of myocardium. Stimulation of the right sympathetic chain (mainly via the recurrent cardiac nerve) generally shortens electrical refractoriness in the anterior left ventricle, and stimulation of the left chain (mainly via the ventrolateral cardiac nerve) shortens the refractoriness of the posterior left ventricle. Sympathetic innervation of the sinus and atrioventricular nodes also has a degree of sidedness, the right sympathetics projecting to the sinus node more than the atrioventricular node, and the left sympathetics projecting more to the atrioventricular node (Zipes, 1990). Thus, left stellate stimulation produces relatively little sinus tachycardia (Armour and Hopkins, 1984).

Sympathetic nerves travel with the coronary arteries in the epicardium before penetrating into the myocardium, whereas vagal nerves penetrate the myocardium after crossing the atrioventricular groove and then continue in the subendocardium. Application of phenol to the epicardium destroys cells about 0.25 to 0.5 mm from the surface (Zipes, 1990; Zipes and Inoue, 1988), enabling tracing of the intracardiac courses of sympathetic and parasympathetic fibers. Epicardial sympathetic nerves provide the main source of noradrenergic terminals in the myocardium, because epicardial application of phenol in dogs markedly decreases tissue catecholamine content and transmitter uptake after 3–14 days (Mori et al., 1989).

Postganglionic noradrenergic fibers reach all parts of the heart. The sinus and atrioventricular nodes and the atria receive the densest innervation, the ventricles less dense innervation, and the Purkinje fibers the least (Dahlstrom et al., 1965; Wikberg and Lefkowitz, 1984). Sympathetic and vagal afferents follow intracardiac routes similar to those of the efferents.

The heart contains high concentrations of NE, compared with concentrations in other body organs. As predicted from the innervation patterns, atrial myocardium possesses the highest concentrations (Angelakos et al., 1970; DeQuattro et al., 1973; Outschoorn and Vogt, 1952; Petch and Nayler, 1979a). In humans, ventricular myocardial NE levels range from 3.5 to 14 nmol/g (Petch and Nayler, 1979a; Pierpont, 1991). Myocardial cells do not store NE; instead, myocardial NE is localized to vesicles in sympathetic nerves (Chang et al., 1990; Eisenhofer, Hovevey-Sion et al., 1989; Goldstein, Chang et al., 1990). NE is by far the main catecholamine in mammalian myocardium (Petch and Nayler, 1979a), with low but present concentrations of EPI and DA.

Although the coronary arteries possess sympathetic noradrenergic innervation, assessing the regulation and physiological role of this innervation has proven very difficult, because several factors complicate neural control of the coronary vasculature. Alterations in myocardial metabolism and systemic hemodynamics change coronary blood flow; coronary vasomotion in response to sympathetic stimulation depends on the functional integrity of the endothelium (Zeiher et al., 1989); and coronary arteries appear to receive less dense innervation than do other arteries.

Vascular Sympathetic Innervation

The body's myriad arterioles largely determine total resistance to blood flow and therefore contribute importantly to blood pressure. Sympathetic nerves enmesh blood vessels in lattice-like networks in the adventitial outer surface that extend inwards to the adventitial–medial border, with the concentration of sympathetic nerves increasing as arterial caliber decreases, so that small arteries and arterioles, the smallest nutrient vessels possessing smooth muscle cells, possess the most intense innervation. The unique architectural association between sympathetic nerves and the vessels that determine peripheral resistance has enticed cardiovascular researchers, particularly in the area of hypertension, for many years.

Sympathetic vascular innervation varies widely among vascular beds, with dense innervation of resistance vessels in the gut, kidney, skeletal muscle, and skin. Sympathetic stimulation in these beds produces profound vasoconstriction, whereas stimulation in the coronary, cerebral, and bronchial beds elicits weaker constrictor responses (Shepherd and Vanhoutte, 1979), consistent teleologically with the "goal" of preserving blood flow to vital organs during stress.

Since endothelium lacks sympathetic nerves, one may speculate that endothelial cells interact with hormones in the vascular lumen and release locally acting paracrine sub-stances, whereas adventitial cells interact with neurotransmitters released from local nerve terminals, both layers therefore modulating delivery of often potent substances to the smooth muscle effector cells in the medial layer. In diseases associated with disruption of endothelial integrity, such as atherosclerosis, an imbalance between neu-rotransmitter-induced vasoconstrictor effects and endothelium-derived relaxing factors could increase the susceptibility to unopposed neurogenic vasoconstriction. Thus, in the coronary circulation of atherosclerotic patients performing the cold pressor test, endothelial dysfunction, indicated by effects of locally-injected acetylcholine, seems to lead to coronary vasoconstrictor rather than the normal vasodilator response (Zeiher et al., 1989). In rat isolated mesenteric and femoral arteries, removal of the endothelium produces analogous augmentation of neurogenic vasoconstriction (Urabe et al., 1990). One may speculate that in diseases associated with vascular smooth muscle hypertro-phy, such as hypertension, distancing of vascular effector cells from both the endothelial and the adventitial layers could render the vessels less responsive to both hormonal (or paracrine) and neuronal influences.

NE released from sympathetic nerve terminals acts mainly locally, with only a small proportion of released NE reaching the bloodstream. The chapter about assessment of catecholaminergic function considers the practical importance of the indirect and distant relationship between plasma NE levels and sympathetic nerve activity.

Norepinephrine: The Sympathetic Neurotransmitter

Norepinephrine Synthesis

Enzymatic steps in NE synthesis have been characterized in more detail than those for any other neurotransmitter. Several years before the identification of NE as the sym-pathetic neurotransmitter, Blaschko (1939) proposed the generally accepted catechol-amine biosynthetic cascade.

Catecholamine biosynthesis begins with uptake of the amino acid tyrosine (TYR) into the cytoplasm of sympathetic neurons, adrenomedullary cells, possibly para-aortic enterochromaffin cells, and specific centers in the brain (Nagatsu et al., 1964). Circu-lating TYR derives from the diet and from hepatic hydroxylation of phenylalanine (Wurtman et al., 1981). Other neutral L-amino acids, including phenylalanine, leucine, valine, isoleucine, and tryptophan, compete with TYR for transport into the brain (Par-tridge and Oldendorf, 1977) and presumably into sympathetic terminals.

Tyrosine Hydroxylase

Tyrosine hydroxylase (TH) catalyzes the conversion of TYR to dihydroxyphenylalanine (DOPA). This is the enzymatic rate-limiting step in catecholamine synthesis (Nagatsu et al., 1964; Udenfriend, 1966). TH also catalyzes the oxidation of phenylalanine (von Euler, 1972).

Because of the slow conversion of TYR to DOPA, compared to the rapid metabolism of DOPA, concentrations of TYR in body fluids and tissues (about 5×10^{-5} M in plasma and brain; Cooper et al., 1991) exceed by far those of DOPA [about 1×10^{-8}

M in human plasma (Goldstein, Stull et al., 1984) and about 5.8×10^{-10} mol/g protein in human brain (Goldstein, Nadi et al., 1988)]. Since the K_m for TYR is in the micromolar range, the enzyme is almost saturated under normal conditions. Thus, alterations in dietary TYR intake normally should not affect the rate of catecholamine biosynthesis, although after prolonged rapid turnover of catecholamines, TYR availability may become a limiting factor (Wurtman et al., 1981).

TH consists of four subunits, each with molecular weight about 60,000 daltons. The subunits contain binding sites for TYR, molecular oxygen, and reduced pteridine (tetrahydrobiopterin) cofactor. The enzyme is stereospecific (Cooper et al., 1991). Concentrations of tetrahydrobiopterin (Brenneman and Kaufman, 1964), Fe^{2+}, and molecular oxygen regulate TH activity. Binding of tetrahydrobiopterin to the enzyme depends in turn on availability of adenosine triphosphate (ATP), cyclic adenosine monophosphate (cAMP), and Mg^{2+} (Lovenberg et al., 1982).

Dihydropteridine reductase (DHPR) catalyzes the reduction of dihydropterin, produced during the hydroxylation of TYR (Cooper et al., 1991; Figure 3–1). Since the reduced pteridine, tetrahydrobiopterin, is a key cofactor for TH, DHPR deficiency decreases the amount of TYR hydroxylation for a given amount of TH enzyme. Both phenylalanine hydroxylase and TH require tetrahydrobiopterin as a cofactor. DHPR deficiency therefore also inhibits phenylalanine metabolism and presents clinically as

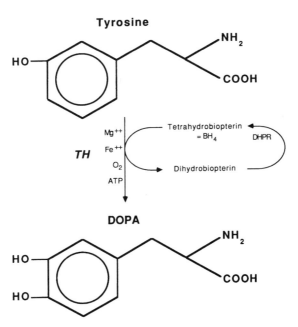

Figure 3–1. Tyrosine hydroxylation. Hydroxylation of the amino acid tyrosine is the enzymatic rate-limiting step in catecholamine biosynthesis. Tyrosine hydroxylase (TH) catalyzes the conversion of tyrosine to DOPA. Tetrahydrobiopterin is a key cofactor for this conversion. The synthesis of tetrahydrobiopterin depends on the enzyme dihydropteridine reductase. Tyrosine hydroxylation depends either directly or indirectly on oxygen, iron, magnesium, and ATP.

an atypical form of phenylketonuria (Classic phenylketonuria results from phenylala-nine hydroxylase deficiency.) DHPR deficiency was the first disorder of tetrahydro-biopterin homeostasis to be described (Kaufman et al., 1975). Treatment of DHPR deficiency includes L-DOPA, bypassing the low rate of TYR hydroxylation.

In common with the other catecholamine-synthesizing enzymes, the 5′-flanking region of TH includes sites for potential regulation of transcription by cAMP and cor-ticotropin (Nagatsu, 1992). In the case of TH, 7 such elements have been identified in the promoter region.

Catecholamines and DOPA feedback-inhibit TH (Nagatsu et al., 1964; Spector et al., 1967), and α-methyl-*para*-TYR inhibits the enzyme competitively (Spector et al., 1965; Figure 3–2). Conversely, exposure to stressors that increase SNS and AHS outflows augments the synthesis and concentration of TH in sympathetic ganglia, sympathetically innervated organs, the adrenal gland, and the locus ceruleus of the pons (Kvetnansky et al., 1970; Kvetnansky, Gewirtz et al., 1971; Kvetnansky, Weise et al., 1971; Miner and Kaplan, 1992; Sabban et al., 1992; Thoenen, 1970; Weiner et al., 1978).

The coupling of catecholamine release with TH activation and the discovery of feed-back inhibition of TH led to the early suggestion that the increase in TH activity attend-ing sympathetic stimulation results from depletion of intraneuronal catecholamines

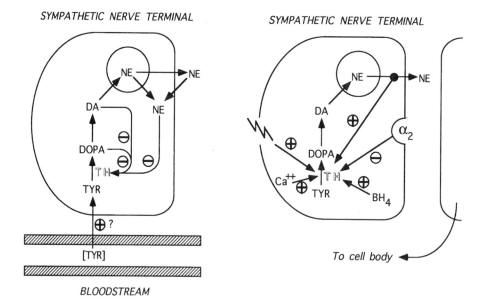

Figure 3–2. Some factors affecting tyrosine hydroxylase activity. The products of tyrosine hydroxy-lation inhibit tyrosine hydroxylase in sympathetic nerve terminals. Tetrahydrobiopterin (BH$_4$) is a required cofactor. Depolarization of noradrenergic terminals, activation of contractile elements involved with exocytosis, and increased axonal ionized calcium concentrations enhance tyrosine hydroxylation, whereas agonist occupation of α$_2$-adrenoceptors on the terminal membrane inhibits tyrosine hydroxylation. Several other membrane receptors, including muscarinic, adenosine, γ-ami-nobutyric acid (GABA) and β-adrenergic receptors, may also modulate tyrosine hydroxylase activity.

(Udenfriend, 1966). Sympathetic stimulation, however, releases NE from the vesicular pool, not the cytoplasmic pool. Moreover, increased ganglionic impulse traffic augments TH activity in the absence of NE release (Anden and Grabowska-Anden, 1985).

Other explanations for increased TYR hydroxylation after stimulation of sympathetic outflow include occupation of nicotinic receptors on postganglionic cell bodies and retrograde transmission from the depolarized terminals. The signal generated by the postganglionic cells has not been identified.

The intracellular mechanism for acute activation of TH probably occurs via phosphorylation catalyzed by a protein kinase (Joh et al., 1978), possibly the cAMP-dependent protein kinase, protein kinase A. Alterations in charges on the catalytic and regulatory subunits would produce conformational changes in the enzyme, increasing the affinities of the enzyme for tetrahydrobiopterin and TYR, increasing the maximal activity of the enzyme, and inhibiting feedback inhibition by reducing the affinity of TH for DA and NE (Lovenberg et al., 1982). A problem with this model is that depolarization of neuronal cells does not always stimulate and actually can inhibit adenyl cyclase and therefore the production of cAMP (Fillenz, 1990). Up to six different protein kinases can phosphorylate TH in vitro (Porter et al., 1992): protein kinase A; calcium–calmodulin-dependent protein kinase; calcium-dependent phospholipid-sensitive protein kinase (probably protein kinase C); protein kinase G; protein kinase N (found in PC12 cells); and TH kinase.

Cytoskeletal elements in the neuronal cytoplasm may participate in the coupling of exocytosis to TH activity, since application of skeletal muscle G-actin markedly increases activity of the enzyme in vitro (Morita et al., 1989).

The normally subsaturating concentration of tetrahydrobiopterin suggests that factors affecting tetrahydrobiopterin synthesis or metabolism may also contribute to regulation of TH activity for a given amount of TH enzyme. Exposure of adrenomedullary cells to reserpine, which increases TH activity, also increases activity of GTP cyclohydrolase, the enzyme that catalyzes the synthesis of the cofactor (Viveros et al., 1981).

Finally, receptors on sympathetic nerve terminals can modulate TH synthesis and activity. Fillenz (1990) has proposed that α_2-adrenoceptors on the terminals inhibit calcium-dependent activation of TH. Thus, the α_2-adrenoceptor agonist clonidine attenuates depolarization-induced increments in TH activity. In rat brain, α_{2B}-adrenoceptors modulate hypothalamic and cerebrocortical TH activity (Pi and Garcia-Sevilla, 1992). Depolarization-induced exocytosis of NE and ATP may lead to occupation of β-adrenoceptors and adenosine receptors, augmenting TH activity, whereas NE reaching α_2-adrenoceptors may act as a brake on the calcium-dependent increases in TH activity. Since a subtype of γ-aminobutyric acid (GABA) receptors and a subtype of muscarinic receptors attenuate cAMP-dependent activation of TH, and another subtype of muscarinic receptors can inhibit calcium-dependent TH activation, six or more different types of receptors on sympathetic nerve terminals may contribute to modulation of the coupling of nerve traffic to the activation of TH in sympathetic nerves.

During acute sympathetic stimulation, increases in TYR hydroxylation peak after about 10 minutes; the increased activity persists after cessation of the stimulation (Cooper et al., 1991). Changes in plasma levels of the immediate product of TYR hydroxylation, DOPA, have about the same rapid time course (Kvetnansky, Goldstein et al., 1992). In contrast, increases of TH mRNA content in the cell bodies occur more gradually—over hours (Fluharty et al., 1985b; Sabban et al., 1992). Increases in concentrations of the enzyme itself in neuronal cell bodies occur with a latency of about 10–18 hours. Since increases in TH immunoreactivity precede increases in enzyme content, as indicated by activity in the presence of saturating amounts of cofactors, the newly synthesized enzyme may exist at first as an inactive precursor (Miner and Kaplan, 1992). In the brain, the enzyme reaches nerve terminals via axoplasmic transport only after several days (Reis and Joh, 1977).

Multiple and complex mechanisms therefore contribute to TH activation during catecholaminergic stimulation. Short-term mechanisms include feedback inhibition and phosphorylation of the enzyme, the latter depending on membrane depolarization, contractile elements, and receptors. Long-term mechanisms include changes in TH synthesis, probably determined by as yet poorly understood mechanisms of trans-synaptic induction and retrograde transport.

During stress-induced sympathetic stimulation, acceleration of catecholamine synthesis in sympathetic nerves helps to maintain tissue stores of NE. Even with diminished stores after prolonged sympathoneural activation, increased nerve traffic can maintain extracellular fluid levels of the transmitter. Thus, in patients with Menkes' disease, who have deficient NE synthesis in sympathetic nerves, plasma and cerebrospinal fluid NE levels often are normal (Kaler et al., 1993). Patients with heart failure have markedly increased cardiac NE spillover (Hasking et al., 1986), despite depletion of myocardial NE (Chidsey et al., 1963; Spann et al., 1964); studies have disagreed about changes in TH activity in this setting. The tissue content and activity of TH therefore seem only indirectly related to the tissue or extracellular fluid content of catecholamines.

L-Aromatic-Amino-Acid Decarboxylase

L-Aromatic-amino-acid decarboxylase (L-AADC, also called DOPA decarboxylase, DDC) in the neuronal cytoplasm catalyzes the rapid conversion of DOPA to DA (Figure 3–3). Many types of tissues contain this enzyme—especially the kidneys, gut, liver, and brain. DDC seems structurally identical in all organs (Albert et al., 1987). Activity of the enzyme depends on pyridoxal phosphate.

Although DDC metabolizes most of the DOPA formed in catecholamine-synthesizing tissues, some of the DOPA enters the circulation unchanged (Eisenhofer, Ropchak et al., 1988; Goldstein, Udelsman et al., 1987). This provides the basis for using plasma DOPA levels to examine catecholamine synthesis, as discussed in the chapter about clinical assessment of catecholaminergic function.

α-Methyl-DOPA, an effective drug in the treatment of high blood pressure, inhibits DDC and therefore NE synthesis. This inhibition does not explain the antihypertensive action of the drug, because α-methyl-DOPA administration decreases blood pressure long before NE stores become depleted. α-Methyl-NE, formed from α-methyl-DOPA in catecholamine-synthesizing tissues, acts in the periphery as a false neurotransmitter, competing with endogenous NE at receptors on vascular smooth muscle cells. Probably

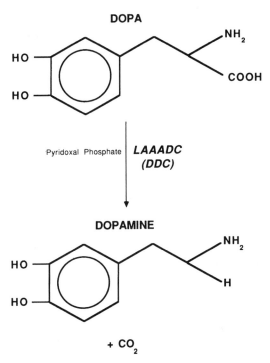

Figure 3–3. DOPA decarboxylation. L-Aromatic-amino acid decarboxylase (LAAAD, also known as DOPA decarboxylase, DDC) is abundant in many organs—especially the kidneys. LAAAD catalyzes the conversion of DOPA to dopamine, producing carbon dioxide as a by-product. This conversion, for which pyridoxal phosphate is a cofactor, is rapid.

more importantly, α-methyl-NE in the brain stimulates $α_2$-adrenoceptors and thereby inhibits sympathetic outflow (Bobik et al., 1986).

Other DDC inhibitors include carbidopa and benserazide. These catechols do not readily penetrate the blood–brain barrier, and by inhibiting conversion of DOPA to DA in the periphery, they enhance the efficacy of L-DOPA treatment of Parkinson's disease.

DDC blockade increases DOPA levels and decreases levels of dihydroxyphenylacetic acid (DOPAC), a DA metabolite. The rates of increase in extracellular fluid DOPA levels and of decrease in DOPAC levels after acute DDC inhibition provide in vivo indices of TH activity (Abercrombie, Nisenbaum et al., 1992; Pacak, Yadid et al., 1993; Robert et al., 1993), as discussed in the chapter about assessment of catecholaminergic function.

In humans, genetic deficiency of DDC produces a severe pediatric neurologic syndrome characterized by hypotonia and oculogyric crises (Hyland et al., 1992).

Dopamine-β-Hydroxylase

Dopamine-β-hydroxylase (DBH) catalyzes the conversion of DA to NE (Figure 3–4). Like TH, DBH is localized to tissues that synthesize catecholamines, such as norad-

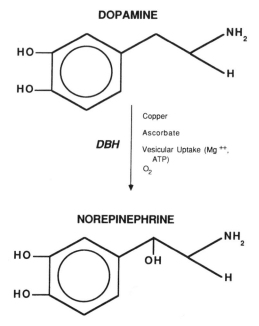

Figure 3–4. Dopamine hydroxylation. Dopamine-β-hydroxylase (DBH) is localized to large dense-core vesicles in noradrenergic cells. After uptake of axoplasmic dopamine into the vesicle, DBH catalyzes the conversion of dopamine to norepinephrine. Although this conversion is rapid in vitro, the combination of translocation and β-hydroxylation in vivo can be rate-limiting in norepinephrine biosynthesis. DBH contains copper, which is required for enzyme activity. The reaction also requires ascorbic acid. Since DBH is in the vesicles, norepinephrine synthesis also requires Mg^{++} and ATP for carrier-mediated translocation of dopamine.

renergic neurons and chromaffin cells. Unlike TH, which is present in the cytoplasm, DBH is confined to the vesicles. Thus, administration of reserpine, which blocks the translocation of amines from the axonal cytoplasm into vesicles, prevents the conversion of DA to NE in sympathetic nerves (Stjarne and Lishajko, 1966). By definition, dopaminergic neurons do not contain DBH.

Like TH, DBH structurally is a tetramer, each subunit with molecular weight about 65,000 daltons (Nagatsu, 1992). DBH occurs in both soluble and membrane-bound forms; the soluble form appears more active. DBH is transported in the axon to the terminals. Additional enzyme may be synthesized in the axonal endoplasmic reticulum.

DBH contains, and its activity depends on, copper (Friedman and Kaufman, 1965). Because of this dependence, children with Menkes' disease, a rare, X-linked recessive inherited disorder of copper metabolism, have neurochemical evidence of concurrently increased catecholamine biosynthesis and decreased conversion of DA to NE, with high plasma and cerebrospinal fluid ratios of DOPA:dihydroxyphenylglycol (DHPG, the neuronal NE metabolite, Kaler et al., 1993). Patients with congenital absence of DBH have virtually undetectable levels of both NE and DHPG and high levels of DA and

DOPAC (Goldstein, Polinsky et al., 1989; Man in't Veld et al., 1987; Robertson, Goldberg et al., 1986).

The copper chelator, disulfiram (Antabuse), used clinically in patients with alcoholism, partially inhibits both DBH (Hoeldtke and Stetson, 1980) and aldehyde dehydrogenase. Alcohol ingestion in patients taking disulfiram causes a syndrome of flushing, vomiting, headache, orthostatic hypotension and occasionally coma and death. Aldehydes are key intermediates in the metabolism of both ethanol and catecholamines; blockade of aldehyde dehydrogenase inhibits metabolism of acetaldehyde after oxidation of ethanol and inhibits metabolism of 3,4-dihydroxyphenylacetaldehyde, the aldehyde intermediate formed after oxidative deamination of DA by monoamine oxidase. Acetaldehyde at high concentrations inhibits dehydrogenation of biogenic aldehydes (Helander and Tottmar, 1987). Thus, by inhibiting both DBH and aldehyde hydrogenase, disulfiram would be expected to increase DA concentrations at receptors in the area postrema in the brain and on noradrenergic terminals, and ingestion of ethanol in the setting of disulfiram treatment would exaggerate these effects. High concentrations of DA in the area postrema, coupled with decreased reflexive NE release, may therefore explain the disulfiram–ethanol syndrome—an as yet untested hypothesis.

Alcoholic patients treated with disulfiram have neither decreased plasma levels of DBH activity nor of NE (Lake, Major et al., 1977). Genetic factors, which determine plasma DBH levels independently of the release of the enzyme from sympathetic nerves (Dunnette and Weinshilboum, 1977; Kopin, 1989), and compensatorily increase sympathetically mediated exocytosis, can explain these findings.

DBH activity requires ascorbic acid, which provides electrons for the hydroxylation. Each molecule of NE synthesized consumes a molecule of intragranular ascorbic acid; loss of granular ascorbic acid stops NE synthesis. Since ascorbic acid does not enter granules, it has been suggested that extragranular ascorbic acid transfers electrons across the granule membrane to regenerate intragranular ascorbic acid from semidehydroascorbic acid formed during the β-hydroxylation of DA (Dhariwal et al., 1991). The exact interaction of DA, oxygen, and ascorbic acid in regulating DBH activity remains poorly understood. Whether vitamin C intake affects DBH activity in vivo is also unknown. Exocytosis during chromaffin cell activation releases soluble DBH. Repeated exposure to stressors such as immobilization apparently compensatorily increases adrenomedullary expression of mRNA for DBH (Sabban et al., 1992).

Phenylethanolamine-N-Methyltransferase

Phenylethanolamine-*N*-methyltransferase (PNMT) catalyzes the conversion of NE to EPI in chromaffin cells. The section below about EPI and the adrenomedullary system discusses this enzyme.

Storage

Varicosities in sympathetic nerves contain two types of cytoplasmic vesicles: small dense-core (diameter 40–60 nm) and large dense-core (diameter 80–120 nm). Vesicles generated near the Golgi apparatus of the cell bodies travel by axonal transport in the axons to the nerve terminals. Noradrenergic vesicles may also form by endocytosis within the axons (Philippu and Matthaei, 1988). Since reserpine eliminates the electron-dense cores of the small but not the large vesicles, the cores of the small vesicles may represent NE, whereas the electron-dense cores of the large vesicles may represent additional components, such as DBH. DBH accounts for about ½ the protein content of the large, dense cores (Klein, 1982). Whether the small dense-core vesicles contain DBH has been unclear.

Cores of both types of vesicle contain adenosine triphosphate (ATP, Blaschko et al., 1956; Aberer et al., 1979). The NE:ATP ratio averages about 1:4 but varies (Cooper et al., 1991). ATP released during sympathetic stimulation can act itself as a neurotransmitter, as discussed below. The vesicles also contain at least three types of polypeptides: (1) chromogranin A, an acidic glycoprotein; (2) enkephalins; and (3) neuropeptide Y (NPY). Extracellular fluid levels of each of these compounds have been considered as an index of exocytosis (e.g., Cryer et al., 1992; Haass et al., 1989a, 1989b); however, physiological manipulations that enhance endogenous sympathetic outflow usually produce much smaller proportionate increases in plasma levels of NPY or chromogranin A than in plasma levels of NE (Takiyyuddin et al., 1990a, 1990b; Tidgren et al., 1990, 1991). The results in intact organisms differ substantially from those in vitro or in isolated organs during electrical stimulation of sympathetic outflow (Haass et al., 1989a; Warner et al., 1991), suggesting that only intense or prolonged increases in sympathetic outflow elicit exocytosis of vesicles containing these polypeptides.

Vesicles in sympathetic nerves actively remove and trap axoplasmic amines (Figure 3–5). Vesicular uptake favors L- over D-NE (von Euler and Lishajko, 1967); Mg^{2+} and ATP accelerate the uptake (Philippu and Matthaei, 1988); and reserpine effectively and irreversibly blocks it (Goldstein, Chang et al., 1990; Kirshner, 1962). Based on studies of chromaffin ghosts, subcellular particles corresponding to chromaffin granules, vesicular uptake of DA seems similar to that of NE (Carty et al., 1985).

According to one model (Philippu and Matthaei, 1988), vesicular trapping of amines depends on cleavage of ATP in the vesicular membrane, translocation of protons into the vesicular matrix, producing an electrochemical gradient (inside positive), and reduction of vesicular pH. The amines, complexed with a carrier molecule, traverse the vesicular membrane, and once inside, protonation prevents back-diffusion of the amine through the vesicular membrane. Dissociation of the hydrogen ion enables the carrier once again to bind amines.

The vesicular uptake carrier protein resembles the neuronal uptake carriers, with 12 hydrophobic and therefore presumably membrane-spanning loops, and with both the amino and carboxy terminals in the cytoplasm. The carrier protein in adrenomedullary cells differs slightly from that in central neural synaptosomes (Hoffman et al., 1992; Liu et al., 1992); both prefer DA over NE. The structure of the carrier protein in sympathoneural vesicles has not yet been reported. In the brain, mRNA for the vesicular transporter is expressed in monoamine-containing cells of the locus ceruleus, substantia nigra, and raphe nucleus, corresponding to noradrenergic, dopaminergic, and serotonergic centers (Erickson et al., 1992). Neurotransmitter specificity therefore appears to

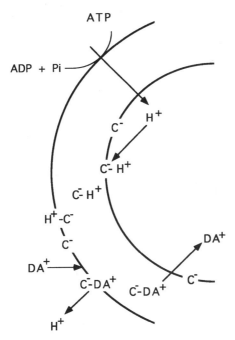

Figure 3–5. Vesicular amine uptake. In this model, an energy-requiring process pumps protons into the vesicle, neutralizing a carrier that traverses the membrane. At the cytoplasmic surface of the membrane, the proton is exchanged for an amine such as dopamine (DA). The carrier–amine complex discharges the amine in the vesicle, where the amine is trapped in protonated form. Thus, according to this model, each molecule of amine taken up into the vesicle is exchanged for a proton leaving the vesicle.

depend more on different transporters in the cell membrane than on different vesicular transporters.

Release

Adrenomedullary chromaffin cells, which are much easier to study than sympathetic nerves, have provided the most commonly used model for studying mechanisms of catecholamine release. Agonist occupation of nicotinic acetylcholine receptors releases catecholamines from the cells. Since nicotinic receptors mediate ganglionic neurotransmission, researchers have presumed that the results obtained in adrenomedullary cells probably apply to postganglionic sympathoneural cells.

The exocytotic theory of NE release (Figure 3–6) includes the following features: Acetylcholine depolarizes the terminal membranes by increasing membrane permeability to sodium. The increased intracellular sodium levels directly or indirectly enhance transmembrane influx of calcium, via voltage-gated calcium channels. The increased cytoplasmic calcium concentration evokes a cascade of as yet incompletely

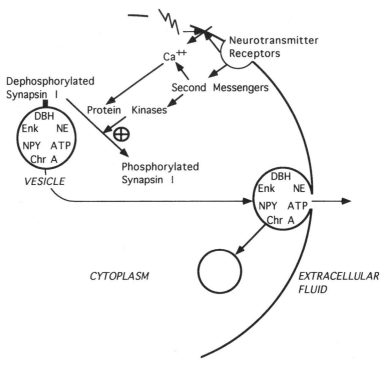

Figure 3–6. Exocytosis. According to the exocytosis theory, depolarization of sympathetic nerve terminals opens membrane calcium channels, increasing intracellular concentrations of ionized calcium. The ionized calcium fosters fusion of the vesicle with the axonal membrane. The mechanism of the fusion may include phosphorylation of synapsin I, freeing the vesicle from a protein complex. A break in the membrane at the site of fusion allows discharge of the soluble vesicle contents (norepinephrine, ATP, DBH, enkephalins, and chromogranin A) into the extracellular fluid. The vesicles reconstitute and may recycle by endocytosis.

defined biomechanical events, resulting in fusion of the vesicular and axoplasmic membranes. The interior of the vesicle exchanges briefly with the extracellular compartment, and the soluble contents of the vesicles diffuse into the extracellular space.

As predicted from this model, manipulations besides application of acetylcholine that depolarize the cell, such as electrical stimulation or increased K^+ concentrations in the extracellular fluid, also activate the voltage-gated calcium channels and trigger exocytosis.

During cellular activation, simultaneous, stoichiometric release of soluble vesicular contents—ATP, enkephalins, chromogranins, and DBH—without similar release of cytoplasmic macromolecules, has provided biochemical support for the exocytosis theory (Slotkin and Kirshner, 1971; Smith, 1973; Weinshilboum et al., 1971). Electron micrographs occasionally have shown an "omega sign," with a gap in the cell membrane at the site of fusion of vesicle with the axoplasmic membrane (Fillenz, 1971; Thureson-Klein et al., 1979). Ultrastructural evidence has suggested release of the contents of large as well as small dense-core vesicles by exocytosis (Thureson-Klein, 1983).

Consistent with transient exposure of the interior of the vesicle to the extracellular fluid, after intravenous injection of fluorescein-labeled antibodies to DBH, labeled antibodies accumulate in the terminals (Jacobowitz et al., 1975); and during stimulation of sympathetic nerves in mouse vas deferens, incubation of the tissue with horseradish peroxidase, an exogenous tracer, leads to retention of the label in small, dense-cored vesicles, although not in large, dense-cored vesicles (Basbaum and Heuser, 1979). The latter suggests that the large vesicles may discharge their contents by exocytosis, and become small vesicles, which recycle back into the neuronal cytoplasm (Winkler, 1988); however, only small vesicles contain a membrane protein called p38 (Navone et al., 1986).

All-or-none release of amines during stimulation would support the exocytosis theory. Discrete "quantal" postjunctional events have been recorded electrophysiologically in vas deferens tissue (Winkler, 1988), and microvoltammetry of readily oxidizable species (presumably catecholamines) in chromaffin cells has provided neurochemical evidence for quantal release (Leszczyszyn et al., 1990, 1991).

Exactly how increased intracellular Ca^{2+} concentrations evoke exocytosis in sympathetic nerves is unknown. By analogy with events in the squid giant synapse, one possibility is that Ca^{2+} activates a protein kinase that phosphorylates a substance called synapsin I (Llinas et al., 1985) on the cytoplasmic surface of vesicle membranes (Nestler and Greengard, 1989). Phosphorylation of synapsin I may free vesicles from an "actin bundling" complex with synapsin I, allowing the vesicles to coalesce with the axonal membrane. Occupation of membrane receptors for catecholamines may also phosphorylate synapsin I by activating cAMP-dependent protein kinases.

Two storage pools of NE appear to exist in sympathetic nerve terminals: a small, readily releasable pool of newly synthesized NE and a large reserve pool in long-term storage. In the isolated, perfused cat spleen loaded with [^{14}C]NE, prolonged sympathetic stimulation decreases the specific activity of [^{14}C]NE in the perfusate; and α-methyl-TYR, which blocks NE synthesis, prevents this decline (Kopin, Breese et al., 1968). In guinea pig vas deferens exposed to [^{3}H]NE or to EPI, fractional release of the exogenous amine during hypogastric nerve stimulation exceeds that of endogenous NE (Moura et al., 1990).

The relationship between the two pools of NE and the two forms of vesicles, large and small dense-core, has not been established. Since only the large vesicles contain chromogranin A and NPY (De Potter et al., 1988; Schwarzenbrunner et al., 1990), and since during physiological changes in sympathoneural outflow, fractional NE release exceeds release of chromogranin A and NPY (e.g., Cryer et al., 1991), whereas during electrical stimulation, the proportionate changes in NE and peptide release seem similar (e.g., Haass et al., 1989b), physiological increases in sympathetic outflow may elicit relatively more exocytosis of the small than the large vesicles, whereas electrical stimulation may evoke exocytosis of both types. Alternatively, different stimuli may elicit differential responses of the vesicle populations.

Sympathetic nerve endings can also release NE by calcium-independent, nonexocytotic mechanisms. One such mechanism probably is reverse transport through the neuronal uptake carrier, because pretreatment with cocaine or desipramine attenuates calcium-independent release of tritiated catecholamines (Graefe and Bonisch, 1988). The indirectly acting sympathomimetic amine, tyramine, releases NE nonexocytotically, since tyramine releases NE independently of calcium and does not release DBH. As predicted from the ionic requirements for neuronal reuptake (see below), increases in intracellular Na^+ concentrations, such as produced by ouabain, enhance carrier-mediated efflux of NE (Stute and Trendelenburg, 1984). Myocardial ischemic hypoxia evokes calcium-independent release of NE (Carlsson et al., 1986; Felder and Thames, 1981; Malliani et al., 1986; Schomig, 1988; Schomig et al., 1987; Staszewska-Barczak, 1971), as discussed in the chapter about cardiovascular diseases.

The hydrophilic nature of catecholamines and their ionization at physiological pH probably prevent NE efflux by simple diffusion.

The occurrence of exocytotic release of NE does not imply that sympathetic neurotransmission is exclusively or even predominantly synaptic. Interactions between synaptic and nonsynaptic neurotransmission are poorly understood (Vizi and Labos, 1991).

Other Sympathetic Transmitters Besides Norepinephrine

As noted above, sympathetic stimulation releases other compounds besides NE. Some of these compounds may function as neurotransmitters. ATP, adenosine, NPY, acetylcholine, and EPI have received the most attention.

According to the cotransmitter hypothesis proposed by Burnstock (1976), ATP released with NE during sympathetic stimulation produces adrenoceptor-independent vasoconstriction (Pelleg and Burnstock, 1990). This can explain sympathetically mediated vasoconstriction that is resistant to blockade of postsynaptic α_1-adrenoceptors but that is attenuated by purine receptor blockade or by bretylium, which inhibits exocytosis (Taddei et al., 1989). The cotransmitter effects of ATP seem prominent during brief bursts of sympathoneural traffic in the mesenteric and hepatic arteries and in the kidney. ATP, rather than NE, may cause the "fast" electrical responses of effector cells (Stjarne, 1988); however, in the rat tail artery, NE release precedes the postsynaptic vascular response to electric nerve stimulation (Gonon et al., 1993).

Ectoenzymes rapidly degrade ATP to form adenosine, which seems to exert antiadrenergic actions, both pre- and postjunctionally, by effects on specific adenosine receptors (White, 1988). Intra-arterial infusion of theophylline, which blunts adenosine-induced vasodilation, augments reflexive vasoconstriction during application of lower-body negative pressure in humans, even during α-adrenoceptor blockade (Taddei et al., 1990), consistent with the view that during reflexive stimulation of sympathetically mediated exocytosis, adenosine, produced from degradation of released ATP, limits vasoconstriction.

Postganglionic sympathetic nerves and adrenal chromaffin cells costore NPY with catecholamines. During some forms of stress, including psychological stress, plasma NPY levels increase, whereas in others, such as exposure to cold, no change in NPY levels occurs, despite increased NE levels (Mormede et al., 1990). Thus, although exogenously administered NPY potently constricts blood vessels, whether the endogenously released peptide modulates sympathetically mediated vasoconstriction or participates in circulatory responses during stress remains unclear.

The physiological roles of enkephalins and chromogranin A in sympathetic neuro-circulatory function are unknown.

In skeletal muscle beds of some species, sympathetic nerves release acetylcholine (Ellison and Zanchetti, 1971; Folkow and Uvnas, 1948). Sympathetic cholinergic mechanisms may contribute to vasodilation during hypothalamic stimulation (Eliasson et al., 1951), exercise (Sanders et al., 1989a), or baroreceptor stimulation (Goldstein and Keiser, 1984; Takeuchi and Manning, 1971). Acetylcholine is the sympathetic transmitter in eccrine sweat glands.

The ''epinephrine hypothesis'' (Majewski et al., 1981; Rand and Majewski, 1984) proposes that after neuronal uptake of circulating EPI, sympathetic stimulation coreleases NE and EPI and that the coreleased EPI binds to β-adrenoceptors on sympathetic terminals to augment further NE release. A section later in this chapter discusses the epinephrine hypothesis in detail.

Local and Reflexive Modulation

Pharmacological stimulation of any of a large variety of receptor types on noradrenergic terminals affects the amount of NE released during cellular activation. Compounds inhibiting NE release include acetylcholine (at muscarinic receptors; Levy and Blattberg, 1976; Muscholl, 1980), DA (Brodde, 1990; Goldberg and Rajfer, 1985), γ-aminobutyric acid (at $GABA_B$ receptors, Fillenz, 1990), prostaglandins of the E series (Hedqvist, 1969), opioids (Szabo et al., 1986), adenosine (Snyder, 1985), and NE itself (Langer, 1974, 1981; Langer et al., 1971). Compounds enhancing NE release include angiotensin II (AII; Hughes and Roth, 1971; Szabo et al., 1990; Zimmerman, 1978, 1981), acetylcholine (at nicotinic receptors), ACTH (Szabo et al., 1989b), GABA (at $GABA_A$ receptors, Fillenz, 1990), and EPI (via stimulation of presynaptic $β_2$-adrenoceptors; Stjarne and Brundin, 1976; Vincent et al., 1982).

In general, whether at physiological concentrations these compounds exert modulatory effects on endogenous NE release remains unproven, especially in humans. For instance, although exogenously administered AII augments plasma NE responses during reflexive increases in sympathetic nerve traffic in anesthetized rabbits, blockade of AII synthesis or effects does not alter the NE responses (Dorward and Rudd, 1991; Szabo et al., 1990). In humans, infusion of a pressor amount of AII does not enhance responses of NE spillover during baroreceptor unloading, indicating an absence of presynaptic modulation of NE release in this setting (Goldsmith and Hasking, 1991); however, brachial intra-arterial infusion of AII, with coadministration of nitroprusside to prevent forearm vasoconstriction, increases forearm NE spillover (Clemson et al., 1994).

Substantial evidence, however, does support inhibitory presynaptic modulation by NE itself, via autoreceptors on sympathetic nerves. Blockade of α-adrenoceptors augments responses of NE overflow during regional sympathetic nerve stimulation (Brown and Gillespie, 1957). This augmentation was at first thought to be due to blockade of α-adrenoceptors on effector cells, increasing NE release by a form of trans-synaptic induction (Brown and Gillespie, 1957). Other explanations included inhibition of neuronal reuptake (Thoenen et al., 1964) or of extraneuronal uptake (Langer, 1970) of NE. In 1971, Starke (Starke et al., 1971) and Langer suggested a prejunctional mechanism for the augmentation of NE release. Subsequent studies, showing differential actions of drugs at pre- and postjunctional α-adrenoceptors, supported the latter explanation. By now, laboratory animal (Brown and Gillespie, 1957; Langer, 1981; Starke et al., 1977; Szabo et al., 1989a; Yamaguchi et al., 1977) and clinical (Grossman, Chang et al., 1991a; Grossman, Rea et al., 1991) evidence has established that endogenous NE can regulate its own release by stimulating inhibitory α_2-adrenoceptors on sympathetic nerves. This modulatory action appears to vary with the vascular bed under study (Docherty and McGrath, 1979; Garty et al., 1990), being prominent in skeletal muscle beds such as the forearm (Grossman, Rea et al., 1991), relatively weak in the kidneys (Garty et al., 1990; Yamaguchi and Brassard, 1988), and virtually absent in the adrenals (Yamaguchi and Brassard, 1988).

Grossman, Rea et al. (1991) reported in humans that systemic administration of the α_2-adrenoceptor blocker, yohimbine, produced much larger proportionate increases in forearm NE spillover than in directly recorded skeletal muscle sympathoneural activity, providing strong evidence that in human limbs, α_2-adrenoceptors on sympathetic nerve endings exert inhibitory modulation of NE release during sympathetic stimulation. Consistent with this suggestion, blockade of local α_2-adrenoceptors during intra-arterial infusion of yohimbine in humans increases forearm NE spillover much more than can be accounted for by concurrently increased regional blood flow (Grossman, Chang et al., 1991a). Thus, endogenously released NE feedback inhibits its own release by occupying α_2-adrenoceptors on sympathetic nerve terminals, even under resting conditions, in humans. Yohimbine administration also increases NE levels in the cardiac venous drainage in humans (Eisenhofer, Esler et al., 1992; Indolfi et al., 1992).

The mechanism of α_2-adrenoceptor-induced inhibition of NE release may involve the ability of cellular activation to increase axoplasmic Ca^{2+} concentrations. α_2-Adrenoceptor stimulation inhibits intracellular generation of cAMP, and cAMP-dependent phosphorylation of calcium channels increases the probability of channel opening during depolarization of the cell membrane (Levitan, 1985). α_2-Adrenoceptor stimulation may also increase potassium conductance or inhibit effects of cytosolic Ca^{2+} at an intracellular site (Fillenz, 1990).

Desipramine-induced blockade of neuronal reuptake of NE augments pressor and plasma NE responses during sympathetic stimulation (Kopin et al., 1984) or yohimbine infusion (Goldstein, Eisenhofer et al., 1988). Systemic administration of desipramine, however, also markedly decreases sympathetic nerve traffic (Cohen et al., 1990; Esler, Wallin et al., 1991; Lavian et al., 1991; Szabo and Schultheiss, 1990). The sympathoinhibition probably offsets the blockade of reuptake, preventing increases in NE spillover.

In addition to local feedback control of NE release, reflexive "long-distance" feedback pathways, via high- and low-pressure baroreceptors, elicit reflexive changes in sympathoneural impulse activity, as discussed in Chapter 2. Alterations in receptor numbers or of intracellular biomechanical events after receptor activation also affect responses to agonists (Bristow et al., 1982, 1986; Fraser et al., 1981), as discussed below in the section about adrenoceptors. These factors may therefore regulate NE release by trans-synaptic local and reflexive long-distance mechanisms.

Disposition of Norepinephrine

Unlike acetylcholine, which is inactivated mainly by extracellular enzymes, NE is inactivated mainly by uptake into cells, with subsequent intracellular metabolism or storage (Figure 3–7).

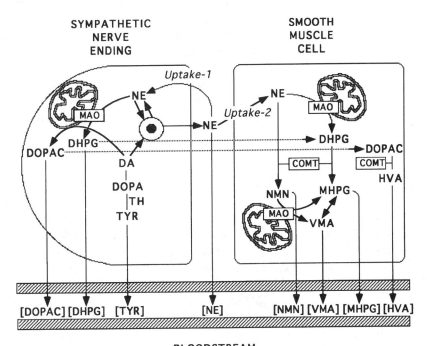

Figure 3–7. Catecholamine removal and metabolism. Endogenously released norepinephrine is taken back up into sympathetic nerve terminals by Uptake-1 and taken up into nonneuronal cells by Uptake-2. Norepinephrine in the axoplasm can be translocated back into the vesicles or converted to dihydroxyphenylglycol (DHPG) by monoamine oxidase (MAO) in the outer mitochondrial membrane. Norepinephrine in nonneuronal cells is converted to normetanephrine (NMN) by catechol-*O*-methyltransferase (COMT). DHPG can diffuse into the bloodstream or can be taken up by nonneuronal cells and converted to methoxyhydroxyphenylglycol (MHPG). MHPG and vanillylmandelic acid (VMA), the latter formed mainly in the liver, are end-products of norepinephrine metabolism. Dopamine in the axoplasm can be translocated into vesicles and converted to norepinephrine or can be converted to dihydroxyphenylacetic acid (DOPAC) by MAO. DOPAC can diffuse into the bloodstream or can be converted extraneuronally to homovanillic acid (HVA), the main end-product of dopamine metabolism. The processes of catecholamine uptake and metabolism are generally independent of actions by adrenoceptors on the nerve terminals or on nonneuronal cells.

Neuronal Re-uptake (Uptake-1)

Reuptake into nerve terminals—Uptake-1 (Iversen, 1973)—is the predominant means of terminating the actions of released NE. Uptake-1 is energy-requiring and carrier-mediated. The carrier is saturable, with a K_m in the micromolar range. Neither diffusion of the catecholamine within the tissue to the carrier sites nor tissue perfusion affects the K_m values, suggesting these factors are not rate-limiting (Graefe and Bonisch, 1988).

The carrier can transport catecholamines against large concentration gradients. In rabbit hearts perfused with L-[^{3}H]NE (in the presence of a monoamine oxidase inhibitor to prevent deamination of cytoplasmic amines), the steady-state tissue/medium ratio of the tracer averages about 100:1 (Bonisch and Graefe, 1976). Vesicular uptake and retention further concentrate neuronal catecholamines, since the myocardial tissue/medium ratio averages 44:1 in hearts of reserpinized animals (Bonisch and Graefe, 1976). When sympathetically innervated tissues remove circulating [^{3}H]DA, the tissue: plasma concentration ratio of [^{3}H]NE exceeds 1000:1 (Hovevey-Sion, Eisenhofer et al., 1989).

The carrier is not stereospecific (Goldstein, Horwitz et al., 1983; Henseling and Trendelenburg, 1978). The only common structural feature of all known substrates for Uptake-1 is an aromatic amine, with the ionizable nitrogen moiety not incorporated in the aromatic system (Graefe and Bonisch, 1988). Uptake-1 does not require a catechol nucleus, since drugs such as metaraminol, tyramine, and octopamine, which have only one phenolic hydroxyl group, are substrates for Uptake-1. Alkylation of the primary amino group decreases the effectiveness of the transport, explaining why sympathetic nerves take up NE more efficiently than they do EPI (Eisenhofer, Esler et al., 1990) and why they do not take up isoproterenol, an extensively alkylated catecholamine, at all (Callingham and Burgen, 1966; Goldstein, Horwitz et al., 1983). Although *N*-methylation decreases susceptibility of a compound to neuronal uptake, α-methylation produces no effect. Sympathetic nerve terminals therefore efficiently remove α-methyl-NE. Methylation of the phenolic hydroxyl groups, however, markedly decreases susceptibility to Uptake-1, and so sympathetic nerves do not take up O-methylated catecholamine metabolites such as normetanephrine.

Neuronal uptake by dopaminergic neurons differs from that by noradrenergic neurons, since the former take up DA more avidly than they take up NE, whereas the latter take up both catecholamines about equally well. Desipramine and other tricyclic antidepressants block uptake by noradrenergic neurons much more effectively than they block uptake by dopaminergic neurons, whereas mazindole is more effective at dopaminergic uptake sites.

These pharmacological differences imply distinct transporters for NE and DA. Recent molecular genetic studies have confirmed this distinction. Expression cloning has revealed the structures of the NE transporter (Pacholczyk et al., 1991) and the DA transporter (Giros et al., 1991; Kilty et al., 1991; Shimada et al., 1991; Usdin et al., 1991). The human NE transporter protein consists of 617 amino acids, with a molecular weight of about 69,000, including 12–13 hydrophobic and therefore probably membrane-spanning domains (Pacholczyk et al., 1991; Figure 3–8). This structure differs

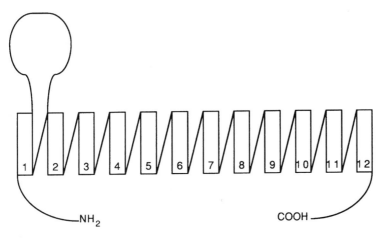

Figure 3–8. Amine transporter structure. Amine transporters, including Uptake-1 and the intracellular vesicular transporter, and transporters for neurotransmitter amino acids such as γ-aminobutyric acid, share several structural features: 12 hydrophobic and therefore presumably membrane-spanning domains, both the amino and carboxyl ends in the cytoplasm, and a large loop between the first and second transmembrane domains.

substantially from that of adrenoceptors and other receptors coupled with G-proteins, as discussed below in the section about adrenoceptors, but is very similar to that of the DA, GABA, serotonin, and vesicular transporters, suggesting a family of neurotransmitter transporter proteins. Transfected cells expressing the NE transporter take up L[^{3}H]NE with a K_m of 0.5 μM, consistent with the above-described pharmacological studies.

Uptake-1 has several metabolic requirements (Eckert et al., 1976; Graefe et al., 1976; Iversen, 1973). Neuronal uptake absolutely requires intracellular K$^+$ and extracellular Na$^+$ and functions most efficiently when Cl$^-$ accompanies Na$^+$. Transport does not directly require ATP; however, maintaining ionic gradients across cell membranes depends on ATP, and the carrier uses the energy expended in maintaining the transmembrane Na$^+$ gradient to cotransport amines with Na$^+$.

Many drugs or in vitro conditions inhibit Uptake-1, including cocaine, tricyclic antidepressants, low extracellular Na$^+$ concentrations, Li$^+$, ouabain, and nitrogen mustards such as phenoxybenzamine (Graefe and Bonisch, 1988). Ouabain probably inhibits Uptake-1 indirectly (Leitz and Stefano, 1970), by decreasing the transmembrane Na$^+$ gradient.

Because phenoxybenzamine can inhibit Uptake-1, administration of the drug in patients with pheochromocytoma can at least theoretically produce false-negative results of nuclear medical scanning procedures that depend on Uptake-1 of radionuclides to localize the catecholamine-secreting tumor.

In laboratory animals, Uptake-1 activity decreases with advancing age. Cocaine administration produces more augmentation of pressor responses to NE in young than in old pithed rats, and in rat atria incubated with [^{3}H]NE, cocaine augments electric stimulation-induced release of the tracer in young but not in old animals (Borton and Docherty, 1989). Whether Uptake-1 activity decreases during normal aging in humans has not been established. Plasma clearance of NE decreases in an age-related manner, whereas plasma clearance of EPI does not (Morrow et al., 1987), and since NE is a better substrate for Uptake-1 than is EPI (Eisenhofer, Esler et al., 1990), the findings suggest an age-related decrease in Uptake-1 in humans. In contrast, compartmental analysis of plasma NE specific activity during [^{3}H]NE infusion has indicated that desipramine administration decreases the clearance of NE from plasma similarly in young and old subjects (Stromberg et al., 1991).

Vesicular Translocation

NE taken up into the axoplasm by the Uptake-1 transporter is subject to two fates: translocation into storage vesicles and deamination by monoamine oxidase. The combination of enzymatic breakdown and vesicular uptake constitute an intraneuronal "sink" (Graefe and Bonisch, 1988), keeping cytoplasmic concentrations of NE very low.

As discussed above, reserpine effectively blocks the vesicular transport of amines from the axoplasm into the vesicles. This not only shuts down conversion of DA to NE but also prevents the conservative recycling of NE. Reserpine therefore rapidly depletes NE stores. After reserpine injection, plasma levels of the neuronal NE metabolite DHPG increase rapidly, reflecting marked net leakage of NE from vesicular stores, and then decline to very low levels, reflecting abolition of vesicular uptake and β-hydroxylation of DA (Eisenhofer, Ropchak et al., 1988). Reserpine does not affect the ability of vesicles to maintain a pH gradient.

Deamination by Monoamine Oxidase

Neural and nonneural tissues contain monoamine oxidase (MAO), which catalyzes the oxidative deamination of DA to form DOPAC and NE to form DHPG. Because of the efficient uptake and reuptake of catecholamines into the axoplasm of catecholaminergic neurons, and because of the rapid exchange of amines between the vesicles and axoplasm (Eisenhofer, Esler et al., 1992), the neuronal pool of MAO, located in the outer mitochondrial membrane, figures prominently in the overall functioning of catecholaminergic systems (Figure 3–9).

Two isozymes of MAO, MAO-A and MAO-B, have been described, based mainly on pharmacological characteristics: clorgyline blocks MAO-A, and deprenyl and pargyline block MAO-B (Youdim et al., 1988). The ability to raise monoclonal antibodies against both subtypes implies that MAO-A and MAO-B have different protein structures (Westlund et al., 1985) and enables tissue localization of the subtypes. MAO-A predominates in neural tissue, whereas both subtypes exist in nonneuronal tissue (Youdim et al., 1988). Thus, inhibitors of MAO-A potentiate the pressor effects of tyramine (discussed below), whereas inhibitors of MAO-B do not (Youdim and Finberg, 1982).

NE and EPI are substrates for MAO-A, and DA is a substrate for both MAO-A and MAO-B. The deaminated products are short-lived aldehydes. For DA, the aldehyde

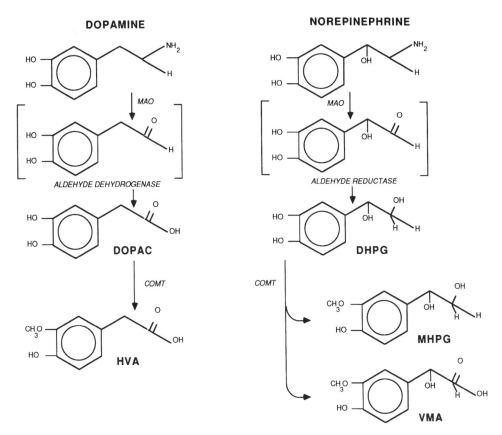

Figure 3-9. Metabolism of endogenous catecholamines. Monoamine oxidase (MAO) catalyzes the oxidative deamination of dopamine and norepinephrine. The aldehydes are converted to dihydroxyphenylacetic acid (DOPAC) and dihydroxyphenylglycol (DHPG). DOPAC and DHPG can enter the extracellular fluid unchanged or can be converted extraneuronally to homovanillic acid (HVA), methoxyhydroxyphenylglycol (MHPG), or vanillylmandelic acid (VMA).

intermediate is converted rapidly to DOPAC by aldehyde dehydrogenase; for NE, the aldehyde intermediate is converted mainly to DHPG by aldehyde reductase.

The formation of the aldehydes reduces a flavine component of the deaminating enzyme. The reduced enzyme reacts with molecular oxygen, regenerating the active form of the enzyme but also producing hydrogen peroxide (Fillenz, 1990), which may be toxic to cells because the peroxidation releases free radicals. MAO-B inhibitors delay neurological degeneration in patients with Parkinson's disease, possibly by limiting this type of oxidative injury (Olanow, 1992).

Since catechol-O-methyltransferase (COMT) in nonneuronal cells catalyzes the O-methylation of DHPG to form methoxyhydroxyphenylglycol (MHPG) and of DOPAC to form homovanillic acid (HVA), plasma levels of DHPG and DOPAC probably mainly reflect neuronal metabolism of NE and DA (Goldstein, Eisenhofer et al., 1988;

Graefe and Henseling, 1983; Halbrugge et al., 1989). The neuronal source of plasma DHPG levels has led to sophisticated techniques to examine aspects of sympathoneural activity by assessing the kinetics of endogenous and [^{3}H]-labeled NE and DHPG (Goldstein, Brush et al., 1988; Eisenhofer, Esler et al., 1992). The chapter about assessment of catecholaminergic function discusses these techniques.

MAO inhibitors are effective antidepressants. A phenomenon known as the "cheese effect" limits their clinical use. In patients taking MAO inhibitors, administration of sympathomimetic amines such as in many nonprescription decongestants, or ingestion of foods such as aged cheese, wine, or meat, which contain tyramine, can produce paroxysmal hypertension (Price and Smith, 1971). Since tyramine and other sympathomimetic amines displace NE from sympathetic vesicles into the axoplasm, blockade of MAO in this setting causes axoplasmic NE to accumulate, and outward transport of the NE, perhaps via the Uptake-1 carrier, stimulates cardiovascular smooth muscle cells, producing intense vasoconstriction and hypertension.

When given alone, MAO inhibitors usually decrease blood pressure and produce orthostatic hypotension. Indeed, until safer and more effective drugs superseded them, MAO inhibitors were used clinically as antihypertensives. To explain the hypotension, Kopin et al. (1964) suggested accumulation of a false neurotransmitter. Since MAO inhibition should increase cytoplasmic concentrations of amines, MAO inhibition may indirectly decrease TH activity; thus, chronic MAO inhibition decreases plasma DOPA levels in humans (Eisenhofer et al., 1986). Whether MAO inhibitors act in the brain to decrease SNS outflow remains unknown.

Brunner and colleagues recently described a point mutation in the structural gene for MAO-A in the p11-p21 region of the X chromosome in a family with X-linked borderline mental retardation and abnormal behaviors such as impulsive aggression. Whether and how MAO-A deficiency causes psychological abnormalities remain to be established. Genetic abnormalities in patients with the Norrie disease, another X-linked disorders characterized by blindness, deafness, and mental retardation, have been mapped to the same region but can involve decreased activities of both MAO-A and MAO-B (Murphy et al., 1991).

Extraneuronal Uptake (Uptake-2) and Metabolism

Nonneuronal cells remove NE actively by a process called Uptake-2 (Iversen, 1983), characterized by the ability to transport isoproterenol, susceptibility to blockade by O-methylated catecholamines, corticosteroids, and β-haloalkylamines, and absence of susceptibility to blockade by the Uptake-1 blockers cocaine and desipramine (Salt, 1972). In contrast with Uptake-1, Uptake-2 functions independently of extracellular Na$^+$. Other extraneuronal transport systems, such as a desipramine-sensitive carrier in pulmonary endothelium, do not have all these characteristics (Trendelenburg, 1988).

The Uptake-2 carrier has little if any stereoselectivity and, unlike Uptake-1, has low affinity and specificity for catecholamines. For instance, extraneuronal cells remove imidazolines such as clonidine by Uptake-2. The affinity of Uptake-2 for dobutamine averages about 100 times that of DA (Trendelenburg, 1988).

Whereas reverse transport via the Uptake-1 carrier requires special experimental conditions, reverse transport via the Uptake-2 carrier can be demonstrated readily, because the V_{max} for Uptake-1 is less than that for the neuronal metabolizing enzyme, MAO, whereas the V_{max} for Uptake-2 exceeds that of the extraneuronal metabolizing enzyme, COMT. Thus, during infusion of a catecholamine at a high rate, the catecholamine can accumulate in extraneuronal cells, with reentry of the catecholamine into the extracellular fluid via the Uptake-2 carrier after the infusion ends.

COMT catalyzes the conversion of NE to normetanephrine (NMN) and EPI to metanephrine (MN; Axelrod, 1966; Axelrod and Tomchick, 1958). Uptake-2 and COMT probably act in series to remove and degrade circulating catecholamines (Trendelenburg, 1988). The methyl group donor for the reaction is S-adenosylmethionine.

Immunohistochemical studies have indicated exclusively extraneuronal localization of COMT (Kaplan et al., 1979), which exists at high concentrations in the liver and kidneys (Graefe and Henseling, 1983). O-Methylation of NE therefore requires extraneuronal uptake. In the cardiovascular system, myocardial and vascular endothelial and smooth muscle cells probably constitute the main sites of O-methylation of catecholamines. Because of the extraneuronal localization of COMT, recently introduced assay methods for metanephrines have enabled refined assessments of extraneuronal metabolism of catecholamines (Lenders et al., 1993), as discussed in Chapter 5.

Vanillylmandelic acid (VMA) and MHPG, the products of the combined O-methylation and deamination of NE, are the two main end-products of NE metabolism, with VMA probably formed mainly in the liver.

Epinephrine and the Adrenomedullary System

EPI, the main adrenomedullary hormone in humans, affects the function of virtually all body organs. Adrenomedullary secretion of EPI figures prominently in neuroendocrine patterns attending distress, as discussed in Chapters 1 and 6.

In the adrenal medulla and certain brain nuclei, the cytosolic enzyme, PNMT, catalyzes the conversion of NE by N-methylation to form EPI (Axelrod, 1966; Kirshner, 1959; Figure 3–10).

Glucocorticoids, present at high local concentrations due to the corticomedullary direction of blood flow, regulate adrenal PNMT activity (Wurtman and Axelrod, 1966). Since genetically different strains of rats have different rates of expression of mRNA for PNMT and corresponding differences in adrenal EPI content (Evinger and Joh, 1989), an intrinsic genetic component probably also regulates adrenal EPI synthesis.

A variety of nonneuronal tissues possess N-methylating activity (Elayan et al., 1990; Kennedy et al., 1990, 1991; Ziegler et al., 1989). Whether these tissues synthesize and release endogenous EPI is unknown.

The Epinephrine Hypothesis

EPI can augment neurogenic vasoconstriction (e.g., Floras et al., 1988a; Tarizzo and Dahlof, 1989). Majewski, Rand, and co-workers (Majewski et al., 1981, 1982) proposed a model to explain this (Figure 3–11). According to the ''epinephrine hypothesis,'':

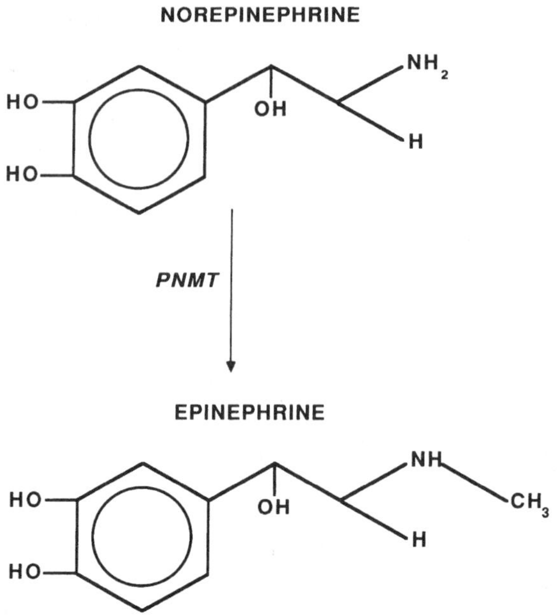

NOREPINEPHRINE

PNMT

EPINEPHRINE

Figure 3–10. Norepinephrine N-Methylation. Phenylethanolamine-*N*-methyltransferase (PNMT) is present in the cytoplasm of epinephrine-synthesizing cells. PNMT catalyzes the conversion of norepinephrine to epinephrine.

1. Sympathetic nerve terminals take up circulating EPI by Uptake-1.
2. Sympathetic stimulation coreleases the removed EPI with NE.
3. Coreleased EPI binds to β-adrenoceptors on sympathetic terminals.
4. Binding of coreleased EPI to β-adrenoceptors augments further NE release.

The EPI hypothesis helps to explain how excessive AHS activity can contribute to the development of essential hypertension by augmenting NE release in the SNS (Majewski et al., 1982; Rand and Majewski, 1984). More generally, the hypothesis provides a model where endogenous compounds taken up into neuronal terminals are coreleased with the transmitter and prolong or exaggerate release of the neurotransmitter by binding to facilitatory presynaptic receptors.

Results from many studies using isolated organs or tissues have supported one or more components of the EPI hypothesis. Sympathetic nerves do possess the capacity to take up exogenously administered, tracer-labeled EPI and to release the tracer-labeled EPI during subsequent sympathetic stimulation (Rosell et al., 1964). Injection of physiologically active amounts of EPI enhances neurogenic vasoconstrictor responses or release of NE during sympathetic stimulation in laboratory animals (Adler-Graschinsky and Langer, 1975; Majewski et al., 1982; Tarizzo and Dahlof, 1989) and in humans (Floras et al., 1988a; Vincent et al., 1982, 1986).

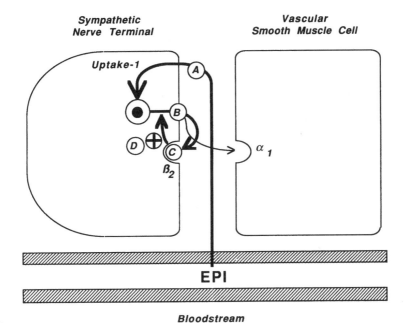

Figure 3–11. The epinephrine hypothesis. According to the epinephrine hypothesis, (A) sympathetic nerve terminals take up circulating epinephrine (EPI) by Uptake-1; (B) sympathetic stimulation co-releases the removed epinephrine with norepinephrine; (C) the coreleased epinephrine binds to β-adrenoceptors on sympathetic terminals; and (D) the binding of coreleased epinephrine to the β-adrenoceptors augments further norepinephrine release.

Studies designed to test the epinephrine hypothesis comprehensively in isolated tissue preparations have failed to confirm it (Abrahamsen and Nedergaard, 1989; Molderings et al., 1988a; Sadeghi and Eikenburg, 1992). In the study of Abrahamsen and Nedergaard, rabbit aortic rings were preincubated in NE or EPI before incubation in [³H]NE. The rings were then stimulated electrically, and the amount of tritium overflow into the medium was measured. β-Adrenoceptor blockade by addition of propranolol or metoprolol to the medium did not inhibit the stimulation-induced overflow of tritium; and neither preincubation with EPI nor withdrawal of EPI after the preincubation affected the stimulation-induced overflow of tritium. In the study of Molderings et al. (1988), venous strips were incubated with [³H]NE and then stimulated electrically. Exposure to EPI, isoproterenol, or β₂-adrenoceptor agonists augmented the stimulation-evoked release of tritium; however, preexposure of the strips to EPI failed to augment the stimulation-evoked release of tritium, with or without propranolol in the medium. When the venous strips were exposed to [³H]EPI, electrical stimulation after withdrawal of the EPI increased overflow of tritium into the medium in a tetrodotoxin-sensitive manner, indicating exocytotic release of the [³H]EPI; however, propranolol failed to inhibit this overflow. Sadeghi and Eikenburg (1992) reported that chronic EPI treatment failed to alter endogenous catecholamine release or prejunctional adrenoceptor modulation of sympathetic neurotransmission by phentolamine in the rat mesentery. Thus, although agonist occupation of β_2-adrenoceptors on sympathetic nerves can augment NE release, thereby potentially facilitating α-adrenoceptor-mediated vasoconstriction, two key elements of the EPI hypothesis—that coreleased EPI augments NE release and that coreleased EPI does so via occupation of the β_2-adrenoceptors—remain unproven.

Indirect evidence suggests that circulating EPI can enhance α-adrenoceptor-mediated vasoconstriction by a postsynaptic effect (Bolli et al., 1983; Vincent et al., 1986); by increasing skeletal muscle sympathetic outflow (Persson et al., 1989); or by augmenting production of AII in vascular smooth muscle cells, with subsequent direct postsynaptic effects of AII and presynaptic facilitation of NE release mediated by AII receptors on the nerve terminals (Molderings et al., 1988b). The finding that β-adrenoceptor blockade can attenuate NE release during sympathetic stimulation without concurrently altering blood pressure or heart rate responses (Draper et al., 1986) provides indirect support for a facilitatory postsynaptic effect.

Dopamine and the Renal DOPA–dopamine System

Until recently, investigators viewed DA as only an intermediary in the biosynthesis of NE in sympathetic nerves and of EPI in adrenomedullary cells (Blaschko, 1939). Research since the 1960s, however, has firmly established DA as a neurotransmitter in the brain. Much more recent evidence has in addition supported a physiological role for DA as an autocrine/paracrine hormone that influences Na^+ disposition in the periphery.

In the 1960s, Goldberg and coworkers described the potent cardiovascular and renal effects of DA (Horwitz et al., 1962; McDonald et al., 1964). Goldberg also introduced the idea of specific vascular receptors for DA (Yeh et al., 1969). In contrast with NE and EPI, injected DA increases renal blood flow and evokes a natriuresis and diuresis, while stimulating the heart. The discovery of this combination of effects led rapidly to the widespread clinical use of DA to treat heart failure and cardiogenic shock.

Despite the potent pharmacological effects of exogenously administered DA, and the presence of specific, functional DA receptors on vascular smooth muscle cells, sympathetic nerve terminals, and renal proximal convoluted tubular cells, the sources and physiological meaning of endogenous DA remain incompletely understood. Histofluorescent studies in the 1970s indicated DA-containing neuronal elements in the kidney (Bell and Land, 1973; Dinerstein et al., 1979); however, because of the relatively slow conversion of DA to NE *in vivo* (e.g., Hovevey-Sion et al., 1989), the results did not exclude detection of DA in noradrenergic nerves. In animals treated with GBR 12909, which blocks catecholamine uptake into dopaminergic terminals, chemical sympathectomy with 6-OHDA does not prevent stimulus-evoked release of DA into the renal venous plasma (Bell and Sunn, 1990).

These histofluorescent and neurochemical findings suggest the presence of renal dopaminergic nerves but do not prove that renal DA production or function depends on this innervation. Renal slices *in vitro* have the capacity to synthesize DA from DOPA in the incubation medium (Soares-da-Silva and Fernandes, 1992), and bilateral renal denervation does not decrease urinary DA excretion (Baines, 1982; Grossman, Hoffman et al., 1990).

In contrast with inconclusive evidence for the existence of renal dopaminergic nerves, substantial evidence has accrued for DA synthesis in renal proximal convoluted tubular cells after uptake of DOPA from the perfusate or incubation medium (Baines and Chan, 1980; Baines et al., 1985; Carey et al., 1990; Hagege et al., 1985; Soares-da-Silva and Fernandes, 1992). *In vivo* studies have agreed that most or all of DA in urine derives from renal uptake and decarboxylation of DOPA (Baines, 1982; Brown and Dollery, 1981; Grossman, Hoffman et al., 1990; Suzuki et al., 1984; Zimlichman et al., 1988; Figure 3–12). A recent study using L-DOPA infusions has confirmed the derivation of virtually all of urinary DA from plasma DOPA in humans (Wolfovitz et al., 1993).

These findings do not exclude the possibility that sparse but critically located dopaminergic nerves release physiologically active DA in the kidney, with urinary DA reflecting a larger but physiologically irrelevant amount of DA. Positive correlations between excretion rates of both DOPA and DA with sodium excretion (Goldstein, Grossman et al., 1993), however, suggest that urinary DA does relate to at least one physiologically important role of DA in the kidneys: enhancement of natriuresis.

Dopaminergic activation in the periphery enhances natriuresis and diuresis by at least four mechanisms. DA acting at DA_1 receptors on vascular smooth muscle cells increases renal blood flow, augmenting glomerular filtration of sodium. DA acting at DA_2 receptors on sympathetic nerve terminals inhibits NE release, increasing renal blood flow indirectly by interfering with sympathetically mediated vasoconstriction. DA in the kidney acts as an autocrine/paracrine hormone at DA_1 receptors on proximal convoluted tubular cells, inhibiting Na/K ATPase and promoting entry of sodium into the tubular lumen, as discussed below. Finally, DA can act in the adrenal cortex, probably at DA_2 receptors, to inhibit aldosterone secretion at baseline or in response to AII (Carey et al., 1980; Lokhandwala and Hegde, 1990; Missale et al., 1988; Porter, Whitehouse et al., 1992). The relative contributions of these mechanisms to DA-induced natriuresis are unknown.

Dietary salt loading increases urinary DA excretion in animals (Grossman, Hoffman et al., 1990, 1992) and humans (Alexander et al., 1974; Gill et al., 1991; Goldstein, Stull et al., 1989). Consistent with sodium-induced compensatory activation of a renal dopaminergic natriuretic system, administration of the DDC inhibitor carbidopa impairs natriuresis acutely, with the magnitude of impairment correlated with the magnitude of decrease in DA excretion (Ball and Lee, 1977; Sowers et al., 1984; Williams et al., 1986; Yoshimura et al. 1987).

Dietary salt loading also increases urinary excretion of DOPA in animals (Grossman, Hoffman et al., 1990) and in humans (Gill et al., 1991; Goldstein, Stull et al., 1989). The increases in DOPA excretion precede the increases in urinary DA excretion, suggesting that during salt loading, increased renal uptake of DOPA produces the increased DA excretion. In rats, increased spillover of DOPA into arterial plasma can explain the DA excretory response during salt loading (Grossman, Hoffman et al., 1990). Salt loading also increases the efficiency of DOPA uptake by proximal tubular cells (Baines, 1990; Soares-da-Silva and Fernandes, 1992). In humans, dietary salt loading may

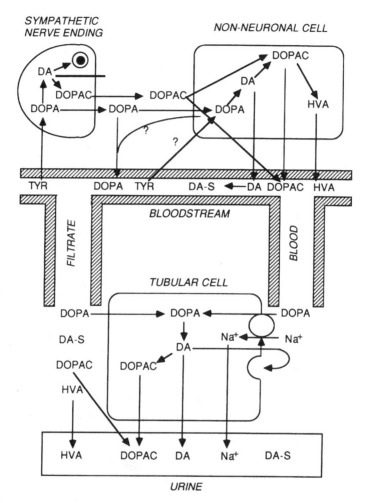

Figure 3–12. Overview of the renal DOPA–dopamine system. According to this model, some of the DOPA synthesized during norepinephrine synthesis in sympathetic nerves exits the nerve terminal and either enters the bloodstream or is taken up by nonneuronal cells. It is possible that DOPA can be formed extraneuronally from tyrosine or phenylalanine. After nonneuronal uptake, DOPA is O-methylated to form O-methylDOPA (not shown) or decarboxylated to dopamine (DA), which can then exit the cell to exert autocrine/paracrine effects (not shown), can be metabolized to dihydroxyphenylacetic acid (DOPAC) and homovanillic acid (HVA), or can enter the bloodstream, where it is rapidly conjugated to form (in humans) DA-sulfate (DA-S). There are two sources of plasma DOPAC in this model: DOPAC formed from oxidative deamination of DA in sympathetic nerves, and DOPAC formed from deamination of DA in nonneuronal cells. In the proximal tubular cells of the kidney, DOPA is taken up from the glomerular filtrate and from the plasma and is decarboxylated to form DA. The renal DA can be excreted unchanged, can be metabolized to DOPAC, or can exit the cell to exert autocrine actions by binding to membrane dopamine receptors. DA receptor occupation inhibits Na/K-ATPase on the abluminal membrane surface, increasing sodium-dependent entry of DOPA from the plasma while decreasing sodium-dependent DOPA uptake from the filtrate. According to the model, urinary DOPAC is derived from both renal dopamine metabolism and filtration of plasma DOPAC;

increase the efficiency of proximal tubular cell uptake of DOPA from the abluminal interstitial fluid or plasma, but probably not from the glomerular filtrate, since this would decrease DOPA excretion (Wolfovitz et al., 1993).

The monitored variables responsible for increased DA excretion during salt loading have not been identified conclusively. Urinary DA excretion increases in response to blood volume expansion with saline but not with 25% albumin (Faucheux et al., 1977), suggesting that the filtered load of Na^+ or Cl^-, rather than increased cardiac filling, is the main factor eliciting augmented DA excretion. In contrast, Cuche et al. (1972) reported that in healthy humans, urinary DA excretion fell while NE excretion increased during orthostasis-induced decreases in cardiac filling. During head-out water immersion in humans, the increases in cardiac filling produce a complex pattern of changes in DA and DOPA excretion (Grossman, Goldstein et al., 1992). Whether blood volume expansion or acute saline administration affects DOPA excretion is unknown.

The dependence of renal DA production on renal uptake of circulating DOPA leads to another issue: sources of circulating DOPA. The chapter about clinical assessment of catecholaminergic function deals with this topic.

Analogous to findings in the kidney, adrenocortical DA appears to derive from DOPA removed from the circulation and decarboxylated in noncatecholaminergic cells (Buu and Lussier, 1990). Stimulation of DA_2 receptors in the adrenal cortex decreases basal aldosterone secretion in the perfused adrenal gland (Porter et al., 1992), attenuates aldosterone responses to AII (Missale et al., 1988), and suppresses aldosterone secretion evoked by sodium depletion in hypertensive patients (Missale et al., 1989). DA also inhibits aldosterone biosynthesis in vitro (Fraser et al., 1989). Whether alterations in dietary salt intake affect adrenocortical uptake and decarboxylation of DOPA is unknown.

If DA acts as an autocrine/paracrine hormone in the kidney and adrenal cortex, then DA may act analogously in other nonneuronal cells. In addition to the classical SNS-noradrenergic and AHS-adrenergic systems, with cellular uptake and metabolism terminating the actions of the neurotransmitter and hormone, there may be a third peripheral catecholaminergic system—an autocrine/paracrine dopaminergic system—with intravascular conjugation preventing systemic effects of the locally formed catecholamine and limiting effector actions to the site of synthesis. Thus, intracardiac and intrapulmonary ganglia in several species possess chromaffin cells (Jacobowitz, 1967; Jacobowitz et al., 1973); substantial amounts of DOPA enter the bloodstream in the human lung (Goldstein, Cannon et al., 1991); myocardial tissue from heart transplant recipients

---

urinary HVA, DA-S, and O-methylDOPA (not shown) are derived mainly from glomerular filtration of plasma HVA, DA-S, and O-methylDOPA. The model considers DA release from sympathetic nerves to be negligibly small. Since circulating DA is extensively conjugated, urinary DA is derived mainly from renal uptake of circulating DOPA. The model does not include the contributions of renal noradrenergic and possibly dopaminergic nerves to proximal tubular cell uptake and metabolism of DOPA and DA, nor the possible occupation of dopamine receptors by neuronally released DA.

has surprisingly high concentrations of DA (Regitz et al., 1990); and DA in the circulation undergoes rapid and extensive conjugation (Ratge et al., 1991).

A paradox of catecholamine neurochemistry is that plasma levels and urinary excretion of metabolites of DA actually exceed those of metabolites of NE. Because of the efficient conversion of DA to NE in sympathetic nerves, and because of the minor contribution of the brain to the circulating and urinary metabolites, neither DA release from noradrenergic terminals nor DA release in the brain accounts satisfactorily for the high rate of DA metabolism in the body. This also leads to the hypothesis that a substantial amount of DA synthesis in the body as a whole occurs in nonneuronal cells.

Nonneuronal cells should not store newly synthesized DA, which would exit the cells by reverse transport via the above-described Uptake-2 carrier or undergo metabolic conversion to DOPAC or HVA. This can explain the high plasma levels and urinary excretion rates of DOPAC (Eisenhofer et al., 1986; Goldstein, Grossman et al., 1993; Kagedal and Goldstein, 1988) and HVA (Hovevey-Sion, Kopin et al., 1989; Kopin, 1985) in laboratory animals and humans. DA production in nonneural cells would also help to explain the very high concentrations of conjugated DA in human and rat plasma (Cuche et al., 1990; Kuchel et al., 1978, 1979). In humans, over 95% of the DA in plasma circulates in sulfoconjugated form. Others have proposed that concentrations of conjugated catecholamines provide markers of long-term sympathetic activity (Kuchel et al., 1984). The foregoing leads to a different hypothesis: Conjugation may have evolved as a means to prevent the buildup of catecholamine concentrations—especially DA concentrations—in the circulation after their release from nonneuronal cells. Catecholamine sulfate levels may therefore reflect not "integrated" sympathoadrenal activity but the synthesis of catecholamines in an independent system.

Is the Sympathoneural System Vital?

Largely as a result of Cannon's persuasive observations, the view has persisted that despite the importance of the SNS in maintaining homeostasis during emergency situations, the maintenance of normal cardiovascular performance under resting conditions does not require a functioning SNS. Thus, within the sheltered confines of a laboratory, animals that have undergone extensive surgical sympathectomies seem entirely normal (Cannon, 1939a; Cannon, Newton et al., 1929).

Cannon did not consider the possibility that loss of the SNS would lead to compensatory recruitment of the AHS, or that destruction of both systems would compensatorily activate other circulatory effector systems. In particular, he did not examine the effects of sympathectomy in adrenalectomized or adrenal-demedullated animals. His son, Bradford Cannon, observed relatively small chronic decreases in blood pressure in dogs that had undergone extensive sympathectomies in three stages, including section of the neural supply of the adrenal glands (Cannon, 1931); however, these procedures would not eliminate hormonal stimulation of adrenomedullary secretion, such as by AII (Zimlichman, Goldstein, Zimlichman et al., 1987), or compensatory activation of the AVP system and RAS, which would mask the effects of the sympathectomy on blood pressure, as discussed below.

The combination of 6-OHDA and adrenal demedullation is so often lethal that few reports about this treatment have appeared. In our experience, administration of 6-OHDA to adrenal-demedullated rats results in hypotension, shock, and death within 24 hours in a large proportion of animals. In the study of Micalizzi and Pals (1979), ganglion blockade in adrenal-demedullated rats and chemical sympathectomy in intact rats decreased blood pressure by about 30% in resting, conscious animals.

Whereas intact, anesthetized dogs undergoing clamping of the adrenal hilar vessels for 10 minutes show no change in blood pressure, chemically sympathectomized dogs undergoing the same clamping, which eliminates adrenomedullary secretion, evince rapid decreases in blood pressure to about 30% of normal (Gauthier et al., 1972) which, if not rapidly reversed, would be expected to produce shock and death. De Champlain and Van Ameringen (1972) reported analogous results in rats. These findings imply a compensatory interaction between the SNS and AHS in tonic regulation of blood pressure.

Adrenalectomized rats (Darlington et al., 1989; Kvetnansky et al., 1993) and hypophysectomized rats (Goldstein, Garty et al., 1993) have much higher basal plasma levels of NE than do sham-operated rats; after hemorrhage, arterial blood pressure recovers normally in adrenalectomized rats, owing to markedly exaggerated responses of NE and renin activity. Mineralocorticoid-replaced, glucocorticoid-pretreated adrenalectomized monkeys have profound increases in plasma NE levels during surgical stress (cholecystectomy) four months later (Udelsman et al., 1987a).

Administration of an AII antagonist or angiotensin-converting enzyme (ACE) inhibitor to sympathectomized animals also produces hypotension. Julien et al. (1990) found that whereas administration of the ACE inhibitor perindopril produced little effect on blood pressure in intact, conscious rats, administration of the drug to rats with guanethidine-induced destruction of peripheral sympathetic fibers produced immediate, marked hypotension. Lo et al. (1991a, 1991b) reported that in genetically hypertensive rats of the Lyon strain that had undergone guanethidine-induced chemical sympathectomy, RAS blockade produced substantial decreases in blood pressure that were about threefold larger than those produced by bilateral adrenalectomy. AVP antagonism augmented the hypotensive response to RAS blockade. These findings led to the conclusion that after sympathectomy, the RAS maintains blood pressure in rats. Chemical sympathectomy produces large increases in plasma AVP levels, and inhibition of AVP effects in chemically sympathectomized animals produces profound, persistent hypotension (Hatzinikolaou et al., 1982).

After recovery from cervical spinal transection, conscious dogs have normal blood pressures, despite low plasma levels of catecholamines. Administration of the ACE inhibitor captopril or (in water-deprived animals) of an AVP antagonist produces hypotension in the sympathectomized animals (Mikami et al., 1983), consistent with the above findings in rats.

The SNS therefore plays a key role not only in circulatory responses during emergency reactions but also in maintaining tonic levels of cardiovascular performance. Sympathetic ablation compensatorily activates other vasoactive systems, including the AHS, RAS, and AVP system, masking the role of the SNS.

Cardiovascular Adrenoceptors

Specific receptors, called adrenoceptors, in the membranes of effector cells such as vascular and cardiac smooth muscle cells, determine the physiological and metabolic effects of catecholamines.

All adrenoceptors identified so far share several structural characteristics (Figure 3–13): an amino-terminal, glycosylated polypeptide chain from the cell membrane extending into the extracellular fluid; 7 polypeptide membrane-spanning domains, each domain consisting of about 20–28 hydrophobic amino acids in an α-helical arrangement, with highly conserved sequences; and a long carboxy-terminal polypeptide chain extending from the internal surface of the cell membrane into the cytoplasm (Raymond et al., 1990).

The structures of adrenoceptors differ markedly from those of the transmembrane carriers responsible for neuronal and vesicular uptake of catecholamines and resemble those of other receptors that use G-proteins, discussed below in the section about intracellular mechanisms.

The membrane-spanning domains determine the ligand binding characteristics of the receptor. The cytoplasmic domains, comprising three loops and the tail ending in the carboxy terminus, regulate the specific coupling with G-proteins and phosphorylating enzymes in the cascade of intracellular events leading to cellular activation or inhibition. The carboxy terminal tail, which contains a serine- and threonine-rich domain, is a site of phosphorylation by protein kinases such as protein kinase C, β-adrenergic receptor kinase (βARK), and cAMP-dependent protein kinase. The extracellular amino terminus is glycosylated. The roles of the N-linked sugars and the three extracellular loops of the receptors are unknown.

Type and Subtypes

NE and EPI differ importantly in their effects on smooth muscle and the heart. Ahlquist (1948) first suggested, based on orders of potency of amines, that differences in the effects of NE and EPI result from different actions at two types of receptor: α and β. Ahlquist defined the α effect by the potency order EPI > NE > isoproterenol and the β effect by the potency order isoproterenol > EPI >> NE. Thus, EPI stimulates both types of receptor, whereas NE stimulates α-adrenoceptors preferentially. The discovery of selective inhibitors of these receptors confirmed the distinction.

In general, β-adrenoceptors mediate the positive inotropic and chronotropic effects of catecholamines in the heart; stimulation of vascular α-adrenoceptors produces vasoconstriction; and stimulation of vascular β-adrenoceptors—especially in skeletal muscle—produces vasodilation.

Nonspecific α-blockers include phenoxybenzamine and phentolamine; nonspecific β-blockers include propranolol and timolol; nonspecific α-agonists include NE; and nonspecific β-agonists include isoproterenol. As noted above, EPI stimulates both α- and β-adrenoceptors. The antihypertensive drug labetalol blocks α- and β-adrenoceptors nonspecifically.

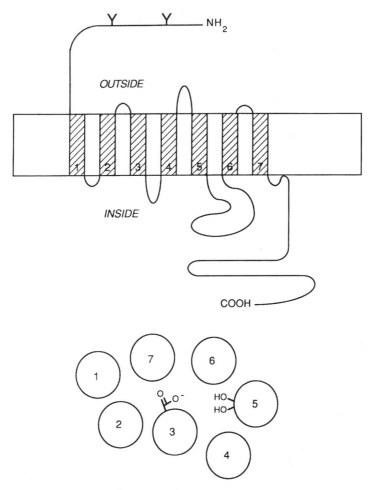

Figure 3–13. Diagram of an adrenoceptor. All adrenoceptors share the same general structure. This is a diagram of the human β_2-adrenoceptor. The receptor has seven hydrophobic and so presumably membrane-spanning domains. The amino terminus is extracellular, and the extracellular tail has glycosylation sites (Y). The long intracellular chain ends in the carboxy terminus. The bottom figure views the β_2-adrenoceptor from above. According to the model of Strader et al. (1989), the carboxyl group of Asp at position 113 on the third transmembrane loop would attract the nitrogen moiety of the catecholamine, and the hydroxyl groups of Ser and positions 204 and 207 of the fifth transmembrane loop would attract the hydroxyl groups of the catechol nucleus.

β-Adrenoceptor Subtypes

Lands et al. (1967), also on the basis of pharmacological evidence, classified β-adrenoceptors into β_1 and β_2 subtypes. Responses of different tissues to β-agonists fell into two categories, with EPI and NE having about equal potency at β-receptors in the heart and adipose tissue (β_1-adrenoceptors) and with EPI having about 20 times greater potency than NE at β-receptors in vascular and bronchial smooth muscle (β_2-adreno-ceptors).

The discovery of selective inhibitors of these receptor subtypes confirmed the pharmacological distinction. Radioligand binding studies demonstrating the simultaneous existence of both β-receptor subtypes in the heart and other tissues led to abandonment of the notion that different tissues contain exclusively β_1- or β_2-adrenoceptors (Minneman et al., 1979).

Molecular cloning techniques have described the primary amino acid sequences of β-adrenoceptor subtypes (e.g., Frielle et al., 1987). β_1-Adrenoceptors consist of about 475–485 amino acids and β_2-adrenoceptors about 410–420 amino acids, β_1-adrenoceptors having about 54% homology with β_2-adrenoceptors.

Dobutamine has relative selectivity for β_1-adrenoceptors and is used as a cardiotonic agent. β_1-Selective antagonists, including atenolol and metoprolol, are used to treat angina pectoris, hypertension, and some arrhythmias. β_2-Selective agonists, including terbutaline, salbutamol, albuterol, and metaproterenol, are used to treat asthma. β_2-Selective antagonists have no established clinical use.

Agonist occupation of the recently identified β_3-adrenoceptor (Emorine et al., 1989) as of all β-adrenoceptors, stimulates adenyl cyclase. The β_3-adrenoceptor seems to participate in lipolytic effects of catecholamines.

α-Adrenoceptor Subtypes

Pharmacologic evidence also provided the first indication that α-adrenoceptors that inhibit release of NE from sympathetically innervated tissues differ from those that produce vasoconstriction and positive inotropic effects on the heart. The former "presynaptic" α-adrenoceptors were subclassified as α_2-adrenoceptors and the latter "postsynaptic" α-adrenoceptors subclassified as α_1-adrenoceptors (Starke, 1972; Wikberg et al., 1975; Wikberg and Lefkowitz, 1984; Wikberg et al., 1975). Evidence that structures other than nerve terminals can possess α_2-adrenoceptors forced modification of this spatial distinction, and subsequent nomenclature based on function replaced that based on location (Berthelson and Pettinger, 1977; Wikberg, 1978), with the α_2-adrenoceptors inhibitory and the α_1-adrenoceptors stimulatory. The functional distinction soon also had to be abandoned, because prazosin, an α_1-adrenoceptor antagonist, and yohimbine, an α_2-adrenoceptor antagonist, both were found to inhibit noradrenergic vasoconstriction (Drew and Whiting, 1979).

The classification of α-adrenoceptor subtypes subsequently came to be based on pharmacological properties, radioligand binding, and finally receptor structures using molecular biologic techniques. The current view is that α_2-adrenoceptors in the periphery are located pre- and extrasynaptically (Langer et al., 1980; Wilffert et al., 1982) and can exert either stimulatory or inhibitory effects, depending on the cell type on which they are located. Thus, occupation of α_2-adrenoceptors on vascular smooth muscle cells elicits muscular contraction, whereas occupation of α_2-adrenoceptors on sympathetic nerve terminals inhibits exocytotic release of NE. Stimulation of either α_1-receptors or α_2-receptors on vascular smooth muscle cells elicits vasoconstriction (Bolli et al., 1983). There is no convincing evidence for presynaptic α_1-adrenoceptors.

α_1-Selective agonists include phenylephrine and methoxamine and α_1-selective antagonists prazosin and terazosin. α_2-Selective agonists include clonidine, guanfacine, guanabenz, and α-methylNE; α_2-selective antagonists include yohimbine, rauwolscine, and idazoxan.

Based on differential affinities for ligands such as prazosin, oxymetazoline, idazoxan, and yohimbine, Bylund et al. (1988) proposed a subclassification of α_2-adrenoceptors into A and B subtypes, α_{2A} and α_{2B}. α_{2A}-Adrenoceptors have low affinity for prazosin and high affinity for oxymetazoline and yohimbine, whereas α_{2B}-adrenoceptors have high affinity for prazosin and low affinity for oxymetazoline and yohimbine. The α_{2A}-adrenoceptor appears to be the sole subtype of α_2-adrenoceptor on human platelets and corresponds to the cloned human α_{2-C10} receptor, named based on its location on chromosome 10 (Kobilka et al., 1987). α_{2B}-Adrenoceptors occur in rat brain and kidney. Evidence from cloning studies has indicated that the brain and kidney α_{2B}-adrenoceptors differ structurally (Flordellis et al., 1991). The cloned human α_{2-C4} receptor, located on chromosome 4 and expressed in the human kidney, may correspond to the α_{2B}-adrenoceptor defined pharmacologically; however, this identification is not yet settled, since the same gene may encode another form of adrenoceptor, α_{2C}, in the opposum kidney (Nichols and Ruffolo, 1991).

Responses to the 3-benzazepine α_2-adrenoceptor antagonist, SKF 104078, can distinguish pre- and postsynaptic α_2-adrenoceptors (Hieble et al., 1988; Ruffolo et al., 1987). This drug blocks postjunctional vascular α-adrenoceptors nonspecifically but does not block presynaptic α_2-adrenoceptors. The putative prejunctional α_2-adrenoceptor does not appear to fit the above A–B classification scheme (Raymond et al., 1990) and may represent a distinct fourth subtype: α_{2D}. Whether the presynaptic α_2-adrenoceptors are structurally unique is unknown, since as of this writing, the receptor has not been cloned.

Imidazolines such as clonidine bind with high affinity not only to α_2-adrenoceptors but also to nonadrenergic, imidazoline binding sites, as discussed in Chapter 4. The adrenal medulla, which possesses relatively few α_2-adrenoceptors, binds imidazolines, and administration of the putative ligand at imidazoline receptors, clonidine binding substance, stimulates release of catecholamines from cultured chromaffin cells (Regunathan et al., 1991).

Evidence provided by Michel et al. (1989, 1990) has complicated the matter further: [^{3}H]Idazoxan, a highly specific ligand at α_2-adrenoceptors, also binds to nonadrenergic receptors in renal cortical membranes. These receptors appear to differ from receptors for the clonidine displacing substance (Ernsberger et al., 1986; Meeley et al., 1986) by not binding clonidine.

Cardiac, Coronary, and Vascular Adrenoceptors

In the intact organism, β-adrenoceptors mediate most of the cardiac effects of catecholamines (Table 3–2). The density of β-adrenoceptors in the heart generally varies inversely with the density of sympathetic innervation, the highest density in the left ventricular apex and the lowest in the atria (Will-Shahab and Schubert, 1991). Whereas

Table 3–2. Responses of Cardiovascular Organs to Catecholamines

Organ	Receptors	Responses
Heart		
SA Node	β_1	Tachycardia
Atria	β_1	Increased contractility and conduction velocity
A-V node	β_1	Increased automaticity and conduction velocity
His–Purkinje	β_1	Increased automaticity and conduction velocity
Ventricles	β_1	Increased contractility, automaticity, conduction velocity, and idioventricular rate
Arterioles		
Coronary	$\alpha_1, \alpha_2; \beta_2$	Constriction (slight); dilation
Skin	α_1, α_2	Constriction
Skeletal muscle	$\alpha_1, \alpha_2; \beta_2$	Constriction; dilation
Cerebral	α_1	Constriction (slight)
Pulmonary	$\alpha_1; \beta_2$	Constriction (slight); dilation (slight)
Abdominal viscera	$\alpha_1; \beta_2$	Constriction; dilation (slight)
Salivary	α_1, α_2	Constriction
Renal	$\alpha_1, \alpha_2; \beta_1, \beta_2$	Constriction; dilation (slight)
Systemic veins	$\alpha_1; \beta_2$	Constriction; dilation

in other species, the total number of cardiac β_1-adrenoceptors exceeds by far that of β_2-adrenoceptors, human myocardium has similar concentrations of the two subtypes. Thus, in humans, EPI probably is not the main endogenous catecholamine acting at cardiac adrenoceptors, because (1) interstitial fluid NE concentrations probably far exceed those of EPI, (2) NE is an agonist at β_1-adrenoceptors, (3) and the heart contains β-adrenoceptors of both subtypes. The β_2-adrenoceptor subtype appears to predominate in vascular smooth muscle cells and on vascular sympathetic nerve terminals. Most cardiac α-adrenoceptors are of the α_1 subtype.

Cardiac effects of β-adrenoceptor stimulation include increased sinus node rate, accelerated AV nodal conduction, decreased refractoriness of the AV node and His–Purkinje system, shortening of the Purkinje fiber action potential, increased His–Purkinje automaticity, and—especially important clinically—increased dispersion of ventricular refractory periods. Stimulation of cardiac β-adrenoceptors of both subtypes increases cardiac contractility, rate, and electrical automaticity. Cardiac β_1-adrenoceptors and α_1-adrenoceptors appear to mediate positive inotropic effects of catecholamines, whereas β_1- and β_2-adrenoceptors appear to mediate chronotropic effects (Minneman et al., 1981), consistent with the predominance of β-adrenoceptors of both subtypes in the atria and α_1- and β_1-adrenoceptors in the ventricles (Hedberg et al., 1980).

Interactions among responses to changes in myocardial metabolism, direct vascular effects, reflexive changes in sympathetic outflow, concurrent release of other neurotransmitters and vasoactive factors, and central effects of adrenoceptor agonists and antagonists all complicate the neural regulation of coronary flow. NE produces only minor net changes in coronary vascular resistance. This results at least partly from a balance between α-adrenoceptor-mediated vasoconstriction and β-adrenoceptor-mediated vasodilation, since β-blockade by propranolol unmasks NE-induced increases in coronary resistance (Beamish and Dhalla, 1985). Since coronary blood flow varies with myocardial metabolism, administration of a β-adrenoceptor agonist that increases myocardial oxygen consumption can decrease coronary vascular resistance without acting directly on coronary adrenoceptors. Analogously, during stimulation of cardiac sympathetic nerves, pronounced increases in myocardial metabolism increase coronary blood flow, masking possible vasoconstrictor effects of NE released from the nerve terminals. Sympathetic stimulation in the setting of β-adrenoceptor blockade, to prevent increased myocardial metabolism, does decrease coronary blood flow, probably because of the above-described unopposed stimulation of α-adrenoceptors of both subtypes (Kopia et al., 1986; Mohrman and Feigl, 1978). During reflexive stimulation of sympathetic outflow by carotid sinus hypotension, β-adrenoceptor blockade unmasks noradrenergic coronary vasoconstriction (Feigl, 1968). Nitric oxide (endothelium-derived relaxing factor) also opposes neurogenic vasoconstriction (Furchgott, 1983; Jones et al., 1993; Urabe et al., 1991), and patients with impaired endothelial function have augmented sympathetically mediated coronary vasoconstriction (Zeiher et al., 1989).

Although presynaptic α_2-adrenoceptors inhibit cardiac release of NE during electrical cardiac sympathetic stimulation (Yamaguchi et al., 1977), the role of α_2-adrenoceptors on cardiac sympathetic nerve terminals in more physiological conditions is poorly understood. In humans, intravenous administration of yohimbine increases skeletal sympathoneural outflow (Grossman, Rea et al., 1991) and blood pressure (Goldberg et al., 1983), decreases baroreflex–cardiac sensitivity (Goldberg et al., 1983), blocks α_2-adrenoceptors on forearm vascular sympathetic nerve terminals (Grossman, Chang et al., 1991a), and increases cardiac NE spillover (Eisenhofer et al., 1992) but produces little or no change in coronary vascular resistance (Vatner et al., 1980). Postsynaptic α_2-adrenoceptor blockade, reflexive sympathoinhibitory effects of increases in systemic pressures, and coronary vasodilator responses to increased myocardial metabolism probably balance the NE-mediated vasoconstrictor effect in this setting.

In skeletal muscle, β_2-, α_1-, and α_2-adrenoceptors contribute to the regulation of regional vascular resistance. Administration of EPI, an agonist at all these receptors, decreases skeletal muscle vascular resistance because of the prominent stimulation of extrasynaptic β_2-adrenoceptors (Wilffert et al., 1982). Neural control of large resistance vessels appears to depend mainly on α_1-adrenoceptors on vascular smooth muscle cells, whereas control of small terminal arterioles appears to depend on α_2-adrenoceptors (Ohyanagi et al., 1991).

Circulatory responses to adrenoceptor agonists or antagonists depend on underlying sympathoneural activity. Thus, depressor responses to clonidine and pressor responses to yohimbine vary as a function of baseline plasma NE levels in patients with hypertension (Goldstein, Grossman, Listwak et al., 1991; Goldstein, Levinson et al., 1985; Grossman et al., 1993), and ganglion blockade attenuates pressor responses to yohimbine (Goldstein, Zimlichman et al., 1986b).

Intracellular Mechanisms

Membrane receptors transmit information via signal-transducing G-proteins (guanine-nucleotide regulatory proteins), located near the receptor on the inner portion of the cell membrane. Details of the intracellular cascade upon activation of G-proteins have been extensively studied for β-adrenoceptors. Gs, the G-protein responsible for cellular activation after occupation of β-adrenoceptors, was isolated by Northrup et al. in 1980.

The G-protein complex consists of an α subunit, responsible for the specificity of the G-protein, and β and γ subunits, the functions of which are largely unknown (Figure 3–14). The heterotrimeric G-proteins constitute a "superfamily," with as many as 15 different α subunits, 2 different β subunits, and 2 different γ subunits (Brown, 1990). Thus, a large variety of receptors appear to work by way of stimulatory or inhibitory G-proteins.

The α subunit of the β-adrenoceptor is designated α_s. Adjacent to the G-protein complex is adenyl cyclase, which spans the cell membrane. Under resting conditions, guanosine diphosphate (GDP) binds to the G-protein. Binding of the agonist to the receptor results in a receptor–ligand complex. In the presence of guanosine triphosphate (GTP), receptor occupation results in substitution of GTP for GDP at the binding site of the G-protein. This activates the G-protein. The activated α_s subunit separates from the β and γ subunits. The activated α_s subunit stimulates adenyl cyclase, which catalyzes the synthesis of cAMP from ATP (Murad et al., 1962). As long as GTP is bound

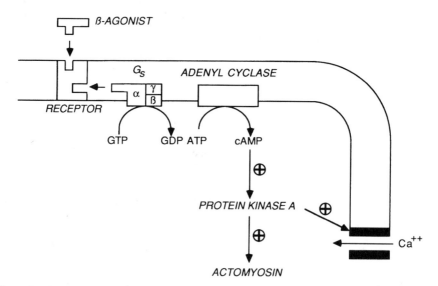

Figure 3–14. Intracellular mechanisms of β-adrenoceptor-mediated smooth muscle cell activation. Occupation of the receptor by an agonist leads to G-protein-coupled activation of adenyl cyclase, increasing generation of cyclic AMP (cAMP) and activating protein kinase A (PKA). PKA phosphorylates calcium channels, and the increased intracellular ionized calcium concentration leads to cellular activation.

to the α_s subunit, cAMP can be generated. The process ceases when the GTP bound to the α_s subunit is converted to GDP, inactivating both the G-protein and the cyclase.

Cyclic adenosine monophosphase, cAMP, an intracellular "second messenger" (the first messenger being the hormone binding to the receptor), stimulates cAMP-dependent protein kinase (CAPK, protein kinase, or PKA), a tetramer including two regulatory and two catalytic subunits. Binding of cAMP to the regulatory subunits of PKA releases them, leading to phosphorylation of many proteins, evoking changes in cellular activity such as contraction or secretion. For instance, cAMP-dependent phosphorylation of phospholamban, located on the sarcoplasmic reticulum, increases both the contractile force and rate of relaxation of the cell, by increasing the flux of Ca^{2+} from the sarcoplasmic reticulum into the cytoplasm and increasing the sensitivity of the contractile apparatus to Ca^{2+}. cAMP-dependent phosphorylation of a component of the membrane calcium channel increases the transmembrane influx of Ca^{2+} into the cell (Trautwein et al., 1987).

PKA also catalyzes phosphorylation of the receptor, desensitizing β-adrenoceptor-mediated processes. The phosphorylation appears to change the conformation of the α_s subunit, interfering with the function of the G-protein. Other mediators of desensitization include β-adrenergic receptor kinase (βARK, Benovic et al., 1986), β-arrestin—an intracellular protein—and protein kinase C (PKC).

Whereas activation of β_2-adrenoceptors on myocardial smooth muscle cells stimulates cellular contraction, activation of β_2-adrenoceptors on vascular smooth muscle cells causes vascular relaxation. The exact basis for this difference has never been identified.

In the heart, at least three mechanisms can explain coronary vasodilation during β-adrenoceptor stimulation (Beamish and Dhalla, 1985). First, neuronally released or circulating catecholamines bind to cardiac β-adrenoceptors, activating adenyl cyclase and increasing cytoplasmic concentrations of Ca^{2+} in coronary vascular smooth muscles cells and in the myocardium. The stimulation of myocardial contraction increases release of metabolic products such as potassium and lactate, which produces local vasodilation. Second, increases in generation of cytoplasmic cAMP in vascular smooth muscle cells may augment sequestration of Ca^{2+} into the sarcoplasmic reticulum or increase the rate of efflux of Ca^{2+} across the cell membrane. Third, activation of PKA in coronary smooth muscle cells may directly inactivate contractile proteins by phosphorylation.

Agonist occupation of α_1-adrenoceptors leads to a different cascade of intracellular events from that consequent to agonist occupation of β-adrenoceptors (Figure 3–15). The α_1-adrenoceptor is linked to a different G-protein, G_p. Occupation of the receptor by the agonist leads to activation of the G-protein by GTP hydrolysis. This stimulates phospholipase C, which catalyzes the hydrolysis of phosphatidylinositol 4,5-diphosphate (PIP_2) to form two active subunits, inositol triphosphate (IP_3; Berridge and Irvine, 1984; Fain and Garcia-Sainz, 1980; Steinberg et al., 1989) and diacylglycerol (DG). There are several different phospholipase C molecules, and it is unclear to which G-proteins they are linked. DG stimulates PKC, leading to cellular activation by as yet unknown mechanisms. IP_3 binds to another receptor on the endoplasmic reticulum,

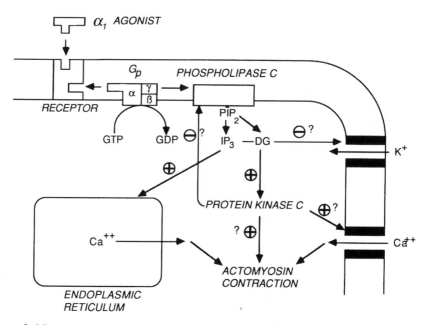

Figure 3–15. Intracellular mechanisms of α_1-adrenoceptor-mediated smooth muscle cell activation. Occupation of the receptor by an agonist leads to G-protein-coupled activation of phospholipase C, which cleaves phosphatidylinositol-4,5-diphosphate (PIP$_2$) to yield two active subunits—inositol triphosphate (IP$_3$) and diacylglycerol (DG). DG activates protein kinase C (PKC), and IP$_3$ binds to a receptor on the endoplasmic reticulum to increase release of ionized calcium into the cytoplasm, leading to cellular activation. The exact mechanism by which α_1-adrenoceptor activation increases entry of calcium into the cell is unknown.

releasing Ca^{2+} from the stores into the cytoplasm (Godfraind, 1976), also activating the cell. IP$_3$ or DG may also activate the cell by inhibiting transient, voltage-activated K$^+$ channels (Fedida et al., 1989).

Agonist occupation of α_2-adrenoceptors inhibits adenyl cyclase by interaction with an inhibitory G-protein, G$_i$ (Lefkowitz et al., 1990). This decreases intracellular formation of cAMP and thereby decreases activity of PKA. Exactly how activated G$_i$ inhibits adenyl cyclase is unclear, and it is possible that G$_i$ works indirectly by interfering with G$_s$-induced activation of the cyclase. The mechanism for vasoconstriction induced by stimulation of α_2-adrenoceptors has also not been established definitively. One possibility is that decreased cAMP concentration attenuates sequestration of cytoplasmic Ca^{2+}.

G-proteins appear to couple receptors to ion channels not only via cytoplasmic second messengers but also by direct pathways (Brown, 1990). G$_i$ proteins mediate activation of K$^+$ transmembrane conductances and inhibit voltage-sensitive channels (Limbird, 1988). Opening of K$^+$ channels via agonist occupation of α_2-adrenoceptors on sympathetic nerve endings may provide a basis for inhibitory modulation of NE release (Zimanyi et al., 1988).

Linkage of individual receptor subtypes to different G-proteins (Raymond et al., 1990) potentially adds another layer of complexity to this already complex subject.

Dopamine Receptors

As of this writing, five structurally distinct DA receptor subtypes have been identified in brain; the existence, localization, and function of DA receptor subtypes in the periphery are less well understood. In the periphery, two DA receptor subtypes have been distinguished pharmacologically: Fenoldapam stimulates and SCH 23390 blocks DA_1-receptors, and N,N-dipropyl-DA stimulates and domperidone blocks DA_2-receptors (Brodde, 1990). These correspond roughly to brain D_1 and D_2 receptors identified by molecular cloning. Renal, mesenteric, coronary, and cerebral arteries possess DA_1-receptors, with DA_1-receptor stimulation producing vasodilation directly. DA_2-receptors located in ganglia and on sympathetic nerve endings exert inhibitory modulation of NE release, producing vasodilation indirectly.

DA receptors occur at high concentrations in the kidneys. Renal DA_1-receptors are localized to the media of microvessels, the cortical collecting ducts, and, perhaps most importantly, the proximal convoluted tubules; whereas DA_2-receptors are thought to be localized to sympathetic nerve terminals in the adventitia and media of renal blood vessels and in the glomeruli.

The expression of mRNA for DA receptor subtypes correlates poorly with the density of the receptors themselves, possibly because of regional differences in turnover of the receptors. Little or no mRNA for the DA_1-receptor was detected in the kidney (Dearry et al., 1990) until Yamaguchi et al. (1993) demonstrated expression of mRNA encoding the DA_{1A}-receptor in proximal tubular cells.

Locally produced DA acts as an autocrine/paracrine substance by a mechanism that includes occupation of DA_1-receptors on the membrane of proximal tubular cells. Agonist occupation of DA_1-receptors inhibits Na/K-ATPase activity (Seri et al., 1988) by cAMP-dependent phosphorylation of an inhibitory protein, the "DA- and cAMP-regulated phosphoprotein of Mr 32,000," or DARPP-32 (Aperia et al., 1991), which is generally expressed only in cells with DA_1-receptors. Activated DARPP-32 inhibits protein phosphatase-1, in turn interfering with activation of the Na/K-ATPase complex. Inhibition of the ATPase allows Na^+ to enter the cell, and the increased cytoplasmic Na^+ concentration augments net Na^+ release into the tubular lumen. Thus, renal administration of Sch 23390, a DA_1-receptor antagonist, produces dose-dependent anti-natriuresis in conscious, uninephrectomized dogs (Siragy et al., 1989), although the ATPase inhibition appears to require simultaneous activation of DA_1- and DA_2-receptors (Bertorello and Aperia, 1990). In contrast with DA and with ANP, NE and AII stimulate renal Na/K ATPase, probably via activation of calcium-calmodulin-dependent protein phosphatase 2B. Several natriuretic and anti-natriuretic factors therefore probably interact complexly in modulating activity of renal Na/K-ATPase and regulating sodium excretion.

The renal DA system mechanism represents a potentially important type of physiological regulator, where an autocrine/paracrine substance formed intracellularly from a circulating precursor affects transmembrane movement of an ion. Since the receptors probably cycle between the membrane surface and the cytoplasm, alterations in the synthesis rate of DA may also influence the numbers of receptors available in the membrane, but this has not been studied directly.

Sensitization

Cannon (1939b) probably was the first to describe in detail the enhancement of responses to catecholamines after section of the sympathetic nerve supply. In his report, he cited the older and preliminary but essentially correct observation of Claude Bernard: "The excitability of all tissues seems to augment when they are separated from the nervous influence which dominates them" (Bernard, cited in Cannon, 1939, p. 748).

Most research about the basis for denervation supersensitivity has focused on changes in the numbers of available adrenoceptors, with relatively little attention to intracellular mechanisms. In general, β-adrenoceptor numbers are thought to be low in spontaneously hypertensive rats, hypothyroidism, diabetes, and heart failure and increased in Dahl salt-sensitive rats, hyperthyroidism, aortic constriction, subpressor NE infusion, and ischemia (Limas and Limas, 1991). α_1-Adrenoceptor numbers are thought to be increased in ischemia and decreased in diabetes and hyperthyroidism, with inconsistent data in spontaneously hypertensive rats, Dahl salt-sensitive rats, and heart failure (Limas and Limas, 1991).

Hormones such as thyroid hormone (Williams et al., 1977) and glucocorticoids (Collins et al., 1988) increase the rate of β-adrenoceptor synthesis; ischemia accelerates the transport of the receptors from the cytoplasm to the membrane (Limas and Limas, 1991); and chronic administration of β-blockers up-regulates membrane β-adrenoceptor numbers (Glaubinger and Lefkowitz, 1977).

Several inconsistencies complicate the literature about mechanisms of sensitization in vivo, especially during cardiovascular manipulations. For instance, studies have disagreed about whether the numbers of adrenoceptors on effector cells increase after blockade of exocytotic release of NE. Conscious dogs with chronically denervated hearts have augmented cardiac inotropic responses to injected NE, without changes in the inotropic response to isoproterenol (Vatner et al., 1985). Since the heart removes NE extensively by Uptake-1, whereas isoproterenol is not a substrate for the transporter, loss of neuronal uptake due to cardiac denervation could explain the supersensitivity to NE. One can demonstrate denervation supersensitivity to isoproterenol, however, after ganglion blockade to abolish opposing reflex effects, suggesting both pre- and postsynaptic mechanisms of denervation supersensitivity. Regional denervation supersensitivity can occur independently of increases in either the number of β-adrenoceptors or the density or affinity of $G_{s\alpha}$ (Warner et al., 1993), consistent with an as yet unidentified intracellular mechanism.

Lymphocyte β_2-adrenoceptor numbers correlate weakly positively with plasma EPI levels, and bicycle exercise produces similar proportionate increases in EPI levels and lymphocyte β_2-adrenoceptor numbers (Graafsma et al., 1990). Since EPI is the main endogenous agonist at β_2-adrenoceptors, the results suggest that acute stimulation of adrenomedullary outflow may increase, rather than down-regulate, β_2-adrenoceptors—which could initiate a positive feedback loop. Similarly, Graafsma et al. (1989) found that during performance of mental arithmetic, groups of hypertensive and normotensive subjects had increases in the density of β_2-adrenoceptors on lymphocytes.

Blockade of ganglionic neurotransmission augments pressor responses to NE and decreases the dose of phenylephrine, an α_1-adrenoceptor agonist, required to maintain mean arterial pressure (Goldstein et al., unpublished observations; Page and McCubbin, 1963). Although these findings are consistent with α_1-adrenoceptor up-regulation after blockade of exocytotic NE release (Davies et al., 1982), interference with baroreflex buffering of blood pressure can also explain them. During acute ischemia, the number of myocardial α_1-adrenoceptors, as assessed by [^{3}H]prazosin binding, increases, and increased α_1-adrenoceptor-mediated responsiveness may contribute to the pathophysiologic changes attending ischemia and reperfusion (Corr et al., 1981), as discussed in the chapter about cardiovascular diseases. Patients with multiple system atrophy and sympathetic denervation have been reported to have markedly increased platelet concentrations of α-adrenoceptors, based on [^{3}H]dihydroergocryptine binding (Davies et al., 1982).

The terms "up-regulation" and "down-regulation" have been used to describe changes in both the numbers of membrane-bound receptors, as quantified from ligand-binding studies, and changes in total numbers of receptors in the cells. This issue is discussed below in the section about desensitization.

Desensitization

One can readily demonstrate desensitization of β-adrenoceptor-mediated responses (e.g., cAMP generation in response to application of a β-adrenoceptor agonist) in in vitro preparations and in in vivo clinical applications, and a large body of research has concentrated on mechanisms of this phenomenon. Relatively few studies have concentrated on desensitization of responses mediated by α-adrenoceptors.

Patients with heart failure, a condition associated with markedly increased cardiac spillover of NE (Hasking et al., 1986), have low numbers of β-adrenoceptors on lymphocytes and in myocardial biopsy tissue (Bristow et al., 1982). β_1-Adrenoceptor numbers seem decreased selectively in this setting (Bristow et al., 1986).

Literature about α-adrenoceptor desensitization has been inconsistent. Desensitization of α_1-adrenoceptor-mediated responses is thought to be analogous to desensitization of β-adrenoceptor-mediated responses, with the receptor uncoupled from the G-protein due to phosphorylation of the receptor by PKA or PKC (Leeb-Lundberg et al., 1987). Whether α_2-adrenoceptor numbers or affinities are subject to up- and down-regulation has been especially unclear. Pfeifer et al. (1984) reported that variations in circulating catecholamine concentrations failed to affect the number or affinity of platelet α_2-adrenoceptors in humans. Hollister et al. (1986) reported that orthostasis, associated with about a doubling of plasma NE levels, decreased the number of high-affinity and decreased the affinity of platelet α_2-adrenoceptors in normotensives. Supiano et al. (1989) found that ingestion of a low-sodium diet, associated with increased plasma NE levels, decreased the number of platelet α_2-adrenoceptors. Motulsky et al. (1986) reported no changes in either the number of α_2-adrenoceptors or the coupling of the receptors to adenyl cyclase in desensitized platelets.

Homologous and Heterologous Desensitization

Homologous desensitization refers to a situation where production of an intracellular second messenger, such as cAMP, decreases in response to stimulation of specific receptors but not in response to stimulation of other receptors using the same second messenger. Homologous desensitization therefore is agonist-specific. Heterologous desensitization entails attenuated responses to all agonists using the same second messenger. Heterologous desensitization is therefore agonist-nonspecific (Sibley and Lefkowitz, 1985).

Several mechanisms of homologous desensitization have been proposed, and whereas evidence for each has been obtained in in vitro systems, the roles of these mechanisms in in vivo are incompletely understood. One mechanism is internalization, where the number of receptor binding sites in the cell membrane decreases and the number in the cytosol increases. Indirect evidence consistent with internalization has been reported in cultured cell lines derived from mammalian astrocytoma tissue (Harden et al., 1980).

A second form of homologous desensitization is by uncoupling, where the receptor dissociates from its G-protein. Uncoupling is an integral part of the normal cascade of events after occupation of receptors that use G-proteins, because after the protein binds GTP, not only is the formation of second messenger enhanced, but also the G-protein–GTP complex decreases the affinity of the receptor for the agonist. Phosphorylation of the receptor can produce this form of desensitization by uncoupling. Benovic et al. (1986) identified a kinase, β-adrenergic receptor kinase (βARK), that phosphorylates the agonist-occupied form of the β-receptor, decreasing the affinity of the receptor for the agonist. Homologous desensitization by βARK is thought to occur only when the receptor is occupied, and the phosphorylation may depend on another endogenous compound, β-arrestin.

Fillenz (1990) has suggested that desensizitation of β-adrenoceptor-mediated responses occurs in three sequential steps: (1) rapid uncoupling of the receptor from the G_s-protein, a process associated with decreased affinity for β-agonists; (2) internalization of the receptor, with reversible loss of receptors at the membrane; and (3) down-regulation, a slowly reversible loss of the total number of functional receptors in the cell. The phenomenon of down-regulation differs from internalization or sequestration in that the numbers of binding sites in both the "light peak" and the membrane fractions of sucrose density gradients decrease. Incubation with GTP or cellular depolarization can reverse down-regulation; in some situations, synthesis of new receptors seems required in order to reverse down-regulation.

Heterologous desensitization has been demonstrated in vitro in astrocytoma cells. Prolonged exposure of the cells to prostaglandins, which stimulate adenyl cyclase, decreases formation of cAMP during subsequent exposure to β-adrenoceptor agonists (Johnson et al., 1978). Whereas frog erythrocytes exhibit homologous desensitization upon prolonged exposure to β-adrenoceptor agonists, turkey erythrocytes exhibit heterologous desensitization, in that the desensitized cells have decreased responsiveness to both isoproterenol and guanine nucleotides, and the turkey erythrocytes do not have internalization of the β-adrenoceptors.

Clinically relevant research about sensitization and desensitization has so far been limited mainly to adaptive responses to exogenously administered pharmacologic agents such as pressor amines, antidepressants, and β-adrenoceptor blockers. Mechanisms of desensitization resulting from chronically repeated episodes of sympathetically mediated NE release, and mechanisms of denervation supersensitivity, originally described by Bernard and Cannon, remain obscure.

Physiological Effects of Catecholamines

Much more is known about the physiological effects of endogenous EPI than of endogenous NE. This is because EPI acts mainly as a hormone in the body and has a single main source—the adrenal medulla—whereas NE acts mainly as a neurotransmitter in the body (Silverberg et al., 1978), and plasma NE derives from myriad sympathetic nerve endings, organs, and glands. Even less is known about neuroendocrine effects of endogenous DA. For DA to exert hormonal effects, plasma DA levels must exceed by far those attained during exposure even to severe stressors (Levinson et al., 1985). The likelihood of endogenous DA acting locally as an autocrine/paracrine substance complicates the study of physiological effects of endogenous DA.

Increases in release of NE and EPI affect the functions of virtually all body systems. Stress-induced, sympathetically mediated cardiovascular adjustments are part of coordinated response patterns involving many effector systems, as discussed in Chapters 2 and 6.

Cardiovascular

Catecholamines affect cardiovascular function by at least three general mechanisms: (1) actions at cardiovascular adrenoceptors, eliciting changes in cardiac and vascular function directly; (2) actions in the nervous system, influencing SNS and AHS outflows and activities of several other stress systems of the body; (3) and actions in the kidney, affecting renal handling of sodium and thereby blood volume and pressure.

All adrenoceptor types participate directly or indirectly in catecholaminergic regulation of vascular smooth muscle. Stimulation of post- or extrasynaptic α-adrenoceptors of both subtypes enhances vascular constriction; β$_2$-adrenoceptor stimulation causes vascular relaxation, especially in skeletal muscle; β$_1$-adrenoceptor stimulation in the kidney increases renin release; presynaptic α$_2$-adrenoceptors exert inhibitory modulation of NE release during sympathetic stimulation; DA$_1$ receptor stimulation elicits vasodilation and natriuresis; and DA$_2$ stimulation inhibits NE release from sympathetic nerves.

Several other types of receptors probably participate in sympathetic–cardiovascular mechanisms, either because the agonists are released from sympathetic nerves or from nonneuronal cells during sympathetic stimulation or because the agonists modulate sympathetic neurotransmission. A section of Chapter 2 considers interactions among stress effector systems in detail; the following mentions these interactions only cursorily. Muscarinic cholinergic receptors mediate active sympathetic vasodilation in skeletal muscle and inhibit cardiac NE release (Folkow and Uvnas, 1948; Levy and Blattberg, 1976); and cholinergic stimulation in the central nervous system increases adrenomedullary secretion (Janowksy et al., 1985; Kennedy et al., 1984). NPY, coreleased with NE during electrical sympathetic stimulation (Warner et al., 1991) and to a lesser extent during manipulations of endogenous catecholaminergic outflow (Tidgren et al., 1991), is a potent vasoconstrictor and when given exogenously inhibits NE release from sympathetic nerve endings. ATP, also coreleased with NE, probably is responsible for rapid postsynaptic cellular electrical activation (Burnstock, 1976, 1990), and adenosine, produced from catabolism of ATP, is a vasodilator that may also modulate NE release from noradrenergic terminals and act postsynaptically to inhibit α-adrenoceptor-mediated vasoconstriction (Smits et al., 1991). Renal sympathoneural stimulation and circulating EPI both stimulate generation of renin, resulting in increases in circulating levels of AII, and AII, in addition to being a powerful vasoconstrictor, may affect SNS outflow by actions in the brain (Cox and Bishop, 1991; Dorward and Rudd, 1991; Harland et al., 1988), augment NE release during sympathetic stimulation (Hughes and Roth, 1971; Szabo et al., 1990; Zimmerman, 1978), or stimulate adrenomedullary secretion (Zimlichman, Goldstein, Zimlichman et al., 1987), via occupation of AII receptors. Enkephalins are coreleased with catecholamines during sympathetic stimulation, and endogenous opioids may affect central autonomic outflow (Morita et al., 1988; Weinstock et al., 1984) or modulate NE release by interactions between opioid receptors and α_2-adrenoceptors (Al-Damluji, Bouloux et al., 1990; Farsang and Kunos, 1979; Szabo et al., 1986).

Circulatory effects of EPI include increased cardiac output, which enhances delivery of oxygen and glucose throughout the body; redistribution of blood volume to the cardiopulmonary area, which preserves perfusion of the heart and brain; and increased skeletal muscle vasodilation and cutaneous, renal, and splanchnic vasoconstriction, which support increased skeletal metabolism during "fight or flight" behaviors. EPI induces relatively small changes in pulmonary, cerebral, and coronary vascular resistance, due to complex interactions between adrenoceptor-mediated actions and effects of alterations in myocardial metabolism, as discussed above.

Systemic injection of NE produces virtually universal vasoconstriction. The increased blood pressure stimulates arterial baroreceptors, and heart rate tends to decrease reflexively. Thus, although in suitable preparations stimulation of α-adrenoceptors increases cardiac contractility, in intact individuals baroreflexes usually mask the cardiac effects of injected α-adrenoceptor agonists.

Cardiac responses to circulating EPI resemble those produced by cardiac sympathetic stimulation: tachycardia related to increased sinoatrial node automaticity, increased cardiac contractility, accelerated atrioventricular conduction, decreased refractory periods, and decreased thresholds for ventricular arrhythmias. The similarity between the hormonal effects of EPI and the neuronal effects of sympathetic stimulation led to Elliot's seminal hypothesis about neurochemical transmission, as discussed above.

Infusion of DA at a low dose (about 5 μ/kg/min) increases cardiac output by a mechanism thought to be mediated by β-adrenoceptors; infusion at higher rates is thought to increase blood pressure by stimulating α-adrenoceptors. DA administration at a low dose increases renal blood flow by interacting with vascular DA_1 receptors (Goldberg and Rajfer, 1985).

Renal

Sympathoneural stimulation augments renal sodium retention, by several mechanisms. Renal vasoconstriction decreases local perfusion and thereby decreases the glomerular filtration of sodium. Stimulation of renal $β_1$-adrenoceptors increases secretion of renin (Weber et al., 1983), increasing production of AII, which both acts as a potent vasoconstrictor and also augments adrenocortical secretion of aldosterone, the latter inducing Na–K exchange in the kidneys and causing further retention of sodium. Finally, NE can exert an antinatriuretic effect by direct actions at renal tubular cells (Osborn et al., 1983).

In contrast with the antinatriuretic actions of NE, DA is a natriuretic catecholamine, evoking natriuresis by increasing renal blood flow, binding to specific receptors on proximal convoluted tubular cells and sympathetic nerve terminals, and inhibiting aldosterone secretion at baseline or in response to AII (Aperia et al., 1991; Baines et al., 1992; Missale et al., 1988; Porter et al., 1992).

Gastrointestinal

Catecholamines generally inhibit gut motility and suspend digestive processes. The usually concurrent splanchnic vasoconstriction shunts blood to the heart, lungs, brain, and skeletal muscle.

Cannon showed that the adrenal effluent and EPI itself relax intestinal muscle (Cannon, 1929a). Indeed, relaxation of intestinal muscle by EPI in bioassays provided the basis for the first demonstration that emotional stress increases adrenal release of EPI (Cannon and de la Paz, 1911). Both α- and β-adrenoceptors mediate the gastrointestinal inhibition, the former located on neurons of the myenteric plexus and the latter ($β_2$ subtype) on smooth muscle cells. Gastroinestinal sphincters possess $α_1$-adrenoceptors.

Gastric mucosal cells possess noradrenergic innervation, and β-adrenoceptor agonists increase gastrin release (Hayes et al., 1972).

Chemical sympathectomy with 6-OHDA and depletion of NE stores with reserpine induce diarrhea.

Dopamine is present at relatively high concentrations in the gastrointestinal tract (Dawirs et al., 1992; Juorio and Chedrese, 1990), where locally produced (Vieira-Coelho and Soares-da-Silva, 1993) or concentrated DA appears to play an autocrine/paracrine role in stimulating duodenal bicarbonate secretion (Flemstrom et al., 1993; Knutson et al., 1993). These findings have led to testing of dopaminergic drugs to prevent gastrointestinal ulceration and to the view that a dopaminergic ''brain-gut axis'' contributes to gastrointestinal mucosal integrity during stress (Glavin, 1991, 1992).

Cutaneous

Pallor, cyanosis, sweating, shivering, and piloerection caused by sympathoneural stimulation constitute major signs of emotional distress and shock. Administration of both NE and EPI produces cutaneous vasoconstriction, due to stimulation of α_1- and α_2-adrenoceptors on vascular smooth muscle cells.

Sympathetic noradrenergic stimulation of apocrine glands induces axillary sweating, whereas combined sympathetic noradrenergic and sympathetic cholinergic stimulation of eccrine glands induces thermoregulatory sweating. In contrast with skeletal sympathoneural activity, which is especially responsive to alterations in baroreflex activity, cutaneous sympathoneural activity is responsive to emotional stressors and to alterations in environmental temperature (Delius et al., 1972a, 1972b).

Facial sweating and flushing associated with body heating or embarrassment depend importantly on active postganglionic sympathetic innervation, since patients with unilateral Horner's syndrome have impaired ipsilateral thermoregulatory sweating and flushing. In contrast, strong gustatory stimulation (such as ingesting peppers) elicits symmetrical sweating and flushing in most patients with Horner's syndrome (Drummond and Lance, 1987). The finding of impaired ipsilateral thermoregulatory flushing in Horner's syndrome patients implies that sympathetic vasodilator fibers accompany sudomotor and vasocontrictor fibers to the face. The identity of the neurotransmitter substance mediating active cutaneous sympathetically-mediated vasodilation is unknown.

Metabolic

Glucose

Administration of EPI increases blood glucose concentrations (Bodo and Benaglia, 1938) by stimulating hepatic gluconeogenesis and glycogenolysis, increasing secretion of glucagon, and inhibiting insulin secretion by the pancreas. α-Adrenoceptors mediate the inhibition of insulin release (Porte, 1969; Porte et al., 1973). Hepatic parenchymal cells possess sympathetic innervation, suggesting that both hormonal EPI and neuronal NE may contribute to glycogenolysis (Himms-Hagen, 1967).

Glucose counterregulation depends importantly on the AHS (e.g., Cryer et al., 1992), as discussed in the chapter about stress response patterns.

Glucose administration increases plasma NE levels even in adrenal-demedullated animals (Levin and Sullivan, 1987), suggesting that glucose stimulates sympathoneural outflows. Since intra-carotid glucose administration increases plasma NE levels (Levin, 1991), the stimulatory effect appears to depend on effects of high circulating glucose levels in the brain.

Lipids

EPI increases plasma levels of free fatty acids, explaining the increases in free fatty acid levels associated with emotional distress (Taggart and Carruthers, 1971). Theoretically, excess free fatty acids can be transformed to triglycerides in the liver (Pauletto et al., 1991), and increases in triglyceride levels follow emotion-associated increases in free fatty acid levels.

EPI administration increases plasma cholesterol levels subacutely in monkeys (Dimsdale et al., 1983) and rats (Kunihara and Oshima, 1983). The mechanisms of this effect are incompletely understood.

In humans, catecholamine levels are unrelated to levels of low-density lipoprotein (LDL) or high-density lipoprotein (HDL) cholesterol (Lundberg et al., 1989). During a three-month preexamination period in medical students, serum total and LDL cholesterol concentrations increased (O'Donnell et al., 1987); however, the increases were unrelated to changes in NE or EPI concentrations. Acute emotional distress does not affect plasma levels of total cholesterol (Taggart and Carruthers, 1971) or LDL or HDL cholesterol (Goldstein, Dionne et al., 1982).

Activation or inhibition of adrenoceptors alters complexly the synthesis and degradation of HDL (Sacks and Dzau, 1986). Extrahepatic lipoprotein lipase activity is blood flow-dependent (Bravo, 1989), so that adrenoceptor-mediated vasoconstriction decreases lipase activity and therefore the formation of HDL cholesterol. Administration of β-adrenoceptor agonists generally stimulates lecithin-cholesterol acyltransferase (LCAT) and extrahepatic lipoprotein lipase, tending to increase HDL levels (Sacks and Dzau, 1986); however, Schauer and Schauer (1989) found that EPI and NE inhibited human LCAT activity in vitro, and patients with pheochromocytoma, which is usually associated with high plasma catecholamine levels, have decreased LCAT activity (Berent et al., 1987).

Thermogenesis

Cannon et al. (1927) noted the importance of adrenomedullary secretion in the chemical control of body temperature. Catecholamine-induced thermogenesis probably results from the lipolytic effect of β-adrenoceptor agonism.

Since physiological increments in plasma EPI levels increase metabolic rate (Himms-Hagen, 1967; Staten et al., 1987), endogenous EPI may participate in maintenance of body weight. Patients with bulemia have decreased sympathetic activity, as indicated by plasma NE levels (George et al., 1990). These patients seem to require less caloric intake than normal to maintain a stable body weight, and the bulemic syndrome could provide a behavioral means to compensate for this tendency. Rates of directly recorded skeletal muscle sympathetic nerve activity correlate positively with energy expenditure in Caucasians but not in Pima Indians, suggesting that a lack of impact of sympathoneural activity on metabolic rate may contribute to obesity in the latter group (Spraul et al., 1994).

Potassium

EPI decreases the serum potassium concentration, by a mechanism dependent on β_2-adrenoceptors (Brown et al., 1983; Jonkers et al, 1987; Struthers et al, 1983). The effect occurs independently of insulin, aldosterone, and renal function (Bravo, 1989). At doses that increase plasma EPI levels by 15- to 30-fold, serum potassium decreases by about

0.5 meq/L (Brown et al., 1983). Whether the hypokalemia results indirectly from EPI-induced hyperventilation and respiratory alkalosis has not been tested.

Calcium

A balance between the actions of parathyroid hormone and calcitonin determines serum calcium concentrations. NE administration increases levels of both hormones, by β-adrenoceptor-mediated stimulation of adenyl cyclase (Chernow and O'Brien, 1984).

Thyroid

Complex interactions among thyroid hormones and the SNS and AHS systems probably determine basal metabolic rate. Hyperthyroidism is generally associated with decreased plasma NE concentrations and hypothyroidism with increased NE concentrations. Hyperthyroidism often presents clinically with signs of cardiovascular sympathetic stimulation, including tachycardia, systolic hypertension, and arrhythmias, perhaps because thyroid hormone increases the numbers of myocardial β-adrenoceptors, as discussed above (Williams et al., 1977).

Blood Components

Platelets

Cannon showed that EPI release during stress responses promotes hemostasis, not only by vasoconstriction but also by accelerated blood clotting (Cannon, 1939a). These effects would have afforded an adaptive advantage in evolution, by minimizing hemorrhage after trauma.

EPI and NE both cause platelet aggregation (EPI is more potent). The concentration of EPI required to produce platelet aggregation directly in vitro is about 10^{-6} M (Gerrard and Peterson, 1985), much higher than the endogenous concentration of about 10^{-10} M in humans under resting conditions. The combination of EPI in vitro with other agents that activate platelets (e.g., thrombin, collagen, adenosine diphosphate, vasopressin) markedly decreases EPI concentrations required to induce platelet aggregation—to about $2-5 \times 10^{-8}$ M (Grant and Scrutton, 1980; Larsson et al., 1990; Mills and Roberts, 1967; Thomas, 1967). EPI administered intravenously to healthy humans at a dose producing a plasma concentration of about 3×10^{-9} M increases platelet aggregability, as indicated by filtragometry readings, whereas at a dose producing a concentration of about 1×10^{-9} M, platelet aggregability remains unchanged (Larsson et al., 1990). Thus, all other things being the same, the plasma EPI concentration must increase by 10- to 30-fold to increase platelet aggregability in vivo in humans. This would occur only during severe adrenomedullary stimulation.

The mechanism of EPI-induced platelet aggregation is thought to be via stimulation of α_2-adrenoceptors, with subsequent transmembrane entry of Ca^{2+} and increased cytosolic Ca^{2+} concentrations. During maximal stress—such as decapitation in rats—the concentration of EPI in arterial blood is in the range of 10^{-7} M, the concentration in adrenal venous blood. Studies about platelet activation in rats rarely have considered the effects of the method of obtaining blood on the experimental results. Decapitation to obtain blood may increase EPI concentrations sufficiently to activate the platelets, increasing intracellular Ca^{2+}.

Hypercholesterolemia augments platelet aggregatory responses to EPI by up to 35-fold (Carvalho et al., 1974; Shattil et al., 1975). Thus, during stress responses involving activation of several neuroendocrine systems simultaneously, relatively small increases in circulating EPI levels may enhance platelet aggregability. During emotional stress in humans, platelet aggregability increases (Haft and Arkel, 1976). Even performance of the color–word conflict test, a laboratory mental challenge, can increase platelet aggregability in healthy humans (Larsson et al., 1990). Whether increased circulating EPI levels actually contribute to the increased platelet aggregability during emotional stress is unknown.

Other Hematologic Parameters

Exogenously administered catecholamines induce a lymphocytosis (Steel et al, 1971), a phenomenon opposite to that produced by exogenously administered corticosteroids. Epinephrine injection changes the relative proportions of lymphocyte subsets in peripheral blood, approximately doubling the percentage of natural killer cells at 30 minutes post-injection (Crary et al., 1983). In humans during acute mental stress, circulating levels of natural killer cells increase, and propranolol treatment to block β-adrenoceptors abolishes these increases (Benschop et al., 1994), consistent with a stimulatory role of endogenous catecholamines in mediating the response of natural killer cells in this setting.

In laboratory animals, sympathetic stimulation contracts the spleen. Splenic contraction expands circulating blood volume and therefore aids in countering effects of traumatic hemorrhage.

EPI-induced vasoconstriction slows the microcirculation in injured regions. This fosters the adhesion of leukocytes to the vascular endothelium (''pavementing''); leukocytes migrate through small blood vessel walls within a few minutes of injury (Cameron, 1967).

Neurobehavioral

Three general mechanisms mediate actions of catecholamines in the nervous system: central neural catecholaminergic pathways; afferent inputs as part of circulatory, metabolic, and behavioral homeostatic systems; and actions of circulating catecholamines in the pituitary gland, hypothalamus, and circumventricular organs. Because of the effective blood–brain barrier for catecholamines (Weil-Malherbe et al., 1959, 1961), circulating catecholamines do not reach most adrenoceptors in the central nervous system.

Many behavioral effects of EPI have been described, including anxiety, increased alertness, trembling, and an energizing effect, with decreased muscular and psychological fatigue. EPI increases the intensity of mental concentration and enhances performance of perceptual-motor tasks, despite EPI-induced tremor. EPI enhances emotional experiences (Schachter and Singer, 1962), as discussed in more detail in the chapter about stress response patterns.

Anti-Fatigue Effect of Adrenaline

Cannon described the anti-fatigue effect of EPI in preparations of skeletal and cardiac muscle.

> Campos, Lundin, Walker, and I have found that when a dog has been extremely fatigued by running a treadmill, the subcutaneous injection of a small amount of dilute adrenin has a striking influence in prolonging the animal's capacity to continue to work. (Cannon, 1929a, p. 129)

The mechanism of the antifatigue effect of EPI is poorly understood, and modern research seems to have ignored the phenomenon. One possibility is that EPI enhances acetylcholine concentrations at cholinergic receptors on skeletal muscle cells, since EPI can inhibit acetylcholinesterase (Benson, 1948). EPI is the only known drug that can reverse cardiac arrest due to asystole.

Strong emotion has an energizing effect. The *Guiness Book of World Records* (1980) includes an extraordinary entry under weight-lifting: A housewife, discovering that her child was pinned under a car, *lifted the car* off the child. Cannon agreed with Charles Darwin and William James that people possess "reservoirs of power" that can be tapped in situations perceived as dire:

> The exploit of John Colter, as reported by a contemporary, exemplifies vividly the reinforcing effects of general excitement. In Montana, in 1808, Colter and a companion were seized by Indians. Colter was stripped naked; his companion, who resisted, was killed and hacked in pieces. The Chief then made signs to Colter to go away across the prairie. When he had gone a short distance he saw the younger men casting aside everything but their weapons and making ready for a chase. "Now he knew their object. He was to run a race, of which the prize was to be his own life and scalp. Off he started with the speed of wind. The war whoop immediately arose; and looking back, he saw a large company of young warriors, with spears, in rapid pursuit. He ran with all the speed that nature, excited to the utmost, could give; fear and hope lent a supernatural vigor to his limbs, and the rapidity of his flight astonished himself." (Cannon, 1929a, pp. 226–227)
>
> And I have heard a football player confess that just before the final game such an access of strength seemed to come to him that he felt able, on the signal, to crouch and with a jump go crashing through any ordinary door . . . [I]t is altogether probable that the critical dangers of adventure have a fascination because fear is thrilling, and extrication from a predicament, by calling forth all the bodily resources and setting them to meet the challenge of the difficulty, yields many of the joys of conquest. (Cannon, 1929a, p. 239)

The mechanism of this effect, analogous to the above-noted antifatigue effect, is unknown. Consistent with participation of EPI in the energizing effect of emotion, Taggart et al. (1978) found that in race car drivers, increases in urinary catecholamine excretion accompanied the tachycardic and emotional responses.

Memory

Relationships between catecholamines in the brain and memory are discussed in detail in the chapter about central function neuroanatomy. Learning appetitive or avoidance behaviors requires recollection of pleasurable and painful experiences. The long-term potentiation of excitatory synaptic inputs in the brain has provided the basis for a cellular model of learning and memory. Bliss et al. (1983) reported that depletion of NE in the brain blocks this long-term potentiation. Skinner (1985) summarized evidence that NE participates in the modulation of three independent types of cortical activity: feature detection, synaptic efficiency, and cerebral event-related responses, suggesting that NE in the brain is related to sensory perception, learning and memory, and psychological stress.

Pupillary Dilation

The iris possesses high concentrations of catecholamine-fluorescent terminals (Malmfors, 1965). The radial muscle contains both α- and β-adrenoceptors. β-Adrenergic blockade produces pupillary constriction. Conversely, pupillary dilation, caused by both EPI and by withdrawal of cholinergic tone, improves distance vision and possibly enhances sexual attraction. The name ''belladonna'' derives from the legendary use of atropine-based concoctions by Italian women to dilate their pupils (Brown, 1990).

Other

Pulmonary effects of EPI include bronchiolar dilation and hyperventilation (Barcroft et al., 1957; Young, 1957). Clinicians exploit the former effect when they inject EPI to abort asthma attacks; and sudden awakening by a noise increases the rate of breathing within a few seconds. The mechanism of ventilatory stimulation by EPI is unknown and seems to have received little recent research attention. The suggestion that EPI directly stimulates a medullary center regulating ventilation must take into account the blood–brain barrier for EPI. Perhaps blood-borne catecholamines reach medullary sites via the area postrema, a circumventricular organ lacking a blood–brain barrier.

Leydig cells of the testes and interstitial cells of the ovaries, the sites of sex steroid synthesis and release in men and women, possess sympathetic innervation. Penile erection in men requires an intact SNS; however, as noted by Cannon (1939a; Cannon et al., 1929), female cats that have undergone complete surgical sympathectomies can nevertheless ovulate, become pregnant, and give birth to normal kittens.

Summary and Conclusions

Catecholaminergic systems determine most of the acute circulatory effects of stressors. The SNS consists of nerve networks, with NE the sympathetic neurotransmitter. The AHS includes the adrenal medulla, which secretes EPI directly into the bloodstream. The renal DOPA–DA system may exemplify a third type of peripheral catecholaminergic system, where nonneuronal cells take up DOPA and convert it to DA, which then acts as an autocrine/paracrine substance.

Sympathetic neuroeffector junctions in the arteriolar walls and in the heart are the main sites for SNS control of cardiovascular function. Sympathetic nerve networks are especially dense in the walls of the body's myriad arterioles, which determine total resistance to blood flow, and in the heart. Other substances (DBH, ATP, NPY, enkephalins, EPI) may be coreleased with NE during sympathetic stimulation; whether any of these act as cotransmitters has not been established firmly.

The rate-limiting enzymatic step in NE synthesis is hydroxylation of TYR to form DOPA. After conversion of DOPA to DA in the sympathoneural axoplasm, DA is translocated into vesicles containing DBH and is converted to NE.

The main means of terminating the actions of endogenously released NE is neuronal reuptake (Uptake-1), which cocaine and tricyclic antidepressants block. Nonneuronal uptake (Uptake-2) is the main means for terminating the actions of circulating EPI. Conjugation appears to be a major means for inactivating DA formed outside sympathetic nerves.

NE removed into the axoplasm can be taken up into the vesicles (a process blocked by reserpine) or deaminated by mitochondrial MAO to form DHPG. DHPG can be O-methylated extraneuronally to form MHPG, an end product of NE metabolism. A small amount of endogenous NE is removed by Uptake-2 and O-methylated to form NMN.

Several endogenous substances and drugs—most notably, α_2-adrenoceptor agonists—modulate release of NE from sympathetic nerve endings. NE may therefore limit its own release.

The SNS is required not only for emergency cardiovascular responses but also for maintaining tonic levels of cardiovascular performance. Failure to monitor or control for compensatory activation of other systems can obscure the latter role.

In the cardiovascular system, α_1-adrenoceptors are located mainly postsynaptically and α_2-adrenoceptors pre- and extrasynaptically. β_1-Adrenoceptor stimulation increases cardiac rate and contractility, and β_2-adrenoceptor stimulation causes arteriolar smooth muscle relaxation in skeletal muscle. Stimulation of dopaminergic receptors increases cardiac output, renal blood flow, urinary volume, and sodium excretion.

All adrenoceptors share the same general structure: a polypeptide chain extending out from the cell membrane; seven polypeptide domains spanning the membrane; and a long polypeptide chain extending into the cytoplasm from the internal surface of the cell membrane.

Intracellular mechanisms of catecholamine action involve membrane G-proteins, which when activated by receptor occupation increase the generation of second messengers (e.g., cAMP) and consequently activate protein kinases (e.g., PKA), resulting in phosphorylation of proteins that influence entry of ions into the cytoplasm via membrane channels or from intracellular storage sites, thereby affecting cellular excitation–contraction processes.

Catecholamines alter the function of virtually all body organs. NE released from cardiac sympathetic nerves and EPI reaching the heart via the bloodstream increase cardiac rate, contractility, and electrical automaticity and produce cutaneous, splanchnic, and renal vasoconstriction and antinatriuresis, whereas DA promotes natriuresis. EPI increases skeletal muscle blood flow, DA increases renal blood flow, and NE is a universal vasoconstrictor. EPI quiets the gut, increases blood glucose levels, exerts an antifatigue effect, augments emotional experiences, and decreases serum potassium concentrations. All the effects of EPI can be understood teleologically in terms of supporting the physiological, behavioral, and experiential changes during distress.

4

Control of Sympathetic Outflow and Functions of Central Catecholamines

This chapter focuses on central nervous mechanisms regulating sympathoneural outflow and on the functions that catecholamines in the brain subserve. Although abundant evidence indicates the participation of brain catecholamines, at several levels of the neuraxis, in the regulation of autonomic outflows, the relationship between release of catecholamines in the brain and release of catecholamines in the periphery is complex, indirect, and poorly understood. An immense literature describes central neuroanatomic pathways directly or indirectly mediating regulation of sympathetic function, and an immense literature deals with central neural catecholamines and their receptors in stress and neurological and psychiatric disorders. This abundance contrasts with a dearth of information specifically about the roles of catecholamines in the central nervous system in the control of sympathetic function.

The organization and contents of this chapter reflect this predicament. After an historical and conceptual introduction, sections follow about central neuroanatomic pathways involved with sympathetic outflow, especially to the cardiovascular system; about noncatecholaminergic endogenous compounds that may act in the brain to modulate sympathetic outflow; and about central catecholamines and adrenoceptors. One can only hope that from this base, future concepts will relate central catecholamines to the SNS.

From a neuroanatomic point of view, despite elucidation of central pathways participating in regulation of sympathetic outflow, knowledge about the functions of the centers those pathways connect lags behind; and despite an explosion of information about neuroanatomical interconnections among cardiovascular "regulatory" centers, little is known about patterned alterations in activity of these centers in diseases. Electrical or chemical stimulation of many brain areas affects sympathetic outflow, but our

164

understanding remains meager about coordination of the sympathoneural with other neuroendocrine systems in the maintenance of cardiovascular homeostasis.

From a neurochemical point of view, although exogenous administration of catecholamines or adrenoceptor-active drugs into the central nervous system can alter sympathetic outflow, the results may not apply to the function of endogenous central catecholaminergic systems, partly because of the likelihood of functional differences based on spatial localization of the receptors with respect to the release sites. The physiological roles of most endogenous neuropeptides and other putative neuromodulators remain obscure, and research to date has failed to decipher a neurochemical ''code'' to explain patterns of colocalization and corelease of catecholamines and other neurotransmitters in the brain.

Historical and Conceptual Introduction

Research about neural circulatory regulation developed along two lines: efferent and afferent, the former involving cardiovascular and neuroendocrine effects of stimulation of sympathetic nerves and the latter involving input from cardiovascular receptors to the brain. Efforts to identify the central neural sites where afferent reflexive pathways terminate and efferent sympathetic pathways originate continue to this day. Only within the past two decades has neurophysiological research traced the neuroanatomic basis for even the simplest neurocirculatory reflex arc.

Regarding efferents, Claude Bernard provided the first demonstration of the sympathetic nervous control of vascular ''tone'' in 1851, when he announced that cutting the ''sympathetic nerve'' in the rabbit neck produced flushing and warmth of the ear on that side and enlargement of the regional network of blood vessels. In 1853, he described the main signs of interference with sympathetic neurotransmission to the head—increased temperature and circulation, constriction of the pupil, ptosis, and recession of the eye into the orbit—a syndrome that bears his name, ''Horner–Bernard syndrome,'' or ''Horner's syndrome.'' (In 1869, Horner described this syndrome for the first time in humans.)

Bernard argued that cutting the sympathetic nerve directly increased local generation of heat. In 1852, he and Brown-Sequard reported skin cooling and blanching during electrical stimulation of the proximal end of the sectioned sympathetic nerve. Brown-Sequard correctly attributed the fall in skin temperature to the constriction of the blood vessels (Brown-Sequard, 1852). Bernard and Brown-Sequard disagreed about priority in this work, the French Academy of Sciences settling the issue in awarding Bernard, for the fourth and last time, its prize for experimental physiology in 1853.

In 1863, Bernard reported that transection of the cervical spinal cord produced immediate, marked hypotension—probably the first evidence that the brain regulates overall cardiovascular ''tone.''

In 1883, Pavlov reported his studies about ''centrifugal nerves of the heart'' that accelerated and augmented cardiac contraction (Pavlov, 1887), and Gaskell (1883–84) traced the source of efferent vasoconstrictor fibers to the lateral horns of the spinal cord.

By the beginning of the 20th century, the anatomy and physiology of the sympathetic innervation of the heart had been described in detail (Cyon, 1907; Keng, 1893).

Approximately contemporaneously with these developments, other investigators noted the indirect, reflexive cardiovascular effects of stimulating afferent neural pathways to the brain. In 1836, Sir Astley Cooper showed that occlusion of the common carotid arteries increased blood pressure and heart rate. He attributed these effects to cerebral ischemia. Experiments reported by Siciliano in 1900 refuted Cooper's explanation and indicated instead a signal to the brain from the region of the bifurcation of the carotid artery. In 1923, Hering found that mechanical stimulation of the wall of the carotid sinus, a small area of dilatation in the region of the carotid bifurcation, produced marked bradycardia and hypotension. Cutting a branch of the glossopharyngeal nerve, the carotid sinus nerve (also known as Hering's nerve), prevented these effects, and stimulation of the nerve reproduced the bradycardia and hypotension (Hering, 1927). This proved the reflexive basis for the effects of carotid occlusion on blood pressure noted by Cooper about a century previously.

From the beginning of the 20th century until now, ideas about the organization of brain mechanisms of neurocirculatory regulation developed in stages (Gebber, 1984). In 1916, Ranson and Billingsley reported that electrical stimulation of a discrete area on the dorsal surface of the medulla of the brainstem produced decreases in blood pressure, and stimulation rostral and lateral to this site produced increases in pressure, suggesting the existence of specific cardiovascular "centers" in the brainstem.

Wang and Ranson (1939); however, found that the dorsal surface area described by Ranson and Billingsley actually constituted apices of large pressor and depressor triangles, extending dorsoventrally through virtually the entire brainstem. According to the generally accepted view from the 1950s until the 1970s, the summed activity of diffusely interconnected fibers of the "reticular activating system" randomly generated sympathoneural outflow (Hilton, 1975), as if an impenetrable neuronal thicket intervened between interoceptive input and neurocirculatory output from the brain.

Several developments forced reconsideration of this position. First, most baroreceptor afferents to the brain were found to terminate in a specific cluster of cells in the dorsomedial medulla, the nucleus of the solitary tract (NTS; Seller and Illert, 1969; Miura and Reis, 1969), a region now known to serve as both a relay and integration center for the baroreflex—that is, the likely location of the arterial "barostat." Second, evidence accumulated that a small collection of neurons in the rostral ventrolateral medulla (RVLM), corresponding in location to EPI-synthesizing C1 neurons, provide a major source of projections to the sympathetic preganglionic neurons in the spinal cord (Reis et al., 1984, 1988). Third, studies using immunohistochemistry and novel anterogradely and retrogradely transported compounds (Bjorklund and Lindvall, 1986; Ciriello and Calaresu, 1981; Lindvall and Bjorklund, 1974) showed that ascending and descending information between the lower brainstem and higher centers travels in tracts of extensively arborized fibers among relatively few clusters of neural cells, rather than in a diffuse reticular system. And fourth, neurophysiological studies in cats demonstrated that preganglionic sympathetic neurons discharge rhythmically, the rhythmic discharges depending importantly on lower brainstem networks of coupled oscillators generating the rhythm inherently—a pacemaker for sympathoneural outflow (Gebber and Barman, 1980).

According to the current view, organized, periodic discharges of relatively few brainstem neurons, particularly in the RVLM, drive activity of the spinal preganglionic neurons in a complexly but not randomly determined manner, with influences by other clusters of cells at several sites in the neuraxis (Barman and Gebber, 1980; Gebber, 1984). Many studies have elucidated the neuronal circuitry connecting these clusters, and a substantial portion of this chapter summarizes those connections.

A web of brain centers therefore seems to determine SNS outflow to the cardiovascular system (Figure 4–1). Although the depicted network appears dauntingly complex, the figure actually substantially oversimplifies the situation. The diagram excludes many other areas and pathways. More than one neurotransmitter can act on or emanate from

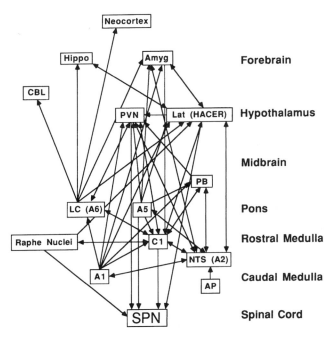

Figure 4–1. Mosaic of central nervous centers involved in sympathoadrenal outflow. Several clusters of cells in the brain contribute to outflow to the spinal pregangionic neurons (SPN). These clusters are interconnected neuroanatomically. Prominent among these clusters are C1 adrenergic cells of the rostral ventrolateral medulla; A1 cells of the caudal ventrolateral medulla; the nucleus of the solitary tract (NTS), the parabrachial area (PB), the midline raphe nuclei, the A6 cells of the locus ceruleus of the pons (LC), the A5 cells of the pons, the paraventricular nucleus (PVN) of the hypothalamus, the posterolateral "HACER" area of the hypothalamus, and the amygdala (Amyg) and hippocampus (Hippo) in the limbic system. The LC provides noradrenergic innervation to much of the telencephalon, including the frontal cortex and cerebellum (CBL). The area postrema (AP), a circumventricular organ, lacks an efficient blood–brain barrier and may be a site of central neural actions of circulating hormones.

the same neurons and can act on more than one type of receptor on the effector cells. Modulatory interneurons within and between areas probably coordinate the functions of the cell clusters. Pathways relaying information in the brain probably use not only neurotransmitters but also hormones and autocrine/paracrine substances. Finally, the static anatomic depiction does not adequately convey dynamic processes, such as conditioning and arousal, development, and degeneration. In particular, resetting of homeostats during stress probably alters the prominence of some centers with respect to others, and the neuroanatomic representation does not portray this likely variability.

The finding of Dahlstrom and Fuxe (1964, 1965) that brainstem catecholaminergic pathways directly innervate large areas of the telencephalon contrasted with the then prevalent view, based on Golgi impregnation and antegrade degeneration techniques, that ascending pathways from the lower brainstem terminate in the hypothalamus, with only indirect connections from the lower brainstem to the cortical mantle (Nauta and Kuypers, 1958). Studies using the glyoxylic acid method (Lindvall and Bjorklund, 1974) confirmed and extended the findings of Dahlstrom and Fuxe. The results demonstrated that, while few in number, central monoaminergic neurons project widely in the central nervous system, with catecholamines present in almost all brain areas. This led to fundamentally new ideas about functional connections in the brain and ushered in an era of "chemical neuroanatomy." Exactly how central catecholaminergic neurochemical pathways jibe with the neuroanatomic web remains incompletely understood, and this chapter includes several examples where clusters of catecholamine-containing cells do not seem confined to neuroanatomically distinct regions.

Based on the presence of brain catecholamine pathways and on the sometimes marked behavioral effects of drugs affecting catecholaminergic function, many theories have proposed how central catecholaminergic pathways participate in a variety of psychological phenomena, such as the state of wakefulness, arousal, emotion, and memory; specific behaviors, such as eating, drinking, thermoregulation, and sexual activity; and disorders in psychiatry (schizophrenia, depression, panic-anxiety, anorexia–bulimia, attention deficit disorder) neurology (Parkinsonism, the Shy–Drager syndrome, disorders of memory and alertness), and cardiology (cardiomyopathy, arrhythmias, neurocirculatory asthenia, hypertension). Sections later in this chapter analyze some of these theories. Nevertheless, no study has proven that any catecholamine in the central nervous system "mediates" any behavior, and no theory has explained how alterations of catecholaminergic function in the brain can account for so many different phenomena. Most remarkably, despite the likely involvement of both the mesotelencephalic DA system and the locus ceruleus NE system in "enabling" the organism's responses to environmental input, no concepts have integrated the functions of these two catecholaminergic systems.

The findings summarized below lead to the proposal that central neural catecholamines participate only indirectly in regulating SNS and AHS outflows, by participating in the elaboration of neuroendocrine response patterns during stress and distress. The bases for these relationships may come to light when researchers consider more the integrated patterns of behavioral, neuroendocrine, and physiological changes that occur in response to stressors, and less the roles of specific cardiovascular "regulatory centers" in the brain.

Hierarchical Neuroanatomic Organization

A hierarchy of central neural circuits regulates sympathetic nerve activity (Figure 4–2). At least three types of input lead to the neurocirculatory responses: afferent nerves from interoceptors and exteroceptors, hormones reaching circumventricular organs that lack an efficient blood–brain barrier, and cognitive simulations in the cortex. The efferent pathways converge at the level of the sympathetic preganglionic neurons.

Folkow (1987) has conceptualized the hierarchical organization of cardiovascular control at three levels: (1) local, involving myogenic activity of the heart and vasculature; (2) bulbar, involving baroreceptor and chemoreceptor inputs to the brainstem and relatively simple homeostatic neurohumoral outputs to regulate blood volume, peripheral vascular resistance, and cardiac output; and (3) higher central neural, involving neocortical, limbic, and hypothalamic expression of integrated behavioral, visceral, and hormonal patterns. The present conception adopts this view (Figure 4–3). Beginning with what is probably a single medullary site of initial termination of input from car-

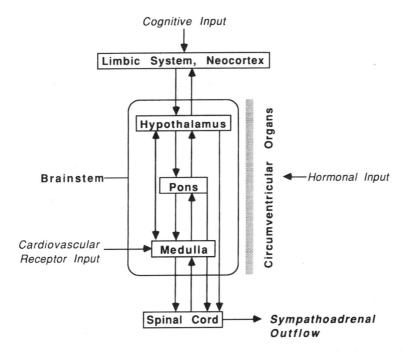

Figure 4–2. Overview of the hierarchy of central neural sites determining neurocirculatory regulation. The main sites of afferent input are via nerves entering the medulla, hormones entering circumventricular organs, and cognitions from the cortex transmitted via the limbic system. Multiple interconnections link each level.

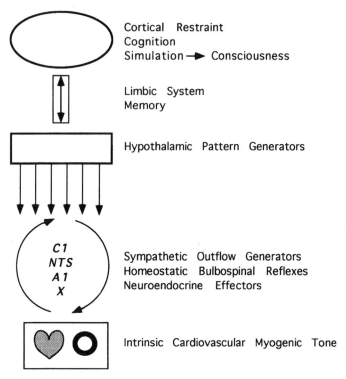

Cortical Restraint
Cognition
Simulation → Consciousness

Limbic System
Memory

Hypothalamic Pattern Generators

C1
NTS
A1
X

Sympathetic Outflow Generators
Homeostatic Bulbospinal Reflexes
Neuroendocrine Effectors

Intrinsic Cardiovascular Myogenic Tone

Figure 4–3. Overview of the hierarchy of central neural sites participating in stress responses. Cardiovascular structures possess intrinsic "tone." Simple homeostatic reflexes maintain appropriate basal levels of cardiovascular performance. The operating characteristics of the homeostats reset as part of hypothalamically elaborated patterns. The limbic and frontal cortices interpret afferent signals about the internal and external environments to determine the occurrence and intensity of the hypothalamically evoked patterns.

diovascular receptors, at each ascending neural level the complexity of interactions increases, with the lower centers subject to modulation by higher centers. At the lowest level, cardiovascular structures possess intrinsic "tone." At the next, simple homeostatic reflexes maintain appropriate "steady-state" cardiovascular performance. The operating characteristics of the homeostats reset as part of hypothalamically elaborated patterns generated at the next higher level. Finally, at the highest level, the limbic and frontal cortices interpret afferent signals about the internal and external environments to determine the occurrence and intensity of hypothalamically evoked patterns. This is the level of memory, learning, simulation (in the sense described in Chapter 1), and consciousness.

Spinal Cord and Sympathetic Nerves

The spinal cord is the most distal site of the central nervous system that generates patterns of sympathetic activity (Figure 4–4). The final common pathway for sympa-

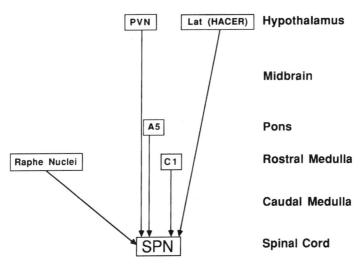

Figure 4–4. Central neural sites projecting to the spinal preganglionic neurons. Same abbreviations as in Figure 4–1.

thetic outflow is the preganglionic neuron. Cell bodies of sympathetic preganglionic neurons (SPNs) are located mainly in the intermediolateral columns of the thoracolumbar spinal cord. SPNs discharge spontaneously at only a slow rate. Their tonic activity depends instead mainly on input from chemoreceptor, somatic, and visceral afferent nerve traffic to the spinal cord, but more importantly on descending input from supraspinal structures—as demonstrated by the marked reduction of activity after cord transection.

Whereas feedback regulation contributes relatively little to direct regulation of SPN activity, feedback becomes a prominent feature at the level of the medulla, where several types of visceral afferents synapse, without direct inputs to higher levels. Medullary cardiovascular centers therefore subserve simple homeostatic reflexes.

Cell groups in the region of adrenergic C1 cells of the RVLM, the "defense" area of the lateral hypothalamus, and the paraventricular nucleus of the hypothalamus (PVN) send direct projections to the intermediolateral columns of the thoracolumbar spinal cord, where the SPNs are situated. Other supraspinal structures projecting directly to this region include medullary and pontine raphe nuclei, A5 and A7 noradrenergic cells, and the Kolliker-Fuse nucleus in the parabrachial nucleus complex (McCall, 1990; Senba et al., 1993).

After exiting the spinal cord, axons from SPNs travel via white rami (from the Latin for "branches") to preaortic and paravertebral chains of sympathetic ganglia (Figure 4–5). A proportion of the axons pass through splanchnic ganglia without synapsing,

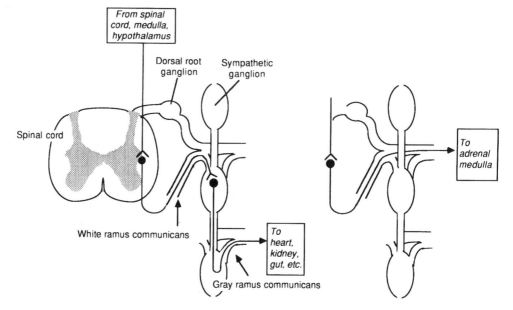

Figure 4–5. Sympathoadrenal ganglionic outflows. Spinal preganglionic neurons in the intermediolateral columns of the thoracolumbar spinal cord exit the cord and enter the sympathetic chain of ganglia. After synapsing in the ganglia, postganglionic sympathetic nerves innervate the heart, blood vessels, kidneys, and glands. The adrenal medulla innervation includes nerves that do not synapse in the ganglia.

providing neural innervation to the adrenal medulla; and a proportion synapses on cell bodies of postganglionic neurons innervating the heart, vasculature, viscera, kidneys, and glands. Adrenal nerve activity therefore at least partly reflects preganglionic outflow, whereas activity in renal nerve reflects postganglionic outflow. Thus, blockade of ganglionic neurotransmission shuts down renal nerve sympathetic activity, with little effect on circulating EPI levels. Adrenomedullary chromaffin cells seem analogous to postganglionic sympathetic neurons, since the adrenomedullary nerves release acetylcholine as the neurotransmitter, as do SPNs synapsing in ganglia.

Medulla

Dittmar (1870) noted that pressor responses to sciatic nerve stimulation persisted after pontine transection but that destruction of the medulla abolished them, demonstrating probably for the first time that medullary vasomotor centers regulate acute blood pressure responses. Owsjannikov (1871) reported that arterial pressure fell successively after cutting the brainstem between the level of the inferior colliculi and the obex. The findings established the importance of the medulla in circulatory regulation.

During the next century, numerous attempts failed to identify specific centers in the medulla where lesions of those centers would reproduce the hypotension caused by spinal cord section. These failures led to the suggestion that projections to SPNs derive from diffusely distributed neurons in the reticular formation (Chalmers, 1975; Hilton, 1975).

More recent studies have established that a discrete group of adrenergic neurons (i.e., neurons containing PNMT), the C1 neurons of the RVLM, constitute a major source of projections determining tonic discharge of SPNs (Reis et al., 1988; Ross et al., 1984a; Figure 4–6).

Rostral Ventral Medulla and the Origin of Sympathetic Outflow

The RVLM region containing the C1 cells is a subdivision of the nucleus paragigantocellularis lateralis (PGi). The nomenclature is confusing, because the neuroanatomic localization does not coincide exactly with the regional neurochemistry: the EPI-containing cells of the RVLM are not confined specifically in this nucleus (Kalia et al., 1985b). Moreover, RVLM cells contain many other potential neurotransmitters besides EPI, including NPY, GABA, glutamate, substance P, acetylcholine, enkephalin, somatostatin, glucagon, and NE (Chalmers and Pilowsky, 1991).

Afferent fibers from receptors sensing blood pressure synapse mainly in the NTS, and neurons in this region project to RVLM neurons, either directly or via cells in the caudal ventrolateral medulla (see below); and bilateral destruction of the RVLM abolishes arterial baroreflexes (Reis et al., 1984, 1988). Thus, the RVLM participates not only in tonic but also in reflexive regulation of sympathetic vasomotor tone.

Since systemic hypoxia activates RVLM cells and stimulates sympathetically mediated vasoconstriction (Sun and Reis, 1994), RVLM neurons respond not only to hemodynamic but also to chemoreceptor input.

Numerous centers in the brain project to the C1 cells or PGi region (Van Bockstaele et al., 1989), including the PVN, the lateral hypothalamic area, the midbrain periaquaductal gray region, the supraoculomotor nucleus of the central gray, the A5 and locus ceruleus (LC) neurons of the pons, the NTS (Ross et al., 1985), A1 neurons of

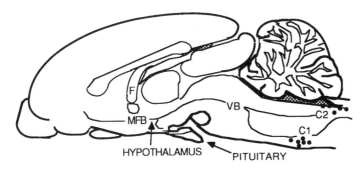

Figure 4–6. Epinephrine pathways in the rat brain. In this schematic diagram of a midsagittal section, the cells containing phenylethanolamine-*N*-methyltransferase are designated C1, C2, etc. C1 cells in the rostral ventrolateral medulla (RVLM) project both rostrally and caudally. The RVLM is thought to be the main site of origin of central nervous outflow to the spinal preganglionic cells.

the caudal ventrolateral medulla (CVLM, Granata et al., 1986), the parabrachial nucleus, the circumventricular area postrema (AP, Blessing et al., 1987), vestibular nuclei, raphe nuclei, and the spinal cord.

Efferents from the C1/PGi region project widely (Aston-Jones et al., 1990; Byrum and Guyenet, 1987; Hilton and Smith, 1984; Li and Lovick, 1985; McCall, 1990; Pieribone et al., 1988; Thor and Helke, 1988; Tucker et al., 1987; van Bockstaele et al., 1989; Figure 4–7). In addition to sending projections to the region of the SPNs, the C1 cells project to the LC, the parabrachial nucleus, the paraventricular and median preoptic nuclei of the hypothalamus, the amygdala, the raphe nuclei, the spinal trigeminal nuclei, the cerebellum, and the NTS. The C1 neurons that project rostrally to the hypothalamus probably differ from those that project caudally to the intermediolateral columns of the spinal cord (Tucker et al., 1987). About 1/3 of the C1 cells project to the intermediolateral columns; about ½ of RVLM projections to the intermediolateral columns contain PNMT; and about ⅓ of the projections from PNMT-containing cells to the intermediolateral columns derive from C1 cells, the remainder from C2 and C3 cells (Chalmers and Pilowsky, 1991), discussed below.

The cells in the PGi region of the RVLM also may play key roles in integrated stress responses, because the cells project to the SPNs and to the LC, electrical stimulation of the PGi area produces analgesia, and PGi neurons discharge during exposure to noxious stimuli (Aston-Jones et al., 1990).

The medial portion of the RVLM contains lateral elements of the B3 region of

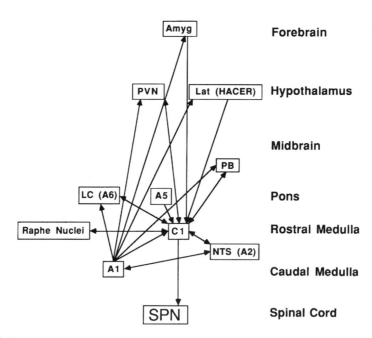

Figure 4–7. Central neural sites connected to the rostral ventrolateral medulla–C1 area. Same abbreviations as in Figure 4–1.

serotonin-containing cells (Chalmers and Pilowsky, 1991). Neurones in this region also can contain excitatory amino acids, substance P, thyrotropin-releasing hormone, enkephalin, somatostatin, cholecystokinin, or GABA. The B3 serotonergic neurones constitute a separate group of sympathoexcitatory cells. As noted below, the more medially located midline raphe cells generally inhibit sympathetic outflow.

Sympathoexcitatory neurons in the rostral ventromedial medulla (RVMM) may function differently from neurons of RVLM in terms of regional blood flow responses, changes in activity of individual sympathetic nerves, susceptibility to changes in respiration, and control of heart rate (Brody et al., 1991). Inactivation of RVLM cells by local microinjection of lidocaine produces larger decreases in lumbar and splanchnic sympathetic activity than does inactivation of RVMM cells (Varner et al., 1989), whereas inactivation of RVMM cells elicits prominent decreases in hindquarters vascular resistance (Cox and Brody, 1989). Stimulation of RVMM cells preferentially increases sympathetic discharges to the cardiovascular system, kidneys, and adrenal glands, with little change in discharges to the sweat glands or to ciliary or gut smooth muscle (McAllen, 1986). The RVMM appears to play a prominent role in regulating hindlimb vascular resistance, whereas the RVLM figures prominently in regulation of renal resistance (Cox and Brody, 1989). Local microinjection of lidocaine into either region decreases blood pressure similarly, and inactivation of cells simultaneously in the two regions virtually abolishes neurogenic maintenance of blood pressure (Varner et al., 1989). One may speculate that differences in the extents of SNS and AHS activation determine the differences in regional hemodynamic responses to RVLM and RVMM stimulation; this has not been tested.

Caudal Ventral Medulla

Below the level of the obex, caudal to the region of C1 cells, the ventrolateral medulla (nucleus reticularis caudoventrolateralis, nCVL) contains A1 noradrenergic cells (Figure 4–8). Just as the RVLM, a neuroanatomical entity, does not correspond exactly with the location of the C1 cells, the caudal ventrolateral medulla (CVLM) does not correspond exactly with the location of A1 cells.

Electrical or chemical stimulation of CVLM neurons produces opposite effects on sympathetic outflow and blood pressure from those produced by stimulation of RVLM neurons (Granata, Kumada et al., 1985). Blood pressure and pulse rate fall, and CVLM stimulation blunts pressor and renal neural responses to hypothalamic stimulation (Blessing and Reis, 1982; McAllen et al., 1982; Willette et al., 1983). Conversely, electrolytic lesions of the CVLM region increase pressure by augmenting SNS outflow and AVP release (Blessing and Reis, 1982; Blessing et al., 1982; Granata, Kumada et al., 1985; Imaizumi et al., 1985; Minson et al., 1986; Sved and Reis, 1985).

Few if any noradrenergic neurons in the CVLM area project directly to the SPNs (Blessing et al., 1981; Chalmers and Pilowsky, 1991), and those that do probably are not catecholaminergic (McKellar and Loewy, 1982). Instead, axons from neurons of the CVLM project to the RVLM, the NTS, and the nucleus ambiguus (NA) and ascend to the Kolliker–Fuse nuclei, the parabrachial nuclei, the periaquaductal gray regions, the intralaminar nuclei of the thalamus, the facial nucleus, the paraventricular and supra-

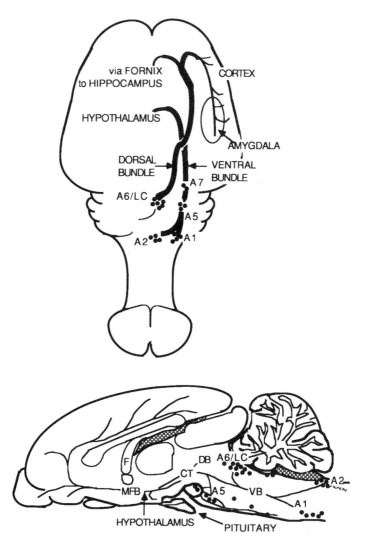

Figure 4–8. Norepinephrine pathways in the rat brain. In these schematic diagrams of the rat brain, the cells containing dopamine-β-hydroxylase but not PNMT are designated A1, A2, etc. A2 cells are localized to the nucleus of the solitary tract (NTS) and A6 cells in the locus ceruleus (LC). Noradrenergic pathways include the ventral noradrenergic bundle (VB), central tegmental tract (CT), the dorsal bundle (DB), and the medial forebrain bundle (MFB). Axons from the medullary A1 and A2 cells ascend via the ventral bundle to provide the main source of noradrenergic innervation of the hypothalamus. Descending axons from the ventrolateral pontine A5 region innervate spinal preganglionic neurons. Axons from the pontine A6 cells ascend via the dorsal bundle to provide the main source of noradrenergic innervation of the cerebral cortex, thalamus, and basal ganglia. The A6 cells also provide the main source of noradrenergic innervation of the cerebellum. The cerebral cortex is the only brain region that receives exclusive noradrenergic innervation from the A6 cells of the locus ceruleus; all other brain regions receive some degree of innervation from the locus ceruleus and lateral tegmental systems.

optic nuclei (PVN and SON) of the hypothalamus, the median eminence, the medial preoptic area, and through the lateral hypothalamus to the bed nucleus of the stria terminalis (BNST) and organum vasculosum of the lamina terminalis (OVLT; Granata et al., 1986; McKellar and Loewy, 1982; Woulfe et al., 1990). The projections to the PVN, BNST, SON, median eminence, dorsal hypothalamus, and dorsomedial hypothalamic nucleus appear to be noradrenergic, since they are sensitive to 6-hydroxydopamine (6-OHDA), which destroys catecholaminergic terminals.

CVLM neurons inhibit sympathetic activity primarily by acting on neurons of the RVLM region (Blessing, 1988; Granata, Kumada et al., 1985; Ross et al., 1985), directly and also indirectly via actions in the hypothalamus. The inhibitory neurotransmitter of the CVLM neurons in the RVLM may be NE, since microinjection of tyramine, which releases amines from storage vesicles, in the RVLM produces hypotension, and destruction of noradrenergic terminals by 6-OHDA prevents both the depressor effect of tyramine and the pressor effect of CVLM lesions (Granata, Kumada et al., 1985, 1986). Effects of the manipulations on EPI neurons of the RVLM, however, can also explain these findings, and tract-tracing studies using double labels have not demonstrated direct connections between the A1 noradrenergic neurons and the RVLM (Chalmers and Pilowsky, 1991). Alternative neurotransmitters for the inhibitory effect of the projection from the CVLM to the C1 (or RVLM) neurons include acetylcholine (McCall, 1990), GABA (Blessing, 1988; Sun and Guyenet, 1985), and glutamate (Blessing and Li, 1989).

Because of extensive projections—many of them noradrenergic—from the CVLM cells to the magnocellular cells of the PVN (Sawchenko and Swanson, 1981a, 1982; Yamashita et al., 1989), many studies have considered the relationship between this medullary region and hypothalamic release of AVP. The results have not supported any simple model. Electrical stimulation of the CVLM increases firing rates of AVP-containing neurons in the PVN and SON and evokes release of AVP (Day, 1989; Day and Renaud, 1984; Mills and Wang, 1964); however, CVLM lesions produce marked hypertension, also associated with increased circulating AVP levels (Blessing et al., 1982; Imaizumi et al., 1985; Minson et al., 1986).

Dorsal Medulla

Electrical stimulation of the dorsomedial medulla elicits large, sympathetically mediated increases in blood pressure (Chai et al., 1963; Wang and Chai, 1967). Since descending pathways from the RVLM to the spinal cord traverse the dorsal medulla, activation of fibers in passage could explain the responses to electrical stimulation of the dorsal medulla; however, microinjection of the neuronal excitant sodium glutamate in the dorsal medulla also produces large pressor responses and increases in plasma catecholamine levels (Chai et al., 1991), suggesting that dorsal medullary cell bodies provide another source of excitatory neuronal outflow from the medulla to the SPNs in the intermediolateral columns.

Near the ventricular surface of the rostral dorsomedial medulla, cells of the nucleus prepositus hypoglossi (PrH) send inhibitory efferents to the LC (Aston-Jones et al., 1990). Reciprocal interconnections of the PrH area with vestibular nuclei, cerebellum, cerebral cortex, and projections to the inferior olive, the superior colliculus and pretectum, and extraocular motor nuclei suggest that the PrH participates in the sense of spatial orientation of the organism and ocular gaze. Aston-Jones et al. (1990) have suggested that the function of the PrH may be related to the "initiation and coordination of holistic orientation responses" (p. 232). The input from the PrH to the LC seems mainly inhibitory; if so, then the activation of LC cells during vigilance or orienting behaviors would appear to depend on phasic disinhibition of input from the PrH.

NUCLEUS OF THE SOLITARY TRACT (NTS)

After Hering's discovery of the reflexive role of the carotid sinus nerve in blood pressure regulation, the discovery of where in the brain this nerve leads took about another half century. It is by now known that afferent impulses from the carotid sinus mechanoreceptors travel via the glossopharyngeal nerve to synapse in the NTS (Ciriello and Calaresu, 1981; Miura and Reis, 1969; Seller and Illert, 1969). Thus, baroreceptor stimulation increases metabolic activity in the NTS, as measured using the $2[^3H]$-deoxyglucose autoradiographic technique to visualize glucose utilization (Ciriello et al., 1983). Metabolic activity also increases in the dorsal motor nucleus of the vagus, the NA, the parabrachial nucleus, the inferior olivary nucleus, and the VLM; in the hypothalamus, increased glucose utilization occurs only in the PVN and SON.

As suggested from the autoradiographic findings, the NTS relays baroreceptor and chemoreceptor information to other brainstem regions involved in relatively simple, "local" reflexive responses of autonomic outflow and to rostral structures, including the hypothalamus, responsible for eliciting "long distance" neuroendocrine and behavioral patterns (Mifflin and Felder, 1990). The efferent projections from the NTS probably define the central neural circuitry of the baroreflexes, and the afferents to the NTS from other central neural sites probably indicate the circuitry for modulation of those reflexes. The NTS receives not only cardiovascular but also other interoceptive afferent information, and termination sites of the efferent projections, such as to the NA, relate not only to cardiovascular reflex regulation but also to respiratory and gastrointestinal function (e.g., Cunningham and Sawchenko, 1989). The anterior portion of the NTS appears to receive gustatory and the posterior portion to receive visceral sensory input.

Many central neural sites interconnect with the NTS (Figure 4–9). These include the PVN, the central nucleus of the amygdala (ACE), the parabrachial nucleus, and catecholamine-containing cell groups in the brainstem. Neurons of the NTS do not appear to project directly to SPNs.

Consistent with the central role of the NTS in reflexive regulation of the circulation, bilateral ablation of the NTS produces fulminant hypertension in rats (Doba and Reis, 1973) and labile hypertension in cats (Nathan and Reis, 1977).

Baroreflex pathways after the initial synapse in the NTS include the VLM and the NA of the medulla (Figure 4–10). In animals with a previous unilateral lesion of the NTS, electrolytic or chemical (kainic acid application) lesion of the contralateral VLM prevents baroreflex-vascular responses (Granata, Ruggiero et al., 1985; Reis et al., 1984).

The NTS probably does not project directly to the LC (Aston-Jones et al., 1990; Thor

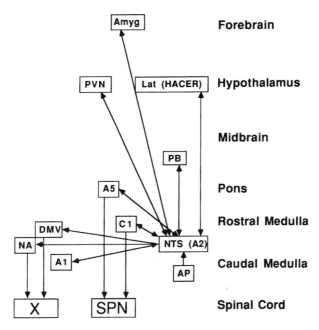

Figure 4–9. Central neural sites connected to the nucleus of the solitary tract–A2 area. Same abbreviations as in Figure 4–1.

and Helke, 1988), the source of most of the NE in the central nervous system. The two regions probably interrelate functionally, since alterations of cardiovascular interoceptive input affect LC neuronal firing (Elam et al., 1984) and release of NE in the hippocampus (Abercrombie et al., 1988), a region with noradrenergic input derived virtually exclusively from the LC.

In the 1960s, several investigators proposed, based on indirect evidence, that baroreceptor afferent activity influences the state of wakefulness or emotional behavior. Bonvallet and Allen (1963) reported that in paralyzed cats, stimulation of the midbrain reticular formation attenuated pupillary constrictor responses, with bilateral electrocoagulation at the head of the NTS prolonging the effect of the mesencephalic stimulation. Bartorelli et al. (1960) reported that increases in carotid sinus pressure led to synchronization of the electroencephalogram and could block or attenuate spontaneously occurring fits of "sham rage" in decorticate cats. Section of the carotid sinus nerve (coupled with vagotomy) eliminated the rage reaction to carotid occlusion, and injection of thiopental into the carotid circulation, in order to produce diencephalic but not medullary anesthesia, dissociated the vasomotor and behavioral responses to carotid occlusion, with normal vasomotor and respiratory responses but with no sham rage behavior. Bartorelli et al. (1960) noted that deafferentiation alone was insufficient to elicit rage in intact animals, suggesting that forebrain structures play at least as important a role as baroreceptor afferents in inhibiting hypothalamic activity.

Lacey (1967) noted that the baroreceptors constituted the first known source of sen-

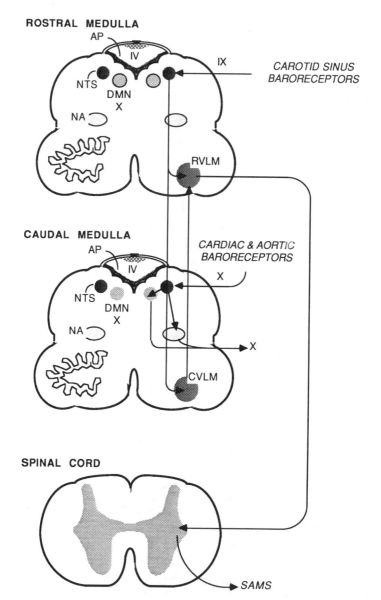

Figure 4–10. Central neuroanatomy of baroreflexes. Afferents from baroreceptors travel via the glossopharyngeal (IX) and vagus (X) nerves and enter the nucleus of the solitary tract. Cardiac vagal outflow is derived from the nucleus ambiguus (NA) and the dorsal motor nucleus of the vagus nerve (X). Sympathoadrenal system (SAMS) outflow is derived from the rostral ventrolateral medullary C1 region. The caudal ventrolateral medullary region containing noradrenergic A1 cells is an intermediary in the baroreceptor–sympathoneural reflex.

sory input to the central nervous system that inhibited cortical activity. Lacey and Lacey (1970) subsequently suggested that the hypertension accompanying acute emotional behaviors may not indicate "arousal" so much as the organism's attempt to restrain further activation by external excitatory processes; that is, that baroreceptor activation evokes a "stimulus barrier" for gating environmental input. Dworkin et al. (1979) expressed this view in the extreme, suggesting that clinical hypertension reflects an attempt to use increased baroreceptor afferent activity to counter the effects of noxious stimulation. These hypotheses did not consider the consequences of acute and chronic baroreflex resetting in acute distress and in chronic hypertension.

Ascending input from the NTS to the hypothalamus probably traverses pathways relatively independently of the LC, such as via the parabrachial nucleus to the PVN or the "HACER" area of the hypothalamus (see below) and then to the ACE and to the BNST (Fort et al., 1990; Kapp et al., 1989). In particular, the parabrachial nucleus appears to serve as the main relay station for ascending interoceptive information from the NTS to the forebrain (Herbert et al., 1990; Herbert and Saper, 1990). Microinjection of clonidine into the NTS attenuates AVP release during depletion of cardiovascular volume, indicating a functional connection between noradrenergic cells in the NTS and the PVN (Iovino et al., 1990).

The baroreceptor–cardiac reflex is not monosynaptic, because the NTS does not contain vagal preganglionic neurons. Injection of the retrograde tracer, fast blue, into the cervical vagus nerve and of the anterograde tracer, wheat germ agglutinin-conjugate horseradish peroxidase, into the NTS, reveals anterogradely labeled terminals from the NTS surrounding retrogradely labeled neurons in the dorsal motor nucleus of the vagus (Ross et al., 1985). This indicates the possibility of a disynaptic baroreceptor–vagal reflex, with one synapse in the NTS, where baroreceptor afferents would terminate, and the other in the dorsal motor nucleus of the vagus, where interneurons from the NTS would terminate.

Baroreceptor–sympathetic reflex arcs may include some direct projections from the NTS to C1 neurons (Ross et al., 1985); however, recent evidence has supported mainly indirect projections via A1 interneurons in the CVLM (Jeske et al., 1993). Analogously, Terui et al. (1990) identified neurons electrophysiologically in the CVLM in a region close to the NA that were activated orthodromically by stimulation of the aortic nerve and antidromically by stimulation of the RVLM. Thus, it appears that arterial barore-ceptor–SNS and baroreceptor–vagal reflexes consist of polysynaptic arcs that often include CVLM interneurons.

Medial Medulla

The midline raphe nuclei of the medulla correspond to the medullary "depressor area" (Alexander, 1946; Wang and Ranson, 1939). Stimulation of the medial medulla typically decreases blood pressure and sympathoneural activity. Some neurons in the medial medulla project directly to SPNs (Morrison and Gebber, 1984). Since electrical stimulation of the paramedian reticular nucleus attenuates or abolishes pressor and plasma catecholamine responses to stimulation of the dorsal or ventrolateral medulla (Chai et al., 1991), the midline nuclei may exert inhibitory modulation of excitatory pathways.

GABA and serotonin (5-HT) appear to interact as the neurotransmitters responsible for inhibition of SNS outflow during activation of this midline area, with the 5-HT neurons exerting a tonic excitatory influence at the level of the SPNs and the GABA-ergic neurons exerting a modulatory, inhibitory interneuronal action at the level of the RVLM (McCall, 1988, 1990). The dorsal raphe does not project directly to the LC; however, caudal raphe nuclei project to the PGi area, which in turn provides a major source of innervation of the LC (Aston-Jones et al., 1990). Increases in the firing rate of dorsal raphe 5-HT neurons after systemic administration of idazoxan (Marsden, 1990) suggest the presence of inhibitory α_2-heteroreceptors or imidazoline receptors on 5-HT cells (Arbilla and Langer, 1990).

The Nucleus Ambiguus (NA)

The nucleus ambiguus (NA) is the main site of origin of vagal efferents mediating reflexive bradycardia. Stimulation of the dorsal motor nucleus of the vagus does not evoke bradycardia, whereas stimulation of the NA does (Seller and Illert, 1969), and most parasympathetic neurons innervating the myocardium derive not from the dorsal motor nucleus of the vagus but from the NA or neurons close to it (Machado and Brody, 1990). A nearby group of neurons identified by Terui et al. (1990) may represent a region in the CVLM that projects to the probable main source of efferents to SPNs. Glutamate stimulation of perikarya of the NA produces vagal bradycardia and increases blood pressure (Machado and Brody, 1990). The pressor response may reflect concurrent activation of RVLM neurons.

Pons

The Locus Ceruleus (LC)

The locus ceruleus (LC), a small cluster of several thousand cell bodies in the dorsal pons, gives rise to most of the NE in the brain. A large body of neurophysiological and neurochemical research has therefore focused on the LC.

Extensive arborization of LC neurons explains how so few cells can project so widely in the central nervous system (Figure 4–11). Noradrenergic neurons of the LC project to the thalamus (especially the anteroventral nucleus), the hypothalamus (including the paraventricular, periventricular, supraoptic, and dorsomedial nuclei), the hippocampus, the septal area (including the BNST, the central and basolateral nuclei of the amygdala, and the olfactory bulb), the cerebellum, and the neocortex, as well as to several brainstem nuclei thought to function as primary sensory or association centers (Levitt and Moore, 1979). LC neurons do not project heavily to NE-containing terminals in the NTS (Ennis and Aston-Jones, 1989; Fritschy and Grzanna, 1990); and although the LC projects to the hypothalamus, NE-containing cell bodies in the medulla constitute the main source of noradrenergic projections to this region.

The LC does not project extensively directly to SPNs and therefore probably participates only indirectly in regulation of sympathoneural outflow. LC fibers do innervate sacral intermediolateral cell columns mediating parasympathetic outflow (Blessing et al., 1981; Westlund et al., 1984) and noradrenergic fibers from the LC and other med-

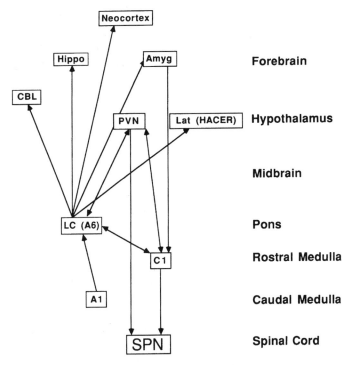

Figure 4–11. Central neural sites connected to the locus ceruleus–A6 area. Same abbreviations as in Figure 4–1.

ullary clusters innervate dorsal horn cells thought to mediate nociception (Basbaum, 1992), but few project to the intermediolateral columns of the thoracic spinal cord (Fritschy et al., 1987; Guyenet, 1980). The LC accounts for about 1/3 of the NE content of the rat spinal cord, the remainder apparently derived mainly from other pontine cell groups (Bjorklund and Lindvall, 1986).

The diffuse projections from the LC contrast with the relatively few sources of afferents to it: the PGi of the RVLM, corresponding neuroanatomically to the neurochemical localization of C1 and A1 EPI- and NE-containing cell bodies near the ventral surface of the brainstem; and the nucleus prepositus hypoglossi of the rostral dorsomedial medulla (PrH), corresponding to the localization of C3 adrenergic neurones near the dorsal surface of the medulla bordering the fourth ventricle (Astier et al., 1990; Aston-Jones et al., 1986, 1990; Bloom et al., 1989; Ennis and Aston-Jones, 1986; Guyenet and Young, 1987; Figure 4–11). Minor inputs to the LC derive from the dorsal cap of the PVN and from the intermediate zone of the spinal gray region. Whereas the ACE and the NTS project heavily to nearby parabrachial area neurons, results using new tract tracing techniques have not confirmed direct innervation of the LC from these two areas. LC cell bodies also receive noradrenergic innervation via collateral axons from other LC cells, helping to explain concerted discharges of LC cells during sensory responses and concerted inhibition of firing during paradoxical sleep (Aston-Jones et al., 1990).

The two sources of afferents to the LC seem to exert different functions mediated by different transmitters. Stimulation of the PGi area predominantly excites LC neurons, possibly via an excitatory amino acid acting at kainate receptors (Aston-Jones et al., 1990). If one considers the presence of C1 cells in the PGi region, PGi stimulation may also release an agonist occupying inhibitory α_2-adrenoceptors in the LC. Stimulation of the PrH area generally inhibits LC firing, possibly by release of an inhibitory amino acid. The neuroanatomic and neurophysiologic findings have led to the suggestion that LC neurons receive phasic, excitatory inputs in response to sensory stimulation and tonic, inhibitory input that modulates LC excitability in different behavioral states (Aston-Jones et al., 1990).

The restricted afferent control of the LC from the lower brainstem indicates no direct forebrain regulation of LC firing, whereas the diffuse forebrain projections from the LC suggest a possible role of the LC in global functions such as ''gating,'' ''enabling,'' and ''vigilance.'' According to one hypothesis (Everitt et al., 1990), the LC exerts a nonspecific influence that affects information processing in discrete terminal regions, with the functional effects depending on the concurrent state of activation in those regions.

Directionally similar changes in LC activity and sympathoneural activity (or plasma NE levels) often occur during a variety of experimental manipulations that have been categorized along two dimensions: internal vs. external and noxious vs. nonnoxious. Manipulations of blood pressure via administration of vasoactive drugs exemplify internal, nonnoxious stimuli. Acute increases in blood pressure decrease both LC and peripheral (splanchnic or renal) sympathoneural activity, and acute decreases in blood pressure induced by nitroprusside administration increase both LC and peripheral sympathoneural activity (Curtis et al., 1993; Elam et al., 1984, 1985). Systemic infusion of phenylephrine to produce arterial hypertension decreases release of NE, measured using a push-pull cannula, in the LC (Singewald et al., 1993). Nitroprusside-induced activation of LC neurons depends at least partly on CRH, since icv administration of the CRH antagonist α-helical CRH$_{9-41}$ attenuates the activation (Curtis et al., 1993). Hemorrhage transiently increases and then often decreases sympathoneural activity, whereas increased LC firing persists (Elam et al., 1985). Bilateral cervical vagotomy abolishes both the central LC and peripheral sympathoneural responses to hemorrhage and abolishes the LC responses but leaves intact the peripheral responses to manipulations of blood pressure, suggesting that the LC responds sensitively to input from the low-pressure cardiopulmonary baroreceptors (Elam et al., 1985; Figure 4–12).

The putative role of the LC in arousal or vigilance may provide a teleological explanation for the sensitivity of LC neurons to information about changes in cardiac filling. In human evolution, orthostasis has been the most common cause of decreases in cardiac filling. When vigilant, we stand erect—we ''*stand* guard.'' When failing to concentrate on our work, we ''lay down on the job.'' When we awaken, we wake *up*.

The LC also responds to changes in input from other interoceptors. Elam, Thoren et al. (1986) reported that stretch of the walls of the bladder, distal colon, or stomach

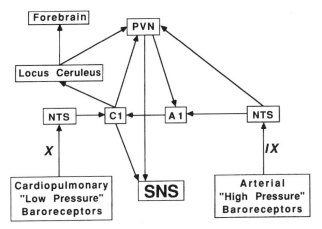

Figure 4–12. Hypothetical schema to explain sensitivity of locus ceruleus to alterations in cardiac filling. Afferents from cardiac low-pressure baroreceptors travel in the vagus (X) nerve, whereas afferents from the carotid high-pressure baroreceptors travel in the glossopharyngeal (IX) nerve. The locus ceruleus (LC) receives innervation from the rostral ventrolateral medullary region corresponding to the C1 cells. Perhaps the LC is more closely linked to the adrenergic C1 cells than the noradrenergic A1 cells of the caudal ventrolateral medulla, whereas the paraventricular nucleus of the hypothalamus (PVN) is more closely linked to the noradrenergic A1 cells of the caudal ventrolateral medulla than to the C1 cells of the rostral ventrolateral medulla.

increased LC firing, even when splanchnic sympathoneural activity was unchanged. These findings lead to the suggestion that the LC may participate in anxiety-induced micturition, irritable bowel syndrome, or the intense alarm reaction associated with vomiting. Patients with nocturnal asthma can report dreaming of suffocating or drowning just before awakening with an attack, and healthy people can dream about rushing to find a bathroom just before they awaken to urinate. One may speculate that in these situations, intense interoceptive input evokes cortical activation via pathways through the LC. Since stimulation of cutaneous nociceptors activates LC neurons in anesthetized rats (Elam, Svensson et al., 1986), LC responses to exteroceptive noxious stimulation do not require consciousness.

LC neurons in cats do not seem responsive to nondistressing exteroceptive input (Jacobs, 1990). LC single-unit activity increases in cats exhibiting defense reactions during exposure to an aggressive cat or to a dog, but LC activity does not increase upon exposure to a nonaggressive cat (Levine et al., 1990). The authors suggested that presenting a cat to another cat would be activating but would not necessarily elicit distress, whereas presenting a barking dog to a cat would be activating as well as distressing to the cat. In contrast, Aston-Jones and Bloom (1981b) reported robust LC responses to nondistressing exteroceptive input in rats. Inconsistencies among studies on this topic may to some extent have resulted from inadequate attention to defining characteristics of distress and to the validity of indices of distress in animals.

During rapid eye movement (REM) sleep, LC firing decreases markedly or disappears

(Aston-Jones and Bloom, 1981a; Aston-Jones et al., 1990), yet heart rate and coronary artery flow increase episodically, stellate ganglionectomy abolishes the hemodynamic responses (Verrier and Dickerson, 1991), and skeletal muscle sympathoneural activity increases (Somers et al., 1993). LC neuronal activity and peripheral sympathoneural activity therefore change differentially in this situation.

Administration of a wide variety of pharmacological agents affects the firing rate of LC neurons. Tricyclic antidepressants, GABA, clonidine, μ-opiate agonists, and cocaine decrease firing rates of LC neurons (Abercrombie and Jacobs, 1987a; Aston-Jones et al., 1990; Bird and Kuhar, 1977; Cedarbaum and Aghajanian, 1977; Pitts and Marwah, 1987; Valentino et al., 1990). The α_2-adrenoceptor antagonist yohimbine, acetylcholine (via stimulation of local muscarinic receptors), and CRH increase LC firing (Rasmussen and Jacobs, 1986; Valentino and Foote, 1988).

The model of a central noradrenergic neuron in Figure 4–13 can explain many drug effects on LC firing and release of NE from terminals of LC neurons. This model includes release of NE not only from synaptic but also from axonal varicosities, so that noradrenergic occupation of α_2-adrenoceptors on the cell bodies inhibits cellular firing, and noradrenergic occupation of α_2-adrenoceptors on the terminals inhibits NE release for a given amount of terminal depolarization. Drugs that block Uptake-1 would increase NE concentrations at the inhibitory α_2-adrenoceptors on the cell body, decreas-

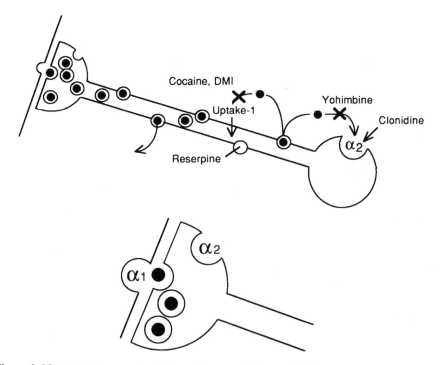

Figure 4–13. Model of a central noradrenergic neuron. This model helps to explain the actions and interactions of drugs commonly used in neurology, cardiology, and psychiatry.

ing cell firing, yet augmenting extracellular fluid NE concentrations in the terminal region. α_2-Adrenoceptor blockers such as yohimbine would elicit large increases in extracellular fluid NE levels in regions innervated by noradrenergic centers such as the LC, due to the combined effects of increased cell firing and augmented NE release.

Electrical stimulation of the LC increases blood pressure (Ward and Gunn, 1976). Since ipsilateral ablation of the RVLM abolishes the pressor response, the pathway mediating the response traverses this region. These findings do not imply a direct neuronal connection from the LC to the RVLM, catecholaminergic mediation of the effect in the RVLM, or dependence of the pressor response on activation of LC cells as opposed to stimulation of fibers in passage. Local administration of glutamate in the LC has been reported to increase (Kawasaki et al., 1991) or decrease (Miyawaki et al., 1991) blood pressure. At intensities or doses that do not affect blood pressure, electrical or chemical stimulation of the LC acutely decreases arterial baroreflex-cardiac gain (Chan et al., 1992).

Because the LC is the main source of NE pathways in the brain, many hypotheses about the role of central neural NE in the state of awakeness, learning and memory, vigilance behavior, physiological stress and coping responses, depression, and panic/anxiety disorders have focused on pathways emanating from the LC. The section about central catecholaminergic pathways later in this chapter considers these hypotheses in detail.

A5 Region

In contrast with the mainly ascending noradrenergic projections from the LC of the pons, more than 90% of the neurons in the A5 noradrenergic region of the ventrolateral pons project caudally to preganglionic neurons in the spinal intermediolateral cell columns (Loewy et al., 1979; McCall, 1990). A5 neurons also project heavily to the perifornical area of the hypothalamus, the midbrain periaquaductal gray region, the parabrachial area, the NTS, and the ACE (Byrum and Guyenet, 1987; Figure 4–14).

Whereas electrical stimulation of the A5 region increases blood pressure, chemical stimulation with glutamate decreases blood pressure. Intracerebroventricular (icv) administration of 6-OHDA abolishes the glutamate-induced depressor response (Loewy et al., 1986). Thus, excitatory fibers of passage may traverse the A5 area, whereas the perikarya may use NE as an inhibitory neurotransmitter. Microinjection of 6-OHDA in the NTS or the intermediolateral cell columns attenuates the depressor response to A5 stimulation, suggesting inhibitory noradrenergic effects mediated by terminals from A5 neurons in these regions.

Blood pressure responses only indirectly reflect sympathoneural responses. Huangfu et al. (1992) assessed effects of the neuronal excitant N-methyl-D-aspartate (NMDA) injected in the A5 region on directly recorded regional sympathetic neural activity in anesthetized rats. NMDA increased splanchnic and renal sympathetic discharges but usually decreased lumbar sympathetic discharges, with splanchnic vascular resistance correspondingly increased and femoral resistance decreased. Baroreflex gain increased, and blood pressure and heart rate decreased slightly. Results of pharmacological studies indicated that the sympathoexcitatory effects of A5 neuronal activation depended on

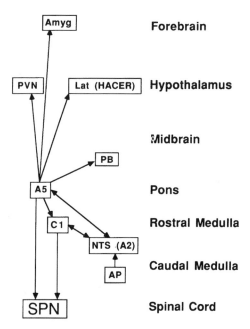

Figure 4–14. Central neural sites connected to the pontine–A5 area. Same abbreviations as in Figure 4–1.

binding of released NE to postsynaptic α_1-adrenoceptors at projection sites in the spinal cord. Thus, in contrast with diffusely increased SNS outflow and vasoconstriction evoked by stimulation of RVLM cells, activation of A5 cells elicits a complex pattern of regional sympathetic and hemodynamic changes. Because of the reliance on anesthetized, paralyzed animals, the relevance of this pattern to neurobehavioral phenomena such as exercise, emotion, and vigilance in conscious individuals is unknown. Also unknown is whether A5 stimulation increases AHS activity.

Hypothalamus

The hypothalamus is the main subcortical center regulating sympathetic activity. The present conception proposes only indirect hypothalamic regulation of sympathetic activity, with the actual "goal" the expression of coordinated, patterned responses of several neuroendocrine systems, including the SNS and AHS, to produce metabolic, circulatory, and behavioral effects. In contrast with Selye's doctrine of nonspecificity, the present stress theory depends importantly on the primitive specificity and adaptive significance of hypothalamically generated response patterns. Learning, memory, attention, and motivational aspects, involving limbic and higher cortical centers, probably modify elicitation of these patterns (Figure 4–3).

    Although most investigators on the topic would agree that clusters of hypothalamic cells determine expression of patterned neuroendocrine responses during stress, little is known about interactions among these clusters during different stress responses. Instead, investigators have usually attempted to identify "regulatory" centers or neurochemical pathways for particular systems or for hemodynamic parameters in anesthetized animals, independent of the behaviors subserved under more naturalistic conditions.

Extirpation of the cerebral cortices of cats or dogs does not eliminate and tends to exaggerate emotional behaviors and the physiological changes accompanying those behaviors (Goltz, 1892). Removal of cortical inhibition explains "sham rage" in decorticate animals (Cannon and Britton, 1925; Bard, 1928). The most rostral portion of the neuraxis required for elicitation of "sham rage" is the posterior hypothalamus (Bard, 1928). Although Cannon and Bard initially ascribed to the thalamus the main role in expression of emotional behaviors, Hess and others subsequently focused on the hypothalamus, distinguishing an anterior "trophotropic" zone, involved with vegetative, inwardly directed, responses and an "ergotrophic" posterior zone, stimulation of which elicits defensive or attack behavior (Hess, 1949). Hess received the Nobel Prize for Physiology and Medicine in 1949.

A key concept follows from the early findings of Cannon and Bard about sham rage in decorticate animals: Whereas medullary mechanisms determining sympathetic outflow subserve relatively simple homeostatic reflexes, higher centers can modify activity of the medullary centers by resetting the reflexes, in essence redefining homeostasis.

One can view the hypothalamus as consisting of several groups of cells that transduce environmental perceptions and emotional experiences into neuroendocrine and autonomic responses. Stimulation or destruction of hypothalamic nuclei produces disturbances of blood pressure, body temperature, drinking, eating, sexual activity, emotional behavior, and sleep, all accompanied by changes in sympathoneural activity (Hess, 1949). The PVN and lateral hypothalamic area have received particular attention as sites of origin for both direct and indirect projections to the SPNs; these hypothalamic regions in turn receive input from several lower brainstem nuclei responsible for homeostatic circulatory regulation (Figure 4–15), as well as from the limbic cortex.

The hypothalamus contains particularly high concentrations of NE. Sources of the noradrenergic projections to the hypothalamus, discussed below, include the medullary A1 and A2 noradrenergic cells and, to a lesser extent, the pontine A6 cells.

Electrical stimulation of different hypothalamic regions can elicit markedly different patterns of responses of plasma NE and EPI levels and associated cardiovascular responses (Stoddard-Apter et al., 1983; Stoddard et al., 1986a). When hypothalamic stimulation elicits "fight or flight" behavior, however, plasma levels of both catecholamines virtually always increase (Stoddard et al., 1986b).

Traditionally, the hypothalamus has been divided neuroanatomically into three longitudinal zones (periventricular, medial, and lateral) and 4 rostrocaudal levels (preoptic, supraoptic, tuberal, and mammillary; Swanson, 1987)—that is, into 12 compartments. This parceling does not correspond well to neurochemical localization. For instance, magnocellular neurons, which synthesize AVP and oxytocin and project to the posterior pituitary gland, cluster in both the PVN and supraoptic nucleus (SON) and are also scattered throughout the rostral hypothalamus (Swanson, 1987).

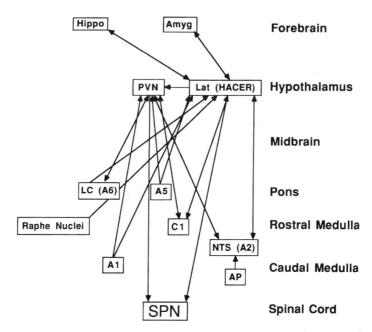

Figure 4–15. Central neural sites connected to the hypothalamus. Same abbreviations as in Figure 4–1.

The periventricular zone contains magnocellular neurosecretory cells that regulate posterior pituitary function and parvocellular cells that project to autonomic centers in the brainstem and spinal cord. This zone also contains the suprachiasmatic nucleus, which receives input from the retina and appears to generate neuroendocrine and behavioral circadian rhythms. Inputs to the periventricular zone derive from the lateral and medial zones; the bed nucleus of the stria terminalis (BNST), a major way-station for fibers from the amygdala and hippocampus; some brainstem cell groups; and the circumventricular subfornical organ (SFO).

The medial zone appears to receive cognitive inputs from the limbic system and, to a lesser extent, visceral inputs from lower brainstem sites, relaying ascending or descending information via the medial forebrain bundle especially to the lateral hypothalamic zone, the amygdala and septum, midbrain central gray region, and portions of the periventricular zone. The mammillary body in the medial zone may participate in learning and memory processes, the ventromedial nucleus in lordosis reflexes, and the medial preoptic area in parental and thermoregulatory behaviors.

The lateral zone is thought to participate in cortical arousal and autonomic and cardiovascular accompaniments of emotional behaviors, as discussed below. Cells in this zone often project to the periventricular zone, the limbic system, the telencephalon, and cells of origin of effector somatomotor and autonomic systems.

Posterolateral Hypothalamus

Hess's work indicated an important role for the posterolateral hypothalamus in the coordinated expression of emotional behaviors such as eating and drinking, aggression, and reproduction. He characterized the feline "defense response" in terms of a constellation of behavioral signs: alerting, turning the head, arching the back, mydriasis, ear flattening, piloerection, hissing, growling, and claw-baring, culminating in sudden, directed attack accompanied by marked cardiovascular changes.

Electrical stimulation of the "defense area" in the posterior hypothalamus increases heart rate and blood pressure by increasing sympathetic outflow to most vascular beds and increasing nerve traffic to the adrenal gland (Yoshimatsu et al., 1987), with preserved skeletal muscle blood flow (Folkow, 1982), probably due to activation of sympathetic vasodilator nerves in skeletal muscle (Eliasson et al., 1951) and to adrenomedullary secretion of EPI. Increases in circulating catecholamines during defense reactions evoked by hypothalamic electrical stimulation in freely moving cats (Stoddard et al., 1986a, 1986b) confirm a relationship between hypothalamically elicited defense behavior and peripheral catecholaminergic activation. Electrical stimulation affects fibers in passage as well as neuronal cell bodies; however, Bandler (1984) found that microinjections of excitatory amino acids to activate neuronal perikarya in the lateral hypothalamus and periaquaductal gray area also evoke somatomotor and autonomic changes characteristic of defensive attack.

Lateral hypothalamic neurons appear to mediate conditioned, sympathetically mediated cardiovascular responses, and the neurocirculatory accompaniments of emotional behaviors depend on this integrative function. Thus, Iwata et al. (1986b) reported that lesions of the lateral hypothalamus attenuated classically conditioned blood pressure responses, whereas unconditioned pressor responses to electric shock and conditioned behavioral responses were preserved.

Smith and co-workers have suggested that in nonhuman primates, the cells determining cardiovascular responses during the defense reaction reside in the lateral hypothalamus–perifornical area (Smith et al., 1990). The authors named this region the "HACER," standing for "hypothalamic area controlling emotional responses." The scattered HACER cells project both to the SPNs (Smith and DeVito, 1984) and to the RVLM, without forming a discrete nucleus. Stimulation of HACER cells produces rapid renal vasoconstriction (followed by a return to baseline and then a second period of vasoconstriction), tachycardia, hypertension, and delayed increases in skeletal muscle blood flow. The late renal vasoconstriction and skeletal vasodilation may result from accumulation of circulating EPI. Injection of the neuroexcitotoxin ibotenic acid into the HACER region attenuates or abolishes the hemodynamic responses (Smith et al., 1990).

In baboons, destruction of the HACER region eliminates the autonomically mediated cardiovascular responses, without altering the behavioral manifestations of conditioned emotional responses (Smith et al., 1980; Smith and DeVito, 1984)—findings analogous to those noted above in rats (Iwata et al., 1986b). HACER cells therefore may link behavioral with autonomic concomitants of emotion.

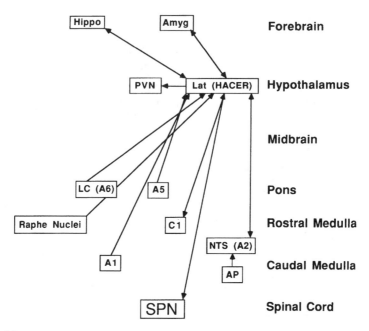

Figure 4–16. Central neural sites connected to the lateral hypothalamic area for controlling emotional responses (''HACER''). Same abbreviations as in Figure 4–1.

Dense descending inputs to the lateral hypothalamus arise from the amygdala, septum, and hippocampus (Swanson, 1987; Figure 4–16), and pontine A6 and A7 and medullary A1 and A2 cells provide ascending noradrenergic input to the posterolateral hypothalamus (Fort et al., 1990; Sakai et al., 1990). The posterior hypothalamus of the cat also receives dopaminergic input from groups A8, A9, and A10, adrenergic input from C1 cells of the RVLM, serotonergic input from raphe nuclei, cholinergic input from the parabrachial pons and PGi, and input from cells containing peptides such as met-enkephalin, substance P, and CRH (Fort et al., 1990; Sakai et al., 1990).

Projections from the lateral hypothalamus reach virtually the entire central nervous system, including the cortical mantle, amygdala and septum, parts of the thalamus, most of the rest of the hypothalamus, at least 20 lower brainstem sites (often with reciprocal innervation of the lateral hypothalamus), and the spinal cord (Swanson, 1987).

Posterior hypothalamic stimulation interferes with arterial baroreflex–cardiac responses (Gebber and Synder, 1970; Hilton, 1963). Conversely, sinoaortic baroreceptor denervation augments pressor, vasoconstrictor, and sympathoneural responses to posterior hypothalamic stimulation (Barron and Heesch, 1990).

Anteroventral Third Ventricle (AV3V) Region

The anteroventral third ventricle region of the hypothalamus (AV3V) participates in neurocirculatory adjustments to regulate body fluids. This rather large area includes the OVLT, the median preoptic nucleus, and the periventricular preoptic nucleus. The median preoptic nucleus receives afferents from the SFO, parabrachial nucleus, and several catecholaminergic nuclei of the brainstem. Efferents project to the parabrachial nucleus, PVN, SFO, NTS, VLM, and the periaquaductal gray, from which relays probably project to brainstem regions regulating sympathoneural outflows.

Stimulation of the AV3V region as a whole produces a pattern of modestly decreased blood pressure, splanchnic and renal vasoconstriction, skeletal vasodilation, and bradycardia—reminiscent of vasovagal reactions. Stimulation of discrete areas within the AV3V region, however, can elicit selective vascular responses (Mangiapane and Brody, 1987).

Acute AV3V lesions cause adipsia, hypernatremia, and dehydration. Upon full recovery, fluid balance, blood pressure, and behavior appear normal. AV3V lesions abolish dipsogenic and pressor responses to centrally administered AII and protect rats from developing one-kidney, low-renin renal hypertension and two-kidney, one-clip, high-renin renovascular hypertension. The median preoptic nucleus in the AV3V appears to be required for the acute pressor and dipsogenic actions of centrally administered AII and for hypertension resulting from sinoaortic deafferentiation (Brody et al., 1986). AV3V lesions also ameliorate or prevent hypertension resulting from NTS lesions or deoxycorticosterone/salt administration but do not affect development of hypertension in the Okamoto strain of spontaneously hypertensive rats. Ventromedial hypothalamic–median eminence lesions produce about the same pattern of antihypertensive effects as do AV3V lesions.

Paraventricular Nucleus (PVN)

The PVN contains noncatecholaminergic, AVP-synthesizing magnocellular neurons that project to the median eminence (a relay center for anterior pituitary release of ACTH), to the posterior pituitary (the site of oxytocin and AVP secretion, Li et al., 1988), and to the lower brainstem and spinal cord. Cells in three locations provide the main innervation of the magnocellular neurons (Sawchenko and Swanson, 1982; Swanson, 1986, 1987)—the A1 region of the CVLM, the SFO, and the median preoptic nucleus (Figure 4–17). Pathways from the A2 medullary region and LC may also reach dendrites of PVN cells (Silverman et al., 1985). The A1 cells of the CVLM provide the main source of ascending baroreceptor information to the PVN magnocellular neurons (Sawchenko and Swanson, 1982).

The PVN also contains parvocellular neurons that synthesize many peptides, including CRH, enkephalins, cholecystokinin, and (in adrenalectomized animals) AVP and AII. AVP, CRH, and AII all can stimulate pituitary release of ACTH, and circulating glucocorticoids feedback-inhibit synthesis of all three peptides. The dorsomedial parvocellular portion of the nucleus contains densely concentrated CRH neurons that project heavily to the median eminence (Swanson, 1987), where CRH is released into the portal circulation to the anterior pituitary. The cerebral cortex provides indirect input to the CRH-synthesizing cells in the PVN, via the hippocampus and amygdala through the BNST (Swanson, 1987). Neurons in this same dorsomedial parvocellular region of the PVN receive noradrenergic, adrenergic, serotonergic, and NPY innervation. The noradrenergic innervation of the parvocellular neurons arises mainly from the A2 cells

PATHWAYS TO PARVOCELLULAR PVN

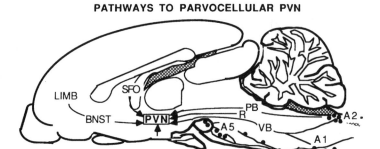

PATHWAYS TO MAGNOCELLULAR PVN

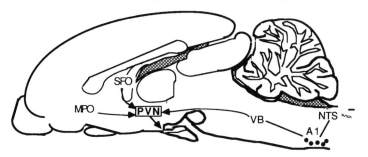

Figure 4-17. Brain pathways to the parvocellular (Top) and magnocellular (Bottom) cells of the paraventricular nucleus (PVN) of the hypothalamus. R = raphe nuclei; VB = ventral noradrenergic bundle; SFO = subfornical organ; BNST = basal nucleus of the stria terminalis; LIMB = limbic system; MPO = median preoptic area. Other abbreviations as in Figure 4–1.

of the NTS, the adrenergic innervation from the C1–C3 cells, and the serotonergic innervation from midbrain raphe nuclei. Afferents from the NTS to the parvocellular region also ascend indirectly via the parabrachial nucleus and A1 and C1 cells (Sawchenko and Swanson, 1981a; Yamashita et al., 1989).

Consistent with an ascending noradrenergic relay of baroreceptor information from the medulla to the PVN, manipulations producing changes in blood pressure elicit reciprocal changes in NE overflow in the PVN, measured using a miniaturized push-pull technique (Qualy and Westfall, 1993). This approach does not distinguish parvocellular from magnocellular sites of release from noradrenergic terminals.

Parvocellular neurons of the PVN send long descending axons to the NTS, to the dorsal motor nucleus of the vagus in the medulla, and directly to SPNs (Sawchenko and Swanson, 1981a, 1981b, 1982; Swanson, 1987; Figure 4–18). Although these cells contain at least nine possible neurotransmitters, the neurotransmitter or transmitters used by the parvocellular PVN cells in producing sympathoexcitation have not yet been identified.

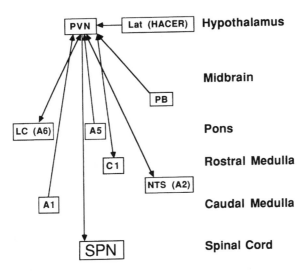

Figure 4–18. Central neural sites connected to the paraventricular nucleus of the hypothalamus. Same abbreviations as in Figure 4–1.

Electrical stimulation of the PVN in rats evokes a circulatory pattern reminiscent of that accompanying the defense reaction in cats, with increased sympathoneural outflow, tachycardia, hypertension, renal and splanchnic vasoconstriction, inhibition of barore-flex-mediated bradycardia, and skeletal muscle vasodilation (Kannan et al., 1989; Porter and Brody, 1985). The hindlimb vasodilator response seems to depend on adrenomed-ullary release of EPI, since bilateral adrenalectomy attenuates the hindlimb vasodilation without affecting the vasoconstriction in other beds. Porter and Brody (1985) suggested that the pathway from the PVN to the NTS may specifically mediate adrenomedullary catecholamine secretion and that the pathway from the PVN to the RVLM may specifically mediate sympathoneural vasoconstriction. This model has not been tested directly by measuring sympathetic and adrenal neural activity or plasma levels of catecholamines. Whereas magnocellular stimulation produces skeletal muscle vasodilation, stimulation of the parvocellular PVN produces skeletal muscle vasoconstriction (Porter and Brody, 1986b). The neurochemical basis for this distinction remains unknown.

Microinjection of glutamate to stimulate cell bodies in the PVN increases blood pressure and renal sympathetic activity. Local application of kainic acid, which also stimulates cell bodies acutely, produces behavioral excitation, increased locomotion, hypertension, tachycardia, and decreased baroreflex–cardiac sensitivity. Local injection of NMDA produces excitotoxic lesions of the PVN. At 26 days after NMDA administration into the PVN of rats, lesioned animals have normal resting blood pressure, heart rate, and baroreflex–cardiac sensitivity (Rockhold et al., 1990), despite extensive loss of parvocellular neurons. In contrast, immediately after recovery from anesthesia, the animals have behavioral excitation, hypertension, and tachycardia, and histologic examination of hearts removed 48 hours after NMDA injection in the PVN reveals catecholamine-induced myocardial necrosis.

PVN stimulation can activate the same cell bodies of the NTS that antidromic vagal stimulation activates, suggesting direct connections between the PVN, NTS, and the dorsal motor nucleus of the vagus. The PVN therefore probably plays a role in modulation of baroreflexes.

Surgical or electrolytic lesions of the PVN attenuate the development of hypertension in spontaneously hypertensive and DOCA-salt hypertensive rats (Ciriello et al., 1984) and prevent increases in blood pressure after aortic baroreceptor denervation (Zhang and Ciriello, 1982).

Although the PVN cells synthesize AVP, and although exogenously administered AVP increases blood pressure, the hypertension produced by PVN stimulation in rats does not depend on AVP release, since PVN stimulation in Brattleboro rats, which lack hypothalamic and spinal AVP, nevertheless produces a pressor response (Brody et al., 1986).

In primates, electrical stimulation in the region of the PVN does not produce increases in blood pressure exceeding 5 mmHg (Smith et al., 1990). Unilateral ablation of the PVN also does not interfere with cardiovascular responses to electrical stimulation of the HACER region. Thus, the extent to which the PVN mediates autonomic outflow and reflexive cardiovascular controls seems to vary among species. The neurotransmitter or neurotransmitters involved have not been identified. Interactions between the PVN and HACER regions of the hypothalamus in mediating emotional behaviors and autonomic activation during stress require more attention.

Limbic System

Papez (1937) suggested that parts of the brain originally called the "rhinencephalon" (fornix, mammillary bodies, anterior thalamic nuclei, and parahippocampal and cingulate gyri) subserve not merely olfaction, as the etymology implies, but emotion.

Soon after Papez published his hypothesis, Kluver and Bucy (1939) reported the effects of partial temporal lobe lesions in monkeys. The lesions included the entire amygdala and large parts of the parahippocampal gyrus, the hippocampus, and the temporal neocortex. The monkeys, previously rather ferocious, became docile, without evidence of fear or rage, developed a persistent apparent compulsion to examine objects orally, exhibited bizarre sexual behavior, including indiscriminate associations with males and females, and had "psychic blindness"—exemplified by an inability to discriminate between food and possibly dangerous objects. The docility, altered sexual behavior, and orality became known as the "Kluver–Bucy" syndrome.

Subsequently, several reports described docility, with little fear or anger, after bilateral lesions of the amygdaloid complex. In humans, bilateral lesioning of the amygdaloid complex decreases aggressive behavior, normalizes antisocial behavior, or reduces emotional excitability (Green et al., 1951; Narabayashi et al., 1963; Pool, 1954), without producing other signs of the Kluver–Bucy syndrome and without affecting memory.

Maclean (1955) proposed that the "limbic system" (from the Latin *limbus,* referring to a border or edge) encircling the brainstem provides the main functional connection between the cerebral cortex and hypothalamus. The limbic system includes the structures of the limbic lobe (the subcallosal, cingulate, and parahippocampal gyri) and associated subcortical nuclei (including the amygdaloid complex, septal nuclei, hypothalamus, epithalamus, anterior thalamic nuclei, and portions of the basal ganglia). Researchers have differed in their definitions for the exact components of the system.

Amygdala

Most recent research about the limbic system and neuroendocrine function during stress has concentrated on the amygdala, in the temporal lobe. Among limbic structures, the amygdala is unique in that it has direct anatomic connections both to neocortex and to brainstem regions involved with autonomic outflow (Gray, 1991a). Efferents from the central nucleus of the amygdala (ACE) descend via the perifornical region of the hypothalamus (Hilton and Zbrozyna, 1963), suggesting a role in conditioned fear responses and defense reactions (Reis and Ledoux, 1987). Direct descending projections from the amygdala to the NTS, the dorsal motor nucleus of the vagus, and the C1 neurons of the RVLM (Cassell and Gray, 1989; Schwaber et al., 1980) provide a potential neuroanatomic substrate for modulatory influences of the amygdala on baroreflex regulation of sympathoneural outflow.

Medullary catecholaminergic cells constitute a potentially important source of ascending innervation of the ACE. Roder and Ciriello (1993) used the retrograde tracer fluorogold, the anterograde tracer *Phaseolus vulgaris* leucoagglutinin, and immunohistochemistry to demonstrate that neurons in the ventrolateral medulla throughout its rostrocaudal extent project predominantly contralaterally to the ACE and that almost 1/2 of the neurons also contain immunoreactive TH or PNMT.

The cell bodies and nerve terminals in the ACE contain at least 16 different neuropeptides (Brown and Gray, 1988; Gray, 1991b), and peptide-containing efferents from the ACE innervate the BNST, the lateral hypothalamus, the PVN, the substantia nigra, the central gray, the raphe nuclei, the parabrachial nucleus, the LC, the VLM, and the NTS (Gray, 1991b). The ACE also receives catecholaminergic and noncatecholaminergic inputs from the A1 region of the CVLM and the A2 cells of the NTS, with relatively few projections from the LC (Due and Schwaber, 1990). Local injection of CRH, thyrotropin-releasing factor, or calcitonin gene-related peptide into the amygdala increases plasma catecholamine concentrations.

The physiological meanings of the numerous peptidergic and catecholaminergic cells and terminals in the amygdala remain obscure. Gray (1991a, 1991b) has proposed a model involving amygdaloid catecholaminergic pathways in autonomic and circulatory responses during stress. According to this model, pathways from the amygdala to A8 and A9 dopaminergic cells participate in startle, locomotor, and thermoregulatory responses; pathways to the LC noradrenergic cells participate in arousal and facilitation; and pathways to the NTS and C1 cells of the RVLM participate in autonomic outflow, both directly and indirectly via alterations in baroreflex function. One problem with this model is that tract-tracing studies have failed to confirm any direct input to the LC from the amygdala. Instead, the amygdala projects to the adjacent parabrachial area (Aston-Jones et al., 1990). Gray (1991b) maintains that innervation of the caudal NTS, the RVLM, and the continuum of dopaminergic cells in the midbrain may still provide a substrate for regulation of autonomic outflow by the amygdala.

In humans, amygdaloid stimulation increases blood pressure, produces pupillary dilation, and can evoke anxiety or fear, although the physiological changes can also occur without changes in mood or somatic responses (Chapman et al., 1954). In animals, amygdaloid stimulation elicits neuroendocrine and circulatory responses reminiscent of the "defense reaction," with depletion of cerebral NE (Reis and Gunne, 1965) and increased plasma levels of NE (Brown and Gray, 1988).

One may hypothesize that the amygdala provides a medium for relaying to the brainstem input based on conscious evaluation and interpretation of stressors (Gray, 1991b)—that is, simulations, as in Dawkins's selfish gene theory discussed in Chapter 1. Thus, amygdaloid destruction blunts measures of fear and anxiety and learned visceral responses to fear-evoking stimuli (Gray, 1991a). During aversive emotional conditioning in rats, blood pressure responses to acoustic stimuli involve transmission of the sensory signal through the amygdala (Reis and Ledoux, 1987). Lesions of the central amygdala blunt pressor and heart rate responses to classically conditioned aversive cues in rats (Iwata et al., 1986a). Cryogenic blockade of the ACE also attenuates conditioned blood pressure and respiratory responses (Zhang et al., 1986). Moreover, the basolateral amygdaloid nucleus, a site of origin of inputs to the ACE, contains a high concentration of benzodiazepine receptors (Niehoff and Kuhar, 1983), suggesting that anxiolytic drugs may work in this region.

Based on Maclean's conceptualization of the "triune brain" (Maclean, 1955, 1970) and on the classic findings of Cannon and Bard about "sham rage" in decorticate animals, it has been thought that the cerebral cortex exerts mainly restraining influences on lower centers regulating autonomic responses (Galosy et al., 1981; Timms, 1977). If the amygdala were the medium for cortical inhibition, this would contrast with the above-cited evidence suggesting an excitatory role of the amygdala in emotional behaviors. In rats and tree shrews, spontaneous changes in extracellular fluid levels of catecholamines obtained using a push-pull cannula in the central amygdala occur concurrently with changes in levels of catecholamines in plasma (Dietl, 1985). Microdialysis studies have indicated that immobilization in rats produces increases in NE release, reuptake, and metabolism in the basolateral nucleus (Tanaka et al., 1991) and ACE (Pacak, Palkovits et al., 1993). Elucidation of the role of the amygdala in stress responses will require more studies of regional neurochemical changes in conscious, behaving individuals.

Hippocampus

The hippocampus receives noradrenergic projections virtually exclusively from the LC. In conscious rats with a microdialysis probe in the hippocampus, immobilization stress, systemic administration of yohimbine, or local blockade of α_2-adrenoceptors increases dialysate NE concentrations (Abercrombie et al., 1988; Thomas and Holman, 1991).

Considering the role of the hippocampus in memory, noradrenergic activation of the hippocampus may facilitate the long-term memory of distressing events. Thus, when chronically stressed rats undergo exposure to a novel stressor, both NE release (Nisenbaum et al., 1991) and tyrosine hydroxylation (Nisenbaum and Abercrombie, 1992) increase markedly in the hippocampus, providing a possible central neurochemical substrate for ''stressor switch hyper-responsiveness,'' or ''dishabituation,'' as discussed in Chapter 1.

Circumventricular Organs

Humoral input in cerebral regions lacking a blood–brain barrier may provide an additional means for central-autonomic neural interactions. These circumventricular sites include the SFO, median eminence, OVLT, and area postrema (AP, Figure 4–19).

Circulating hormones can act at these sites. AII receptors seem particularly concentrated in circumventricular organs. Injection of AII into blood supplying the head produces rapid increases in blood pressure (Bickerton and Buckley, 1961). AP ablation blunts the pressor effect of intravascular AII and blocks the chronic hypertension produced by long-term systemic administration of AII (Cox and Bishop, 1991). AII administered at very low doses into the SFO or OVLT of rats evokes thirst, AVP release, diffuse increases in sympathoneural traffic, and increased blood pressure, suggesting a role for circulating AII acting at these organs in countering hypotension or depletion of blood volume (Barnes and Ferrario, 1987). In cats, dogs, and rabbits, the AP constitutes the main site responsible for the pressor response to circulating AII; in rats, the AV3V (OVLT) and SFO are the main sites (Brody et al., 1991).

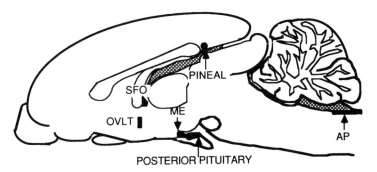

Figure 4–19. Circumventricular organs. SFO = subfornical organ; ME = median eminence; AP = area postrema; OVLT = organum vasculosum of the lamina terminalis.

Injection of AVP into the vertebral artery increases baroreflex–cardiac sensitivity and augments reflexive sympathoinhibition. AP lesions abolish the enhancement of baro-receptor–sympathoneural reflex gain (Bishop et al., 1987). Increases in endogenous AVP levels during osmotic stimulation also appear to augment baroreflex sensitivity by an action in the AP (Hasser et al., 1988). Suzuki et al. (1989) have suggested that circulating AVP inhibits renal sympathetic nerve activity indirectly via a pathway from the AP to the NTS.

Studies using the [^{14}C]deoxyglucose radioautographic technique in halothane-anes-thetized rats have revealed that electrical stimulation of the dorsocentral AP decreases blood pressure and increases medullary metabolic activity in the NTS, the dorsal motor nucleus of the vagus, and the A1 area; increases pontine metabolic activity in the LC and parabrachial nuclei; increases hypothalamic metabolic activity in the magnocellular and parvocellular regions of the PVN, the supraoptic and suprachiasmatic nuclei, and the median eminence; and increases metabolic activity in the pituitary gland (Gross et al., 1990). AP stimulation therefore appears to activate, directly or indirectly, many centers in the neuraxis involved with neurocirculatory and neuroendocrine regulation, with the net effect augmentation of baroreflexes (Hasser et al., 1987).

In rabbits, the AP appears to be the only source of catecholaminergic input to the C1 cells of the RVLM (Blessing et al., 1987).

The SFO interconnects extensively with other brainstem sites involved in autonomic oiutflows, including the NTS and dorsal motor nucleus of the vagus. SFO stimulation produces diffuse, sympathetically mediated vasoconstriction and increases in blood pressure, mediated at least partly by the PVN (Mangiapane and Brody, 1986; Ferguson and Renaud, 1984).

The OVLT, in the circumventricular portion of the AV3V region, probably contains osmoreceptors that relay through the AV3V region to effect AVP release.

Higher Cortical Centers

The neocortex has relatively few connections with the hypothalamus or other centers involved with autonomic outflow. Cannon hypothesized that the most "encephalized" parts of the brain regulate the experience and physiological manifestations of emotion (Cannon, 1931), determining the character and intensity of autonomic output.

Skinner (1985) has proposed that three output pathways from the orbitofrontal cortex participate in the autonomic activation following exposure to a stressor: The first proj-ects to the thalamus and influences sensory channels; the second projects to the temporal lobe and amygdala; and the third projects via the dorsal hypothalamus to the the lower brainstem. Consistent with the clinical relevance of these pathways to the cardiovascular consequences of stress, in pigs with myocardial ischemia, blockade of frontocortical-brainstem outflow prevents ventricular fibrillation (Skinner and Reed, 1981).

As noted in Chapter 1, Skinner (1985) has also suggested that stress is a cerebral reaction to a stimulus event, rather than an inherent feature of the stressor itself; this view affirms the importance of interpretive processes in the elaboration of stress response patterns. Patients with damaged frontal lobes have blunted conditioned visceral responses (Rochstroh et al., cited in Skinner, 1985); and in patients with frontal lobotomies, verbal reports and observed behaviors indicate attenuation or absence of the experience of distress (Teuber, 1964), with a corresponding lack of autonomic responses to stimuli expected to be emotionally arousing (Heilman et al., 1978).

Neuropeptides and Other Central Neurotransmitters in the Regulation of Sympathetic Outflow

If relationships between central and peripheral catecholaminergic function seem complex and incompletely understood, relationships between other neurotransmitters in the brain and sympathoneural and adrenomedullary outflows seem even more so.

The list of neuropeptides and other compounds as candidate central neurotransmitters or neuromodulators potentially mediating sympathetic outflow has grown rapidly over the past decade and includes, but is by no means limited to acetylcholine, adenosine, AII, bombesin, cholecystokinin, clonidine-displacing substance, CRH, enkephalin, galanin, GABA, glutamate, NPY, neurophysin, nitric oxide (NO), substance P, thyrotropin-releasing hormone, and AVP.

Colocalization

Catecholamines and other neurotransmitters can occur in the same cells—a phenomenon first noted in peripheral sympathetic neurons and later in the central nervous system. Transmitters colocalized with NE include enkephalin, galanin, N-acetyl-aspartyl glutamate, NPY, neurophysin, and AVP (Holets, 1990).

This colocalization appears to have a degree of spatial differentiation among brain regions. For instance, NPY coexists with NE in medullary tegmental nuclei (Blessing et al., 1987; Hokfelt et al., 1983), relatively little in the LC, and virtually not at all in the A5 and A7 regions; and galanin, neurophysin, N-acetyl-aspartyl glutamate, and AVP coexist with NE in LC and lateral tegmental cell groups to varying extents (Holets, 1990). Although the LC contains GABA-ergic terminals, GABA does not appear to coexist with NE in the same cells.

Many studies have determined by immunohistochemical techniques the presence of putative neurotransmitters in projections to regions known to participate in cardiovascular regulation. For instance, NTS projections to the ACE, the BNST, and parabrachial and hypothalamic nuclei all contain somatostatin, met-enkephalin, dynorphin, NPY, and neurotensin (Riche et al., 1990). Projections from the NTS to the parabrachial nucleus also contain cholecystokinin, galanin, and CRH (Herbert and Saper, 1990); and projections from raphe nuclei to the NTS contain 5-HT and substance P (Thor and Helke, 1987). In the C1 region of the RVLM, thought to be a major source of outflow to the SPNs, potential neurotransmitter candidates identified immunohistochemically include GABA, acetylcholine, NPY, and substance P.

A technique combining transneuronal viral infection with immunohistochemistry can identify neurotransmitter candidates in brain regions projecting to SPNs (Strack et al., 1989a, 1989b). Infected cells in the raphe nuclei and ventromedial medulla contained

5-HT, substance P, thyrotropin-releasing hormone, met-enkephalin, and somatostatin. In the ventromedial and RVLM, infected cells contained PNMT, substance P, NPY, somatostatin, and enkephalin. In the A5 region, noradrenergic and somatostatin-containing cells become infected. In the dorsal parvocellular PVN, TH- and substance P-immunoreactive cells become infected.

The colocalization of catecholamines with other neurotransmitter candidates obviously leads to the possibility of functional specificity—neurochemical "coding." Peptide-containing LC neurons project preferentially to the hypothalamus compared with the spinal cord and cerebral cortex (Holets, 1990), and Sawchenko (1991) has suggested chemical coding of visceral sensory afferents to the PVN. No comprehensive theory about neurochemical coding, however, has emerged so far. This probably will require much more information about colocalization of NE and other neurotransmitters in nerve terminals as opposed to cell bodies and about corelease during neuronal activation.

Intracerebroventricular Administration

A commonly used experimental approach involves administration of compounds by the intracerebroventricular (icv) route and assessing the effects on efferent sympathetic nerve activity or plasma levels of catecholamines. Icv administration of several types of peptide affects plasma levels of catecholamines. These include releasing hormones such as CRH (Brown and Fisher, 1984) and thyrotropin-releasing hormone (Feuerstein et al., 1983), opiates (Siren et al., 1989), and peptides that are vasoactive in the periphery. Brown and Fisher (1984) reported that central administration of any of several neuropeptides (e.g., bombesin, CRH, thyrotropin-releasing hormone, β-endorphin, AII, AVP, cholecystokinin, met-enkephalin, and substance P) increases plasma catecholamine levels.

For most peptides that increase SNS outflow or plasma catecholamine levels when injected icv, the specific site or sites of central action remain unknown. Brown (1991) proposed that bombesin selectively increases plasma EPI concentrations when injected icv at low doses. In conscious rats, injection of as little as 5.7 pmol of bombesin into the rostral NTS produces marked increases in plasma EPI concentrations, suggesting the NTS may be a central neural site of action of this peptide.

Somatostatins constitute a peptide family including somatostatin-14 (SS-14), somatostatin-28 (SS-28), and des $AA^{1,2,3,4,5,12,13}[D\text{-}Trp^8]$-SS-14 (ODT8-SS). Originally noted for their growth hormone-inhibiting properties, somatostatins inhibit secretion by several types of neuroendocrine cells, and they appear to inhibit AHS outflow. Icv SS-14 decreases adrenal nerve activity (Somiya and Tonoue, 1984), and icv SS-28 or ODT8-SS selectively inhibits plasma EPI responses to CRH, bombesin, carbachol, insulin-induced hypoglycemia, and inhalation of ether vapor (Brown, 1991). Moreover, administration of cysteamine, which depletes brain somatostatins, augments adrenomedullary outflow (Brown, Fisher et al., 1985). These findings are also consistent with different central neural mechanisms of regulation of SNS and AHS outflows, a theme repeated in the chapter about stress response patterns.

Nitric oxide (NO) functions not only as the endothelium-derived relaxing factor but also possibly as a novel type of gaseous neurotransmitter in the brain and periphery. Systemic or icv administration of *N*-methylarginine, which inhibits NO synthase, increases blood pressure and sympathoneural traffic (Togashi et al., 1992), and intravenous arginine or cervical spinal cord transection abolishes these effects, suggesting that NO in the brain may restrain SNS vasoconstrictor outflow.

Results of studies using compounds injected icv are usually difficult to interpret. Effects of pharmacological doses may be unrelated to effects of the much smaller amounts of the endogenous compounds; icv administration results in unknown amounts of the drug at effector sites in the brain; drug concentrations at extrasynaptic receptors would be expected to exceed those at postsynaptic receptors, the reverse of the physiological situation; and the drug may diffuse to brain regions normally not exposed to active concentrations of the endogenous compound.

Baroreflex Transmitters

Likely neurotransmitter candidates in medullary baroreflex pathways include substance P, glutamate, opioids, and GABA (Blessing, 1988; Chalmers and Pilowsky, 1991; Guyenet et al., 1987; Helke et al., 1980; McCall, 1990; Humphrey and McCall, 1984; Reis et al., 1988; Sun and Guyenet, 1985). Other possibilities include acetylcholine, 5-HT, AVP, AII, and thyrotropin-releasing hormone.

Somogyi et al. (1989) reported that after VLM injection of [³H]aspartate, a tracer for radiolabeling excitatory amino acid (e.g., glutamatergic) pathways, more than 90% of the retrogradely labeled neurons were localized in the NTS. Since injection of an NMDA receptor antagonist into the CVLM prevented depressor responses evoked by stimulation of the NTS in rats or the aortic depressor nerve in rabbits, the results suggested that an excitatory amino acid released by NTS cells that terminate in the CVLM may mediate reflexive depressor responses. These results, consistent with findings by other groups (e.g., Guyenet et al., 1987; Reis et al., 1988), do not necessarily imply, however, that the excitatory amino acid is glutamate (Leone and Gordon, 1989).

Enkephalin-containing neurones project from the NTS to the RVLM, and local application of naloxone in the RVLM increases blood pressure (Chalmers and Pilowsky, 1991). Endogenous opioids may therefore play an inhibitory modulatory role in the RVLM. The sources of opioid-containing terminals in the RVLM are unknown.

Whereas an excitatory amino acid seems to mediate stimulatory effects of increased arterial baroreceptor afferent traffic on cells in the NTS and CVLM, release of the inhibitory neurotransmitter GABA may mediate the inhibitory effects of increased arterial baroreceptor afferent traffic on cells in the RVLM (Blessing, 1988; Sun and Guyenet, 1985). Afferents from cardiopulmonary baroreceptors also appear to inhibit RVLM neurons by a GABA-ergic mechanism (Sun and Guyenet, 1987). GABA may also mediate baroreflex inhibition of neurosecretion in the SON and PVN (McCall, 1990).

Glutamate and acetylcholine, glutamate and substance P, and acetylcholine and substance P may interact synergistically in determining baroreflex-mediated alterations in firing of RVLM neurons (Agarwal and Calaresu, 1992).

Despite high concentrations of NE-containing A2 cells of the NTS, and pharmacological evidence indicating participation of α_2-adrenoceptors in the NTS in baroreflex-mediated bradycardia and depressor responses (Gurtu et al., 1982; Kubo and Misu, 1981), the exact role of catecholamines in the NTS in mediating baroreflexes remains unclear. Microinjection of NE or EPI into the NTS decreases heart rate and inhibits NTS cell firing (Feldman and Moises, 1988; Gurtu et al., 1982; Howe, 1985), and the effects on blood pressure are inconsistent. Destruction of catecholaminergic terminals in the NTS, by bilateral microinjection of 6-OHDA, does not abolish reflexive bradycardia (Snyder et al., 1980) but does decrease baroreflex–cardiac gain by about 1/2 and produces chronically labile blood pressure.

Corticotropin-Releasing Hormone (CRH)

Interest in the coordination of hypothalamic–pituitary–adrenocortical (HPA) and autonomic responses during stress has led to many studies about CRH, first identified by Vale and co-workers (Vale et al., 1981). Icv administration of CRH not only increases plasma levels of ACTH but also evokes large increases in plasma levels of catecholamines (Brown and Fisher, 1984, 1985; Kurosawa et al., 1986). The central neural site of action of CRH that mediates the peripheral catecholaminergic activation has not been identified (Brown, 1986).

Brown et al. (1986) reported that icv administration of a CRH antagonist (α-helical CRH_{9-41}) suppressed responses of plasma EPI levels during insulin-induced hypoglycemia, supporting a role of endogenous CRH in the adrenomedullary response to this classic stressor. Goldstein, Garty et al. (1993), however, failed to replicate this finding. Icv administration of α-helical CRH_{9-41} also has been reported to suppress adrenal EPI release induced by ether vapor or 30% hemorrhage but not by sodium nitroprusside, electrical stimulation of the ACE, or electrical stimulation of the anterior hypothalamus in rats (Brown, 1991). Icv α-helical CRH_{9-41} does attenuate responses of LC neurons to nitroprusside (Curtis et al., 1993). Thus, results using this antagonist have not yet delineated the exact role of CRH in the mediation of SNS and AHS responses to different stressors.

CRH releases NE not only in the periphery but also in the brain. Local administration of CRH increases LC firing rates (Valentino and Foote, 1987), and icv CRH increases NE concentrations in microdialysate obtained from the anterior and medial hypothalamus or the medial prefrontal cortex (Emoto et al., 1993; Lavicky and Dunn, 1993).

Conversely, noradrenergic pathways ascending from the medulla via the ventral noradrenergic bundle (VNB) probably modulate hypothalamic secretion of CRH. In humans, peripheral administration of the α_1-adrenoceptor agonist methoxamine increases ACTH levels, α_1-adrenoceptor blockade with prazosin abolishes this effect (Al-Damluji and Francis, 1993), and patients with hypothalamic dysfunction can fail to have methoxamine-induced increments in ACTH levels (Al-Damluji and Francis,

1993). In rats, icv administration of NE increases hypophyseal–portal concentrations of CRH, with α_1-adrenoceptor blockade by corynanthine preventing this effect (Plotsky, 1987); and icv NE increases plasma ACTH levels, with α_1-adrenoceptor blockade by prazosin preventing this effect (Szafarczyk et al., 1987). Depletion of central NE by icv 6-OHDA attenuates stress-induced release of ACTH (Feldman et al., 1988) and attenuates ACTH responses to combined icv administration of a catecholamine precursor and an α_2-adrenoceptor blocker (Al-Damluji and White, 1992). 6-OHDA injection into the VNB markedly decreases PVN concentrations of NE and attenuates adrenalectomy-induced ACTH responses (Weidenfeld and Feldman, 1991). According to one model, stimulation of central postsynaptic α_1-adrenoceptors augments release of AVP (Al-Damluji et al., 1990), AVP in turn facilitating CRH release or permitting CRH effects at pituitary corticotrophs (Gwinup et al., 1967; Plotsky et al., 1985).

Vasopressin (AVP)

Since Brattleboro rats, deficient in endogenous AVP, have high plasma NE and EPI levels (Zerbe et al., 1982), and since brain knifecuts or lesions that disconnect the mediobasal hypothalamus or PVN increase plasma catecholamine levels (Makara et al., 1986), AVP in the brain appears to inhibit SNS and AHS outflows, probably via augmentation of baroreflex-mediated sympathoinhibition (Bishop et al., 1987; Guo et al., 1982, 1986; Hasser et al., 1988). As discussed above, systemically administered AVP exerts similar effects by reaching cells in the AP, which lacks an efficient blood–brain barrier. AVP-containing cells of the PVN project to the LC and spinal cord and may inhibit activity of SPNs (Gilbey et al., 1982).

In contrast with the view that central neural AVP inhibits SNS outflow, icv AVP increases plasma catecholamine levels and blood pressure (King et al., 1985; Martin et al., 1988). Local administration of NE in the PVN has produced inconsistent effects, increasing AVP release into the systemic circulation (Benetos et al., 1986) but decreasing PVN cell firing (Barker et al., 1971). As noted previously in this chapter, destruction of A1 noradrenergic projections to the PVN evokes marked hypertension and AVP release, suggesting tonic noradrenergic inhibition of AVP secretion; however, CVLM stimulation also increases AVP release. Thus, although substantial literature indicates AVP–catecholaminergic interactions in the brain, studies have disagreed remarkably about what those interactions are.

Angiotensin II (AII)

All the elements of the RAS are present in the central nervous system (Ganten et al., 1983). When injected icv, AII increases drinking behavior, blood pressure, and sympathoneural activity (Steele et al., 1991), with the pressor response resulting from increased sympathetic outflow (Camacho and Phillips, 1981). In rats, the central neural site for the pressor action of icv AII appears to be in the periventricular AV3V region (Bellin et al., 1987). Circulating AII may act at circumventricular organs to inhibit baroreflex function, since ablation of the AP blocks hypertension elicited by chronic systemic administration of AII (Cox and Bishop, 1991). In AVP-deficient, water-deprived animals, icv administration of AII fails to increase blood pressure (Harland et al., 1988), suggesting complex mechanisms relating AII to blood pressure.

Whereas icv injection of sarthran, an AII receptor blocker, or captopril, which inhibits synthesis of AII, decreases mean arterial pressure, these drugs do not affect renal sympathetic nerve activity in anesthetized rats with sinoaortic denervation (Steele et al., 1991). In conscious rabbits, icv injection of saralasin, an AII receptor blocker, does not affect renal sympathetic nerve activity, either at baseline or during baroreflex-mediated changes in sympathetic activity (Dorward and Rudd, 1991). Thus, although icv AII stimulates sympathetic activity, this may not indicate a role for endogenous AII in the central regulation of SNS outflow, at least to the kidneys.

Since renal sympathetic neural activity importantly influences activity of the RAS, and since AVP augments baroreflex inhibition of sympathetic outflow, several potential peripheral as well as central mechanisms exist by which AVP and AII can interact in affecting sympathoneural responses (Steele et al., 1991).

Endogenous Opioids

Three endogenous opioid systems have been described in brain (Bennett, 1990). Enkephalin-containing cells and fibers are distributed diffusely in the limbic system, basal ganglia, hypothalamus, periaquaductal gray, and substantia gelatinosa of the spinal cord. Endorphins are synthesized in the arcuate nucleus of the hypothalamus and in pituitary corticotrophs, and the arcuate cell bodies project to the limbic system, thalamus, periaquaductal gray, LC, and medulla. The dynorphins are present in magnocellular cells of the PVN and the SON, in medullary cells, and in the dorsal horn of the spinal cord. These compounds probably interact with all four known types of opioid receptors in the brain, but there appears to be no matching anatomically of the agonists with particular receptor types.

Much more research attention has focused on opioid–NE interactions in the brain and spinal cord—especially in anti-nociception—than on the role of endogenous opioids in regulation of sympathoneural outflow. Icv administration of agonists at receptors for opioids—that is, the μ-selective agonists D-Ala^2, MePhe^4, Gly-ol^5-enkephalin (DAGO), and dermorphin and the δ-selective agonist D-Pen^2, D-Pen^5-enkephalin (DPDPE)—increase plasma catecholamine levels (Marson et al., 1989; Siren et al., 1989), and treatment with the opioid antagonist naloxone augments catecholamine responses to several forms of stress. Since naloxone does not alter plasma catecholamine levels in animals at rest, endogenous opioids probably contribute little to basal SNS or AHS outflow. In humans, naloxone does not augment plasma catecholamine responses to stressors that do not evoke pain (Morris et al., 1990).

Naloxone increases responses of heart rate, LC single unit activity, and plasma catecholamine levels to noxious stimuli such as immobilization (Abercrombie and Jacobs, 1988; Stepanovic et al., 1989). Conversely, local application of opioid agonists in the LC usually decreases cellular firing, and at LC terminal regions opiates usually inhibit release of NE. In the rat cortex and hippocampus, opioids inhibit release of [^{3}H]NE; however, the effects of opioid receptor agonists on [^{3}H]NE release vary substantially across species (Bennett, 1990).

In rats undergoing prolonged, continuous restraint, LC firing rates tend to adapt. Administration of naloxone during the restraint increases LC firing to about double the initial rate (Abercrombie and Jacobs, 1988). Naloxone produces no effect on central noradrenergic activity under baseline conditions. These results suggest that endogenous opioids inhibit the organism's responses to noxious stimulation (Jacobs, 1990). The excessive response to naloxone suggests a mechanism for dishabituation: Exposure of an adapted organism to a novel stressor may interfere with endogenous opiate restraint of LC firing. Although several reports have confirmed that iontophoresis of morphine decreases LC firing, studies have not determined whether the dishabituation effects of naloxone depend on actions in the LC.

Much research attention has focused on the interaction of endogenous opioids and α_2-adrenoceptors in the brain. The effects on anxiety, sedation, and anti-nociception of agonists at opioid receptors and at α_2-adrenoceptors seem similar. Clonidine has been used successfully for opiate withdrawal (Gold et al., 1978), and noradrenergic agonists may prove useful in the treatment of pain (Besson and Guillbaud, 1992). Administration of yohimbine, which blocks α_2-adrenoceptors, often produces tremor, restlessness, increased salivation, hypertension, and insomnia—a syndrome resembling that during opiate withdrawal. Administration of naloxone can reverse the antihypertensive effect of clonidine in some circumstances (Farsang and Kunos, 1979); however, administration of naloxone to hypertensive patients treated with clonidine does not increase blood pressure.

If μ-opioid receptors and α_2-adrenoceptors were colocalized on the same neurons, agonists at either type of receptor would elicit the same intracellular effects (Fornai et al., 1990). Alternatively, inhibitory opioid receptors could decrease firing of noradrenergic cells, and α_2-adrenoceptors on the terminals could decrease NE release for a given amount of cell firing (Al-Damluji, 1991). Since local blockade of α_2-adrenoceptors both increases LC firing and enhances evoked NE release from terminals (Mermet et al., 1990), another model proposes inhibitory α_2-adrenoceptors and opioid receptors both on noradrenergic cell bodies and nerve terminals.

Acetylcholine

Icv administration of cholinesterase inhibitors such as neostigmine augments acetylcholine concentrations at muscarinic cholinergic receptors in the central nervous system and usually increases values for indices of SNS and AHS outflows, blood pressure, and heart rate, associated with a respiratory pattern of increased tidal volume and decreased respiratory rate. Central cholinesterase inhibition also enhances catecholamine responses to immobilization stress (Stepanovic et al., 1989).

In humans, administration of physostigmine in the setting of methscopolamine treatment, to block the peripheral effects of physostigmine, increases plasma EPI levels (Kennedy et al., 1984).

Although these results suggest that central cholinergic stimulation increases peripheral catecholamine release, the extremely rapid metabolic breakdown of the transmitter and the lack of availability of drugs to block acetylcholine release have impeded research about the physiological role of endogenous acetylcholine.

Benzodiazepines

Benzodiazepines exert behavioral effects by facilitating the binding of the inhibitory central neurotransmitter, GABA, to its receptor. Administration of diazepam or other benzodiazepines inhibits sympathetic outflow (Sigg and Sigg, 1969), decreases plasma levels of NE (Hossmann et al., 1980), and attenuates plasma EPI responses to several forms of stress (e.g., Dionne et al., 1984). Conversely, administration of β-CCE, a β-carboline thought to act as a "reverse antagonist" at benzodiazepine receptors, increases plasma catecholamine levels and produces behaviors suggesting anxiety in conscious monkeys (Ninan et al., 1982).

Adrenal Corticosteroids

The HPA system, the SNS, and the AHS constitute major stress effector systems, and Chapter 2 discusses several of their interactions in the periphery. The following focuses on catecholamine–steroid interactions in the brain.

Glucocorticoid receptors (type 2, low-affinity corticosterone receptors) occur at high concentrations in the PVN and SON, the arcuate nucleus, the limbic system, cortical and thalamic neurons, and cells of the ascending catecholaminergic pathways in rat brain. The vast majority of noradrenergic and adrenergic cells in the rat brain possess nuclear glucocorticoid receptors (Harfstrand et al., 1986). Mineralocorticoid receptors (type 1, high-affinity corticosterone receptors) occur mainly in the hippocampus.

Studies using in vivo microdialysis in conscious rats have indicated that chronic hypercortisolemia decreases hypothalamic extracellular fluid concentrations of NE and attenuates yohimbine-induced NE release (Pacak et al., 1992a), findings analogous to those in the periphery (Szemeredi et al., 1988a, 1990). Glucocorticoids probably also suppress catecholamine biosynthesis in the brain (Pacak et al., unpublished observations).

Consistent with inhibitory effects of glucocorticoids on brain mechanisms mediating SNS outflow to the cardiovascular system, icv administration of a glucocorticoid receptor antagonist increases blood pressure (van den Berg et al., 1990). Effects of central glucocorticoid antagonism on SNS and AHS outflows have not yet been assessed.

Central Catecholaminergic Pathways

In the presence of formaldehyde, catecholamines form intensely fluorescent by-products, a phenomenon exploited by Falck (1962) and Hillarp (Falck et al., 1962) to visualize catecholaminergic areas in tissue slices by exposing the slices to formaldehyde vapor and examining the slices by fluorescence microscopy. A modification uses gly-oxylic acid, which enhances the sensitivity of the procedure and produces more stable fluorescence.

The fluorescence techniques do not distinguish easily among the three endogenous catecholamines. The purification of catecholamine synthetic enzymes led to specific immunohistological techniques to identify separately noradrenergic, dopaminergic, and adrenergic pathways. In this approach, the tissue slice is incubated with the antibody—for example, rabbit antiserum to DBH. The section is incubated with another antibody linked to a detectable marker, such as fluorescein or horseradish peroxidase, that rec-ognizes the rabbit immunoglobulin. Dopaminergic neurons contain TH but do not con-tain DBH; noradrenergic neurons contain DBH but not PNMT; and adrenergic neurons contain all three enzymes.

Subsequent autoradiographic techniques exploited the avid neuronal uptake processes for catecholamines. Most recently, in situ hybridization has visualized regions express-ing mRNA encoding catecholamine-synthesizing enzymes; and microdialysis has ena-bled assessments of regional catecholamine synthesis, release, and metabolism in vivo.

Monoaminergic neurons have several unusual characteristics. They possess numerous collaterals; they exhibit functional plasticity and can even regenerate (Bjorklund and Stenevi, 1979); they lead to nonjunctional as well as junctional terminal connections; and they often degenerate very slowly. A single catecholaminergic cell can have from 10 to 100,000 nerve terminals and can innervate cells in several different portions of the central nervous system (Palkovits and Brownstein, 1989). Unlike neurotransmitters that directly alter ion channels to effect rapid, transient discharges of discrete neurons, monoamines appear to exert mainly neuromodulatory actions by affecting intracellular concentrations of second messengers, resulting in slower but amplified and prolonged responses (Stricker and Zigmond, 1986).

Virtually all neurohistochemical research about adrenergic cells in the brain has been conducted in rats; however, the distribution of central monoamine-synthesizing neurons in the humans seems generally similar to that in rats (Halliday et al., 1988). Catechol-aminergic cells in rat brain have been grouped into five main systems (Bjorklund and Lindvall, 1986): a noradrenergic system based in the pons, with LC cells projecting especially rostrally to the hypothalamus, limbic system, and telencephalon; a lateral medullary noradrenergic and adrenergic system, with noradrenergic cells projecting mainly rostrally to the hypothalamus and adrenergic cells projecting both rostrally and distally to the sympathetic preganglionic neurons; a mesencephalic dopaminergic sys-tem innervating the corpus striatum, limbic system, and cortex; a periventricular, mainly dopaminergic system innervating the hypothalamus by short projections and also pro-jecting caudally in long tracts; and a short system of dopaminergic pathways within the hypothalamus and from the hypothalamus to the pituitary gland. NE-containing peri-karya occur only in the pons and medulla, whereas dopaminergic perikarya occur more rostrally (Figures 4–8, 4–20).

Dahlstrom and Fuxe (1964) identified 12 groups of catecholaminergic cells, desig-nated A1 to A12 in ascending anatomic order from the medulla to the hypothalamus,

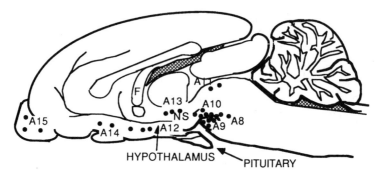

Figure 4–20. Dopamine pathways in the rat brain. In this schematic diagram of a midsagittal section, the cells containing tyrosine hydroxylase but not DBH are designated A8, A9, etc. A9 cells are localized to the substantia nigra, the main source of dopamine pathways in the brain. NS = nigrostriatal pathway.

olfactory bulb, and retina of rats. An A13 group was identified later in the rostral zona incerta, an A14 group in the anterior periventricular nucleus of the hypothalamus and preoptic region, and an A15 group in the periglomerular portion of the olfactory bulb.

Dopamine

The sources of DA pathways in the brain are in the midbrain and hypothalamus (Figure 4–20). Three main dopaminergic systems in the brain have been described: nigrostriatal, mesocortical, and tuberohypophysial. Palkovits and Brownstein (1989) subdivided these into eight DA pathways: mesocortical, mesostriatal, mesolimbic, incerto-hypo-thalamic, periventricular, descending, olfactory, retinal interneuronal. Cooper et al. (1991) classified dopaminergic pathways in terms of the lengths of the efferent fibers: ultrashort systems, including the interplexiform amacrine-like neurons of the retina and the periglomerular DA cells of the olfactory bulb; intermediate length systems, includ-ing the tuberohypophysial DA cells, the incertohypothalamic neurons, and the medul-lary periventricular group; and long-length systems, including pathways from the ven-tral tegmental area and substantia nigra to three main target regions—the neostriatum, the limbic cortex, and other limbic structures (e.g., septum, nucleus accumbens, and amygdala).

The most prominent dopaminergic pathway, the nigrostriatal, courses from the zona compacta of the substantia nigra (SN) of the midbrain (A9 cells) to the corpus striatum (the caudate and putamen). The terminal fields of the nigrostriatal projections contain almost 80% of all the DA in brain. Depletion of striatal DA characterizes Parkinson's disease, associated with and thought to be due to degeneration of the SN.

The mesocortical dopaminergic pathway extends from cell bodies of the SN and ventral tegmentum to terminal areas in the amygdala, ventral entorhinal area, and per-irhinal and piriform cortex; the septal nuclei, nucleus accumbens, and interstitial nucleus of the stria terminalis; the medial frontal and anterior cingulate cortex; and the olfactory tubercle, anterior olfactory nucleus, and olfactory bulb (Bloom et al., 1989). This pathway may be dysfunctional in schizophrenia, since many effective neuroleptics appear to work by blocking effects of DA released in the mesocortical system.

The tuberohypophysial dopaminergic pathway originates from A12 cells in the arcuate and periventricular nuclei of the hypothalamus and projects to the median eminence and to the intermediate lobe of the pituitary. This pathway plays a neuroendocrine role in modulating release of prolactin.

Although dopaminergic neurons in the rat brain outnumber noradrenergic neurons by about 4:1, the total content of DA averages only about twice that of NE. This implies that the total amount of NE in noradrenergic neurons is 2–3 times the amount of DA in dopaminergic neurons—about 30 pg for the average dopaminergic neuron and about 75 pg for the average noradrenergic neuron (Bjorklund and Lindvall, 1986). For average half-lives of 2 h and 4 h for DA and NE in brain, both types of neuron would synthesize about 10 pg of catecholamine per hour (Bjorklund and Lindvall, 1986).

Complete, bilateral lesioning of brain DA systems in rats produces a behavioral syndrome of akinesia, sensory inattention, aphagia, and adipsia, giving the appearance of generalized behavioral unresponsiveness. This "DA deficiency syndrome" applies to all voluntary acts requiring motivation, sustained alertness, and receptiveness to sensory input. DA-deficient animals fail to initiate coordinated motor responses and fail to orient to sensory stimuli. Motivated behaviors are not eliminated, but there appears to be an increase in the arousal threshold before the behaviors are elicited (Stricker and Zigmond, 1986). Most research in this area has depended on administration of 6-OHDA to produce chemical ablation of dopaminergic cells; however, 6-OHDA also destroys noradrenergic cells. Whereas nigrostriatal DA depletion elicits the DA deficiency syndrome, mesolimbic DA depletion does not (Bloom et al., 1989).

Stricker and Zigmond (1986) have proposed that the DA system regulates behavioral responsiveness indirectly, by inhibitory modulation of an inhibitory striatal control mechanism. Patients with Parkinson's disease therefore experience particular difficulty in initiating and terminating motor activity. Conversely, increased dopaminergic activity, such as produced by L-DOPA, amphetamines, or DA receptor agonists, produces hyperactivity and stereotypy in rats and choreiform movements, dystonia, agitation, or psychosis in humans.

Bloom et al. (1989) have conceptualized the behavioral role of ascending dopaminergic pathways from the midbrain as follows. Activation of the system as a whole increases spontaneous locomotor activity and induces species-specific stereotypic motor behaviors, and inactivation of the system produces general behavioral inactivation, decreased spontaneous locomotion, reduced responsiveness to sensory input, and, in severe cases, aphagia and adipsia. The nigrostriatal component appears to mediate the stereotypy, whereas the mesolimbic component appears to mediate the increased locomotion and reinforcement produced by psychomotor stimulants—due not so much to pleasurable "reward" sensations as to an "enabling action" that decreases the threshold for initiating responses.

Exposure to intermittent tail shock increases DA release diffusely but differentially in several brain regions. Microdialysate concentrations of DA, DOPAC, and HVA increase in the striatum, nucleus accumbens, and ·medial frontal cortex, with the proportionate DA responses largest in the frontal cortex (Abercrombie, Keefe et al., 1989).

The mesocorticolimbic dopaminergic system constitutes a major brain system involved in "drug reward", where an animal learns to self-administer an agent that increases DA levels in extracellular fluid in the brain or learns an operant behavior where the reinforcement arises from administration of a drug that increases DA levels. Three different transmitters-the catecholamine DA, an endogenous opiate peptide, and the amino acid GABA-may interact in the nucleus accumbens and ventral tegmental area, key areas in "reward pathways" (Koob, 1992); however, as noted above, one cannot easily separate "reward" from "enabling" in laboratory animals.

Norepinephrine

Noradrenergic cell bodies in the brain are localized to the medulla and pons (Figure 4–8). The CVLM, extending from the level of the AP to the caudal portion of the facial nucleus, contains A1 cells; A2 cells occur in the region of the medial subnucleus of the NTS, along the dorsal borders of the dorsal motor nucleus of the vagus nerve, with about the same rostrocaudal extent as A1 cells; A6 cells occur in the LC of the pons; and A5 cells of the pons lie ventral to the LC.

Kalia et al. (1985a) have considered A2 neurons to occur both within the NTS and in the adjacent AP and dorsal motor nucleus of the vagus. A2 cells in the AP have been designated A2d cells. The LC has been suggested to contain A6 cells, A4 cells (a dorsolateral extension of the A6 group in the lateral part of the roof of the fourth ventricle), and a subceruleus group located just ventral to the A6 cells (Holets, 1990).

A1 cells of the RVLM that contain PNMT have been presumed to be adrenergic and have been designated C1 cells (Hokfelt et al., 1974). In the rostral portion of the A2 cell group in the region of the NTS, PNMT-positive cells have been designated C2.

Neuroanatomically, the most distinctive feature of central noradrenergic neurons is their tremendous arborization throughout the forebrain from relatively few perikarya. It has been estimated that each noradrenergic neuron can give rise to 100,000 varicosities and 30 cm of axonal branches (Jarrott, 1991; Bjorklund and Lindvall, 1986). From about 10^4 cells, about 10^9 varicosities bud from the axonal twigs, providing a morphologic basis for the hypothesized global functions of central noradrenergic neurons.

Three main noradrenergic systems have been described in brain: the LC–subceruleus system, the dorsal medullary system, and the lateral tegmental system. Bjorklund and Lindvall (1986) have divided the noradrenergic groups into the LC–subceruleus complex, containing A6 cells; the dorsal medullary region, containing A2 cells; and the lateral tegmental region, containing A1 and A5 cells. The lateral tegmental group has also been divided into two parts, medullary and pontine, and subdivided again, into a medullary subgroup including the ventrolateral caudal medullary A1 neurons and the dorsomedial A2 neurons, and a pontine subgroup containing the A5 and A7 cells (Holets, 1990).

About half the noradrenergic cell bodies are in the LC and about 1/3 in the lateral tegmental system. The main source of NE in brain, and the sole source of NE in the frontal cortex and cerebellum, is the LC, which contains 45–50% of the brain's noradrenergic neurons; the subceruleus contains another 10–15%; the lateral tegmental system (including the A1, A3, A5, and A7 regions) about 30%; and the dorsal medullary group (A2) about 10% (Jarrott, 1991).

Noradrenergic cells in these regions project differentially, with the LC innervating the forebrain, cerebellum, and brainstem, the lateral tegmental system innervating the hypothalamus, limbic system, brainstem, and (in the case of the A5 and A7 neurons) spinal cord, and the dorsal medullary group innervating the hypothalamus and limbic system. Thus, most noradrenergic pathways ascend in the neuraxis rather than descend to the spinal cord. The pathways of the dorsal medullary and lateral tegmental noradrenergic systems have not been completely differentiated, and they often are considered together.

Noradrenergic pathways ascend in four axon bundles: the dorsal tegmental bundle (dorsal noradrenergic bundle, DNB, also called dorsal bundle, DB), the medial forebrain bundle (MFB), the central tegmental tract (CT), and the ventral medullary catecholamine bundle (ventral noradrenergic bundle, VNB; Holets, 1990). The most prominent pathway from the LC is via the DNB, through the central gray and via the dorsal longitudinal fasciculus and central tegmental tract to terminate diffusely throughout the telencephalon. The MFB carries most of the ascending dopaminergic and noradrenergic fibers from the pons and midbrain to the hypothalamus and telencephalon, including the hippocampus. At the border of the midbrain and diencephalon, the DB joins the MFB. The CT carries most of the noradrenergic and adrenergic fibers from the medulla and pons outside the LC. After fanning out complexly in the tegmentum, the CT joins the MFB in the midbrain. The VNB constitutes a caudal extension of the central tegmental tract. Another pathway descends to the ventral portion of the intermediolateral column of the spinal cord (Bloom et al., 1989).

These different pathways imply spatial differentiation of the sources of noradrenergic innervation of brain regions. In particular, most of the noradrenergic innervation of the cortex, basal forebrain, thalamus, cerebellum, and hippocampus (especially the pyramidal and molecular cell layers) derives from the LC, whereas most of the noradrenergic innervation of the hypothalamus and brainstem derives from the lateral tegmental cell groups. Noradrenergic innervation of the hypothalamus and medial preoptic area emanates especially from ventrolateral A1 and dorsal A2 neurons (Bjorklund and Lindvall, 1986). As noted above, most of the adrenergic innervation of the SPNs derives from the lateral tegmental groups, not the LC (Fritschy et al., 1987; Holets, 1990).

Transection of the brain caudal to the hypothalamus markedly attenuates release of catecholamines in the posterior hypothalamus (Dietl et al., 1981) and PVN (Pacak, Palkovits, Kvetnansky, Kopin et al., 1993), demonstrating the lower brainstem source of noradrenergic terminals in the hypothalamus. About 40% of all the cells in the SON and PVN contain TH immunoreactivity (Li et al., 1988). The dense noradrenergic innervation of the PVN derives from A1 and A2 cells of the medulla and to only a minor extent from the LC. A1 and A2 projections innervate the parvocellular division of the PVN, with A2 projections to CRH-containing neurons particularly prominent (Cunningham and Sawchenko, 1988), whereas A1 projections predominate in the innervation of the magnocellular division of AVP-synthesizing cells (Sawchenko and Swanson, 1981a, 1982). The SON receives innervation from A1 cells, with massive noradrenergic projections to portions of the nucleus populated by vasopressingergic cells. Noradrenergic afferents to the arcuate nucleus and median eminence also arise partly from A1 cells. Medullary noradrenergic cells contribute to the innervation of the septal area (especially the BNST) and ACE.

In the lower brainstem, noradrenergic projections of non-LC origin innervate primary motor and visceral nuclei such as the motor trigeminal, hypoglossal, and ambiguus nuclei, the dorsal motor nucleus of the vagus, the NTS, and the nucleus commissuralis. Other noradrenergic innervation sites include the ventral mesencephalic central gray region, the parabrachial nuclei, the principal inferior olivary nucleus, and the raphe nuclei.

Sites of origin of the noradrenergic terminals in the lower brainstem have not yet been established conclusively. In contrast with a previous suggestion that the nucleus commissuralis is the source of noradrenergic terminals in the NTS (Takahashi et al., 1979), Thor and Helke (1988) reported that about 60% of the projections to the NTS derive from A1 and C1 cells of the VLM and 20% from the pontine A5 cell group. The pontine lateral tegmental noradrenergic neurons (A5 and A7) project mainly caudally to the spinal cord.

In summary, the LC is the main source of noradrenergic innervation of the neocortex, some thalamic nuclei, the tectum, and cerebellum. The pontine A5 cells and medullary C1 cells of the lateral tegmental system are the main sites of origin of catecholaminergic descending projections to the spinal cord. The dorsal medullary A2 and ventrolateral A1 cells groups are the main sources of noradrenergic innervation of the hypothalamic and preoptic areas.

Functions of Norepinephrine in Brain

Substantial research in psychoneuroendocrinology has so far failed to delineate the exact roles of brain NE in regulation of sympathetic outflow to the cardiovascular system and more generally in the elaboration of stress responses. When Vogt (1954) described the presence of catecholaminergic neurons in the brain, she suggested a general relationship between central release of NE and peripheral catecholaminergic activation, since pharmacological manipulations evoking adrenomedullary secretion depleted NE in the brain. Subsequent work attempted to identify effects of NE in the regulation of specific behaviors, such as ingestion of food and water. Most of the studies were flawed by inadequate controls, use of drugs with multiple concurrent effects, neurochemical changes in widely separated regions, lesions of neurons as well as fibers in passage, and lack of consideration of other neurochemical mediators (Stricker and Zigmond, 1986).

There is no convincing evidence for a direct role of central neural NE in the regulation of sympathetic outflow and therefore in the release of catecholamines from sympathetic nerve terminals or the adrenal glands. Instead, although the evidence is incomplete, NE in the central nervous system seems to play several indirect roles. First, ascending pathways from the LC noradrenergic neurons participate complexly in psychological processes such as vigilance behavior, memory, extinction of conditioned responses, anxiety, and distress. Alterations in SNS outflow virtually always accompany these phenomena. Second, in the hypothalamus, NE, derived mainly from lower brainstem cell bodies, participates in secretion of releasing hormones, such as thyrotropin-releasing hormone and CRH, which in turn secondarily affect SNS and AHS outflows. Indeed, NE has been considered as an intermediary in virtually every neuroendocrine system (Bennett, 1990). Third, noradrenergic (or adrenergic) pathways emanating from medullary cell groups appear to modulate transmission of interoceptive information, such as from baroreceptors, to the LC, hypothalamus, and limbic system. Fourth, noradrenergic terminals in the dorsal horn of the spinal cord and on sensory afferents may gate ascending nociceptor information to the brain, influencing distress-induced recruitment of SNS and AHS responses during exposure to painful stimuli.

Factors that regulate homeostasis of central monoaminergic systems resemble those regulating homeostasis of NE concentrations at noradrenergic receptors in the periphery: (1) presynaptic modulation by short- and long-distance feedback and autoreceptors; (2) conservation of releasable stores by neuronal reuptake; (3) coupling of transmitter release with catecholamine synthesis, both by rapid alterations in TH activity and by slower increases in the amount of TH enzyme; and (4) adaptive changes in postsynaptic adrenoceptors (Stricker and Zigmond,1986). As a result, further analyses of factors regulating catecholaminergic function in the periphery are likely to yield information relevant to regulation of catecholaminergic function in the brain.

Differences among noradrenergic projection systems in the brain probably relate to functional differences in mechanisms of neural circulatory regulation. As discussed above, the pontine noradrenergic cell clusters (LC and A5) seem responsive to both exteroceptive and interoceptive sensory stimuli (Cedarbaum and Aghajanian, 1978a), whereas the medullary A2 neurons respond more to visceral interoceptive (e.g., carotid sinus baroreceptor) than to somatic sensory exteroceptive (e.g., sciatic nociceptor) input (Bjorklund and Lindvall, 1986). Thus, chemical or surgical destruction of ascending catecholaminergic pathways to the hypothalamus via the VNB, with sparing of the LC, does not attenuate plasma catecholamine or ACTH responses to handling, footshock, or immobilization—that is, to somatic sensory input perceived as noxious (Castagne et al., 1990; Pacak, Palkovits, Kvetnansky, Kopin et al., 1993; Rivet et al., 1990).

Local application of NE in regions innervated by the LC produces a slowly progressive *inhibition* that differs in several respects from the inhibition produced by the classic inhibitory neurotransmitter of the brain, GABA (Foote et al., 1983). Activation of the LC during stress might therefore attenuate the organism's responses (Amaral and Sinnamon, 1977), such as in seizures (Goldstein, Nadi et al., 1988; Mason and Corcoran, 1979); however, since locally applied NE stimulates inhibitory α_2-adrenoceptors, both pre- and extrasynaptically, the inhibition may not indicate the physiological role of endogenously released NE at postsynaptic receptors.

More frequently, it has been suggested that LC activation during stress is *stimulatory*, mediating vigilance behavior and possibly the accompanying increases in autonomic outflows. Exposure to any of a large variety of stressors (e.g., cold, footshock, aggregation, hypoxia, exercise) depletes brain NE, increases NE turnover, and increases tissue concentrations of NE metabolites. All these findings indicate that stress responses often include activation of central noradrenergic neurons. Microdialysis studies have confirmed rather diffuse activation of noradrenergic centers in the brain during distress. Hemorrhagic hypotension, which elicits large increases in circulating AVP levels, increases dialysate concentrations of NE and MHPG, in the SON (Kendrick and Leng, 1988), in the PVN-anterior hypothalamic area (van Huysse and Bealer, 1991), and in the dorsomedial medulla (van Huysse and Bealer, 1991). Hypotension elicited by systemic administration of a vasodilator also increases dialysate NE concentrations in the PVN and dorsomedial medulla (van Huysse and Bealer, 1991). In conscious rats, immobilization produces large-magnitude increases in extracellular fluid concentrations of NE, DHPG, and MHPG in the PVN (Pacak et al., 1992b) and amygdala (Pacak, Palkovits, Kvetnansky, Fukuhara et al., 1993; Tanaka et al., 1991) and of NE in the hippocampus (Abercrombie et al, 1988). In rats studied 1–2 months after 6-OHDA lesions of NE terminals, extracellular fluid concentrations of NE, while decreased, remain detectable, but with abolition of NE responses to handling (Kalen et al., 1988). Classical aversive conditioning also increases NE concentrations in hypothalamic microdialysate (Yokoo et al., 1990).

Thus, whereas studies involving icv or local injections of NE or adrenoceptor agonists have led to the view that NE is an inhibitory neurotransmitter that decreases sympathetic outflow and blood pressure (McCubbin et al., 1960; Share and Melville, 1963), studies using microdialysis or single-cell electrophysiological recordings have indicated that stressors activate noradrenergic pathways from the LC and lower brainstem centers as part of an arousal mechanism (Aston-Jones and Bloom, 1981b; Bloom et al., 1989; Foote et al., 1980, 1983).

The function of NE may vary with the *level of the neuraxis* at which the neurotransmitter is released. According to this view, in the brainstem below the LC, endogenous NE plays mainly an inhibitory role in the regulation of blood pressure and sympathetic outflow (Head, 1991). In a suitable preparation (vagally blocked, baroreceptor denervated, decerebrate), intracisternal administration of 6-OHDA to release endogenous NE acutely decreases blood pressure and cardiac sympathetic outflow, whereas chronic depletion of spinal NE by local injections of the neurotoxin increases blood pressure. Destruction of ascending noradrenergic pathways does not appear to affect baseline blood pressure. NE released from the posterior hypothalamus, spinal cord, or peripheral sympathetic nerve endings increases blood pressure, whereas NE released near the NTS or in the anterior hypothalamus has the opposite effect (Conlay, 1988).

Most of the studies that have led to this concept have been based on effects of exogenous administration of NE or agonists at noradrenergic receptors. These manipulations may not exert the same effects as those produced by endogenously released NE. A neuropharmacologic method to assess the role of endogenous NE in the regulation of sympathetic outflow is based on icv or local injection of tyramine, which displaces NE from noradrenergic vesicles. Local injection of tyramine in the A2 area decreases blood pressure (Zandberg et al., 1979), and injection of tyramine into the C1 area decreases blood pressure, pulse rate, and renal sympathetic nerve activity (Granata, Numao et al., 1986), consistent with an inhibitory as a role of NE as a neurotransmitter in these medullary regions. In contrast, Sun and Guyenet (1990) reported that tyramine increased the firing rate of RVLM pacemaker neurons in tissue slices. Several MEDLINE searches failed to locate studies about effects of icv injected tyramine or of local injections of tyramine in other areas on sympathetic nerve activity. The availability of in vivo microdialysis should enable future studies about effects of locally administered tyramine on NE release in particular brain regions and on autonomic outflows.

Beginning with the suggestions of Brodie and Costa (1962), other concepts about NE in the brain have emphasized a *neuromodulatory* role, where NE functions neither as a direct inhibitor nor stimulator but alters responsiveness to other synaptic inputs (Woodward et al., 1979). By decreasing "background" discharges and enhancing phasic excitatory or inhibitory inputs, NE would increase the "signal-to-noise" ratio, by effects on responsiveness of target neurons or by effects on interneurons. The enhancement of signal-to-noise ratios would participate in processes such as attention, memory, and learning. Consistent with the noradrenergic modulation hypothesis, presentation of a neutral cue tends to decrease evoked hippocampal firing during LC stimulation, and NE enhances this inhibition, whereas when hippocampal neuronal activity increases as a classically conditioned response to an appetitive unconditioned stimulus (food reward), NE enhances the excitatory response (Segal and Bloom, 1976).

Another explanation for inconsistencies about the role of NE in the brain proposes that exogenously administered NE or adrenoceptor-active agents preferentially stimulate "safety valve" receptors that limit—and generally produce effects opposite from—stimulation of postsynaptic receptors actually mediating physiological responses. In essence, this view explains the different functions of NE on the basis of *types and localization of adrenoceptors.* Based on ultrastructural immunocytochemical localization of DBH, about 3/5 of the noradrenergic varicosities in the hypothalamus, limbic system, and cerebellum are actually axodendritic (Olschowka et al., 1981). Administration of NE exogenously, such as by the icv route, might therefore stimulate mainly receptors that normally inhibit endogenous NE release, and the relative balance of pre- and post-synaptic adrenoceptors would determine the responses to endogenously released NE.

LEARNING AND MEMORY

Rats learn to press a bar when the behavior leads to electrical stimulation of the LC or pathways from it, consistent with the hypothesis that NE in the brain participates in mechanisms of positive reinforcement. Studies in the 1970s and early 1980s demonstrated, however, that lesions of the LC or DNB fail to abolish intracranial self-stimulation or the acquisition of positively reinforced behaviors (Amaral and Foss, 1975; Mason and Iversen, 1977).

The LC and its ascending projections, while not involved directly with reward or acquisition, may nevertheless participate in the retention and more specifically with the extinction of learned behaviors. Rats with bilateral 6-OHDA-induced lesions of ascending projections from the LC fail to extinguish previously learned behaviors (Mason and Iversen, 1979). Lesions of the DNB generally interfere with the acquisition of new, motivation-related behaviors and with the extinction of learned behaviors after removal of reinforcement contingencies, rather than with the retention of previously learned behaviors or the acquisition of simple discrimination tasks.

This phenomenon, called the "dorsal bundle extinction effect" or the "dorsal bundle effect," has in turn suggested involvement of the LC system in filtering out irrelevant stimuli (Mason and Iversen, 1979) or in inhibiting learned behaviors no longer rewarded or else punished (Gray, 1982). The dorsal bundle effect may only occur in learning paradigms involving distress or aversive reinforcement contingencies, rather than paradigms involving both appetitive and aversive behaviors (Bloom et al., 1989). Thus, Rasmussen and Jacobs (1986) reported classical conditioning of LC firing using an aversive UCS (air puff to the face) but not using an appetitive UCS (food). Since destruction of the hippocampus impairs extinction of conditioned behaviors, and since the hippocampus receives dense noradrenergic innervation from the LC, one may speculate that interference with hippocampal mechanisms subserving extinction mediates the dorsal bundle effect.

Consistent with involvement of noradrenergic pathways from the LC in memory processing, patients with senile dementia of the Alzheimer's type have a loss of pigmented NE-synthesizing cells in the LC (Iversen et al., 1983) and a loss of noradrenergic fibers in the hippocampus (Powers et al., 1988). Perhaps treatment with deoxyphenylserine (DOPS), an amino acid converted directly to NE by DDC, may affect memory in patients with this disease.

In rats, cats, and monkeys, repetition of simple sensory stimuli progressively diminishes responses of firing rates of LC neurons. This habituation implies memory processing. In the hippocampus, a terminal field of LC noradrenergic neurons, stress-related increases in microdialysate NE concentrations also habituate (Abercrombie et al., 1992). In animals repeatedly exposed to the same stimulus, exposure to a *novel* stimulus produces exaggerated responses of dialysate NE levels (Abercrombie et al., 1992).

The habituation of LC neurons after repeated exposure to the same sensory cue may reflect not simple adaptation but a more complex process, where the organism continually assesses the motivational significance of cues and adjusts the responsiveness of attention, memory, vigilance, and emotional processes. LC firing does not habituate with repeated exposure to stimuli persistently evoking distress. For instance, in monkeys, 3- to 10-fold increases in LC firing during human imitations of agonistic social signals do not habituate (Grant and Redmond, 1984). Analogously, responses of neither plasma nor hypothalamic microdialysate NE levels habituate during repeated immobilization stress (Pacak et al., 1992b).

ATTENTION AND VIGILANCE

Natural selection would have favored the evolution of mechanisms fostering memory consolidation during distressing situations, so as to avoid similar situations in the future, and selective attention to cues from the internal or external environment, so as to recognize and respond rapidly to those situations. Perhaps the LC noradrenergic system subserves these processes.

Alterations in LC discharge accompany awakening, orienting, and electroencephalographic spindling (Aston-Jones and Bloom, 1981a, 1981b; Foote et al., 1980; Jacobs,

1990). Arousing stimuli that interrupt behaviors such as sleep, grooming, and eating produce bursts of activity of LC neurons, indicating increased attentiveness to the external environment. Bloom et al. (1989) have therefore suggested that LC activation may enhance neural activity in terminal fields concurrently receiving transient bursts of input stimuli (e.g., environmental events) and attenuate activity in regions receiving only inhibitory inputs (e.g., tonic biological homeostats). Thus, the LC system may bias attention towards novel, rapidly changing external signals and away from tonic internal signals. Analogously, Aston-Jones (1985) has proposed that the LC functions as a gate for the overall orientation of the organism toward attention to novel features of the environment and away from elicitation of vegetative behavior patterns. As noted above, LC neurons also respond to novel interoceptive cues, even if innocuous (e.g., Elam et al., 1985).

If the function of the LC noradrenergic cells were to increase attentiveness to motivationally relevant, phasic environmental or internal sensory cues, then one would predict that lesions of the LC or DNB would decrease attentiveness and therefore decrease distractibility to external stimuli; however, animals with LC lesions appear generally to have increased distractibility to phasic stimuli (Everitt et al., 1990). The deficit therefore seems subtle—in a way analogous to the clinical pediatric condition "attention deficit disorder," characterized by a failure to attend persistently to those environmental cues that actually are motivation-relevant, thereby interfering with the ability to carry out assigned tasks. Sympathomimetic amines often improve patients with attention deficit disorder, perhaps by increasing extracellular NE concentrations in the brain.

Jacobs (1990) has hypothesized that just as the sympathetic nervous system regulates the functioning of numerous body systems during stress, the LC functions globally in the brain as an emergency or alarm system. Thus, repetition of sensory stimulation, even if somewhat stressful, produces habituation of LC neuronal responses, whereas responses to persistently agonistic social signals do not habituate (Abercrombie and Jacobs, 1987c; Grant and Redmond, 1984). LC neuronal activity is subject to classical aversive but not classical appetitive conditioning (Rasmussen and Jacobs, 1986), and LC firing tends to decrease during "vegetative" behaviors such as grooming, eating, and sleep (especially REM sleep). Jacobs (1990) therefore has supported a role of the LC in vigilance—that is, the transition in behavioral state to an increased level of activation, especially in an aversive situation, rather than in determining the level of activation itself. Thus, exposure of a cat to albino rats, while arousing in the cat, does not increase LC firing or plasma catecholamine levels in the cat (Abercrombie and Jacobs, 1987b; Rasmussen et al., 1986), consistent with elicitation of instinctive predatory behavior without distress. In contrast, exposure of a cat to another aggressive cat or to a dog markedly increases LC firing and plasma catecholamine levels in the cat (Levine et al., 1990).

As noted in the discussion about the LC as a neuroanatomic entity, stimuli that affect LC firing have been considered along two continua—noxiousness vs. nonnoxiousness and internal vs. external. The literature has disagreed about LC responses to internal, noxious stimuli; stressor-specificity of central noradrenergic responses may explain the discrepancies. Elam et al. (1985) reported stimulatory effects of nitroprusside or hemorrhage, as well as stimulation in response to stretching of the walls of the bladder, colon, or stomach (Elam, Thoren et al., 1986). In contrast, Morilak et al. (1987) reported that hemorrhagic hypotension produced no significant increase in LC unit activity, and Jacobs (1990) noted that hypoglycemia increased LC firing only at the nadir of blood glucose levels. Differential AHS activation during hemorrhagic hypotension and hypoglycemia, with relatively less mediation by central NE release, could resolve these inconsistencies; however, information is lacking about whether different stressors differentially activate noradrenergic centers in the brain.

If the LC served as a channel or gate to vigilance, then the LC could regulate the ability of discrepancies between afferent sensations—from sense organs and interoceptors—and setpoints for responding to reach consciousness and thereby to elicit experiential sensations, behaviors, and neuroendocrine patterns. Both external and internal perturbations can activate the LC, the latter after sensory processing in medullary nuclei. Perhaps if a stimulus were perceived as novel, severe, or threatening, LC activation would foster transmission of the signal to higher brain centers, facilitating active attention and memory consolidation and further orienting the organism to the stimulus. A psychological positive feedback loop could develop easily in this setting, where the organism would focus more and more on the particular perturbation to the exclusion of all other afferent information to the brain—a temporary obsession.

ANXIETY

Redmond and co-workers have proposed that the somatic manifestations of anxiety result from activation of LC neurons. In unanesthetized primates, electrical stimulation of the LC evokes a behavior pattern suggesting anxiety, increased vigilance, and decreased exploration; and spontaneous firing rates of LC neurons increases during threatening situations and decreases during sleep, eating, and grooming behavior (Aston-Jones, 1985; Foote et al., 1980, 1983; Redmond and Huang, 1979).

It has been hypothesized further that the LC is also important for the *experience* of anxiety (Redmond and Huang, 1979; Redmond et al., 1976). Charney and Redmond (1983) suggested that the anxiolytic effect of α_2-adrenoceptor agonists results from suppression of LC firing. Bloom et al. (1989) have questioned this suggestion, arguing that the anti-anxiety effects of decreased LC activity may reflect decreased responsiveness to novel or aversive stressors rather than direct involvement of the LC in the experience of anxiety.

The LC possesses a high concentration of α_2-adrenoceptors, and in individuals predisposed to anxiety or panic, interference with the function of inhibitory α_2-adrenoceptors can evoke emotional experiences and accompanying neuroendocrine patterns. Goldstein, Grossman, Listwak et al. (1991) found that in young patients with mild or moderate hypertension, a subgroup had excessive pressor and plasma catecholamine responses to intravenously infused yohimbine. Patients with excessive sympathetic responses often had a positive psychiatric history. The yohimbine-induced emotional experiences varied markedly across patients: Patients with a history of depression became depressed, with a history of anxiety or panic became anxious, with a history of aggressive behavior became angry, and with a history of hypomania became elated. These largely anecdotal findings merit prospective study.

Central or peripheral administration of three types of drugs can elicit panic or anxiety: α_2-adrenoceptor antagonists, such as yohimbine (Charney et al., 1983, 1984); β-carbolines, such as β-CCE, which act as "inverse agonists" at benzodiazepine receptors (Ninan et al., 1982); and CRH (Brown and Fisher, 1985). Increases in plasma catecholamine levels accompany the behavioral effects. Several lines of evidence have also indicated important modulation of α_2-adrenoceptor-mediated effects by endogenous opioids, as discussed above, and clonidine can block effectively the symptoms and signs of opioid withdrawal (Gold et al., 1978). Interrelationships among catecholamines, benzodiazepines, CRH, and opioids in the production of anxiety remain poorly understood. Patients with excessive responsiveness to yohimbine can respond to alprazolam, a benzodiazepine. Since diazepam attenuates yohimbine-induced anxiety (Charney et al., 1983), and since the two main sources of afferent pathways to the LC appear to use α_2-adrenoceptors and GABA receptors (Aston-Jones et al., 1990), the interaction of GABA and α_2-adrenoceptors in the LC also merits further study.

DEPRESSION

The high frequency of depression in patients treated with reserpine, and the therapeutic effects of tricyclic antidepressants, which inhibit reuptake of NE in the brain, provided early support for the monoamine theory of depression, imputing a pathophysiological role of depletion of NE (or 5-HT) in the brain.

The role of endogenous NE in the etiology of depression has aroused persistent controversy. Since chronic treatment with desipramine can down-regulate β- and α_2-adrenoceptors (Green, 1990; Stanford et al., 1983), it remains unclear whether the underlying problem is the depletion of amines, hypersensitivity of postsynaptic β-adrenoceptors, excessive activity of α_2-autoreceptors, excessive responsiveness of postsynaptic α_2-adrenoceptors—or none of these. Uncontrollable, inescapable shock in animals can produce behavioral depression—"learned helplessness" (Seligman and Maier, 1967)—a model of depression. The extent of decrease in NE content in the LC correlates with the extent of depression (Weiss et al., 1981).

Repeated exposure to noxious stimuli, such as repeated immobilization in rats, decreases β-adrenoceptor numbers and β-adrenoceptor-mediated cellular responses (U'Prichard and Kvetnansky, 1980). Since several effective treatments for depression (MAO inhibitors, tricyclic antidepressants, and electroconvulsive shock) increase catecholamine levels in extracellular fluid and decrease β-adrenoceptor numbers, the changes in β-adrenoceptor numbers may represent an adaptive response; however, there is no convincing evidence that β-adrenoceptor down-regulation, or habituation of LC noradrenergic cells during repeated stimulation, actually relate to behavioral adaptation (Sanford, 1990). Long-term antidepressant treatment also decreases TH mRNA expression in the LC (Brady et al., 1991), and one can conceptualize an *increase* rather than a decrease in amine turnover as an etiologic neurochemical process in depression. This would explain reserpine-induced depression, since reserpinization increases amine turnover.

Two contrasting hypotheses therefore may be offered about the possible pathophysiological link between NE depletion in the LC and depression. One is that NE pathways derived from the LC are important for coping processes, such as vigilance behavior, and loss of NE causes a loss in adaptive responsiveness. The second is that the NE depletion decreases inhibitory feedback by α_2-autoreceptors on LC neurons, thereby increasing cellular firing rates and increasing adrenoceptor-mediated processes in the terminal areas.

Gold et al. (1988) have proposed that systems involving CRH and NE in the brain reinforce each other's activities. NE stimulates release of CRH from rat hypothalamus in vitro (Hillhouse and Milton, 1989; Joanny et al., 1989; Widmaier et al., 1989) and in vivo (e.g., Plotsky, 1987), and as noted above, CRH increases LC firing rates and NE levels in hypothalamic microdialysate (e.g., Emoto et al., 1993). In cerebrospinal fluid of patients with major depression, concentrations of CRH correlate positively with concentrations of NE and MHPG (Roy et al., 1987).

Gold et al. (1988) have hypothesized that, in essence, depression represents a maladaptive form of Selye's General Adaptation Syndrome, due to inadequate restraint of both the CRH and NE–LC systems. This theory assumes direct functional connections between the PVN and the LC. As noted above, most of the noradrenergic innervation of the PVN derives from medullary cell groups, and autonomic outflow from PVN parvocellular regions can traverse the same medullary cell groups or impinge directly on SPNs. The theory appears to be too restrictive neuroanatomically, but the notion of an abnormality of coregulation of NE and CRH in the central nervous system of depressed patients merits further testing, especially since chronic antidepressant treatment decreases both CRH mRNA expression in the PVN and TH mRNA expression in the LC (Brady et al., 1991; Nestler et al., 1990).

PAIN

Accumulating evidence implicates a descending noradrenergic system in modulating transmission of nociceptive afferents to the brain. Iontophoretic application of NE inhibits discharges of spinal nociceptive neurons (Belcher et al., 1978), and intrathecal NE in the lumbar subarachnoid space produces dose-dependent analgesia (Reddy and Yaksh, 1980). DBH-containing perikarya in the LC and A5 regions project to cells in the dorsal horn of the spinal cord (Tavares et al., 1993). Neurons in the CVLM mediate an antinociceptive action by attenuating the responsivess of dorsal horn cells to painful stimulation; this action probably occurs indirectly via LC and A5 cells to which CVLM neurons project, rather than directly via noradrenergic projections from A1 cells to dorsal horn cells (Tavares et al., 1993).

α_2-Adrenoceptors on dorsal horn neurons appear to mediate this noradrenergic analgesia (Yaksh, 1985). Administration of agonists at α_2-adrenoceptors synergistically enhances analgesia produced by opiates (Meert et al., 1993), and epidural infusions of clonidine or the α_2-adrenoceptor agonist medetomidine are being studied as possible treatments for intractable cancer pain (DuPen et al., 1993). Epidural clonidine produces analgesia similar to that produced by the potent opioid alfentanil (Eisenach et al., 1993).

NON-LC SYSTEMS

Interest by psychologists and neurologists in cortical mechanisms of learning, memory, and attention has led to extensive literature about the organization and function of the LC noradrenergic system. Neurophysiologists, neuroanatomists, and neurochemists have also concentrated on the LC because of the localization of the noradrenergic cell bodies in a discrete, approachable area with well-defined terminal fields. The organization, regulation, and functions of lower brainstem catecholaminergic neurons remain less well understood. Nevertheless, neuroendocrine and peripheral catecholaminergic responses during different forms of stress probably depend importantly on activation of ascending catecholaminergic inputs from the lower brainstem. Lachuer et al. (1991) found that exposure to any of a variety of stressors (immobilization, ether inhalation, insulin-induced hypoglycemia) rapidly increases concentrations of DOPAC in the A1/C1 and A2/C2 areas, consistent with rapid increases in TH activity and therefore with increased catecholamine synthesis in these areas. The extents of the increases appear to vary with the type of stressor, but this notion requires further testing.

Epinephrine

EPI is present only at low concentrations in the central nervous system. In the rat medulla, only about 4,500 cells contain PNMT (Jarrott, 1991). PNMT is cytoplasmic, whereas the EPI precursor, NE, is synthesized by DBH in the vesicles. For EPI to act as a neurotransmitter, NE must escape the vesicles and undergo N-methylation in the cytoplasm, with the vesicles then taking up and storing the resulting EPI. Whether EPI and NE release are subject to differential regulation in PNMT-containing cells in the brain is unknown.

Epinephrinergic (adrenergic) systems have been divided into two or three cell groups: a ventral C1 group, a dorsal C2 group, and a dorsal midline C3 group underlying fourth ventricular ependymal cells (Jarrott, 1991; Figure 4–6). The C1 and C2 neurons intermingle with the A1 and A2 noradrenergic neurons in the VLM and the NTS. Most adrenergic pathways in brain probably emanate from the C1 cells in the RVLM. As discussed previously in the section about this brainstem region, C1 cells project both rostrally to the LC, hypothalamus, and periaquaductal gray, and distally to the intermediolateral columns of the spinal cord.

Extracellular fluid in the hypothalamus has been reported to contain relatively high concentrations of EPI. Consistent with the notion of differential regulation of catecholamine release, electrical stimulation of C1 neurones increases microdialysate concentrations of EPI but not of NE in the posterior hypothalamus (Routledge and Marsden, 1987). This does not necessarily mean that adrenergic rather than noradrenergic pathways from the VLM determine the hypothalamic modulation of sympathetically mediated pressor responses during stress.

EPI-containing neurons of the RVLM project to the intermediolateral cell columns (Ross et al., 1984a; Tucker et al., 1987); however, this does not imply that EPI acts as a neurotransmitter at the synaptic connections with the SPNs. Only about ½ of the neurons of the RVLM that project to the intermediolateral columns contain either immunoreactive TH or PNMT. Sun et al. (1988) reported that the "pacemaker" cells of the RVLM are not catecholaminergic and that cells containing catecholamine-synthesizing enzymes do not have pacemaker activity. Two populations of cells with different pacemaker properties have been described, one with a rapid conduction velocity (about 3.5 m/sec) and one with a slow conduction velocity (about 0.7 m/sec). The slower conducting neurons send both ascending projections in the CT and descending projections to the spinal cord; their activity is sensitive to changes in baroreflex afferent activity and to clonidine and is pulse-synchronous. In contrast, the rapid-conducting neurons have exclusively descending projections and, while also pulse-synchronous and barosensitive, are not inhibited by clonidine. It is possible that the slow-conducting neurons are at least indirectly catecholaminergic and that the second population includes nonadrenergic cells of the RVLM (Haselton and Guyenet, 1989).

Probably the most frequently cited evidence against a sympathoexcitatory role of endogenous EPI from C1 cells is that local administration of exogenous EPI or adrenoceptor agonists usually decreases the discharge rate of SPNs (Guyenet and Cabot, 1981; Guyenet and Stronetta, 1982); however, spatial localization of pre-, post-, and extrasynaptic adrenoceptors can explain this finding. Catecholamines released from terminals of C1 cells may also bind to receptors on interneurons in the intermediolateral columns. It is also of course possible that EPI is irrelevant to the regulation of sympathetic outflow by RVLM neurons. Connor and Drew (1987) found that inhibition of PNMT by intrathecal LY134046 did not alter the tachycardia or hypertension produced by stimulation of the RVLM; and effective depletion of central and peripheral EPI stores, by combined inhibition of DDC and PNMT, does not affect resting levels of blood pressure, nor the pressor response to electrical stimulation of the RVLM, in stroke-prone spontaneously hypertensive rats (Rogers et al., 1991). These studies did not include more direct indices of sympathoneural activation.

Thus, despite establishment of a neuroanatomic link between C1 cells of the RVLM and the intermediolateral columns, the excitatory neurotransmitter producing activation of SPNs during RVLM stimulation remains unidentified. Other candidate neurotransmitters for the excitatory projections from the RVLM neurons include substance P, 5-HT, acetylcholine, met- and leu-enkephalin, and glutamate (McCall, 1990).

Adrenoceptors in the Brain

Most ideas about adrenoceptor localization, agonism and antagonism, and intracellular mechanisms of action in the brain have been generated based on studies of these receptors in the periphery. Receptors for each of the three endogenous catecholamines, NE, EPI, and DA, have been described in brain. NE and EPI exert actions at adrenoceptors of both the α and β types. EPI concentrations in most brain areas are very low, and thus it is likely that NE is the main agonist at α- and β-adrenoceptors in brain. The following discussion concentrates on the α-receptors, because drugs that act at these receptors are well-known to affect sympathoneural outflow and cardiovascular variables.

Research about adrenoceptors in the brain has had several major limitations. One has been the limited pharmacological specificity of receptor ligands. Thus, clonidine binds to imidazoline receptors as well as to α_2-adrenoceptors (Ernsberger et al., 1986); idazoxan can bind to nonadrenergic receptors in addition to α_2-adrenoceptors (Michel et al., 1989, 1990); and β-adrenoceptor ligands can bind to 5-HT$_{1B}$ receptors (Jones et al., 1990). Brain tissue often substantially binds ligands nonspecifically. Poor penetration of the blood–brain barrier by several adrenoceptor ligands has resulted in insufficient in vivo information. Molecular genetic techniques have identified receptor subtypes for which ligands have not yet been developed. Localization of some adrenoceptor subtypes varies markedly across species. Finally, for some types of adrenoceptors, such as α_1-adrenoceptors, glaring and inadequately explained discrepancies have been noted between the intensity of catecholaminergic innervation and the regional distribution of the receptors.

As in the periphery, responses to an adrenoceptor agonist may depend importantly on the type, location, and functions of the adrenoceptors. Rather than NE acting universally as an inhibitory or stimulatory neurotransmitter (recall the issue about the existence of "sympathin I" and "sympathin E," in the chapter about peripheral catecholaminergic systems), or even as a neuromodulator, the actions of NE in the brain may depend on the localization and functions of the receptors on effector cells. Virtually nothing is known about how endogenous catecholamines and their receptors interact in the brain to produce physiologically relevant changes in sympathoneural outflow.

α-Adrenoceptors

α_1-Adrenoceptors

Several reports have implicated brain α_1-adrenoceptors in integrative functions of the central nervous system, including cardiovascular regulation (e.g., Huchet et al., 1983), nociception, movement, arousal, sudomotor activity, and release of hormones (Szabadi and Bradshaw, 1987).

The unavailability of adequately potent and specific ligands retarded until recently understanding of the localization of α_1-adrenoceptors. [3H]Prazosin, [3H]HEAT (2-[β-(4-hydroxyphenyl)-ethylaminomethyl]tetralone; Unnerstall, 1987), and a radioiodinated form of HEAT, [125I]BE 2254, or 2-[β-(4-hydroxy-3-iodo-phenyl)-ethylaminomethyl]tetralone have been used. The specificity of ligands for α_1-adrenoceptor subtypes remains limited, since both [3H]prazosin and [125I]BE 2254 are ligands at both α_1-adrenoceptor subtypes α_{1a} and α_{1b} (Jones et al., 1990), and prazosin binds to a subtype of α_2-adrenoceptors.

In rat brain, α_1-adrenoceptor concentrations bear little relationship to the intensity of noradrenergic innervation as indicated by [3H]desipramine binding to label NE uptake sites (Rainbow and Biegon, 1983). Highest levels of [3H]HEAT binding have been reported in the external plexiform layer of the olfactory bulb; lamina I and lamina V of the frontal and parietal cortex; the medial septal nucleus and the BNST; several thalamic nuclei; the molecular layer of the cerebellum; in the midbrain, the dorsal lateral tegmental nucleus, dorsal raphe, and median raphe nuclei; and pontine and medullary nuclei, including the dorsal LC, parabrachial nucleus, trigeminal nuclei, NTS, inferior olive, external cuneate nucleus, and raphe nuclei (Unnerstall, 1987). [^{3}H]HEAT binding is rather low in the hypothalamus, and there does not appear to be concentration of [^{3}H]HEAT binding in the VLM. Instead, the entire medulla, pons, and thalamus seem to have diffusely increased [^{3}H]HEAT binding compared to other brain areas (Unnerstall, 1987). Rainbow and Biegon (1983) similarly found [^{3}H]prazosin binding in rat forebrain concentrated in layer V of the motor portion of the frontoparietal cortex and in all nuclei of the thalamus, with moderate binding in the limbic system and little binding in the caudate putamen or nucleus accumbens.

The apparently high concentrations of α_1-adrenoceptors in the thalamus and lamina of the cortex and low concentrations in the hypothalamus would be consistent with the view that the receptors predominate in terminals emanating from the LC, since the LC projects via the DNB to the neocortex, hippocampus, thalamus, and cerebellum, whereas the lateral tegmental noradrenergic pathway ascends in the VNB to the hypothalamus, brainstem, basal ganglia and descends to the spinal cord (Szabadi and Bradshaw, 1987). In rats, however, Unnerstall (1987) found little [^{3}H]HEAT binding in the hippocampus. The neuroanatomic localization also suggests a role of α_1-adrenoceptors in transmission of sensory information, such as by nociceptors.

Human brain possesses high concentrations of [^{3}H]prazosin binding in the hippocampus, especially in the dentate gyrus (Gross-Isseroff et al., 1990). The discrepancy between the results in rat hippocampus using [^{3}H]HEAT binding and in human hippocampus using [^{3}H]prazosin binding has not been explained. Relatively high concentrations of α_1-adrenoceptors are found also in the human SON and PVN, compared to corresponding regions in other species, suggesting a role of α_1-adrenoceptors in regulation of AVP release and water homeostasis in humans (Jones et al., 1990). Unnerstall (1987) has concluded that α_1-adrenoceptors are not specific for any particular presynaptic sources of noradrenergic innervation.

As in the periphery, increased IP$_3$ formation is thought to be a major means by which α_1-adrenoceptor agonists increase cytoplasmic concentrations of Ca^{++} and activate cells. Whereas the association between noradrenergic pathways and α_1-adrenoceptor densities is weak, there is a strong relationship between a drug's ability to bind to α_1-adrenoceptors and its ability to increase the formation of IP$_3$. In brain, unlike in the periphery, stimulation of α_1-adrenoceptors also increases generation of cAMP (Szabadi and Bradshaw, 1987).

In the neocortex, NE applied by microelectrophoresis can produce excitatory, depressant, or biphasic responses. Selective activation of α_1-adrenoceptors in neocortex is excitatory and β_2-adrenoceptors inhibitory, whereas α_2-adrenoceptors appear not to be involved (Szabadi and Bradshaw, 1987). In the SON, NE also appears to exert a mainly excitatory action due to effects on α_1-adrenoceptors. In the brainstem, the situation is complex, with both excitatory and inhibitory effects of NE described. Application of α_1-adrenoceptor agonists is excitatory in the dorsal raphe nucleus.

In summarizing cellular responses mediated by adrenoceptors in brain regions, Szabadi and Bradshaw (1987) suggested that A1, A2, and A6 neurons of the lower brainstem possess only inhibitory α_2-adrenoceptors, whereas areas of the forebrain receiving noradrenergic innervation can possess a variety of adrenergic receptors. Excitatory α_1-

adrenoceptors predominate in the lateral geniculate and dorsal raphe nuclei and inhibitory β-adrenoceptors on cerebellar Purkinje cells.

Central administration of α_1-adrenoceptor agonists stimulates ACTH release, by a mechanism that appears to depend on AVP (Al-Damluji, Thomas et al., 1990; Al-Damluji, White et al., 1990). In humans, peripheral administration of α_1-adrenoceptor agonists increases ACTH secretion (Al-Damluji and Francis, 1993; Al-Damluji et al., 1987).

The hypothesis that α_1-adrenoceptors are stimulatory and α_2-adrenoceptors inhibitory in many brain regions resembles that about the functions of α-adrenoceptor subtypes in the periphery. Since in the periphery the spatial localization of α-adrenoceptors at sympathetic neuroeffector junctions importantly determines the physiological roles of the receptors, the same may be the case in the central nervous system. To date, as in the periphery, in the brain no convincing evidence has accrued for the existence of functional presynaptic α_1-adrenoceptors (Arbilla and Langer, 1990).

α_2-Adrenoceptors

α_2-Adrenoceptors in the brain have been suggested to participate in a variety of homeostatic phenomena, such as regulation of blood pressure and gastrointestinal activity, neuroendocrine activity, the sleep–waking cycle, analgesia, and anxiety (Fornai et al., 1990).

α_2-Adrenoceptors are concentrated in several regions involved with sympathoneural outflow, including the anterior and posterior hypothalamus and dorsomedial caudal medulla (Morris and Woodcock, 1982). In general, the distribution of α_2-adrenoceptors in the brain corresponds roughly to the distribution of noradrenergic cells. In rat forebrain, the receptors are concentrated in lamina of the cortex, the lateral septum, the hippocampus, the thalamus, and especially in the entorhinal cortex and ACE (Jones et al., 1990; Kuhar and Unnerstall, 1984). In the hypothalamus, α_2-adrenoceptors are prominent in the arcuate and periventricular areas (Jones et al., 1990). In the lower brainstem, α_2-adrenoceptors are concentrated in the central gray area, the dorsal and ventral pons and medulla along tracts that include the LC, A5 region, NTS, dorsal motor nucleus of the vagus, NA, raphe pallidus, and VLM, with lower levels in the SN (Jones et al., 1990; Kuhar and Unnerstall, 1984). In the spinal cord, α_2-adrenoceptors are concentrated in the intermediolateral columns, ventral horns, and particularly in the dorsal horns in the region of the substantia gelatinosa.

In human postmortem material, forebrain α_2-adrenoceptors visualized by autoradiography and membrane binding of [^{3}H]bromoxidine ([^{3}H]UK-14304) are concentrated in the neocortex, ventral hypothalamus, hippocampus, and some thalamic nuclei (Pascual et al., 1992; Pazos et al., 1988). Using p-[^{3}H]aminoclonidine or [^{3}H]bromoxidine, high concentrations of α_2-adrenoceptors have been reported in the visual cortex, the dorsal motor nucleus of the vagus, the LC, the NTS, the midbrain gray region, and the substantia gelatinosa of the spinal cord. Human brain appears to have higher concentrations of p-[^{3}H]aminoclonidine binding sites in the NTS and fewer sites in the raphe nuclei than in the corresponding regions in rats (Probst et al., 1985). The basal ganglia, substantia nigra, and raphe nuclei contain only sparse α_2-adrenoceptors, suggesting an association between α_2-adrenoceptors and noradrenergic, as opposed to dopaminergic or serotonergic, centers (Pascual et al., 1992). In the study of Pascual et al. (1992), several hypothalamic nuclei, the superior colliculus, the lateral periaquaductal area of the midbrain, the LC, the dorsal motor nucleus of the vagus, the stratum granularis and Purkinje molecular layer of the cerebellum, and the substantia gelatinosa of the spinal cord had particularly high concentrations of α_2-adrenoceptors.

In contrast with the often excitatory actions of α_1-adrenoceptor stimulation in brain regions, α_2-adrenoceptor stimulation virtually always results in neuronal depression (Szabadi and Bradshaw, 1987). Systemic administration of α_2-adrenoceptor agonists produces sedation, dry mouth, decreases in blood pressure and heart rate, decreased gastrointestinal secretion and motility, hyperphagia, and increases in pituitary release of growth hormone and thyroid-stimulating hormone. Systemic administration of clonidine prolongs barbiturate anesthesia, and yohimbine shortens anesthesia duration (Mason and Angel, 1983). Prior depletion of brain NE by 6-OHDA prevents these effects, indicating that α_2-adrenoceptors modulating release of NE in brain participate in the state of wakefulness.

Intracellular mechanisms of action of α_2-adrenoceptors in the nervous system have not been well characterized and have been presumed to be similar to those in the periphery, where α_2-adrenoceptor stimulation inhibits generation of cAMP. In rodent astrocytes, α_2-adrenoceptor stimulation does not decrease cAMP production but does attenuate cAMP responses to β-adrenoceptor stimulation (Korn and McCarthy, 1981). Considering the inhibition of cAMP responses by α_2-adrenoceptor stimulation, inhibition of cAMP-dependent phosphorylation of voltage-sensitive Ca^{2+} channels may provide a basis for inhibitory modulation at noradrenergic terminals (Arbilla and Langer, 1990).

Data have been inconsistent about whether α_2-adrenoceptor agonists or antagonists affect plasma levels of ACTH or β-endorphin. Central administration of the α_2-adrenoceptor antagonist idazoxan does not alter ACTH secretion (Al-Damluji, Bouloux et al., 1990), in contrast with the stimulatory effect of α_1-adrenoceptor agonists (Al-Damluji and Francis, 1993). Idazoxan administration does enhance ACTH responses to naloxone. Pettibone and Mueller (1981) reported that clonidine increased plasma immunoreactive β-endorphin levels in rats, whereas Goldberg et al. (1986) reported no effects of α_2-adrenoceptor blockade by yohimbine on plasma levels of ACTH or β-endorphin in humans.

Al-Damluji, Bouloux et al. (1990) have presented a model for an interaction of central α_2-adrenoceptors and opioid receptors on noradrenergic neurons in the regulation of pituitary ACTH release. According to this model, inhibitory opioid receptors decrease noradrenergic cellular activity, and inhibitory α_2-adrenoceptors on the terminals inhibit NE release and occupation of postsynaptic stimulatory α_1-adrenoceptors. Consistent with this model, idazoxan enhances ACTH and cortisol responses to naloxone without affecting basal levels of these compounds.

As in the periphery, in the brain α_2-adrenoceptors occur both pre- and post- or extrasynaptically. Early findings by Haeusler (1974) indicated that the depressor effect of clonidine persisted even after depletion central neural catecholamines, suggesting that the fall in blood pressure resulted mainly from stimulation of postsynaptic α_2-adreno-ceptors. Lesions of the DNB fail to decrease α_2-adrenoceptor numbers in most brain areas (U'Prichard et al., 1980), indicating mainly postsynaptic localization. This does not imply that behavioral and neuroendocrine effects of α_2-adrenoceptor stimulation result only from actions at postsynaptic receptors, despite the abundance of those recep-tors. Heal (1990) has concluded that mydriasis produced by α_2-adrenoceptor stimulation depends on actions at postsynaptic receptors, whereas hypoactivity depends on presyn-aptic receptors. The location of α_2-adrenoceptors mediating sedation has not been settled.

Systemically administered yohimbine increases microdialysate concentrations of NE, its main intraneuronal metabolite DHPG, and the prominent noradrenergic metabolite MHPG in the hypothalamus and in the pontomedullary area of the brainstem in rats (Szemeredi, Komoly et al., 1991), indicating that at least in these brain regions, blockade of α_2-adrenoceptors releases endogenous NE. The microdialysis results have generally confirmed the findings of Dietl et al. (1981), who used a push–pull cannula in the posterior hypothalamus of cats.

As in the periphery, α_2-adrenoceptors in the hypothalamus and cerebral cortex, regions containing noradrenergic projections from the lower brainstem and LC, inhibit TH activity in vivo (Pi and Garcia-Sevilla, 1992). The mechanisms linking α_2-adren-oceptor-induced inhibition of NE release with α_2-adrenoceptor-induced inhibition of catecholamine biosynthesis in the brain remain obscure.

Administration of yohimbine icv into conscious rabbits increases blood pressure and plasma levels of NE and DHPG (Eisenhofer, Cox et al., 1991), and intravertebral arterial injection of yohimbine increases blood pressure in anesthetized dogs (Huchet et al., 1982), suggesting that blockade of central neural α_2-adrenoceptors increases sympa-thoneural outflow to the cardiovascular system. Confirming a relationship between NE release in the brain and periphery would require assessing the effects of depletion of central neural NE on yohimbine-induced increments in sympathoneural outflow.

α-MethylDOPA and clonidine, effective antihypertensive agents, act in the brain to decrease sympathetic nerve activity (Doxey and Everitt, 1977; Guyenet et al., 1981; Haeusler, 1973; Heise and Kroneberg, 1973). α-MethylDOPA is converted to the "false neurotransmitter" α-methylNE, which stimulates α_2-adrenoceptors. The depressor effect of clonidine depends on actions in the central nervous system, since in humans with tetraplegia, clonidine fails to decrease blood pressure (Reid et al., 1977); however, whether clonidine decreases SNS outflow by stimulating α_2-adrenoceptors specifically has been controversial. Since midcollicular transection does not attenuate clonidine's sympatholytic effect, clonidine is thought to act in the brainstem or spinal cord (Korner and Angus, 1982). On the other hand, stereotaxic application of clonidine in the hypo-thalamus produces hypotension (Struyker-Boudier and van Rossum, 1972). Studies combining lesions and microinjection of clonidine in anesthetized animals have led to the conclusion that the drug's main site of antihypertensive action in the brain is in the RVLM (Bousquet and Feldman, 1987; Granata et al., 1986; Guyenet and Cabot, 1981; Reis et al., 1988).

The depressor effect of clonidine in the RVLM may not depend on occupation of local α_2-adrenoceptors, since local administration of neither NE nor any other catecholamine or phenylethylamine decreases blood pressure, and local administration of α_2-antagonists does not consistently increase blood pressure (Bousquet and Feldman, 1987). Clonidine is an imidazoline, and it has been suggested that clonidine may elicit hypotension by stimulating imidazoline receptors in the RVLM (Bousquet et al., 1984). A substantial proportion of clonidine binding sites in this region appear to be receptors for imidazolines, not for catecholamines, and an imidazoline- or imidazoline-like substance, ''clonidine-displacing substance,'' has been suggested as an endogenous ligand (Bousquet et al., 1989; Meeley et al., 1986). The use of anesthetized animals in these studies may have masked hypotensive effects of clonidine by other mechanisms or at higher levels of the neuraxis. Thus, microinjection of clonidine into the LC produces behavioral sleep and electroencephalographic synchronization, and injection of yohimbine or phentolamine produces behavioral arousal (De Sarro et al., 1987).

Clonidine not only causes sympathoinhibition but also evokes vagally mediated bradycardia. As noted above, α_2-adrenoceptors are concentrated in the dorsal motor nucleus of the vagus and the NA, intermediary centers for arterial baroreflex-mediated parasympathetic activation. Intravertebral arterial injections of α_2-adrenoceptor agonists potentiate, whereas α_1-antagonists inhibit, baroreflex-induced vagal bradycardia (Huchet et al., 1982). Clonidine also is an effective analgesic, probably because agonist binding to α_2-adrenoceptors on sensory terminals or in the substantia gelatinosa of the spinal cord inhibits ascending transmission of nociceptor information (Basbaum, 1992; Jones and Gebhart, 1986).

In some brain areas, such as the LC and midbrain periaquaductal gray region, α_2-adrenoceptors appear to be colocalized with opiate receptors; in other areas, α_2-adrenoceptors appear to be localized on cells containing 5-HT, CRH, AVP, growth hormone, or thyrotropin-releasing hormone (Jones et al., 1990). This colocalization may affect the responses to drugs acting at α_2-adrenoceptors. Langer has emphasized inhibitory α_2-heteroreceptors on serotonergic cells (Arbilla and Langer, 1990). Other examples of adrenoceptors that are thought to be heteroreceptors include inhibitory α_1-adrenoceptors on peripheral cholinergic neurones in rat atria and inhibitory α_2-adrenoceptors on cholinergic neurones in guinea pig Auerbach's plexus. Whether endogenous NE stimulates α_2-heteroreceptors on serotonergic cells is unknown.

Since α_2-adrenoceptor agonists seem to function primarily as inhibitory modulators, elucidating the physiological role of α_2-adrenoceptors may depend on experiments involving alterations in NE release. For instance, as noted above, PGi cells of the RVLM send excitatory projections to the LC and to SPNs. In both terminal regions, stimulation of α_2-adrenoceptors may limit the excitation but may not affect cellular firing at baseline.

β-Adrenoceptors

As with α_1-adrenoceptors, the distribution of β-adrenoceptors in the brain appears to correlate only weakly with the distribution of NE. For instance, the caudate nucleus has a relatively low concentration of NE but a high concentration of β-adrenoceptors.

Both β_1 and β_2 subtypes of β-adrenoceptors have been described in brain (Rainbow et al., 1984). In rats, high concentrations of β_1-adrenoceptors have been detected in the cingulate cortex, lamina I and II of the cerebral cortex, the hippocampus, and nuclei of the thalamus (gelatinosa, mediodorsal, ventral). High concentrations of β_2-adrenoceptors have been reported in the molecular layer of the cerebellum, over pia mater, and in thalamic nuclei (central, paraventricular, caudal lateral posterior). Nuclei of the medulla appear to possess about equal concentrations of the two subtypes. Virtually all the β-adrenoceptors in the cerebellum are of the β_2 subtype, whereas in the cortex β_1-adrenoceptors predominate.

In contrast with rat brain, human brain contains high concentrations of β-adrenoceptors in the caudate, nucleus accumbens, and putamen (Jones et al., 1990). High levels are also detected in the hippocampus, globus pallidus, and neocortex. Ocular β-adrenoceptors seem remarkably conserved across species, whereas in the pituitary there is substantial interspecific variation in the density and localization of the receptors. In the rat pituitary, the highest concentration of β-adrenoceptors is in the intermediate lobe.

The functional significance of the spatial localization of β_1- and β_2-adrenoceptors in brain is unknown. Since β_2-adrenoceptors appear to be dispersed rather homogeneously in brain, whereas β_1-adrenoceptor concentrations can vary by 20-fold in different brain areas, β_2-adrenoceptors may be associated with diffusely distributed glial cells or blood vessels and may not be located on neural cells (Minneman et al., 1979, 1981); however, even for β_1-adrenoceptors there is no close correlation between the regional concentration of the receptors and the density of noradrenergic innervation.

Dopamine Receptors

The distribution of DA receptors in the brain generally corresponds with the distribution of dopaminergic terminals. An exception appears to be that the D_3-receptors are not highly concentrated in the corpus striatum, as noted below.

There are at least five distinct types of DA receptors in brain (Cooper et al., 1991; Sibley and Monsma, 1992), as determined by using molecular biologic techniques in addition to the more traditional pharmacological approaches (Dearry et al., 1990; Rao et al., 1990; Sokoloff et al., 1990). The receptors have been separated into two general classes, D_1 and D_2, with three D_2 subtypes (D_2, D_3, and D_4) and two D_1 subtypes (D_1 and D_5).

Postsynaptic stimulatory receptors in the D_1 group are coupled to the stimulatory G-protein, G_s (Cooper et al., 1991), whereas postsynaptic, low-affinity receptors in the D_2 group inhibits adenylate cyclase by interacting with the inhibitory G-protein, G_i, and presynaptic, high-affinity D_2 receptors on dopaminergic terminals also interact with G_i. D_1 receptors, however, not only stimulate adenylate cyclase but also stimulate phosphoinositide turnover (Cooper et al., 1991), and D_2 receptors not only inhibit adenylate cyclase but also inhibit transmembrane entry of Ca^{2+} via voltage-sensitive calcium channels, enhance K^+ conductance, and possibly modulate phosphoinositide metabolism.

For the D_1 receptor subtype, the highest concentrations of mRNA expression are in the caudate, nucleus accumbens, and olfactory tubercle, with little or no mRNA detectable in the SN (Dearry et al., 1990). The D_5-receptor, in the D_1 family, is expressed to a much smaller extent than is the D_1 receptor, with highest expression in the hippocampus and hypothalamus. Postsynaptic D_1 receptors in the central nervous system may work synergistically with D_2 receptors in "enabling" behavioral and locomotor effects of dopaminergic pathway activation (Cooper et al., 1991).

In general, D_2 receptors exert inhibitory actions in a wide variety of cell types and regions (Cooper et al., 1991; Sibley and Monsma, 1992). D_2 autoreceptors in the striatum and nucleus accumbens inhibit DA synthesis in and DA release from dopaminergic terminals. In the SN and ventral tegmental area, D_2 receptor stimulation inhibits firing of dopaminergic cells. In the corpus striatum, D_2 stimulation inhibits acetylcholine release from cholinergic interneurons. In the pituitary gland, D_2 receptor stimulation inhibits release of prolactin and α-MSH. Stimulation of D_2 receptors on peripheral sympathetic nerve terminals inhibits NE release (Langer and Lehmann, 1989). The physiological functions of the subtypes of D_2 receptors remain to be established.

The D_3-receptor, one of the D_2 subtypes, is expressed predominantly if not exclusively in the limbic area (Sokoloff et al., 1990) and has a relatively high affinity for the dopaminergic agonist, quinpirol. The D_4-receptor, another D_2 subtype, is expressed predominantly in the frontal cortex, midbrain, amygdala, and medulla has relatively high affinity for the atypical neuroleptic clozapine (Sibley and Monsma, 1992).

Summary and Conclusions

Catecholaminergic pathways in the brain probably participate in arousal, memory, and vigilance behavior, and in psychiatric, neurological, and cardiovascular disorders; however, how central neural catecholamines contribute to these complex behaviors and disorders remains obscure. In particular, very little is known about the basis for the relationship between release of NE the brain and sympathetically mediated release of NE in the periphery. This relationship probably is indirect, reflecting the variable participation of central neural NE in the elaboration of complex behaviors with neuroendocrine components. Thus, despite improved delineation of central neuroanatomic pathways, knowledge about the functions of the centers they connect has lagged behind. Almost nothing is known about central neural coordination of peripheral catecholaminergic systems with other neuroendocrine systems in cardiovascular homeostasis.

At the level of the end organs, cardiovascular structures possess intrinsic "tone." SPN activity depends importantly on excitatory input from lower brainstem centers that mediate simple homeostatic reflexes, maintaining appropriate "steady-state" cardiovascular performance. At the next higher level, hypothalamically elaborated patterns reset homeostats. At the highest level, limbic and frontal structures use memory, learning, simulations, and consciousness to interpret afferent signals about the internal and external environments and to determine the occurrence and intensity of the hypothalamically evoked patterns.

Organized, periodic discharges of neurons in the RVLM generate SNS outflow in a complexly but not randomly determined manner, with important influences by clusters of cells at several more rostral sites in the neuraxis, especially during stress, and influences by more caudal medullary sites that receive interoceptive input. A network of brain centers therefore determines sympathetic neurocirculatory regulation. Prominent in this network are noradrenergic A2 cells in the NTS, the main site of termination of baroreceptor input to the brain; EPI-synthesizing C1 cells of the RVLM, which projects caudally to the SPNs and rostrally to several brainstem areas; noradrenergic A1 cells of the CVLM, which projects to AVP cells of the PVN and to the RVLM; noradrenergic A6 cells in the LC, the main source of NE in the brain; the PVN and posterolateral HACER area in the hypothalamus, the latter the apparent main subcortical center responsible for the generation of instinctive emotional behaviors in primates; and the ACE in the limbic system, a way-station between cortical centers and the brainstem.

Catecholaminergic cells in the brain occur in two noradrenergic and three dopaminergic pathways. Almost 80% of brain DA is in the terminal field of the nigrostriatal projection. Central neural DA seems to enable action, decreasing the threshold for initiating responses. Parkinson's disease, associated with degeneration of the SN, probably results from depletion of striatal DA; and schizophrenia probably results from dysfunction of the mesocortical dopaminergic system.

Rather than acting as a direct inhibitor or stimulator of neuronal function, NE seems mainly to modify responsiveness to other synaptic inputs. By decreasing background discharges and enhancing phasic excitatory or inhibitory inputs, the signal-to-noise ratio of neuronal responsivity increases. LC discharge biases attention towards novel, rapidly changing external and interoceptive signals. Despite the apparent involvement of both the mesotelencephalic DA system and the LC noradrenergic system in determining responses to environmental and interoceptor input, no concepts have explained whether and how the two catecholaminergic systems work together.

If the association between central catecholaminergic and peripheral SNS function seems complex and incompletely understood, the relationship between neuropeptides in the brain and sympathoneural outflow appears to be even more so.

Receptors for all three endogenous catecholamines have been described in brain. α_1-Adrenoceptors in the brain may mainly be stimulatory and α_2-adrenoceptors inhibitory; however, the functions of adrenoceptor subtypes probably depend on their cellular localization. Blockade of presynaptic α_2-adrenoceptors in the brain increases sympathetic outflow. The depressor effect of clonidine, an α_2-adrenoceptor agonist, in the RVLM may result from stimulation of a type of imidazoline receptor where "clonidine-displacing substance" acts as an endogenous ligand.

The literature about central catecholaminergic pathways and adrenoceptors is expanding rapidly; however, the role of central catecholamines specifically in regulation of SNS and AHS outflows remains poorly understood. This role probably will prove to be indirect and complex, with catecholamines in the central nervous system gating afferent information from exteroceptors and interoceptors, modulating hypothalamic secretion of releasing hormones and elaboration of neuroendocrine response patterns, and facilitating long-term memory of distressing events, vigilance, and initiation of motor behaviors.

5

Clinical Assessment of Catecholaminergic Function

Comprehending the mass of experimental literature about stress response patterns and the role of catecholaminergic systems in cardiovascular diseases requires acquaintance with clinical approaches to assess catecholaminergic function. This chapter discusses these assessment techniques.

The Concept of Sympathetic "Activity"

Walter Cannon considered catecholaminergic systems to function as a neuroendocrine unit: the sympathoadrenal system. If this view were correct, then a straightforward means to measure sympathoadrenal activity would be to record sympathetic nerve traffic directly. Even assuming congruence between SNS and AHS activities, and assuming homogeneity of sympathoneural outflows throughout the body, direct microneurographic recording of sympathetic nerve traffic would still not describe comprehensively the events at neuroeffector junctions that determine sympathoneural regulation of cardiovascular performance, because many processes intervene between the transmission of the nerve impulse and the responses of the smooth muscle effector cells.

Most clinical investigators have used neurochemical rather than neurophysiological means to examine sympathoadrenal "activity," such as by measurements of plasma levels of EPI, the adrenomedullary hormone, of NE, the sympathetic neurotransmitter (Lake et al., 1976), or of total catecholamines. Differential SNS and AHS responses during exposure to different stressors (e.g., Robertson, Johnson et al., 1979; Young and Landsberg, 1979; Young et al., 1984), and heterogeneous alterations in sympathoneural outflows to the heart, vasculature, organs, and glands as components of response patterns during stress, not only imply that neither plasma NE nor plasma EPI levels can indicate overall sympathetic "activity" but also call into question the meaning of the term. Since stress responses include patterned activation of neuronal, hormonal, and autocrine/paracrine catecholaminergic effectors, no single physiological or biochemical measurement can assess adequately the contributions of these effectors to homeostasis.

Clinical investigators have used noradrenergic "activity," "turnover," "spillover," "tone," and "function" largely interchangeably:

> Calculations based on steady-state infusion studies of either labelled or unlabelled catecholamines have increased the sensitivity of measurements of sympathetic nervous activity turnover. (Izzo, 1989, p. 305S)

These processes are not the same, and the differences are more than semantic. The rate of entry of NE into the bloodstream (NE spillover) relates only indirectly to the rate of exocytotic release of the transmitter from sympathetic nerve terminals, because the terminals extensively recycle endogenously released NE for re-use. The rate of exocytosis, if it could be measured, would relate only indirectly to the rate of turnover of NE in sympathetic nerve endings, because under resting conditions most of the irreversible loss of the transmitter results from leakage from storage vesicles and subsequent metabolism, not from exocytosis. Finally, the turnover rate of NE in the terminals relates only indirectly to the synthesis rate of NE; uncoupling of the two processes causes depletion of tissue NE stores.

This chapter emphasizes that neurochemical measurements can indicate distinct aspects of catecholaminergic function. For instance, whereas renal production of NE depends importantly on renal sympathetic nerve activity, renal production of DA, the natriuretic catecholamine, depends mainly on removal and decarboxylation of circulating DOPA, a process largely independent of renal sympathoneural activity; under baseline conditions, spillover of DHPG, the main intraneuronal metabolite of NE, depends mainly on leakage of NE from storage vesicles and therefore on noradrenergic turnover, a process different from the rate of sympathetically mediated release of NE; and changes in regional spillovers of DOPA and DOPAC probably reflect changes in regional rates of catecholamine biosynthesis, which, while usually closely linked with catecholamine turnover, relate only indirectly to changes in the rate of regional sympathetic nerve traffic.

Chemical Methods

Biochemical measurements have been the mainstay of clinical research about sympathetic cardiovascular regulation. Later sections describe other recently introduced clinical methods, including direct sympathetic nerve recording, spectral analysis of heart rate variability, and nuclear scanning. None of these other techniques alone can assess sympathetic "activity" comprehensively; combined measurements are required.

Terminology

Catecholamine terminology is confusing. A catechol is a chemical that contains an aromatic benzene ring and two adjacent hydroxyl groups on the ring (Figure 5–1) A specific chemical, "catechol," has this structure. In general, assays for "plasma catechol levels" refer to all the endogenous compounds that contain a catechol nucleus, not to the single chemical, "catechol," which probably is not an endogenous substance. A "catecholamine" consists of a catechol nucleus and a short hydrocarbon chain that ends in an amine group. The three endogenous catecholamines in human plasma are NE, EPI, and DA. "Adrenalin" is the brand name used by Parke-Davis for EPI. Since the description by Takamine (1901), reports in British journals have used "adrenaline" and "noradrenaline," whereas reports in American journals have used "epinephrine" and "norepinephrine," according the nomenclature of Abel (Abel and Crawford, 1897; Abel, 1902).

The other endogenous catechols consistently found in human plasma are DOPA, the precursor of the catecholamines; DHPG (or DOPEG), a deaminated metabolite of NE; and DOPAC, a deaminated metabolite of DA. In all body fluids, concentrations of the metabolites exceed by far concentrations of the parent amines. Partly because of

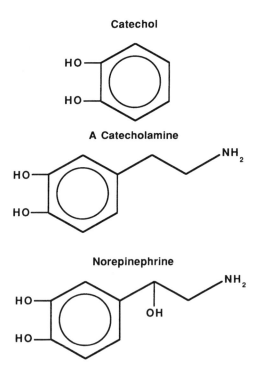

Figure 5–1. Chemical structures of catechols. A catechol contains an aromatic ring and two adjacent hydroxyl groups. A catecholamine contains a catechol and a hydrocarbon tail that includes an amine group. Norepinephrine is an example of a catecholamine.

the relative ease technically of measuring levels of the metabolites, many studies have reported levels of the metabolites rather than of the catecholamines themselves.

Early Methods

Soon after the identification of EPI as the vasoactive principal of the adrenal gland (Abel and Crawford, 1897; Oliver and Schafer, 1895) and the description of the profound cardiovascular effects of sympathetic nerve stimulation (Cyon, 1907; Pavlov, 1887), clinical investigators began to attempt to measure sympathoadrenal "activity." Observations of the effects surgical sympathectomy or adrenalectomy, measurements of physiological parameters, and administration of various drugs that interfere with sympathetic function all had their day. All have important theoretical and practical limitations. Sympathectomies and adrenalectomies could be done only in patients with underlying pathology justifying the operations, and values for no cardiovascular physiological parameter were found to correlate specifically with SNS activity. Moreover, since sympathectomy, adrenalectomy, or administration of sympatholytic drugs elicits compensatory changes in adrenoceptor numbers or activates other homeostatic systems, results of studies using these techniques tend to underestimate the sympathetic contribution to values for cardiovascular parameters.

Attention therefore turned early to chemical means for assessing catecholaminergic function. Since EPI was known to be secreted by the adrenal medulla, and since EPI, or a substance closely related to it (originally called "sympathin" and finally identified as NE), was thought to be released during sympathetic stimulation, attempts to measure endogenous EPI levels began early in the twentieth century. Bioassay preparations, such as used by Walter Cannon, exploited the extraordinarily potent effects of EPI on circulatory and other physiological parameters. In one of Cannon's early experiments (Cannon and de la Paz, 1911), he used the extent of relaxation of gastrointestinal smooth muscle to measure increases in adrenomedullary secretion during emotional stress. Later, Cannon and others used the magnitude of the increase in heart rate in animals with denervated hearts to reflect the circulating level of the cardioactive hormone, with abolition of the tachycardia in adrenalectomized animals confirming the hormone's adrenal source.

The potency of catecholamines explains their very low endogenous concentrations in the bloodstream. In antecubital venous plasma of resting humans, EPI levels can be less than 5 pg/ml, or less than about 3×10^{-11} M. Early attempts failed to measure endogenous levels of these compounds chemically. Assays for plasma catecholamine concentrations remain difficult, and EPI concentrations in arm venous plasma of healthy subjects at rest still strain the sensitivity of current methods.

The first chemical method for detecting catecholamines was colorimetric (Battelli, 1902), based on the unusual susceptibility of catecholamines to oxidize, forming a brownish solution, "adrenochrome." In 1949, von Euler and Hamberg introduced a colorimetric method where the adrenochrome was converted chemically to 1-methyl-3,5,6-trihydroxyindole. Trihydroxyindole has characteristic fluorescent properties, and detection of the fluorescence provided the basis for several methods that proved adequate to measure the small amounts of catecholamines in tissues (von Euler, 1959). Another type of fluorimetric assay was based on the condensation of oxidized cate-cholamines with ethylenediamine (Weil-Malherbe, 1956). Generally more sensitive radiometric procedures subsequently supplanted the fluorimetric methods, became the standard approach in the 1970s, and still are widely used.

Radioenzymatic Methods

The approach for all radioenzymatic techniques for measuring endogenous catechol-amine concentrations is the same: The catecholamine of interest in the sample is reacted with an enzyme that transfers a radioactive methyl group from a donor compound to the catecholamine. The radioactive derivative is then partially purified and the radio-activity counted. In the first methods for measuring plasma NE (e.g., Henry et al., 1975; Saelens et al., 1967; Weise and Kopin, 1976), based on the use of PNMT, NE in the sample was N-methylated by PNMT in the presence of radiolabeled S-adenosylmethio-nine (SAM), the donor of the radioactive methyl group. The resulting radioactive EPI was separated chromatographically before liquid scintillation counting. In 1968, Engel-man et al. described a radioenzymatic assay method using COMT. Two isotopes were included, [^{14}C]SAM as the methyl donor and [^{3}H]NE as an internal standard. The meth-ylated (methoxylated) derivatives were separated by cation-exchange chromatography and converted to vanillin before liquid scintillation counting. Purification of the deriv-atives using thin layer chromatography (Engelman and Portnoy, 1970) improved the sensitivity of the procedure. Passon and Peuler (1973) and Peuler and Johnson (1977) added other improvements that resulted in about a 10-fold increase in sensitivity and increased selectivity.

Liquid Chromatography with Electrochemical Detection

Since about 1980 (Allenmark and Hedman, 1979; Goldstein, Feuerstein et al., 1981; Hjemdahl et al., 1979), methods using liquid chromatography, usually coupled with electrochemical detection (LCED or HPLC methods) have rapidly gained popularity. The HPLC approaches have two important advantages: They do not involve radioac-tivity, and they can detect simultaneously several compounds related to catecholamin-ergic function besides the catecholamines themselves. Injection of fluorescent deriva-tives of the catecholamines enables assays of catecholamine levels by HPLC coupled with fluorimetric detection. This approach can be very sensitive and specific (van der Hoorn et al., 1989), but it cannot be used for simultaneous measurements of levels of DOPA, catecholamines, and metabolites.

The basis for electrochemical detection is the same as for the early colorimetric techniques—the tendency of catecholamines to oxidize at very low oxidizing potentials. The oxidation generates electric current. The compounds of interest are separated by passage through a high-pressure (high-performance) liquid chromatographic column (hence the designation, HPLC), and the compounds are identified based on character-istic retention times of standards on the column.

LCED assays for plasma catecholamines always include a sample preparation step to purify the catecholamines partially, in order to obtain interpretable chromatographic recordings. This step usually is an alumina extraction. Alumina (also called aluminum oxide) has the property of binding to the hydroxyl groups of catechols under basic conditions and freeing catechols under acidic conditions (Anton and Sayre, 1962). Alumina extraction has proven to be a remarkably simple, reliable, and effective way to purify plasma catechols. Another sample preparation procedure uses cation exchange chromatography, based on attraction of the positively charged amine group of catecholamines to negatively charged residues (e.g., sulfonate or carboxylic acid residues) on a cation exchange resin. Addition of a counter-ion with a positive charge, which competes with the amine group for binding sites on the resin, or of an acidic eluent, which neutralizes the anions of the resin, releases the amines from the resin. An advantage of the alumina method is its specificity, allowing direct injection of the eluent into a liquid chromatograph, whereas ion exchange methods alone often are inadequate for preparation of urine specimens. More important, the alumina procedure allows detection not only of the catecholamines but also of the precursor of the catecholamines, DOPA, which is a catechol amino acid; of the catechol intraneuronal metabolite of NE, DHPG; and of the catechol metabolite of DA, DOPAC. Since these metabolites are deaminated, they are not detected in samples after cation exchange chromatography.

Norepinephrine and Sympathoneural "Activity"

By far the most commonly used clinical approach for assessing sympathoadrenal "activity" has been to assay plasma concentrations of NE and EPI in arm venous blood. Plasma NE levels have been used to indicate activity of the neuronal sympathoneural component and EPI levels to indicate activity of the hormonal adrenomedullary component of the sympathoadrenal system.

No direct neurochemical index of sympathetically mediated exocytosis has been established. Although DBH is coreleased with NE during exocytosis, genetic factors independent of sympathetic activity determine individual differences in plasma levels of the enzyme, so that antecubital venous NE concentrations are unrelated to DBH concentrations (Lake, Ziegler et al., 1977). Although chromogranin A and NPY probably are also coreleased with NE during exocytosis, plasma levels of these peptides change relatively little during physiological changes in sympathoneural outflow that produce large changes in plasma NE levels (Cryer et al., 1991; Dimsdale and Ziegler, 1991; Tidgren et al., 1991).

Abundant clinical and laboratory evidence has confirmed a generally close relationship between plasma levels of NE and sympathetically mediated exocytosis. Patients with quadriplegia due to spinal cord transection or orthostatic hypotension due to pure autonomic failure have low plasma levels of NE (Goldstein, Polinsky et al., 1989; Mathias et al., 1976; Polinsky et al., 1981), and patients with a regional sympathectomy have a decreased arteriovenous increment of the plasma NE concentration in the sympathectomized limb (Goldstein, Bonner et al., 1986). The amount of directly recorded skeletal muscle sympathetic activity (SMSA) at baseline correlates positively with NE concentrations in antecubital venous blood (Anderson et al., 1989; Leimbach et al., 1986; Morlin et al., 1983; Seals et al., 1988; Victor et al., 1987; Wallin et al., 1981; Yamada et al., 1989), and during reflexive stimulation of sympathoneural outflow, increases in regional venous NE levels correlate fairly well with increases in directly recorded SMSA (Rea, Eckberg et al., 1990). In animals, sympathetic stimulation evokes release of NE into the bloodstream (Brown and Gillespie, 1957; Yamaguchi and Kopin, 1979; Yamaguchi et al., 1977); and physical ablation of sympathetic pathways decreases plasma NE levels (Kopin et al., 1984; Yamaguchi and Kopin, 1979). Reflexive changes in directly recorded renal sympathoneural activity relate closely to changes in plasma NE levels (Garty, Deka-Starosta, Chang et al., 1989).

The validity of plasma NE levels in indicating sympathetic nerve traffic or sympathetically mediated exocytosis depends importantly on several factors (Figure 5–2). First, plasma levels of any endogenous biochemical represent the ratio of the rate of release (spillover) of the substance into the bloodstream and the clearance of the substance from the bloodstream. This kinetic fact is especially important for NE because of the continuous release of NE into and rapid removal of NE from plasma. Second, the SNS consists of myriad nerve networks throughout the body, and stress responses often include patterned, heterogeneous changes in sympathetic outflow to different vascular beds. Because sympathetic nervous activity in the arm influences levels of NE in arm venous plasma, these levels may not reflect sympathetic nervous activity elsewhere in the body, especially during stress (Folkow et al., 1983). Third, only a small proportion of NE released from sympathetic nerve endings reaches the circulation, the majority being removed back into the axonal cytoplasm by neuronal reuptake (Iversen, 1973). If Uptake-1 were inhibited pharmacologically, such as by a tricyclic antidepressant, or were decreased as part of a pathophysiological process, then for a given amount of sympathetically mediated exocytosis, the rate of entry of NE into the bloodstream would increase. Fourth, any of several endogenous biochemicals—including NE itself—have the potential to modulate the rate of release of NE for a given amount of sympathetic nerve traffic. In particular, clinical studies have indicated that α_2-adrenoceptors on vascular sympathetic nerve endings tonically inhibit regional NE spillover in the forearm (Grossman, Chang et al., 1991a; Grossman, Rea et al., 1991). Factors affecting this modulation alter the amount of exocytotic release of NE for a given amount of sympathetic nerve traffic. Fifth, although NE in plasma derives to only a very small extent from the adrenal medulla under resting conditions, the adrenomedullary contribution to plasma NE levels can change during stress responses (Garber et al., 1976; Goldstein, Breier et al., 1992; Goldstein, McCarty et al., 1983; Yamaguchi et al., 1989). Moreover, at least in laboratory animals, the relative proportions of NE and EPI in the adrenal venous drainage can vary in response to different stimuli (Feuerstein and Gutman, 1971; Folkow and von Euler, 1954). Sixth, NE spillover into the venous drainage of a given vascular bed can vary with regional blood flow (Grossman, Chang et al., 1991b). Seventh, because of the homeostatic nature of catecholaminergic systems, drugs, dietary factors, and physiologic and pathologic states increase interindividual variability in catecholamine levels, resulting in the possibility of Type I (false negative) errors. Table 5–1 lists some of these factors. Two of the most commonly used of all drugs—nicotine

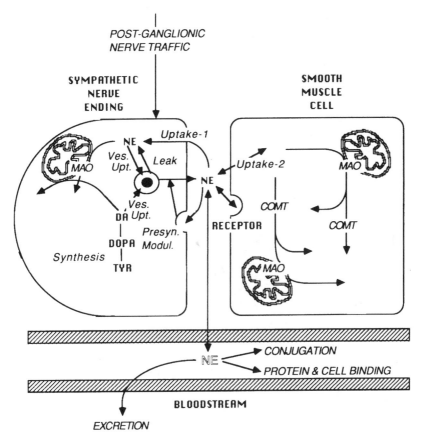

POST-GANGLIONIC
NERVE TRAFFIC

SYMPATHETIC
NERVE
ENDING

SMOOTH
MUSCLE
CELL

Figure 5–2. Factors affecting the relationships between sympathetic nerve activity and plasma norepinephrine. Many factors intervene between the rate of postganglionic sympathoneural activity and the concentration of norepinephrine in the bloodstream. Presynaptic factors include Uptake-1, modulation by receptors on the nerve terminals, net leakage of amines from storage vesicles, synthesis, and metabolism by oxidative metabolism. Postsynaptic factors include Uptake-2 and metabolism by O-methylation and deamination. Intravascular factors include sulfate-conjugation and binding to plasma proteins and cell membranes. Extravascular factors include renal excretion.

and caffeine—increase catecholamine levels acutely in humans (Cryer, 1980; Cryer et al., 1976; Curatalo and Robertson, 1983; Robertson, Johnson et al., 1979; Robertson et al., 1978, 1981). And eighth, sympathomimetic drugs or pathological states can disrupt the relationship between sympathetically mediated exocytosis and neuronal NE release; for instance, administration of tyramine increases plasma NE levels (Goldstein, Nurnberger et al., 1983) by a mechanism independent of exocytosis, and during anoxic myocardial ischemia, NE appears to leak at an increased net rate from storage vesicles into the axoplasm, entering the extracellular fluid by reverse transport through the Uptake-1 carrier (Schomig et al., 1987).

This is not to say that plasma NE levels in antecubital venous blood are invalid in

Table 5-1. Some Factors Affecting Plasma Catecholamine Concentrations

Conditions of Sampling

Posture (increased NE)
Exercise (increased NE and EPI)
Time of day (early AM peak of NE and EPI)
Room temperature (increased NE in cool room)
Postprandial state (increased NE after meal)
Calorie intake (increased NE with caloric excess; increased EPI with glucoprivation)
Salt intake (increased NE during salt restriction)
Normal aging (increased NE in normotensive subjects)
Ovulation or luteal phase (increased NE)
Barbiturate anesthesia (decreased NE)

Diseases or Pathological Conditions

Cardiovascular
Myocardial infarction (increased NE and EPI)
Congestive heart failure (increased NE)
Pulmonary edema (increased EPI and NE)
Cardiac arrest (increased EPI and NE)
Shock (increased EPI and NE)
Hemorrhage (increased NE early, increased EPI with hypotension)
Intravascular volume depletion (increased NE)
Early essential hypertension (increased NE or EPI in some patients)
Hyperdynamic circulation syndrome (increased NE)
Early essential hypertension (increased NE or EPI in some patients)
Mitral valve prolapse syndrome (increased NE or EPI in some patients)
Vasodepressor syncope (increased EPI, no change in or decreased NE)

Endocrine
Hypoglycemia (increased EPI)
Pheochromocytoma (increased NE)
Hyperthyroidism (decreased NE)
Ketoacidosis (increased NE and EPI)

Neurological
Stroke due to intracranial bleeding (increased NE and EPI)
Pure autonomic failure (decreased NE)
Multiple system atrophy (decreased NE response to standing)
Dopamine-β-hydroxylase deficiency (absent NE and EPI)
Neuroblastoma (variably increased NE)
Sympathectomy (decreased NE)

Psychiatric
Distress (increased EPI, increased NE if locomotion)
Anxiety (variably increased EPI)

Drugs (See also Tables 5–2 and 7–3)

Diuretics (increased NE)
α_2-Adrenoceptor agonists, e.g., clonidine, guanabenz, guanfacine, α-methylDOPA (decreased NE)
α_2-Adrenoceptor antagonists, e.g., yohimbine, rauwolscine (increased NE)
Isoproterenol (increased NE)
α-Methyltyrosine (decreased NE)
Sympathomimetic amines, e.g., dextroamphetamine, tyramine (increased NE)
Ganglion blockers, e.g., trimethaphan (decreased NE)
Reserpine (decreased NE)
Tricyclic antidepressants, e.g., desipramine (usually no change in NE—see text)
Glucocorticoids, e.g., prednisone (decreased NE)
Sedatives, e.g, diazepam, barbiturates (decreased NE)

diagnosis, treatment, or prognosis in neurocardiology. One must interpret plasma NE levels carefully, however, keeping in mind the purpose of the test, the characteristics of the patient, the possible interacting effects of medications, and the above-described other factors that can influence the obtained results.

Sources of Plasma Norepinephrine

NE in the bloodstream emanates mainly from the networks of sympathetic nerve endings that enmesh blood vessels—especially arterioles—throughout the body and pervade parenchyma of the heart, viscera, and endocrine glands. Because the average caliber of the arterioles determines total peripheral resistance to blood flow, the sympathetic innervation of arteriolar smooth muscle represents a focal point in neural regulation and dysregulation of the circulation.

NE released in arterial walls appears to reach the bloodstream mainly by diffusion into capillary networks at the adventitial surface. Although the path in arterioles from the sympathetic nerve endings to the circulation has not been defined, a proportion of released NE probably diffuses directly into the vascular lumen.

Under basal conditions in humans and laboratory animals, little if any circulating NE in mixed venous blood derives from the adrenal medulla (Planz and Planz, 1979) because of the very small proportion of the cardiac output distributed to the adrenal glands. Adrenalectomized patients and rats have normal urinary excretion of NE (Price, 1957; von Euler et al., 1954); however, compensatory SNS activation in adrenalectomized subjects may lead to underestimation of the adrenomedullary contribution. In some species the catecholamine content of adrenal venous plasma includes a substantial amount of NE; in cats, for instance, NE accounts for about 50% of the catecholamines in the adrenal venous drainage (Chai et al., 1991).

The vas deferens contains a high density of noradrenergic terminals. The small blood flow to this organ, coupled with the narrow width of the synaptic clefts (about 10–30 nm compared with 60–4000 nm in blood vessels; Bevan et al., 1980; Richardson, 1962), imply that the contribution of this densely innervated structure to NE concentrations in mixed venous plasma is negligibly small.

In the heart, sympathetic nerves run alongside the myocardial cells, forming a latticelike network in close proximity to capillaries. This morphological arrangement helps to explain why about 20% of NE in the myocardium derives from uptake of circulating NE (Kopin and Gordon, 1963) and why the myocardial nerves remove in one pass about ⅔ of NE in the coronary arterial supply (Goldstein, Brush et al., 1988).

Most of NE released from sympathetic nerves does not reach the bloodstream unchanged, because, as noted in the chapter about peripheral catecholaminergic systems, the major route of inactivation of endogenously released NE is by reuptake into the nerve terminals. The extent of diffusion of NE from the synaptic clefts into the circulation varies with the width of the clefts (Bevan and Su, 1974; Bevan et al., 1980; Hume and Bevan, 1984). Nonvascular sites of sympathetic innervation, such as the vas deferens, have very narrow clefts, whereas arterioles generally have wide clefts. Cleft widths in walls of arteries vary markedly. If one considers the heavy sympathetic innervation of arterioles and the wide synapses in vascular walls, most of the circulating NE probably derives from release from nonjunctional varicosities and from neuroeffector junctions in arteriolar walls. Stjarne (1988) has emphasized that most sympathetic varicosities are nonjunctional. The relative contributions to plasma NE levels from NE released into synapses and NE released nonjunctionally are unknown.

In virtually all vascular beds, sympathetic nerves release NE into the venous drainage (Goldstein, McCarty et al., 1983). In most beds, the rate of NE spillover exceeds the rate of removal, resulting in a net arteriovenous increment in the plasma NE concentration. An exception is found in the liver, which extensively removes portal venous NE, diminishing the contribution of gut sympathetic activity to NE concentrations in mixed venous blood. Another exception is found in the heart, which removes such a large proportion of coronary arterial NE that the arteriovenous increment in plasma NE levels across the heart can be virtually zero, grossly underestimating the substantial spillover of NE into the cardiac venous drainage (Goldstein, Brush et al., 1988).

One can estimate the contribution of a particular vascular bed to NE in mixed venous plasma, from the regional venous NE concentration and the proportion of the cardiac output distributed to that bed. Thus, the adrenal gland has a very large arteriovenous increment in plasma NE, but since only a very small proportion of the cardiac output is distributed to the adrenal gland, the contribution of the adrenal to NE in arterial blood is small in humans—2% or less (Brown, Jenner et al., 1981; Planz, 1978; Planz and Planz, 1979). The contribution of the heart to arterial plasma NE is also small because of the relatively small proportion of the cardiac output distributed to the heart. In contrast, the kidneys, which receive about ⅕ of the cardiac output, and skeletal muscle contribute substantially to plasma NE levels in arterial or mixed venous blood (Esler, Jennings, Korner et al., 1984b; Esler, Jennings, Leonard et al., 1984; Esler et al., 1990).

The relative contributions of these beds to arterial plasma NE levels during physiological manipulations remain incompletely understood. Renal nerve stimulation and clinical renovascular hypertension both are associated with increased renal production of NE; however, neither situation is consistently associated with increased NE concentrations in arterial plasma (Brown, Jenner et al., 1981; Oliver et al., 1980). Bilateral carotid artery occlusion increases arterial NE levels via increased estimated renal NE release, apparently without increased net release in the femoral, splanchnic, or pulmonary beds (Reison et al., 1983); however, this conclusion was based on regional arteriovenous differences in NE concentrations and did not take into account possible changes in regional NE clearance.

Modulation of Norepinephrine Release

Presynaptic receptors influence the relationship between sympathetic nerve traffic and NE release (Langer, 1974, 1981; Langer and Lehmann, 1989) and therefore the accuracy of plasma NE levels in indicating sympathetic nerve activity. The chapter about peripheral catecholaminergic systems discusses these processes in detail, and the following presents only salient features related to the sources and meanings of plasma NE levels.

Endogenously released NE can inhibit its own release, by stimulating inhibitory α_2-

adrenoceptors on sympathetic nerve endings. Blockade of α_2-adrenoceptors by intravenous yohimbine administration increases blood pressure and arterial plasma NE levels in humans (Goldberg et al., 1983; Goldstein, Zimlichman et al., 1986b). Brachial intra-arterial infusion of yohimbine increases forearm NE release into the bloodstream proportionately much more than can be attributed to concurrently increased forearm blood flow (Grossman, Rea et al., 1991), and intravenous infusion of yohimbine increases arterial NE levels in humans proportionately much more than can be attributed to increased skeletal muscle sympathetic activity (Rea, Eckberg et al., 1990). Yohimbine does not affect blood pressure or plasma NE levels in unstimulated pithed rats (Kopin et al., 1984) or in ganglion-blocked humans (Goldstein, Zimlichman et al., 1986b). Systemic administration of another α_2-adrenoceptor blocker, rauwolscine, also increases directly recorded sympathetic activity (McCall et al., 1983). These results suggest that increases in sympathoneural outflow (elicited via direct drug actions in the brain and via reflexive responses to systemic vasodilation) and blockade of presynaptic α_2-adrenoceptors on sympathetic terminals combine to produce the increases in plasma NE levels attending α_2-adrenoceptor blockade.

EPI can stimulate presynaptic β-adrenoceptors and thereby augment release of NE during sympathetic stimulation (Tarizzo and Dahlof, 1989). In humans, intravenous administration of the nonselective β-adrenoceptor agonist isoproterenol increases plasma NE levels (Goldstein, Zimlichman et al., 1986a; Vincent et al., 1986), probably by augmenting NE release from sympathetic nerve endings. Other possible mechanisms for this effect, such as decreased NE clearance and baroreceptor unloading, seem unlikely, because β-blockade with propranolol decreases NE clearance (Cryer et al., 1980), and isoproterenol administration increases systolic and pulse pressures (Gero and Gerova, 1967).

During reflexive stimulation of sympathetic outflow, EPI taken up into from the circulation into sympathetic nerve terminals can theoretically be coreleased with NE and stimulate β-adrenoceptors on the terminals to augment further NE release. These are the key elements of the ''epinephrine hypothesis,'' discussed in the chapter about peripheral catecholaminergic systems.

Occupation or blockade of any of several other types of receptors on sympathetic nerves has the potential to modulate NE release. The receptors include those for acetylcholine (Levy and Blattberg, 1976), AII (Zimmerman, 1978, 1981), adenosine (Snyder, 1985), and prostaglandins (Hedqvist, 1969). For most of these, direct clinical evidence for such modulation is lacking. Since stimulation-induced release of NE depends on increases in cytoplasmic Ca^{2+} concentrations, drugs or circulating factors that affect transmembrane movement of Ca^{2+} or release of Ca^{2+} from intracellular stores should also influence NE release; however, concurrent circulatory effects that alter sympathetic outflow reflexively may obscure these influences.

Endothelium-derived relaxing factor (NO) may also modulate sympathetically mediated release of NE. Interference with NO production or disruption of endothelial integrity augments neurogenic vasoconstriction (Furchgott, 1983; Urabe et al., 1991; Zeiher et al., 1989) and coronary vasoconstrictor responses to α-adrenoceptor agonists (Jones et al., 1993). Endothelial denudation of rabbit carotid arteries studied in vitro augments release of NE from the luminal and adventitial surfaces (Cohen and Weisbrod, 1988); however, whether interference with NO production causes this augmentation is unknown.

Indirectly acting sympathomimetic amines release NE from sympathetic nerve endings by a nonexocytotic mechanism, increasing plasma NE levels (Goldstein, Nurnberger et al., 1983; Scriven et al., 1983). Replacement of endogenous catecholamines by false neurotransmitters such as octopamine helps to explain the development tachyphylaxis of pressor responses after repeated administration of sympathomimetic amines such as tyramine.

Pharmacologic agents that affect activities of catecholamine biosynthetic or degradative enzymes in sympathetic nerve terminals also alter NE release. α-Methyltyrosine (α-MT) inhibits TH, depleting NE stores by blocking competitively the rate-limiting enzyme in catecholamine biosynthesis. Repeated administration of α-MT decreases plasma NE levels (Goldstein, Udelsman et al., 1987). Since the drug also diminishes synthesis of DA in the brain, prolonged administration of α-MT can evoke parkinsonian signs (Imperato-McGinley et al., 1987).

α-MethylDOPA is an effective antihypertensive drug. In neuronal and nonneuronal cells, α-methylDOPA is decarboxylated to form α-methylDA. In sympathetic nerves, the α-methylDA is taken up into storage vesicles and converted to α-methylNE. α-MethylNE acts as a false transmitter and is less potent than NE at α-adrenoceptors on vascular smooth muscle cells. The false transmitter mechanism was initially accepted as the basis for the antihypertensive action of α-methylDOPA. In the brain, however, α-methylNE inhibits central sympathetic outflow by stimulating α_2-adrenoceptors, and this central sympathoinhibitory effect is now thought to be the main mechanism for the antihypertensive action of the drug.

Reserpine inhibits vesicular uptake of DA, and since DBH is localized to the vesicles, reserpine inhibits synthesis of NE from DA, resulting in depletion of releasable NE stores. The blockade of formation of NE from DA leads to a buildup of axoplasmic DA, which is metabolized by MAO to form DOPAC, and the DOPAC is O-methylated extraneuronally to form HVA. Thus, in rats treated with reserpine, the rate of urinary excretion of the DA metabolite HVA increases to the same extent that the excretion of the major NE metabolite, MHPG, decreases (Kopin and Weise, 1968), and plasma levels of DOPAC increase to high values, whereas plasma levels of DHPG eventually decrease to very low values (Eisenhofer, Ropchak et al., 1988).

Clonidine Suppression and Yohimbine Challenge Tests

Neurochemical evidence indicating increased sympathoneural outflow does not itself imply an augmented noradrenergic contribution to blood pressure. Clonidine decreases and yohimbine increases sympathoneural outflows and plasma NE levels. A lack of suppression of plasma NE levels after clonidine administration constitutes a positive finding in the diagnostic evaluation of pheochromocytoma, as discussed in the chapter about cardiovascular diseases; and the combination of a high plasma NE level and a large depressor response to clonidine may identify patients with "hypernoradrenergic hypertension" more accurately than either measure alone (Goldstein, Levinson et al., 1985). Yohimbine challenge testing may distinguish patients with excessive pressor responsiveness for a given increment in sympathetic activity (i.e., postsynaptic hyper-responsiveness) from patients with excessive pressor responsiveness due to excessive NE release (i.e., presynaptic hyperresponsiveness), as also discussed in the chapter about cardiovascular diseases.

Plasma Norepinephrine Kinetics

The pharmacokinetic term "spillover" refers to the appearance rate of an endogenously released substance in the plasma, and "clearance" refers to the volume of plasma emptied of that substance per unit time. As noted above, the steady-state plasma level of NE does not indicate NE spillover or clearance, only their net result. Pharmacokinetically, the concentration of NE in arterial plasma (NE_a) is determined by the ratio of the spillover rate of NE into the arterial plasma and the clearance of NE from the arterial plasma:

$$NE_a = \text{Spillover} / \text{Clearance}$$

The relationship between "total body spillover" of NE and the spillover rate of NE into arterial plasma can be confusing. If one were to add together the rates of release of NE in all the vascular beds of the body, the sum would exceed the rate of spillover of NE into the arterial plasma, because some release sites are arranged in series, such as in the splanchnic–portal system and the lungs. Within a given vascular bed, the estimated spillover rate of NE into the venous drainage underestimates the regional total rate of release of the transmitter into the bloodstream within the organ, because some of the released NE is removed before it can reach the venous drainage. Quantifying the contribution of the lungs to arterial NE spillover is an especially complex problem, because the lungs do not remove NE from the systemic arterial plasma.

One can estimate the clearance of an endogenous compound, such as NE, from the plasma by measuring the steady-state concentration of the compound during its infusion. At a given infusion rate, the more rapid the clearance, the lower the steady-state concentration. NE is a potent drug, and early methods to measure clearance of NE from plasma required physiologically active NE concentrations. The use of infusions of tracer amounts of [³H]NE avoids the problem (Esler, 1982). The steady-state clearance (ml/min) of NE from arterial plasma can therefore be calculated from the infusion rate of the [³H]NE (dpm/min) divided by the steady-state concentration of [³H]NE (dpm/ml) in the plasma.

Since the ratio of the spillover rate to the clearance defines the arterial plasma level of endogenous NE, the spillover rate of NE into the plasma (pmol/min) can be calculated from the product of the plasma NE concentration (pmol/ml) and NE clearance (ml/min), the latter determined from the above-described tracer method. In mathematical terms,

$$\text{Arterial NE Clearance} = \frac{\text{Infusion Rate of } [^3\text{H}]\text{NE}}{[^3\text{H}]\text{NE}_a}$$

$$\text{NE Spillover Rate into Arterial Plasma} = \text{Arterial NE Clearance} \cdot \text{NE}_a$$

where $[^3\text{H}]\text{NE}_a$ is the arterial plasma concentration of $[^3\text{H}]\text{NE}$ and NE_a the arterial plasma concentration of endogenous NE.

Healthy people release about 0.3–0.5 μg/min (1.8-3.0 nmol/min) of NE into arterial plasma (Esler, Jennings, Korner et al., 1988; Goldstein, Eisenhofer et al., 1987), a rate too slow for endogenously released NE to exert hormonal effects (Silverberg et al., 1978).

In early studies of tracer NE kinetics, the rate of NE spillover into antecubital venous plasma, as opposed to arterial plasma, was presumed to reflect "total body" spillover of NE; however, during intravenous infusion of $[^3\text{H}]\text{NE}$, tissues of the arm remove about one-half the labeled catecholamine in the arterial plasma (Chang et al., 1986; Goldstein, Zimlichman et al., 1985), indicating that NE clearances calculated from arterial concentrations of $[^3\text{H}]\text{NE}$ average about one-half those calculated from antecubital venous $[^3\text{H}]\text{NE}$ concentrations. Thus, NE clearances based on samples of antecubital venous blood overestimate NE clearances from arterial blood (Christensen et al., 1984; Hilsted et al., 1983). Because of the usually small arteriovenous increment in plasma NE concentrations in the forearm, these findings also indicate substantial local release of endogenous NE into the forearm venous drainage.

Inhibition of Uptake-1 increases the proportion of released NE that enters the circulation, obscuring the relationship between the rate of sympathetic nerve traffic and the rate of NE spillover. Without other neurochemical information, one cannot distinguish increased arterial NE spillover due to increased sympathetically mediated NE release from increased spillover due to decreased neuronal reuptake of NE.

Assessing the kinetics of simultaneously infused $[^3\text{H}]\text{NE}$ and $[^3\text{H}]$isoproterenol provides a way to make this distinction, since sympathetic nerves do not remove isoproterenol. After cessation of a simultaneous infusion of $[^3\text{H}]\text{NE}$ and $[^3\text{H}]$isoproterenol, the ratio of $[^3\text{H}]$isoproterenol to $[^3\text{H}]\text{NE}$ in plasma increases rapidly, because the $[^3\text{H}]\text{NE}$ concentration decreases faster than does the $[^3\text{H}]$isoproterenol concentration. Desipramine treatment abolishes this increase in the $[^3\text{H}]$isoproterenol:$[^3\text{H}]\text{NE}$ ratio, indicating that the difference in clearances of the two tracer reflects neuronal uptake of NE. Thus, the rate of increase in the isoproterenol:NE ratio, expressed as a function of the ratio in the infusate, can provide an index of Uptake-1 activity (Goldstein, Horwitz, Keiser et al., 1983; Polinsky et al., 1985). This approach assumes equal removal of NE and isoproterenol by Uptake-2. The technique seems valid in the human arm (Goldstein, Zimlichman et al., 1985), the canine hindlimb (Zimlichman et al., 1986), and the human heart (Goldstein, Brush et al., 1988), but not in the canine kidney (Zimlichman et al., 1986).

Measurements of plasma levels of radiolabeled and endogenous NE and DHPG provide another means to assess Uptake-1 activity, as discussed below in the section about regional NE kinetics. A third approach compares NE clearances before and after

Uptake-1 blockade using desipramine. Desipramine-induced inhibition of sympatho-neural outflow (Eisenhofer, Saigusa et al., 1991; Lavian et al., 1991; Szabo and Schultheiss, 1990) complicates this method and explains why desipramine administration often does not increase plasma NE levels in humans, despite decreased NE clearance (Cohen et al., 1990; Eisenhofer, Esler et al., 1990; Goldstein, Zimlichman et al., 1985).

Any manipulations, drugs, or diseases that affect Uptake-1 can alter the apparent spillover rate of NE into plasma. Esler, Jennings, Korner et al. (1988) summarized situations where alterations in removal of NE from the bloodstream can distort the relationship between SNS activity and plasma levels of NE. In heart failure, orthostasis, autonomic insufficiency, hypertension, or treatment with β-adrenoceptor blockers, tricyclic antidepressants, cocaine, or digitalis glycosides (Leitz and Stefano, 1970), plasma NE concentrations exceed those expected from NE release. Decreased NE spillover during β-blockade in humans can offset the prolongation of NE clearance, mitigating the increase in plasma NE levels (Rosen et al., 1990). During high dietary intake of calories, plasma NE concentrations are lower than expected from NE release. Plasma NE concentrations and release agree (i.e., NE clearance is normal) in most patients with essential hypertension, depression, cirrhosis, hypothyroidism, hyperthyroidism, multiple system atrophy, diabetes, dietary salt restriction, and during treatment with diuretics, clonidine, insulin, MAO inhibitors, and hydrocortisone. General anesthesia with pentobarbital markedly decreases NE spillover, and since NE clearance decreases concurrently, decreases in plasma NE levels in barbiturate-anesthetized subjects probably underestimate substantially the extent of sympathoinhibition (Best et al., 1984). In parenchymal failure of the heart, lungs, liver, or kidneys, plasma NE clearance can decrease (McCance and Forfar, 1990; Ring-Larsen et al., 1982; Sole et al., 1979), augmenting plasma NE levels for a given rate of NE release from sympathetic nerve terminals.

Restriction of dietary salt intake tends to increase plasma NE levels, especially in elderly people and in patients with hypertension (Luft et al., 1979; Zimlichman, Goldstein, Stull et al., 1987). Salt restriction increases directly recorded skeletal sympathetic nerve activity (Anderson et al., 1989); however, on the basis of application of a two-compartment model to results of NE kinetics, Linares et al. (1988) suggested that the increase in plasma NE levels during dietary salt restriction results from a decreased volume of distribution of circulating NE.

Orthostasis increases antecubital venous NE levels by about two-fold and increases the estimated rate of release of NE into the extravascular compartment (Linares et al., 1988; Supiano et al., 1990). Directly recorded SMSA increases concurrently to about the same extent (Burke et al., 1977; Delius et al., 1972b).

Antecubital venous NE levels generally increase with increasing subject age (Goldstein, Lake et al., 1983; Ziegler et al., 1976), although several studies have reported an absence of this relationship in hypertensives (Goldstein and Lake, 1984; for review see Goldstein, 1983b). Directly recorded skeletal muscle sympathetic activity also increases with increasing subject age (Morlin et al., 1983; Sundlof and Wallin, 1978a; Yamada et al., 1989). Whether plasma NE clearance declines with aging has been controversial. Whereas Esler (1982) reported decreased NE clearance, other investigators have reported age-related increases in NE spillover (Hilsted et al., 1985a; Hoeldtke et al., 1985; MacGilchrist et al., 1989; Veith et al., 1986). Supiano et al. (1990) used compartmental analysis to conclude that the basal supine rate of release of NE into the extravascular compartment in elderly subjects exceeds that in young subjects.

During mental challenge (playing a video game), arterial NE spillover increases substantially, with the increment related directly to the magnitude of the pressor and cardiac output responses; in contrast, antecubital venous NE levels can fail to increase and therefore can be unrelated to the systemic hemodynamic responses (Goldstein, Eisenhofer et al., 1987). These findings show that if one ignores the effects of a stressor on NE clearance, one can reach erroneous conclusions from antecubital venous NE levels about the contribution of sympathoneural activation to the hemodynamic responses (Dimsdale and Ziegler, 1991; Todd et al., 1984).

As cardiac output can be viewed as representing the sum of blood flows in many parallel vascular circuits, total body NE spillover can be viewed as representing the sum of regional spillovers of NE into the bloodstream in several parallel innervated regions. As such, "total body" NE spillover, reflected by arterial NE spillover, seems a useful theoretical construct; however, because of the serial arrangement of release and removal sites in the lungs and portal–hepatic beds, the sum of regional NE spillovers exceeds arterial NE spillover. More importantly, because of the frequently heterogeneous responses of sympathetic outflow in different vascular beds during exposure to stressors, assessments of arterial NE spillover can fail to detect changes in sympathetically mediated NE release in particular beds such as the heart, kidneys, and gut.

Regional Norepinephrine Kinetics

Measurements of cardiac output can fail to detect localized derangements in blood flow (e.g., arteriovenous fistula, arterial thrombosis), and analogously, measurements of arterial NE spillover can fail to detect localized derangements in sympathetically mediated release of NE. This limitation would not be important in stress responses involving diffuse, directionally similar changes in sympathetic nerve traffic (e.g., reflexive SNS stimulation during nitroprusside-induced hypotension) but would be important in stress responses involving differential and heterogeneous changes in nerve traffic (e.g., postprandial, thermoregulatory, and possibly defense responses).

The chapter about stress response patterns discusses in detail this patterning of sympathetic outflows, and so the following presents only a few examples. Orthostasis, isometric exercise, exposure to cold, and depletion of extracellular volume elicit reflexive, sympathetically mediated shifts in blood flow distribution; plasma NE normally increases in these situations (Robertson, Johnson et al., 1979). Stimulation of arterial "high pressure" baroreceptors inhibits sympathetic outflow rather diffusely, although there are quantitative differences in the responses among regional beds (Ninomiya et al., 1971). Sympathetic responses to unloading of "low pressure" baroreceptors are more heterogeneous (Karim et al., 1972), with prominent increases in sympathoneural outflow to skeletal muscle. Responses to increased afferent activity from both types of baroreceptors include skeletal muscle and renal sympathoinhibition. Stimuli that influence sympathetic outflow to the skin differ from those that influence sympathetic outflow to skeletal muscle. External cooling or warming markedly affects skin sympathetic outflow but not skeletal muscle outflow, whereas stimuli that elicit baroreceptor-sympathetic responses exert little effect on skin sympathetic activity (Delius et al., 1972a, 1972b).

Measurements of regional NE spillover avoid the lack of sensitivity and specificity of measurements of arterial or ''total body'' spillover. Assessments of regional NE kinetics distinguish clearance from spillover as factors determining arteriovenous differences in plasma NE levels.

The most common approach for measuring regional NE spillover uses intravenous infusion of [^{3}H]NE, with measurements of regional plasma flow and of arterial and regional venous plasma concentrations of total and [^{3}H]NE. A second approach uses intra-arterial infusion of [^{3}H]NE into the organ of interest, with measurements of the regional plasma flow and venous plasma concentrations of total and [^{3}H]NE. The first approach offers the potential for examining simultaneously NE spillovers in more than one organ; the latter does not; however, the first approach entails potentially larger errors of measurement and requires much more radioactivity. The calculations include values for regional plasma flow, not regional blood flow, because [^{3}H]NE traverses red cell membranes relatively slowly.

One may view the regional spillover rate of NE as the sum of two processes that determine the arteriovenous difference in the plasma NE concentration. The first is the rate of release of NE into the circulation within the organ, and the second is the rate of removal of NE from the circulation within the organ. If these two processes balanced each other exactly, the arteriovenous difference in the plasma NE concentration would be zero. If NE were released into the circulation within the organ, but none of the NE in the circulation were removed, then the arteriovenous increment in the plasma NE concentration (multiplied by the regional plasma flow) would equal the regional spillover rate. If no NE were released into the circulation within the organ, but the organ removed a proportion of circulating NE, then the regional spillover rate would be zero, and the proportionate arteriovenous decrement in the plasma NE concentration (multiplied by the regional plasma flow and the arterial NE concentration) would equal the regional removal rate of circulating NE. Thus, the regional spillover rate of NE is the sum of the arteriovenous production rate of NE and the removal rate of NE. In mathematical terms,

$$\text{Regional Extraction Fraction of NE} = E_{NE} = \frac{[^3H]NE_a - [^3H]NE_v}{[^3H]NE_a}$$

$$\text{Regional Removal Rate of NE} = RRR = Q \cdot E_{NE} \cdot NE_a$$

$$\text{Regional Arteriovenous Production Rate of NE} = AVPR = Q \cdot [NE_v - NE_a]$$

$$\text{Regional Spillover Rate of NE} = RRR + AVPR$$

where Q is regional plasma flow and NE_v the concentration of NE in regional venous plasma. Rearrangement leads to:

$$\text{Regional NE Spillover} = [Q \cdot (NE_v - NE_a)] + (Q \cdot E_{NE} \cdot NE_a)$$

$$\text{Regional NE Spillover} = Q \cdot \{NE_v - [NE_a \cdot (1 - E_{NE})]\}$$

These relationships have several implications: (1) Regional NE spillover increases when regional plasma flow increases, unless regional extraction of arterial NE decreases correspondingly. (2) Regional NE spillover relates only indirectly and complexly to the regional venous NE concentration; and (3) In the presence of substantial regional removal of circulating NE, the arteriovenous increment in plasma NE levels, multiplied by regional plasma flow, underestimates regional NE spillover.

Using the second approach for measuring regional NE spillover, E_{NE} is calculated from the proportion of the [³H]NE infused into the artery that does not appear as [³H]NE in the regional venous drainage:

$$E_{NE} = [I_{[^3H]NE} - (Q \cdot [^3H]NE_v)]/I_{[^3H]NE}$$

where $I_{[^3H]NE}$ is the rate of intra-arterial infusion of [³H]NE. The second method for measuring regional NE spillover assumes that the tissues remove all the [³H]NE infused into the artery that does not appear as [³H]NE in the regional venous drainage. Since some of intra-arterially infused [³H]NE binds rapidly to blood cells (Grossman, Chang et al., 1991b), applying the second method yields higher estimated clearances and therefore higher estimated spillover rates of NE than does applying the first method.

Esler and coworkers have applied the technique of measuring the regional kinetics of intravenously infused [³H]NE to identify abnormalities of regional NE spillover in several cardiovascular diseases, including essential hypertension, congestive heart failure, and autonomic failure, as discussed in the chapter about cardiovascular diseases (for review see Esler et al., 1990).

Not only increased firing of regional sympathetic nerves but also decreased regional Uptake-1 activity or decreased presynaptic inhibitory modulation of NE release increases estimated regional spillover of NE. Comparisons of regional removal rates of [³H]isoproterenol and [³H]NE, combined measurements of regional spillovers of NE and DHPG, or assessments of effects of blockade of neuronal uptake or adrenoceptors can distinguish among these possibilities (e.g., Eisenhofer, Esler et al., 1992).

If some of an endogenously released compound were removed within the organ before the compound entered the venous drainage, then the regional spillover calculated from the above equations would underestimate the actual rate of entry of the compound into the bloodstream within the organ. This sort of problem applies not only within an organ, where release sites and removal sites can be viewed as arranged in series, but also among organs in portal systems, such as in the splanchnic portal vascular bed, where the organs are arranged in series. Figure 5–3 depicts the problem schematically. For simplicity, we assume no release of endogenous NE in the liver and no release or removal of NE in the lungs. NE concentrations are in italics, with concentrations in terms of radioactivity per unit of volume, dpm/ml, in plain italics and concentrations in terms of mass per unit of volume, pg/ml, in boldface italics. The model includes

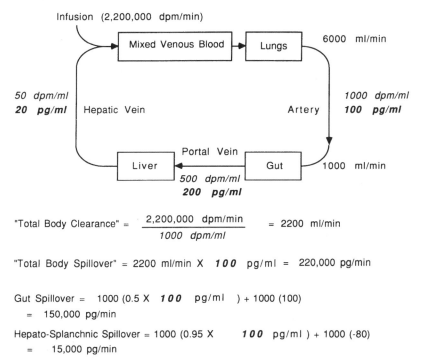

$$\text{"Total Body Clearance"} = \frac{2,200,000 \ dpm/min}{1000 \ dpm/ml} = 2200 \ ml/min$$

"Total Body Spillover" = 2200 ml/min X *100* pg/ml = 220,000 pg/min

Gut Spillover = 1000 (0.5 X *100* pg/ml) + 1000 (100)
= 150,000 pg/min

Hepato-Splanchnic Spillover = 1000 (0.95 X *100* pg/ml) + 1000 (-80)
= 15,000 pg/min

Figure 5–3. Norepinephrine kinetics in the gut. Norepinephrine concentrations in terms of radioactivity per unit of volume (dpm/ml) are in plain italics and concentrations in terms of mass per unit of volume (pg/ml) are in boldface italics. As the portal venous blood passes through the hepatic vascular bed, the liver removes circulating catecholamines with an extraction fraction of 0.90. Applying the equations in the text, the spillover rate of norepinephrine in the gut is a large fraction of the "total body spillover," as indicated by the spillover rate of norepinephrine into arterial plasma; however, the extensive hepatic extraction renders the substantial splanchnic spillover inapparent in the quantification of the spillover rate into arterial plasma.

substantial release of NE into the splanchnic venous plasma, as indicated by the arteriovenous increment of 100%, from 100 pg/ml in the artery to 200 pg/ml in the portal vein. As the portal venous blood passes through the hepatic vascular bed, the liver removes circulating catecholamines very efficiently, with an extraction fraction of 0.90. From the above equations, the spillover rate of NE in the gut constitutes a large fraction of the "total body spillover," as indicated by the spillover rate of NE into arterial plasma; however, the extensive hepatic extraction renders the substantial splanchnic spillover inapparent in the quantification of the spillover rate into arterial plasma. In fact, according to the model, if the hepatosplanchnic extraction of NE averaged 80%, calculated hepatosplanchnic spillover would be zero, and therefore, the hepatosplanchnic contribution to the spillover of NE into arterial plasma would be zero, despite the large arteriovenous increment in NE levels across the gut.

Uptake-1 contributes much more to removal of endogenously released than of circulating NE. Eisenhofer and colleagues have developed tracer techniques to examine neuronal reuptake of endogenous NE based on spillovers of NE and DHPG, as described below in the section about DHPG. These investigators have provided a comprehensive model of neurochemical events at sympathetic neuroeffector junctions (Figure 5–4).

Recent studies have detected cerebrovascular NE spillover, based on arteriovenous differences in plasma NE concentrations and extraction of [^{3}H]NE between a systemic artery and the internal jugular vein (Esler, Jennings and Lambert, 1988; Goldstein, Cannon et al., 1991). The sources of cerebrovascular NE spillover have not yet been identified conclusively; they may include release of NE in the brain and release of NE from postganglionic sympathetic nerves innervating cerebral blood vessels or the choroid plexus.

Norepinephrine Levels at Vascular Neuroeffector Junctions

The several removal processes for NE at nerve terminals and in tissues produce a concentration gradient between the effector sites on smooth muscle cells and the plasma (Kopin et al., 1984). Because of the series of removal processes, during an infusion of NE to achieve a given pressor response, the steady-state NE concentration in the plasma must exceed that at the average vascular neuroeffector junction. Similarly, during release of endogenous NE into the synapse to achieve the same pressor response, the steady-state NE concentration in the plasma must be less than that at the average vascular neuroeffector junction. The mean ''junctional'' NE concentration associated with a given pressor response must therefore lie between the steady-state plasma concentrations measured during NE release and during NE infusion. Assuming a similar gradient in both directions, one can estimate the concentration of NE at the effector sites from the geometric mean of the two values (Kopin et al., 1984). In rats, the geometric mean is about 600 pg/ml, or about 3.5×10^{-9} M.

The ''window'' for estimating NE concentrations at effector sites on vascular smooth muscle cells is quite large. In humans, in order to increase mean arterial pressure 20 mm Hg by infusing NE, the venous NE concentration usually must exceed 2000 pg/ml (Bianchetti et al., 1982; Silverberg et al., 1978), whereas during pressor responses of similar magnitude induced by release of endogenous NE, the venous NE concentration increases by only a few hundred pg/ml or less (Bianchetti et al., 1982; Goldstein, Nurnberger et al., 1983).

Blockade of Uptake-1 decreases the width of this ''window.'' Kopin et al. (1984) observed a marked shift to the left in the pressor–log plasma NE relationship during NE infusion and a symmetric shift to the right in this relationship during sympathetic stimulation. During blockade of circulatory reflexes, of α_2-adrenoceptors—which as noted previously appear to be situated extrasynaptically—and of Uptake-1, estimates of cleft NE were obtained in rats. Applying an analogous method in healthy people, a 20 mm Hg sympathetically mediated pressor response was estimated to be associated with an average of about a 560 pg/ml (3×10^{-9} mol/L) concentration of NE at the

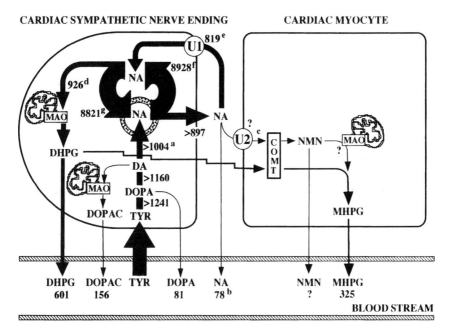

CARDIAC SYMPATHETIC NERVE ENDING   CARDIAC MYOCYTE

DHPG   DOPAC TYR   DOPA   NA   NMN   MHPG
601   156   81   78[b]   ?   325

BLOOD STREAM

Figure 5–4. Estimated rates of neurochemical processes in the human heart. Note the very rapid exchange between norepinephrine in the vesicles and in the cytoplasm and the derivation of DHPG from norepinephrine leaking from the vesicles and from norepinephrine removed by neuronal reuptake. According to this model, clinical disorders affecting vesicular storage would be much more likely to lead to depletion of endogenous norepinephrine stores than would disorders increasing sympathetically mediated exocytosis; drugs or disorders affecting Uptake-1 markedly alter norepinephrine concentrations at vascular effectors; and kinetics of tissue levels of radiolabeled norepinephrine do not estimate regional sympathoneural activity so much as the net rate of leakage of vesicular norepinephrine—that is, vesicular turnover of norepinephrine. (Illustration provided by G. Eisenhofer.)

vascular effector sites, corresponding to about a threefold cleft–plasma concentration gradient (Goldstein, Zimlichman et al., 1986b).

This approach has a several limitations. The method does not distinguish NE released from nonjunctional varicosities from NE released in synaptic regions. Blockade of Uptake-1 may not decrease the concentration gradient from the effector sites to the plasma but instead decrease the clearance of circulating NE, so that for a given amount of sympathetic traffic, the arterial concentration would increase. Moreover, desipramine, the drug used to block Uptake-1, decreases sympathoneural outflow by a central effect (Eisenhofer, Smolich et al., 1992; Esler, Wallin et al., 1991; Szabo et al., 1989; van der Hoorn et al., 1991). Despite these limitations, application of an analogous method based on simultaneous measurements of NE and DHPG concentrations has led to a similar estimated three- to five-fold concentration gradient between neuronal uptake sites and plasma in humans (Goldstein, Eisenhofer et al., 1988; Ludwig et al., 1990, 1992) and rabbits (Halbrugge et al., 1989).

Norepinephrine in Cerebrospinal Fluid

An effective blood–brain barrier excludes catecholamines from most of the central nervous system (Weil-Malherbe et al., 1959, 1961), explaining the absence of EPI in cerebrospinal fluid (CSF). The CSF–blood barrier for catecholamines, however, is not very effective. Glowinski et al. (1965) showed that a proportion of tracer-labeled NE administered into the CSF space enters plasma unchanged. Whether this means that NE released in brain tissue can enter plasma via the CSF is unknown.

Despite the blood–brain barrier for catecholamines, CSF NE levels average about ⅔ those in plasma (Goldstein, Zimlichman et al., 1987; Kagedal and Goldstein, 1988), and plasma and CSF concentrations of NE are highly correlated among individual subjects (Eide et al., 1979; Lake, Gullner et al., 1981; Lake, Polinsky et al., 1980; Lake, Wood et al., 1978; Vlachakis et al., 1981; Ziegler, Lake et al., 1977b). Moreover, in response to most physiological or pharmacological stimuli, including exposure to a variety of stressors, CSF and plasma NE levels change in the same direction (Table 5–2).

Two mechanisms can explain the relationship between CSF and plasma NE in the presence of an effective blood–brain barrier for catecholamines. First, CSF NE may reflect "central noradrenergic tone" (DeQuattro et al., 1984; Lake, Gullner et al., 1981; Ziegler, Lake et al., 1977b), with manipulations affecting central noradrenergic tone also affecting SNS outflow. As discussed in the chapter about central functional neuroanatomy, alterations in NE release in the brain may participate in several ways in alterations of SNS outflow during stress responses. Several groups of investigators have therefore interpreted elevated CSF levels of NE in patients with hypertension (Cubeddu et al., 1984; DeQuattro et al., 1984; Eide et al., 1979; Kawano et al., 1982; Lake, Gullner et al., 1981; Lake, Polinsky et al., 1980; Ziegler et al., 1982) or in patients with schizophrenia (Lake et al., 1980) as indicating increased release of NE in the brain.

Consistent with a central noradrenergic source of CSF NE, Matsumoto et al. (1991) reported that central administration of the catecholaminergic neurotoxin 6-OHDA decreased CSF NE levels. The proportionate decrease in the CSF NE concentration, however, was smaller than the proportionate decrease in the cerebral tissue concentration, and the investigators did not assess effects of centrally administered 6-OHDA on plasma NE levels.

A contribution to CSF NE from postganglionic noradrenergic nerves can also potentially explain the relationship between CSF and plasma NE levels. In pentobarbital-anesthetized dogs, intravenous administration of the ganglion blocker trimethaphan decreases CSF NE levels (Goldstein, Zimlichman et al., 1987) and produces hypotension. Intravenous infusion of nitroprusside to produce an identical amount of hypotension produces significant increases in CSF NE levels; simultaneous infusion of trimethaphan with the direct-acting vasoconstrictor phenylephrine, to prevent trimethaphan-induced hypotension, decreases CSF NE levels to virtually exactly the same extent as during infusion of trimethaphan alone. Since nitroprusside probably does not cross the blood–brain barrier, the stimulatory effect of nitroprusside on CSF NE seems reflexive. The decrease in CSF NE levels during ganglion blockade, and the

Table 5-2. Pharmacological or Pathophysiological Stimuli Affecting CSF Norepinephrine and Plasma Norepinephrine

Pharmacological	Δ CSF NE	Δ Plasma NE	Reference
Alcohol withdrawal	Increase	Increase	Hawley et al., 1981; Eisenhofer et al., 1985
Amphetamine	Increase	Increase	Goldstein et al., 1983; Ziegler et al., 1979a
Angiotensin II	Increase	Increase	Chevillard et al., 1979; Rowe and Nasjlettia, 1981
Bromocriptine	Decrease	Decrease	Ziegler et al., 1979b
Clonidine	Decrease	Decrease	Cubeddu et al., 1984; Cubeddu et al., 1986; DeQuattro et al., 1984; Martin et al., 1984
Clonidine withdrawal	Increase	Increase	Cebeddu et al., 1986
Hydrochlorothiazide	No change	No change	Cubeddu et al., 1986
Pentobarbital	Decrease	Decrease	Takemoto, 1992
Probenecid	Increase	Increase	Lake et al., 1978
Propranolol	Increase	Decrease	Lerner et al., 1981
Propranolol	No change	Slight increase	Cubeddu et al., 1986
Pathophysiological			
Cerebral vasospasm	Increase	Increase	Shigeno, 1982
Post-carotid endarterectomy	Increase	Increase	Ahn et al., 1989
Chronic sodium depletion	Increase	Increase	Brosnihan et al., 1981
Dorsal column stimulation	Increase	Increase	Levin and Hubschmann, 1980
Early essential hypertension	Increase	Increase	DeQuattro et al., 1984; Eide et al., 1979; Kawano et al., 1982
Early renal hypertension	Increase	Increase	Suzuki et al., 1983
Encephalitis	No change	No change	Ratge et al., 1985
Hemorrhage	Little change	Little change	Cameron et al., 1984
Hemorrhage	Increase	Increase	Elam et al., 1984
Hemorrhagic brain infarction	Slight increase	Slight increase	Ratge et al., 1985
Insulin hypoglycemia	Increase	Decrease	Radosevich et al., 1988
Meningitis	Increase	Increase	Ratge et al., 1985
Seizures during hemodialysis	Increase	Increase	Ratge et al., 1985
Subarachnoid hemorrhage	Increase	Increase	Dilraj et al., 1992
Normal aging	Increase	Increase	Ziegler et al., 1980

absence of reflexive increases in CSF NE during hypotension in ganglion-blocked animals, support the suggestion that CSF NE may emanate at least partly from postganglionic sympathetic nerve endings. Since epithelial cells of the choroid plexus possess substantial postganglionic noradrenergic innervation from the superior cervical ganglion (Lindvall et al., 1978), and since choroid plexus cells secrete CSF, postganglionic noradrenergic terminals on choroid plexus cells could provide a source of CSF NE, via extraneuronal uptake and subsequent secretion of the transmitter with the CSF.

Although a blood–brain barrier prevents circulating catecholamines from entering most regions of the brain, an exception is the hypothalamus, which accumulates intravenously injected radioactive EPI (Weil-Malherbe et al., 1959). No studies have determined whether circulating catecholamines can exert effects at circumventricular organs (such as the AP and SFO) to influence central neural processes involved with either release of NE in the brain or with regulation of SNS outflow.

Peskind et al. (1986) reported that peripheral sympathectomy using guanethidine in rats at one week of age, followed by adrenal medullectomy at seven weeks, did not affect CSF NE concentrations measured at 12 weeks but did decrease plasma NE levels, suggesting that peripheral sources of NE do not contribute to CSF NE in rats. The study design did not exclude the possibility that peripheral sympatholysis stimulated LC activity and thereby increased NE release in the brain. Since the CSF was obtained from the cisterna magna, trauma to the dorsal brainstem, which contains high concentrations of NE, could have increased NE concentrations artifactually. Finally, no assessment was made of reflexive increases in CSF NE levels in the sympathectomized and control rats.

The source and meaning of CSF NE therefore remain incompletely understood. This issue is important, for at least two reasons. If CSF NE were derived partly from postganglionic sympathetic nerves, this would force reconsideration of inferences about central noradrenergic "tone" based on CSF levels of NE. This would also introduce the possibility that postganglionic sympathetic nerve activity can provide afferent information to the brain directly, rather than via afferents from interoceptors.

Norepinephrine in Urine

NE in urine has a complex source. Only 10% or less of circulating NE appears unchanged in the urine (Henry et al., 1979; Ziegler et al., 1990). A proportion of urinary NE therefore probably derives from renal noradrenergic nerves (Lappe et al., 1982). Recipients of transplanted—and presumably denervated—kidneys have increased urinary excretion of intravenously infused [3H]NE but decreased excretion of endogenous NE, compared to values in control patients (Ziegler et al., 1990), suggesting a renal neural source of endogenous NE in urine. Effects of chemotherapeutic agents administered to the renal transplant patients, however, could have led to overestimation of the magnitude of the renal neuronal contribution to urinary NE excretion. For instance, transplant patients often receive high doses of adrenal corticosteroids, and glucocorticoids inhibit SNS and AHS outflows (Brown and Fisher, 1986; Szemeredi, Bagdy, Stull et al., 1988a) and inhibit extraneuronal uptake of circulating catecholamines (Salt, 1972). These drug effects could decrease endogenous NE excretion and increase excretion of [3H]NE independently of renal denervation.

Norepinephrine in the Heart

NE concentrations in the heart—especially in the atria—exceed those in most other organs. Since reserpinization markedly decreases myocardial NE concentrations and prevents tissue accumulation of injected radiolabeled catechols (Chang et al., 1990; Eisenhofer, Hovevey-Sion et al., 1989), virtually all the NE in the heart is confined to the vesicles in sympathetic nerves.

The slow turnover of NE in myocardium (replacement time about 1 day in rats, Kopin and Gordon, 1963) contrasts markedly with the rapid removal of NE from plasma (half-time about 1.5 minutes). The rate of decline of myocardial radiolabeled NE has been used as an index of cardiac sympathetic "activity" (Johnson et al., 1983; Rappaport et al., 1982; Young and Landsberg, 1979); however, this approach ignores the important contribution of vesicular leakage to myocardial NE turnover, as discussed below.

Dihydroxyphenylglycol (DHPG, DOPEG) and Norepinephrine Turnover

DHPG, formed from oxidative deamination of axoplasmic NE by MAO, is probably the main neuronal metabolite of NE (Goldstein, Eisenhofer et al., 1988; Graefe, 1981; Graefe and Bonisch, 1988; Halbrugge et al., 1989; Ludwig et al., 1988). Axoplasmic NE, and therefore DHPG production, has two sources: reuptake of NE from the neuroeffector junctions after NE release, and leakage of NE from storage vesicles.

Since DHPG is a glycol, it traverses cell membranes readily to enter the circulation. Plasma levels of DHPG average about 5 times those of NE (Eisenhofer et al., 1986). The finding that healthy subjects have a small arteriovenous increment in plasma DHPG levels in the arm, whereas sympathectomized patients have no arteriovenous increment in plasma DHPG levels, provides clinical evidence that plasma DHPG derives at least partly from sympathetic nerve endings (Goldstein, Eisenhofer et al., 1988). Patients with orthostatic hypotension due to sympathetic dysfunction or denervation have low plasma DHPG levels (Goldstein, Polinsky et al., 1989) and have virtually no cardiac DHPG spillover (Meredith et al., 1991).

During sympathetic stimulation, increments in plasma DHPG levels generally parallel increments in plasma NE levels (Goldstein, Eisenhofer et al., 1988), because sympathetic nerve endings remove a large proportion of the released NE, and some of the removed NE is metabolized by mitochondrial MAO.

Increments in plasma DHPG levels during sympathetic stimulation depend on neuronal reuptake of the released NE, because treatment with desipramine, which blocks Uptake-1, prevents increases in plasma DHPG levels during manipulations that release endogenous NE (Eisenhofer, Cox et al., 1990, 1991; Goldstein, Eisenhofer et al., 1988; Ludwig et al., 1988). Desipramine also prevents increments in plasma DHPG levels during intravenous infusion of NE (Goldstein, Eisenhofer et al., 1988).

Reserpine, which blocks translocation of catecholamines from the axoplasm into the vesicles, produces a biphasic effect on plasma DHPG levels (Eisenhofer, Ropchak et al., 1988). At first, increased net leakage of NE from vesicles into the cytoplasm produces large increases in plasma DHPG levels, reflecting the high rate of exchange of amines across the vesicular membrane. As vesicular NE stores becomes depleted, DHPG levels decline, and fully reserpinized animals have very low plasma DHPG levels. These findings confirm the neuronal source of circulating DHPG.

Since extraneuronal cells remove NE by Uptake-2, and since both neuronal and nonneuronal cells possess MAO, one might expect DHPG in plasma to have a mixed neuronal and extraneuronal source; however, extraneuronal DHPG seems to be metabolized rapidly by COMT to form MHPG. Studies of rats have indicated that a substantial proportion of MHPG production is derived from DHPG that emanates from sympathetic nerve terminals and is converted to MHPG in extraneuronal cells before the DHPG enters the bloodstream (Eisenhofer, Goldstein et al., 1988). Thus, inhibition of COMT increases plasma levels of DHPG (Halbrugge et al., 1993).

The clinical meanings of plasma DHPG and NE levels differ because of their related but distinct sources. Uptake-1 blockade produces only small decreases in plasma DHPG levels and regional DHPG spillover (Eisenhofer, Esler et al., 1992; Eisenhofer, Goldstein et al., 1988; Halbrugge et al., 1989; Ludwig et al., 1988), and administration of clonidine, which decreases sympathetic outflow and plasma NE levels, decreases plasma DHPG levels only modestly (Goldstein, Eisenhofer et al., 1988), consistent with derivation of plasma DHPG not so much from reuptake of endogenously released NE as from net leakage of NE from storage vesicles into the axoplasm. Thus, under basal conditions, plasma DHPG levels reflect the turnover of NE stores more than they do the reuptake of released NE.

Combined measurements of regional spillovers of NE and DHPG can yield unique clinical information about sympathoneural function (Eisenhofer, Esler et al., 1992; Eisenhofer, Goldstein et al., 1989). For instance, when sympathetically mediated exocytosis increases, plasma levels of NE and DHPG both increase; however, Uptake-1 blockade augments plasma NE responses but attenuates or abolishes DHPG responses during sympathetic stimulation. Conversely, α-MT-induced inhibition of TH decreases plasma DHPG levels acutely, whereas plasma NE levels remain unchanged (Goldstein, Udelsman et al., 1987; Kvetnansky, Armando et al., 1992).

The different sources and meanings of plasma DHPG and NE levels have provided a means for estimating NE concentrations at Uptake-1 sites and Uptake-1 activity. The estimated average NE concentrations at Uptake-1 sites appear to be about the same as those at vascular effector sites, as discussed above. In conscious rats, the total body rate of neuronal uptake of endogenous NE averages 1.45 nmol/kg/min and in humans about 0.40 nmol/kg/min (Eisenhofer, Esler et al., 1992; Eisenhofer, Goldstein et al., 1989). In both species this represents about 10 times the total body rate of release of NE into the bloodstream, confirming that sympathetic nerves remove most of endogenously released NE, with only a small fraction of released NE diffusing into the bloodstream.

In patients undergoing cardiac catheterization, Eisenhofer, Esler et al. (1992) used regional spillover rates of NE and DHPG, before and during desipramine-induced Uptake-1 blockade, to estimate in vivo rates of most of the sympathetic intraneuronal processes determining NE release, reuptake, turnover, and synthesis (Figure 5–4). A few aspects of these estimates merit emphasis: the tremendously high exchange rate of amines between the axoplasm and the vesicles; the efficient reuptake of endogenously released NE; and the prominence of net leakage of NE from vesicles in the determination of tissue NE turnover. These considerations imply that interference with vesicular storage is much more likely to lead to depletion of NE stores than is increased sympathetically mediated exocytosis; that interference with Uptake-1 exaggerates increments in NE concentrations at cardiovascular adrenoceptors during sympathetic stimulation; and that the rate of decline of tissue levels of radiolabeled NE reflects net leakage from vesicles more than it reflects regional sympathoneural activity.

O-Methylated Metabolites and Extraneuronal Metabolism of Norepinephrine

Consistent with efficient reuptake of endogenously released NE and extraneuronal localization of COMT, plasma levels of the O-methylated metabolite of NE, NMN, are much smaller than those of DHPG (Lenders et al., 1992, 1993), and NMN levels provide a marker of extraneuronal metabolism of NE. Plasma NMN levels in humans average about 0.4 nM. Patients with pheochromocytomas, tumors that release NE into the bloodstream, virtually always have high plasma NMN levels, reflecting extraneuronal metabolism of the secreted NE (Lenders et al., 1993), in contrast with often normal or slightly increased DHPG levels (Brown, 1984; Grossman, Goldstein et al., 1991). In rats undergoing NE infusion, the plasma NMN response, relative to the plasma NE response, exceeds by about threefold that in rats undergoing immobilization, further supporting the mainly extraneuronal source of plasma NMN and leading to the estimate that 30% of plasma NMN derives from circulating NE and 70% from NE diffusing from sites of release before entering the circulation (Lenders et al., in press).

Plasma levels of metanephrine (MN), the O-methylated metabolite of EPI, average about 0.2 nM (Lenders et al., 1993) and reflect extraneuronal metabolism of EPI (Axelrod et al., 1959). Relatively larger increases in plasma MN than NMN levels during infusion of NE and EPI suggest preferential extraneuronal uptake or O-methylation of EPI over NE or more efficient metabolism of NMN than MN (Lenders et al., in press). Only a minority of patients with pheochromocytoma have increased plasma MN levels.

In plasma, CSF, urine, and brain microdialysate, concentrations of metabolites resulting from the combined actions of MAO and COMT on catecholamines exceed by far metabolites resulting from the actions of either enzyme alone. Thus, in human plasma, levels of NE, the O-methylated metabolite NMN, and the deaminated metabolite DHPG average less than about 5 nM, whereas levels of the O-methylated, deaminated metabolites MHPG and vanillylmandelic acid (VMA) exceed 20 nM (Kagedal and Goldstein, 1988; Kopin, 1985). Analogously, plasma DA levels normally average less than 0.5 nM, DOPAC levels 10–20 nM, and homovanillic acid (HVA) levels higher than 50 nM (Kagedal and Goldstein, 1988; Kopin, 1985).

Plasma levels of MHPG have a mixed source. In rats undergoing infusions of [³H]NE, Uptake-1 blockade with desipramine markedly decreases plasma levels of [³H]DHPG, whereas [³H]MHPG levels decline by slightly over ½ (Eisenhofer, Goldstein et al., 1988). This suggests that a small proportion of MHPG in plasma derives from deamination and O-methylation of NE in nonneuronal cells, whereas most of plasma MHPG derives from intraneuronal deamination of NE, release of DHPG, and O-methylation of DHPG in nonneuronal cells.

The rate of conversion of DHPG to MHPG appears to vary among vascular beds, and so the validity of plasma MHPG levels to indicate regional NE turnover depends on the vascular bed under study. In the heart, relatively little MHPG is produced from DHPG, and the large cardiac arteriovenous increment in plasma DHPG levels exceeds that of plasma MHPG levels (Eisenhofer, Brush et al., 1989; Eisenhofer, Esler et al., 1992; Eisenhofer, Goldstein et al., 1988; Goldstein, Brush et al., 1988). In contrast, in the forearm, there is only a small arteriovenous increment in plasma DHPG levels (Eisenhofer, Brush et al., 1989).

Epinephrine

Since the adrenal medulla secretes EPI directly into the bloodstream, plasma EPI levels generally reflect neural outflow to the adrenal medulla. Thus, increments in adreno-medullary secretion of catecholamines resulting from manipulations of circulatory reflexes or from icv administration of drugs correlate with increments in directly recorded adrenal nerve activity (e.g., Ito et al., 1984). A few qualifications limit this generalization, however, as discussed below.

Plasma levels of adrenaline are very low in antecubital venous plasma of healthy volunteers at rest—as little as 3×10^{-11} mol/L. This contrasts with plasma levels of NE, which normally exceed 6×10^{-10} mol/L.

In innervated organs including the heart, sympathetic nerves can remove circulating EPI and subsequently release it during regional sympathetic stimulation (Eisenhofer, Smolich et al., 1992; Peronnet et al., 1988; Rosell et al., 1964). In humans, the arterial–great cardiac vein proportionate decrease in plasma [^{3}H]NE levels exceeds that in plasma EPI levels (Goldstein, Cannon et al., 1991). This does not necessarily indicate cardiac EPI spillover, because circulating EPI is less susceptible than is NE to neuronal uptake in the heart (Eisenhofer, Esler et al., 1990). With the possible exception of strenuous bicycle exercise (Esler, Eisenhofer et al., 1991), there has been no convincing evidence of cardiac EPI release in humans.

AHS activity increases markedly in response to hypoglycemia, hemorrhage, asphyxiation, circulatory collapse, and distress. In these situations plasma EPI concentrations increase to a much greater extent than do NE concentrations (Cryer, 1980; Kopin, 1989; Robertson, Johnson et al., 1979). As discussed in the chapters about stress and about stress response patterns, circulatory, metabolic, and visceral homeostatic responses serve to maintain delivery of oxygen and glucose to vital organs (Garber et al., 1976; Johnson et al., 1983), and the large increases in plasma EPI levels in response to these stressors reflect the prominence of the AHS effector. Even mild, asymptomatic hypoglycemia elicits larger increases in EPI than NE levels, and in the relatively benign form of circulatory failure represented by fainting, plasma EPI concentrations increase without increases in plasma NE concentrations (Goldstein, Spanarkel et al., 1982; Ziegler et al., 1986).

Adrenalectomized patients have detectable urinary excretion of EPI (von Euler et al., 1954, 1961) and have small but consistent increases in plasma EPI levels during insulin-induced hypoglycemia (Garber et al., 1976). Whether these findings indicate EPI synthesis in sympathetic nerves in adrenalectomized patients or a contribution of extra α-adrenal chromaffin tissue to plasma EPI levels during hypoglycemia in these patients has not been established. In either case, the results suggest that sources other than the adrenal medulla can release EPI into the bloodstream.

PNMT-like enzymatic activity, enabling conversion of NE to EPI, has been identified in nonneuronal tissues, including parenchyma of the lung (Kennedy et al., 1990), kidneys (Ziegler et al., 1989), and cardiovascular system (Elayan et al., 1990; Kennedy et al., 1991). Whether nonneuronal cells synthesize endogenous EPI and, if so, whether nonneuronal EPI diffuses appreciably into the bloodstream are unknown.

Dopamine

Plasma Dopamine

Detailed understanding about the sources and meanings of plasma NE and EPI levels contrasts with meager understanding about the sources and meanings of plasma levels of DA. DA circulates at very low free (unconjugated) concentrations—about those of EPI. In humans, sulfoconjugated DA circulates at concentrations 20–100 times that of free DA. Exposure to severe stressors such as surgery in adrenalectomized animals or nitroprusside-induced hypotension increases plasma DA levels (Udelsman et al., 1987a); less severe stressors do not. Thus, DA does not appear to be coreleased with NE during exocytosis except under extreme conditions.

Effects of manipulations of dietary salt intake on plasma DA are unclear, in contrast with consistent changes in urinary DA excretion, as discussed below. Carey et al. (1981) reported decreases in plasma DA levels during dietary sodium depletion in humans; Romoff et al. (1978) reported the opposite, with plasma DA levels inversely related to urinary sodium excretion.

Most of the catecholamine content in human plasma consists of sulfoconjugated DA. In humans, over 95% of circulating DA is in the form of DA sulfate. In rats, DA glucuronidation is the major route of conjugation of DA (Wang et al., 1983). Sulfo-conjugated DA has a much longer plasma half-life (several hours) than does unconjugated DA (less than about 2 minutes). During infusion of DA into humans, plasma concentrations of sulfoconjugated DA increase gradually over a few hours (Ratge et al., 1991).

Whereas acute exposure to stressors often evokes large, rapid increases in plasma levels of free catecholamines, concentrations of conjugated catecholamines increase relatively little and slowly. Thus, electroconvulsive shock in humans markedly increases plasma free NE and EPI levels and to a much smaller extent increases free DA levels, with no changes in levels of sulfated catecholamines (Cuche et al., 1990).

The sources of conjugated DA are unclear (Cuche et al., 1990). Ingestion of catecholamine-containing foodstuffs fails to increase plasma or urinary levels of unconjugated catecholamines but does increase levels of the sulfate conjugates. Analogously, oral administration of L-DOPA produces large increases in plasma levels of DA sulfate (Cuche et al., 1985). These findings suggest mural sulfoconjugation of DA in the gastrointestinal system. Since infusion of DA into humans rapidly increases plasma levels of DA sulfate (Ratge et al., 1991), however, sulfoconjugation cannot occur only in the gut wall. Platelets contain abundant phenolsulfotransferase (PST), which catalyzes the sulfoconjugation of catecholamines. This suggests intravascular sulfoconjugation of catecholamines; however, severely thrombocytopenic patients can have normal circulating levels of DA sulfate (Kuchel et al., 1985), possibly because granulocytes also contain thermostable PST (Anderson et al., 1991). Although the adrenal gland contains

DA sulfate, in humans there is no arteriovenous increment in plasma levels of DA sulfate across the adrenal glands, kidneys, or tissues drained by the inferior vena cava (Kuchel et al., 1984). Uremic patients have high plasma levels of sulfoconjugates, and the levels decrease during hemodialysis (Cuche et al., 1986), whereas anhepatic liver transplant patients have approximately normal plasma levels of sulfoconjugates (Tyce et al., 1987). These findings suggest that the liver is not a major source of conjugated catecholamines and that excretion of the conjugates depends on glomerular filtration.

The physiological meaning of the conjugation of catecholamines such as DA is also unclear. Since conjugated catecholamines appear to be inactive metabolites, rapid conjugation may prevent buildup of catecholamine levels—especially of DA—in extracellular fluid. Alternatively, since even a very small amount of deconjugation of DA sulfate could maintain the low resting plasma levels of free DA in humans, DA sulfate could act as a slow generator of circulating free DA, providing an alternative source of substrate for NE synthesis in sympathetic nerves. Buu and Kuchel (1979) reported conversion of DA sulfate to NE; the physiological significance of this conversion in vivo is unknown.

One may speculate that sulfoconjugation in the gastrointestinal wall constitutes part of a "gut–blood" barrier, preventing toxic effects of ingested catecholamines or of similar compounds in foodstuffs. Intravascular conjugation of DA could have evolved as a means for preventing diffusion of DA into the bloodstream from sites where the catecholamine would act as an autocrine/paracrine substance. Consistent with this hypothesis, hypertensives with low plasma levels of conjugated catecholamines can have dopaminergic "surges" mimicking pheochromocytoma (Kuchel et al., 1981). The evolution of nerve networks, with much more efficient means of localizing, inactivating, and recycling neurotransmitters, could have superseded this more primitive autocrine/paracrine conjugation system, as discussed in the chapters about stress and about peripheral catecholaminergic systems.

Urinary Dopamine

Urine contains substantially higher concentrations of free and conjugated catecholamines and catecholamine metabolites than does plasma. Renal mechanisms determining urinary excretion of these compounds include both glomerular filtration and active secretion by the renal tubular epithelium (Rennick and Pryor, 1965).

The predominant free (unconjugated) catecholamine in human urine is DA (Kagedal and Goldstein, 1988). Since in humans the excretion rate of DA exceeds by far the rate of delivery of free (unconjugated) DA to the kidney, a substantial proportion of DA excreted by the kidney must be produced locally. Potential sources include renal dopaminergic nerves, DA released from noradrenergic nerve terminals in the kidneys, renal uptake and deconjugation of conjugated DA, and renal uptake and decarboxylation of circulating DOPA.

Studies of DA excretion after injection of DA sulfate have excluded renal uptake and deconjugation of DA sulfate in the kidney as a source of urinary DA (Buu et al., 1986).

The existence and function of renal dopaminergic nerves have been controversial. Renal nerve stimulation increases release of both NE and DA into the renal venous drainage (e.g., Ball et al., 1982a, 1982b), and renal denervation decreases renal venous DA concentrations. These findings, while consistent with renal dopaminergic innervation, do not separate DA released from noradrenergic nerves from DA released from putative dopaminergic nerves. After renal denervation, DA secretion continues into the renal venous plasma, although at a decreased rate, and rats with bilateral renal denervation excrete normal amounts of DA in the urine (Grossman, Hoffman et al., 1990). These findings question the importance of renal dopaminergic nerves as a source of urinary DA, but they do not rule out the possibility that release of DA from such nerves can play a physiological role in the kidneys. For at least one function of DA in the kidneys, however—sodium homeostasis—evidence presented below supports uptake and decarboxylation of circulating DOPA as the main source of physiologically active DA. Stimulation of renal DA production during acute volume expansion does not require intact renal nerves (Hegde and Lokhandwala, 1992).

Urinary DA derives mainly from renal uptake and decarboxylation of circulating DOPA (Baines and Drangova, 1984; Ball and Lee, 1977; Brown and Dollery, 1981; Grossman, Hoffman et al., 1992; Suzuki et al., 1984; Williams et al., 1986; Wolfovitz et al., 1993; Zimlichman et al., 1988). Histofluorescence studies of DA production in rat kidney slices incubated in DOPA-rich medium (Hagege et al., 1985), biochemical studies of isolated, perfused kidneys (Baines and Drangova, 1984) and kidney slices (Soares-da-Silva and Fernandes, 1992), and micropuncture studies of proximal tubules injected with radioactive DOPA (Baines and Chan, 1980)—all have indicated production of DA from DOPA in proximal convoluted tubular cells of the kidney. Renal DA is highly localized to the proximal tubular cells, and production of DA from DOPA occurs mainly in those cells. The production of DA from DOPA in the tubular cells does not require renal innervation (Baines and Chan, 1980) but does require DDC and Na^+, the latter apparently cotransported with DOPA into the cells (Soares-da-Silva and Fernandes, 1992).

In vivo studies involving L-[^{3}H]DOPA infusion in dogs (Zimlichman et al., 1986) and rats (Grossman, Hoffman et al., 1992) or L-DOPA infusion in humans (Wolfovitz et al., 1993) have confirmed the derivation of urinary DA from plasma DOPA. Rats chemically sympathectomized by 6-OHDA injection have decreased urinary DA excretion, whereas rats with bilateral renal denervation have normal DA excretion. This difference results from decreased delivery of DOPA to the kidneys in chemically sympathectomized animals. In healthy volunteers undergoing L-DOPA infusion, about 30% of the drug removed in the kidneys is excreted as unconjugated DA (Wolfovitz et al., 1993). Applying this percentage to the delivery rate of endogenous DOPA to the kidneys, renal uptake and decarboxylation of circulating DOPA can account for all of endogenous DA excretion in humans.

In patients with renal transplants, Ziegler et al. (1990) reported decreased urinary excretion of DA to about ⅓ the value in uninephrectomized control subjects, suggesting a renal neuronal source of urinary DA; however, the transplant patients, but not the control subjects, underwent treatment with prednisone and cytotoxic drugs. Since glucocorticoids decrease sympathoneural activity (Brown and Fisher, 1986; Szemeredi, Bagdy et al., 1988a) and shunt amino acids to the liver for gluconeogenesis, transplant patients could have had decreased renal delivery or uptake of DOPA.

If urinary DA were formed from uptake and decarboxylation of circulating DOPA, then inhibition of the decarboxylation should decrease urinary DA excretion. Williams et al. (1986) reported exactly this. After acute oral administration of the DDC inhibitor carbidopa to humans, urinary DA excretion decreased by 70%. Yoshimura et al. (1987) reported similar results in rats. Ball and Lee (1977) reported that carbidopa administered for several days caused significant (although smaller-magnitude) decreases in urinary DA excretion, and Jeffrey et al. (1987) reported virtually complete suppression of urinary DA excretion. In the study of Williams et al. (1986), carbidopa also caused about a twofold increase in plasma DOPA levels, consistent with continuous release of DOPA into the bloodstream and decreased removal from it during DDC inhibition. Analogously, Goldstein, Stull et al. (1989) reported that administration of carbidopa increased urinary DOPA excretion by about 10-fold and decreased urinary DA excretion by about ½.

Dietary salt loading increases urinary excretion of DA (e.g., Alexander et al., 1974; Gill et al., 1988; Goldstein, Stull et al., 1989) and DOPA (Gill et al., 1991; Goldstein, Stull et al., 1989; Wolfovitz et al., 1993), and interference with conversion of DOPA to DA can inhibit natriuresis acutely (Nowicki et al., 1993; Sowers et al., 1984; Williams et al., 1986; Yoshimura et al., 1987). These findings indicate that an increase in the filtered load of sodium activates a homeostatic dopaminergic mechanism involving increased DOPA uptake by proximal tubular cells of the kidneys, relatively independently of alterations in renal sympathoneural outflow. In rats, increased spillover of DOPA into the bloodstream can explain the increased renal uptake of DOPA during dietary salt loading (Grossman, Hoffman et al., 1990; however, in humans, this explanation does not suffice (Wolfovitz et al., 1993). Increased efficiency of DOPA uptake from the tubular lumen would be expected to decrease DOPA excretion, and DOPA excretion consistently increases rather than decreases during salt loading in humans. One may therefore hypothesize that salt loading increases the efficiency of DOPA uptake across the basolateral membrane of proximal tubular cells.

Dihydroxyphenylalanine (DOPA)

Sympathoneural and Adrenomedullary Contributions to Plasma DOPA Levels

DOPA is the precursor of all the endogenous catecholamines and the immediate product of the rate-limiting step in catecholamine biosynthesis—hydroxylation of tyrosine. DOPA therefore occupies a pivotal position in catecholaminergic function.

Until recently it was thought that all of the DOPA synthesized from TYR in sympathetic nerve endings is rapidly converted to DA in the axoplasm, due to the abundance of DDC. Traditional concepts about catecholamine biosynthesis therefore would not predict that DOPA synthesized in sympathetic nerve endings would enter the bloodstream.

In humans, plasma levels of DOPA exceed those of NE by about 10-fold (Goldstein, Stull et al., 1984). Since DOPA is an amino acid, plasma DOPA could theoretically derive from trace amounts of DOPA as a dietary constituent; however, studies in dogs (Banwart et al., 1989) and rats (Garty, Deka-Starosta, Stull et al., 1989) have refuted this hypothesis, and several lines of evidence discussed below have supported at least partial derivation of plasma DOPA from sympathetic nerves.

Healthy humans virtually always have an arteriovenous increment of plasma DOPA levels in the arm, whereas patients with sympathectomized limbs have no arteriovenous increments in DOPA levels (Goldstein, Udelsman et al., 1987), indicating that the normal arteriovenous increment in plasma DOPA depends on release of DOPA from sympathetic nerve endings. Arteriovenous increments in plasma DOPA levels also occur across the human heart, head, and leg (Goldstein, Cannon et al., 1991; Goldstein, Udelsman et al., 1987; Meredith et al., 1991), and patients with sympathetic failure have an absence of an arteriovenous increment in plasma DOPA in the heart (Meredith et al., 1991).

Substantial arteriovenous increments in plasma DOPA levels in the limbs and substantial total blood flow to skeletal muscle suggest that skeletal muscle provides an important source of plasma DOPA in humans (Goldstein, Cannon et al., 1991) and rats (Grossman, Hoffman et al., 1992). Another major source appears to be the lungs, mainly because the entire cardiac output flows through them, resulting in a high rate of estimated DOPA spillover (Goldstein, Cannon et al., 1991).

In conscious dogs, administration of α-MT, which competitively inhibits TH, decreases plasma DOPA levels by about 60% (Goldstein, Udelsman et al., 1987). Kvetnansky, Armando et al. (1992) reported analogous findings in rats. Because of the localization of TH in catecholamine-synthesizing cells, these findings support a sympathoneural contribution to plasma DOPA. Electrical stimulation-evoked release of DOPA from canine portal vein in vitro depends on extracellular Ca^{2+}, suggesting release rather than simple diffusion as the mechanism of increased DOPA overflow in this setting (Hunter et al., 1992). Hunter et al. (1992) estimated that under control conditions, about 80% of DOPA enters the catecholamine biosynthetic cascade, 8% is released from the vein, and 14% remains unchanged in the tissue.

In rats, detectable regional spillover of DOPA has been reported in the adrenal gland, hindlimb, and kidney (Grossman, Hoffman et al., 1992). The kidneys extract a large fraction of circulating DOPA (Ball et al., 1982a, 1982b; Garty et al., 1989; Goldstein, Udelsman et al., 1987; Grossman, Hoffman et al., 1992; Zimlichman et al., 1988), with renal venous DOPA levels typically about ⅓ less than arterial. During systemic intravenous infusion of L-[³H]DOPA into rats, the renal extraction fraction of the tracer averages about 40% (Grossman, Hoffman et al., 1992). Since the extraction fraction of the tracer slightly exceeds the proportionate arteriovenous decrement in DOPA levels in the kidney, the kidney also releases DOPA into the bloodstream. The adrenals have by far the largest arteriovenous increment in plasma DOPA concentrations (Grossman, Hoffman et al., 1992), and adrenal demedullated rats have slightly but significantly decreased arterial plasma DOPA levels (Garty, Deka-Starosta, Stull et al., 1989).

Chemical sympathectomy with 6-OHDA virtually abolishes regional DOPA spillover in the hindlimb and kidney in rats and decreases the adrenal arteriovenous increment in plasma DOPA levels by about ½ (Grossman, Hoffman et al., 1992). In pithed rats, stimulation of the spinal cord rapidly increases arterial plasma DOPA levels (Szemeredi, Pacak et al., 1991), and ganglion blockade with chlorisondamine virtually abolishes these increases, confirming the dependence of the DOPA release on postganglionic nerve traffic. Curarization, which prevents skeletal muscle contraction, attenuates by about ½ the increments in arterial plasma DOPA levels, suggesting DOPA release during electrically evoked skeletal muscle contraction.

Acute immobilization also rapidly increases plasma DOPA levels in rats (Kvetnansky, Goldstein et al., 1992). Since ganglion blockade or treatment with α-MT markedly attenuates these increases (Kvetnansky, Armando et al., 1992), they probably reflect increased tyrosine hydroxylation related to increased depolarization of postganglionic sympathetic neurons. Anden et al. (1989a, 1989b) found that ganglion blockade inhibited the tissue accumulation of DOPA in the pancreas, kidney, and spleen after DDC inhibition.

All these findings point to a substantial sympathoneural contribution to plasma DOPA. Nevertheless, this issue is not settled (Eldrup, Christensen et al., 1989; Eldrup, Richter et al., 1989).

In rats, dietary salt loading increases TH activity in sympathetic ganglia and the brain (Wang et al., 1988). Thus, the renal DOPA–DA natriuretic system may serve as an effector for a homeostatic loop, where salt loading increases tyrosine hydroxylation, increasing DOPA production and release, augmenting renal DA synthesis and release in the kidney, and in turn enhancing natriuresis by local autocrine/paracrine effects.

Arterial plasma DOPA levels do not decrease to zero in chemically sympathectomized rats, and since chemical sympathectomy does not affect the clearance of L-[^{3}H]DOPA from arterial plasma, estimated DOPA spillover into arterial plasma also does not decrease to zero after chemical sympathectomy (Grossman, Hoffman et al., 1992). In dogs, 6-OHDA fails to decrease arterial plasma DOPA levels (unpublished observations). These findings suggest a nonneuronal—or more accurately a 6-OHDA-insensitive—source of plasma DOPA. Moreover, after continued α-MT treatment in dogs, plasma DOPA levels increase toward baseline values (Goldstein, Udelsman et al., 1987), and during immobilization of rats treated with α-MT, plasma DOPA levels increase from the low levels produced by the blockade of TH, at a time when plasma DOPA levels in similarly treated control rats remain low (Kvetnansky, Armando et al., 1992).

The source of this residual DOPA is unknown. 6-OHDA generally spares adrenomedullary cells, since administration of the neurotoxin decreases adrenal DOPA spillover by only about 1/2 (Grossman, Hoffman et al., 1992) and tends to increase plasma levels of EPI (Micalizzi and Pals, 1979); however, only a very small proportion of plasma DOPA derives from the adrenals.

A proportion of ingested DOPA must enter the circulation unchanged, since oral L-DOPA is a mainstay in the treatment of Parkinson's disease; however, 2 hours after an oral dose of L-DOPA in humans, only about 0.5% of the administered dose is present in plasma (Sandler, 1972). Moreover, neither feeding rats laboratory chow after a 24-

hour fast (Garty, Deka-Starosta, Stull et al., 1989) nor feeding dogs canned dog food after a 24-hour fast (Banwart et al., 1989) affects plasma DOPA levels.

Another potential source of endogenous DOPA is skin melanocytes. DOPA formed from the action of tyrosinase on TYR is an intermediate in the biosynthesis of melanin. Black Americans have slightly higher rates of DOPA and DA excretion than do Caucasian Americans (Goldstein, Grossman et al., 1993); however, since albino humans have plasma DOPA levels similar to those of Black and Caucasian Americans (Garty, Stull et al., 1989), melanocytes probably contribute relatively little to circulating DOPA.

Although phenylalanine hydroxylase catalyzes the hydroxylation of phenylalanine to form TYR, phenylalanine hydroxylase is thought not to recognize TYR as a substrate. Thus, DOPA probably cannot be formed from phenylalanine without the intervening activity of TH. Phenylalanine hydroxylase is expressed in liver, pancreas, and kidney but not in neurons (Proud et al., 1989). To date, no convincing evidence has been obtained for synthesis of DOPA by tyrosine hydroxylation in other than chromaffin cells.

The relationship between tissue DOPA stores and plasma DOPA levels is unclear. In anesthetized rats undergoing infusion of L-[³H]DOPA, the femoral venous specific activity of L-[³H]DOPA is less than the arterial specific activity, that is, the venous/arterial ratio of specific activity of L-[³H]DOPA is less than 1.0 (Grossman, Hoffman et al., 1992). This indicates release of endogenous DOPA into the venous drainage of the leg. In chemically sympathectomized animals, the specific activity ratio is increased to a mean value of about 1.0, implying that release of endogenous DOPA into the venous drainage of the leg depends on intact sympathetic innervation. Despite these findings, tissue DOPA concentrations decrease only fractionally in sympathectomized animals. Eldrup, Richter et al. (1989) reported that muscle tissue of regionally sympathectomized limbs contained normal DOPA concentrations, whereas Grossman, Hoffman et al. (1992) found that chemical sympathectomy decreased tissue DOPA concentrations in most organs, including skeletal muscle. If there were pools of parenchymally stored DOPA, circulating DOPA could maintain them after uptake of DOPA released into the bloodstream from local sympathetic nerve endings.

DOPA can form from demethylation of *O*-methylDOPA (OMeDOPA, methoxytyrosine) in red blood cells (Tyce, 1977). Since plasma OMeDOPA concentrations average about 10 times those of DOPA (Armando et al., 1991), even a small amount of demethylation could maintain plasma DOPA levels. 6-OHDA stimulates TH in the adrenal medulla and sympathetic ganglion cells (Fluharty et al., 1985), and increased DOPA release from surviving adrenomedullary or sympathetic postganglionic cells could partly maintain arterial DOPA levels.

The possibility of tyrosine hydroxylation in nonneuronal cells that are insensitive to 6-OHDA and even of nonenzymatic hydroxylation of TYR must also be considered.

Plasma DOPA and TH Activity

The sympathoneural contribution to plasma DOPA and the fact that DOPA is the immediate product of the rate-limiting step in catecholamine biosynthesis lead to the hypothesis that changes in regional DOPA spillover provide an in vivo index of changes in regional NE synthesis in sympathetic nerves. Thus, in every situation examined so far where TH activity changes acutely, plasma DOPA levels have been found to change in the same direction (Eisenhofer, Ropchak et al., 1988; Goldstein, Udelsman et al., 1987; Kvetnansky, Goldstein et al., 1992; Table 5–3).

Since NE synthesis usually balances NE turnover, positive correlations between production of DHPG, which reflects noradrenergic turnover, and of DOPA would support the view that the latter reflects catecholamine biosynthesis. In patients undergoing cardiac catheterization, regional arteriovenous production rates of DOPA across the heart and brain correlate positively with those of DHPG (Eisenhofer, Brush et al., 1989). Antecubital venous DOPA levels correlate positively with antecubital venous DHPG levels (Goldstein, Polinsky et al., 1989), and urinary excretion of DOPA correlates

Table 5–3. Factors Affecting Plasma DOPA Concentrations

Conditions of Sampling

Exercise (increased)
Salt intake (no change)
Advanced age (decreased)
Tilt or orthostasis (no change)
Postprandial (no change)

Diseases or Pathological Conditions

Cardiovascular
Shock (increased)
Hemorrhage (increased)

Endocrine
Hypoglycemia (usually no change)
Pheochromocytoma (increased in malignant pheochromocytoma)

Neurological
Pure autonomic failure (decreased)
Multiple system atrophy (usually normal)
Dopamine-β-hydroxylase deficiency (increased)
Menkes disease (increased)
Neuroblastoma (increased)
Sympathectomy (decreased)
Spinal cord stimulation in pithed rats (increased)

Psychiatric
Distress, e.g., immobilization in conscious rats (increased)

Drugs

Resperpine (increased)
α-Methyl-para-tyrosine (decreased)
α_2-Adrenoceptor agonists, e.g., clonidine (decreased)
Desipramine (decreased)
Vasodilators, e.g., nitroprusside (increased)
Ganglion blockers, e.g., trimethaphan, chlorisondamine (decreased)
MAO inhibitors (decreased)

positively with those of DHPG (Goldstein, Grossman et al., 1993; Wolfovitz et al., 1993). Patients with pure autonomic failure have decreased plasma levels of both catechols, whereas patients with multiple system atrophy, thought to result from abnormal central neural regulation of sympathetic outflow without loss of sympathetic nerve terminals, usually have normal plasma DOPA levels (Goldstein, Polinsky et al., 1989).

One must distinguish TH activity from tissue content of the enzyme. Acute exposure to stressors increases TH activity rapidly by phosphorylation of the enzyme (Masserano et al., 1989). During immobilization stress in rats, plasma DOPA levels begin to increase within 1 minute, whereas even after 120 minutes of immobilization, the adrenal content of TH remains unchanged (Kvetnansky, Goldstein et al., 1992; Sabban et al., 1992). In contrast, after repeated episodes of immobilization, baseline plasma DOPA levels are normal, whereas the adrenal content of TH is increased (Kvetnansky, Armando et al., 1992).

Plasma levels of NE tend to increase with normal aging, as discussed above, whereas plasma levels of DOPA tend to decrease. Thus across healthy individuals, the plasma NE/DOPA ratio increases significantly as a function of age (Garty, Stull et al., 1989). Whether this corresponds to an age-related decline in TH activity is unknown.

Urinary DOPA and Renal Dopamine Production

Circulating DOPA can influence catecholamine synthesis and cellular function in tissues lacking TH, via uptake and conversion by decarboxylation to DA. DOPA may therefore act indirectly as a neurohormone, with a unique mechanism of action: uptake into cells that cannot synthesize it, with conversion to an active metabolite that acts as an autocrine–paracine substance.

The kidneys extensively remove DOPA from the plasma, and as noted above, in proximal tubular cells, DOPA is converted by DDC to DA. DA, in turn, probably contributes to regulation of extracellular fluid volume and blood pressure by stimulating natriuresis, causing renal vasodilation, inhibiting adrenocortical production of aldosterone, and inhibiting NE release from sympathetic nerve terminals.

In humans and rats, urinary DOPA excretion rapidly increases during dietary salt loading (Gill et al., 1991; Goldstein, Stull et al., 1989; Grossman, Hoffman et al., 1992). In Dahl rats, DOPA excretion increases by six fold within 1 day after initiation of high salt intake (Grossman, Hoffman et al., 1990). Urinary DA excretion tends to lag behind, consistent with DOPA serving as the precursor for DA excreted by the kidneys. Proportionate increases in DOPA excretion during dietary salt loading are similar to or larger than increases in DA excretion, implying that the DA excretory responses to dietary salt loading result mainly if not exclusively from increased DOPA uptake by proximal tubular cells. Among healthy individuals, daily urinary DOPA excretion correlates strongly positively with DA excretion (Goldstein, Grossman et al., 1993).

Species differ substantially in patterns of urinary excretion of DOPA and catecholamines. In humans, the daily rate of DOPA excretion is similar to that of NE and about $\frac{1}{10}$ that of DA. In rats, very little DOPA is excreted in urine, due to extremely efficient renal uptake and decarboxylation of DOPA. Dogs have relatively less DA excretion than DOPA excretion, due to less conversion of circulating DOPA to urinary DA (Zim-lichman et al., 1988). In baboons, preliminary evidence suggests substantial metabolism of renal DA to urinary DOPAC (unpublished observations).

Since the renal DOPA–DA system appears to be activated compensatorily to maintain sodium homeostasis during alterations of dietary salt intake, Gill et al. (1991) studied whether patients with salt-sensitive hypertension have an abnormality of this system. Regardless of dietary salt intake, salt-sensitive inpatients had a significantly higher urinary DOPA/DA ratio than did salt-resistant inpatients, suggesting either decreased efficiency of uptake of DOPA into renal proximal tubular cells or decreased renal conversion of DOPA to DA, as discussed in the chapter about cardiovascular diseases.

DOPA in Cerebrospinal Fluid

DOPA concentrations in CSF exceed those of NE. The source and meaning of DOPA in CSF are unknown.

Dihydroxyphenylacetic Acid (DOPAC)

Dihydroxyphenylacetic acid (DOPAC) is formed from the deamination of DA by MAO. The deamination results in the formation of an aldehyde, which is then converted rapidly to a carboxylic acid. This contrasts with the fate of the aldehyde of NE, which is converted mainly to the glycol, DHPG.

The concentration of DOPAC in antecubital venous plasma in humans averages about $15–20 \times 10^{-9}$ mol/L (Eisenhofer et al., 1986; Kopin, 1985), about 50 times that of DA.

Sources of DOPAC in plasma have rarely been studied. Several lines of evidence suggest that plasma DOPAC is derived at least partly from metabolism of DA in nor-adrenergic nerves. In rats and dogs treated with reserpine to block vesicular translo-cation of catecholamines and thereby NE synthesis, plasma DOPAC levels increase markedly (Eisenhofer, Ropchak et al., 1988; Goldstein, Grossman, Tamrat et al., 1991). In contrast, interference with tyrosine hydroxylation results in rapid, persistent decreases in plasma DOPAC levels, with the decreases preceding those in NE levels (Goldstein, Udelsman et al., 1987). In rats, treatment with α-MT to block TH or chlorisondamine to block ganglionic neurotransmission attenuates plasma DOPAC responses to immo-bilization (Kvetnansky, Armando et al., 1992), and treatment with desipramine to block Uptake-1 attenuates but does not abolish plasma [³H]DOPAC responses after [³H]DA injection (Hovevey-Sion, Eisenhofer et al., 1989). Desipramine pretreatment or chem-ical sympathectomy with 6-OHDA also markedly attenuates responses of plasma levels of 6-[¹⁸F]fluoroDOPAC after systemic intravenous injection of 6-[¹⁸F]fluoroDA into dogs (Chang et al., 1990; Goldstein, Grossman, Tamrat et al., 1991). Selective inhibition of MAO-B, thought to be localized in nonneuronal cells, does not produce large falls in DOPAC levels in rats, whereas inhibition of MAO-A, thought to be present in both neuronal and nonneuronal cells, decreases plasma DOPAC levels substantially (Hov-evey-Sion, Kopin et al., 1989).

Patients with pure autonomic failure usually have low plasma DOPAC levels, whereas patients with DBH deficiency have high plasma DOPAC levels (Goldstein, Polinsky et al., 1989). Individual values of plasma DOPAC and DHPG levels correlate positively in rats (Eisenhofer, Ropchak et al., 1988) and humans (Goldstein, Polinsky et al., 1989). In humans, chronic treatment with the MAO-B inhibitor deprenyl decreases plasma DOPAC levels (Eisenhofer et al., 1986), but this may reflect indirect effects of deprenyl on sympathoneural outflow or TH. Debrisoquin, thought to inhibit MAO in sympathetic nerves, markedly decreases plasma DOPAC levels in rats (Hovevey-Sion, Kopin et al., 1989).

DOPAC Levels and Catecholamine Synthesis

As noted above, blockade of catecholamine biosynthesis by α-MT decreases plasma DOPAC and DHPG to very low levels (Goldstein, Udelsman et al., 1987). Plasma DOPAC levels decline more rapidly than do DHPG levels (Kvetnansky, Armando et al., 1992). Leakage of NE from storage vesicles may temporarily maintain plasma DHPG levels in this setting, whereas the much smaller vesicular pool of DA cannot maintain DOPAC levels. The rate of DOPAC production therefore seems to reflect the rate of tyrosine hydroxylation.

Rats chronically exposed to cold stress have normal baseline TH activity at baseline but have augmented increments in enzyme activity in response to a novel stressor, acute tail-shock; hippocampal extracellular fluid DOPAC concentrations, assessed by microdialysis, show the same pattern (Nisenbaum et al., 1991). Partial destruction of central noradrenergic neurons sufficient to decrease tissue NE contents and extracellular fluid concentrations of DOPAC does not decrease extracellular fluid concentrations of NE (Abercrombie and Zigmond, 1989), suggesting a link between DOPAC production and catecholamine turnover, even when transmitter release is maintained.

The contribution of cerebrospinal fluid DOPAC to plasma DOPAC is unknown but is probably small, because as noted above, debrisoquin, a MAO inhibitor that does not enter the brain, produces large decreases in plasma DOPAC levels. In humans, plasma levels of DOPAC exceed cerebrospinal fluid levels (Devinsky et al., 1992).

Urinary excretion rates of DOPAC exceed by several-fold the excretion rates of all other free (unconjugated) catechols combined (Goldstein, Grossman et al., 1993). The sources and meaning of DOPAC in urine are poorly understood. Wolfovitz et al. (1993) have obtained evidence suggesting that DOPAC in urine derives from both circulating DOPAC and from metabolism of DA in the kidneys.

If renal DA and plasma DOPAC shared the same ultimate source—DOPA synthesized in sympathetic nerves—then neither classical concepts about catecholamine biosynthesis in sympathetic nerves, nor observations indicating that most of axoplasmic DA is translocated into vesicles containing DBH (Eisenhofer, Esler et al., 1992), would explain the high plasma DOPAC levels and high rates of excretion of DOPAC in humans. These concepts also do not explain the high plasma levels of DA sulfate and the high rate of urinary excretion of HVA in humans, leading one to speculate that a substantial amount of DA may be synthesized in nonneuronal cells.

Clinical Uses of Catechol Levels

Since levels of catechols in biological fluids have related but distinct sources, indicating different aspects of catecholaminergic function, combined measurements of catechol levels have many uses in clinical diagnosis, therapeutics, and prognosis. This section summarizes some of these applications. The chapter about cardiovascular diseases includes more detailed discussions of catechol levels in specific cardiovascular disorders.

Diagnosis

Measuring levels of catechols in biological fluids can aid in the diagnostic evaluation of tumors of neural crest origin, dysautonomias, panic/anxiety, hypernoradrenergic essential hypertension, and inherited disorders of catecholamine metabolism.

Pheochromocytomas are catecholamine-secreting tumors that constitute a rare but curable cause of hypertension. Since patients harboring pheochromocytomas virtually always have increased plasma levels or urinary excretion rates of NE and its metabolites (Duncan et al., 1988; Grossman, Goldstein et al., 1991; Lenders et al., 1993), the diagnostic evaluation always includes these measurements. Measuring the ratio of plasma NE:DHPG (Brown, 1984) does not greatly improve diagnostic accuracy (Grossman, Goldstein et al., 1991; Lenders et al., 1992). The chapter about cardiovascular diseases discusses plasma levels of metanephrines and clonidine suppression and glucagon stimulation testing, which enhance substantially the diagnostic evaluation of pheochromocytoma.

Neuroblastoma is the most common malignant solid tumor of children. The tumor cells contain TH and synthesize DOPA. Whereas plasma levels of catecholamines often are not increased, plasma levels of DOPA almost always are (Boomsma et al., 1989; Goldstein, Stull et al., 1986).

Different forms of dysautonomia produce characteristic abnormalities of plasma levels of catechols (Goldstein, Polinsky et al., 1989; Meredith et al., 1992; Ziegler et al., 1977b). Dysautonomia in adults commonly presents clinically as orthostatic hypotension, discussed in the chapter about cardiovascular diseases. Patients with pure autonomic failure or multiple system atrophy have a failure to increase NE spillover into arterial plasma during orthostasis.

The hyperdynamic circulation syndrome includes high baseline plasma levels of NE and EPI, increased cardiac output, labile or systolic hypertension, and excessive circulatory responses to the β-adrenoceptor agonist isoproterenol (Frohlich, 1977; Frohlich et al., 1969; Goldstein and Keiser, 1985).

During attacks of vasodepressor syncope, patients have increased plasma EPI levels and an absence of increased plasma NE levels despite the hypotension (Goldstein, Spanarkel et al., 1982; Ziegler et al., 1986). Between episodes, the patients have normal responses of plasma NE levels during orthostasis. Chapter 6 discusses the distinctive neuroendocrine pattern attending vasodepressor syncope.

Reflex sympathetic dystrophy (RSD) is a painful, dysesthetic disorder of extremities. Whether this condition actually involves abnormal sympathoneural function, as indicated by regional spillover of NE, is unknown. RSD patients have, if anything, decreased plasma NE and DHPG levels in the affected limb (Drummond et al., 1991) and have augmented hand vein constrictor responses to NE (Arnold et al., 1993), suggesting denervation-supersensitivity or dysregulation of adrenoceptors on nociceptors.

"Autonomic epilepsy" can be associated with hypertension, flushing, and high circulating catecholamine levels that decrease during clonidine treatment (Metz et al., 1978).

Patients with panic/anxiety disorders appear to have normal levels of plasma catecholamines at rest. Elicitation of symptoms by infusion of lactate or yohimbine often increases plasma levels of catecholamines or NE metabolites (Carr et al., 1986; Charney et al., 1984; Goldstein, Grossman, Listwak et al., 1991). Panic in naturalistic settings, such as during flying in flight-phobic patients, increases plasma catecholamine levels (Ekeberg et al., 1990).

The possible etiologic role of increased SNS or AHS activity in clinical essential hypertension has aroused persistent controversy (Goldstein, 1983b). The chapter about cardiovascular diseases discusses this issue. Plasma catecholamine levels are normal in most patients with essential hypertension; however, a hypernoradrenergic subgroup has increased PRA and cardiac output, with anger or anxiety (Esler et al., 1977).

Considering the role of endogenous DA in sodium homeostasis, an abnormality in the renal DOPA–DA system may play a pathophysiologic role in salt-sensitive hypertension (Gill et al., 1988, 1991).

As noted in the chapter about catecholaminergic systems, since tetrahydrobiopterin is a key cofactor for TH, deficiency of dihydropteridine reductase (DHPR) decreases the amount of tyrosine hydroxylation for a given amount of TH enzyme. This produces an atypical form of phenylketonuria, where dietary restriction of phenylalanine fails to correct the neurological deterioration. Whether endogenous plasma, urine, or cerebrospinal fluid levels of DOPA are decreased in patients with DHPR deficiency is unknown.

Menkes' disease is another inherited disorder producing neurological deterioration in infants. The disease results from abnormal copper metabolism. Since DBH is copper-dependent, levels of NE would be expected to be low in plasma or cerebrospinal fluid; however, Menkes' patients actually have normal or only slightly decreased NE levels (Kaler et al., 1993), apparently because of compensatory activation of sympathetic outflow and catecholamine biosynthesis. Thus, Menkes' patients have high ratios of DOPA/DHPG and DOPAC/DHPG in plasma and CSF.

Aromatic L-amino acid decarboxylase deficiency is a relatively recently described inborn error of metabolism. Consistent with low DDC activity, affected patients have high levels of DOPA and low levels of HVA in plasma, urine, and CSF (Hyland and Clayton, 1992).

Clinical Therapeutics

Many commonly used drugs affect catecholaminergic function, explaining their clinical effects. One can use measurements of levels of catechols and catecholamine metabolites to monitor the drug effects.

Drugs inhibiting SNS function are effective antihypertensive agents. Reserpine blocks vesicular translocation of amines, markedly increasing net leakage of NE into the axonal cytoplasm and depleting NE stores. Guanethidine and tyramine act as false neurotransmitters, displacing NE from the vesicles; the former also interferes with NE release. Bretylium inhibits NE release, with less depletion of NE stores. Hexamethonium and trimethaphan block ganglionic neurotransmission.

These drugs produce different patterns of plasma levels of catechols, as discussed above. Reserpine acutely increases plasma levels of DHPG and DOPAC, as DA and NE leak from the vesicles; when NE stores become depleted, plasma levels of DHPG fall markedly, whereas high plasma levels of DOPAC persist, and stimulation of catecholamine biosynthesis increases plasma DOPA levels. Ganglion blockade decreases plasma NE levels, with only slight decreases in DHPG and DOPA levels, possibly due to alterations in plasma clearance of these compounds (Garty, Deka-Starosta, Chang et al., 1989) or to ongoing catecholamine biosynthesis and vesicular turnover.

Drugs acting at adrenoceptors are also important antihypertensives. β-Adrenoceptor blockers tend to increase plasma NE levels by decreasing NE clearance (Cryer et al., 1980). α_2-Adrenoceptor agonists inhibit sympathoneural outflow and stimulate inhibitory autoreceptors on sympathetic nerve terminals, attenuating exocytosis and thereby decreasing plasma NE and DHPG levels (Goldstein, Eisenhofer et al., 1988).

Antihypertensive agents that do not affect sympathoneural function directly can affect plasma levels of catechols reflexively. Hydrochlorothiazide, a diuretic, tends to increase plasma NE levels in hypertensives (Lake et al., 1979), and nitroprusside, a vasodilator, increases plasma NE, DHPG, and DOPA levels (Garty, Deka-Starosta, Chang et al., 1989).

L-DOPA, converted in the brain to DA, is a mainstay in the treatment of Parkinson's disease. Serial measurements of plasma DOPA levels may aid in the diagnostic evaluation of causes of the "on-off" phenomenon in Parkinsonian patients (Eriksson et al., 1988). The catechol carbidopa inhibits DDC in the periphery, the combination of carbidopa and L-DOPA increasing the delivery of DOPA to the brain. Because carbidopa inhibits renal DDC, the ratio of urinary excretion of DOPA to that of DA increases markedly during carbidopa treatment (Goldstein, Stull et al., 1989). This could provide a simple index of the extent of DDC inhibition in patients taking the drug combination.

Most of L-DOPA administered therapeutically is not decarboxylated but is O-methylated. Treatment with a COMT inhibitor should augment DA production from L-DOPA. One could monitor the extent of COMT inhibition from the increased ratios of DOPA:OMeDOPA and DOPAC:HVA in plasma or urine (Nissinen et al., 1992).

The cause or causes of the nigrostriatal degeneration that is the hallmark of the disease are a subject of active research. One possible mechanism is neurotoxic. Since injection of a dopaminergic neurotoxin produces sustained decreases in plasma levels of DHPG and DOPAC (Johannessen et al., 1990), screening tests for dopaminergic neurotoxins may include plasma levels of catechols.

Treatment with deprenyl, a MAO-B inhibitor, delays the progression of Parkinson's disease (The Parkinson Study Group, 1993), perhaps by decreasing deamination-induced oxidative injury to nigral cells. MAO-B inhibition may (Eisenhofer et al., 1986) or may not (Hovevey-Sion, Kopin et al., 1989) affect plasma DHPG levels but should increase the plasma NMN/DHPG ratio.

The classical antidepressant agents, MAO inhibitors and tricyclics, produce characteristic changes in plasma levels of catechols. Global or MAO-A inhibitors decrease plasma DOPAC and DHPG levels (Eisenhofer et al., 1986; Hovevey-Sion, Kopin et al., 1989), with little or no effect on plasma NE levels. Tricyclic antidepressants, which inhibit Uptake-1, augment responses of concentrations of NE at effector cells during sympathetic stimulation, with small or absent increases in DHPG levels (Goldstein, Eisenhofer et al., 1988). Analogously, cocaine, a classical inhibitor of Uptake-1, accentuates plasma NE responses during sympathetic stimulation (Bayorh et al., 1983).

Amphetamine, a sympathomimetic amine that probably also inhibits catecholamine reuptake, increases plasma NE levels (Goldstein, Nurnberger et al., 1983). Benzodiazepines such as diazepam usually decrease plasma NE and EPI levels and inhibit catecholamine responses during exposure to emotional stressors (Dionne et al., 1984).

Since patients with neuroblastoma have high DOPA levels, plasma or urinary DOPA can be used to monitor the tumor burden during therapy and to detect relapse (Boomsma et al., 1989).

Sympathectomy attenuates or abolishes regional release of NE into the circulation (Goldstein, Bonner et al., 1986). Measurements of NE spillover can assess the extent of sympathectomy or reinnervation.

Prognosis

The SNS and AHS are two of the body's most potent and rapidly acting homeostatic effectors. Cardiac decompensation, associated with left ventricular failure or myocardial infarction, is usually associated with elevated plasma catecholamine levels (e.g., Thomas and Marks, 1978). In heart failure as well as in acute myocardial infarction, patients with high plasma catecholamine levels have a worse long-term prognosis than those with normal plasma catecholamine levels (Cohn et al., 1984; Karlsberg et al., 1981). Whether the elevated catecholamine levels in patients with poor prognoses indicate greater recruitment of sympathetic activity to maintain cardiovascular performance, or whether the elevated levels are themselves pathogenic, is unclear (Packer, 1990), as discussed in the chapter about cardiovascular diseases.

Intracranial bleeding increases plasma levels of catecholamines, and patients with poor clinical outcome (death or severe disability) have higher plasma catecholamine levels than do patients with good clinical outcome (moderate or no disability, Dilraj et al., 1992).

In patients with pheochromocytoma, elevated plasma DOPA levels suggest malignancy (Goldstein, Stull et al., 1986). Plasma NE levels can be used to follow the course of patients with pheochromocytoma. In patients with catecholamine-induced cardio-myopathy due to pheochromocytoma, tumor excision can reverse the cardiomyopathy and normalize NE levels (Imperato-McGinley et al., 1987).

Direct Sympathetic Nerve Recording

Microneurography can record sympathetic nerve activity directly in skin and skeletal muscle in humans (Hagbarth and Vallbo, 1968). Under resting conditions, these regions contribute relatively little to overall circulatory regulation; however, cutaneous and skeletal muscle sympathetic activity reflect processes that do underlie systemic neuro-circulatory changes. Skin sympathetic activity increases during emotional provocation and exposure to cold, decreases during exposure to warmth, and remains generally unchanged during exposure to hemodynamic perturbations that alter baroreflex activity (Mark, 1990). In contrast, pulse-synchronous skeletal muscle sympathoneural activity (SMSA) increases as part of baroreflex-mediated patterns of neural activation, such as during changes in blood pressure, cardiopulmonary filling, and exercise.

Whether SMSA increases during psychological stress has been unclear. Anderson et al. (1987) and Hjemdahl et al. (1989) reported that laboratory mental challenges increased SMSA in the leg, in contrast with earlier findings of Delius et al. (1972a, 1972b). If skeletal sympathoneural outflow increased during the ''defense reaction,'' as described by Folkow (1982), then EPI, other circulating factors, local metabolic products, or active cholinergic vasodilation could explain the prominent skeletal vaso-dilator component of the reaction.

Decreased cardiac baroreceptor afferent activity during application of lower body negative pressure (LBNP) rapidly increases peroneal SMSA (Rea and Hamden, 1990; Rowell and Seals, 1990; Sundlof and Wallin, 1978b), as does decreased cardiac and arterial baroreceptor afferent activity during infusion of nitroprusside (Rea, Eckberg et al., 1990). Systemic injection of EPI also increases SMSA (Persson et al., 1989), pos-sibly via baroreflex responses to vasodilation.

Under baseline conditions, antecubital venous NE concentrations correlate positively with SMSA (Floras et al., 1991; Morlin and Wallin, 1983; Wallin et al., 1981, 1987), supporting the validity of plasma NE levels in indicating sympathetic outflow, at least in the limbs.

In all circumstances tested so far where SMSA has been found to change, antecubital venous levels of NE have been found to change in the same direction. For instance, dietary salt loading tends to inhibit SMSA (Anderson et al., 1989) and to decrease plasma NE levels (Luft et al., 1979). Insulin- or 2-deoxyglucose-induced glucopenia increases SMSA (Fagius and Berne, 1989; Frandsen et al., 1989) and plasma NE levels (Garber et al., 1976; Goldstein, Breier et al., 1993). Both SMSA and plasma NE levels increase with normal aging (Yamada et al., 1989; Ziegler et al., 1976), and both decrease—despite orthostatic hypotension—during fainting (Wallin and Sundlof, 1982; Ziegler et al., 1986). During orthostasis, plasma NE levels and SMSA rapidly increase by about two-fold (Burke et al., 1977; Lake et al., 1976; Mueller et al., 1974).

These findings suggest that either sympathetically mediated release in the forearm determines NE levels in antecubital venous plasma or that these stressors evoke diffuse increases in SNS outflows. In contrast with the suggestion that SMSA determines *arterial* levels of NE (Folkow et al., 1983), Esler and co-workers have demonstrated that skeletal muscle NE spillover constitutes only a minor source of the total spillover of NE into arterial plasma (for reviews see Esler, Jennings et al., 1984b, 1990; Esler, Jennings, Korner et al., 1988). More likely, although sympathoneural responses can be heterogeneous during stress, under resting conditions sympathoneural activity in several body regions probably is regulated to some extent as a unit—for example, via baroreflexes and medullary "generators" (Gebber, 1984). This can explain why SMSA correlates positively not only with antecubital venous NE levels but also with arterial NE spillover (Hjemdahl et al., 1989), pulse rate, and PRA (Floras et al., 1991).

Several reports have related directly recorded sympathoneural activity to regional NE spillover. In laboratory animals, nitroprusside-induced hypotension and phenylephrine-induced hypertension produce correlated changes in renal sympathetic nerve activity and renal NE spillover (Deka-Starosta et al., 1989; Noshiro et al., 1991; Sano et al., 1989). In humans, LBNP increases peroneal SMSA proportionately more than it does forearm NE spillover (Goldstein et al., unpublished observations). Inhibitory modulation of NE release by α_2-adrenoceptors on the nerve terminals may explain this discrepancy.

Simultaneous measurements of sympathetic nerve activity and plasma NE spillover allow examination of presynaptic receptors that may modulate NE release. For instance, intravenous administration of the α_2-adrenoceptor blocker yohimbine increases forearm NE spillover proportionately much more than the drug increases SMSA, suggesting tonic regulation of NE release by α_2-adrenoceptors on sympathetic terminals in humans (Grossman, Chang et al., 1991a; Grossman, Rea et al., 1991).

Spectral Analysis of Heart Rate Variability

Heart rate variability generally has two frequency components—a high frequency component (corresponding to vagally mediated respiratory sinus arrhythmia), and a low frequency component. Since the power of the low-frequency component increases during stimuli that probably augment cardiac sympathetic drive and decreases during β-adrenoceptor blockade, the low-frequency component may reflect cardiac SNS "tone" (Malliani, 1990; Malliani et al., 1990, 1991; McCance, 1991; Pagani et al., 1986).

Although the high-frequency component probably does reflect cardiac parasympathetic "tone," the low-frequency component depends only partly on cardiac SNS outflow. Sinus nodal parasympathectomy decreases the low-frequency peak by about 50% in conscious dogs (Randall et al., 1991), demonstrating that the low-frequency peak reflects activity of both divisions of the autonomic nervous system. To date, no study has correlated low-frequency power with cardiac NE spillover.

Visualization of Sympathetic Innervation and Function

Nuclear medical imaging techniques can visualize tissue sympathetic innervation, especially in the heart. One technique has used ^{123}I-labeled *meta*-iodobenzylguanidine (MIBG, Dae and Botvinick, 1990; Dae et al., 1989; Glowiniak et al., 1989; Sisson and Wieland, 1986), a radioactive analogue of guanethidine. This technique has sufficient resolution to visualize sites of cardiac regional denervation in dogs (Dae et al., 1989) and humans (Wichter et al., 1994) but entails relatively long imaging times and limited spatial resolution. Moreover, MIBG is not a substrate for catecholamine-metabolizing enzymes.

Scanning by positron emission tomography (PET) affords better resolution and allows assessments of radioactivity concentrations over time. Schwaiger and co-workers (Schwaiger et al., 1990a, 1990b; Wieland et al., 1990) have developed 6-[18F]fluorometaraminol and [11C]hydroxyephedrine, positron-emitting analogues of sympathomimetic amines, as PET imaging agents to visualize cardiac sympathetic innervation. Schwaiger et al. (1990b) conducted PET scanning of the heart after injection of [11C]hydroxyephedrine into healthy humans and patients with recent cardiac transplantations. The transplant recipients had 82% less myocardial retention of [11C]hydroxyephedrine-derived radioactivity than did the healthy subjects, indicating relatively little nonneuronal binding of the agent. These investigators subsequently obtained evidence for sympathetic reinnervation of the transplanted human heart (Schwaiger et al., 1991).

MAO and COMT do not metabolize 6-[18F]fluorometaraminol or [11C]hydroxyephedrine, so that analysis of PET myocardial radioactivity–time curves (time–activity curves, TACs) after injection of these agents yields little functional information. Goldstein and co-workers have developed 6-[18F]fluoroDA ([18F]-6F-DA) as a PET imaging agent that has the potential to visualize sympathetic innervation and function.

[18F]-6F-DA, a positron-emitting analogue of DA (Figure 5–5), is a substrate for all the known removal and metabolic processes that affect the disposition of endogenous catecholamines. Studies of rats (Chang et al., 1990; Chieuh et al., 1983; Hovevey-Sion, Eisenhofer et al., 1989), dogs (Goldstein, Chang et al. 1990; Goldstein, Grossman, Tamrat et al., 1991), and humans (Goldstein, Eisenhofer et al., 1993) have shown that neuronal and nonneuronal cells take up the tracer, by Uptake-1 and Uptake-2 (Figure 5–6). In nonneuronal cells, MAO and COMT convert [18F]-6F-DA to [18F]-6F-HVA.

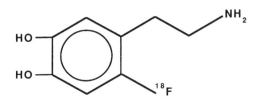

Figure 5–5. Structure of 6-[18F]fluorodopamine.

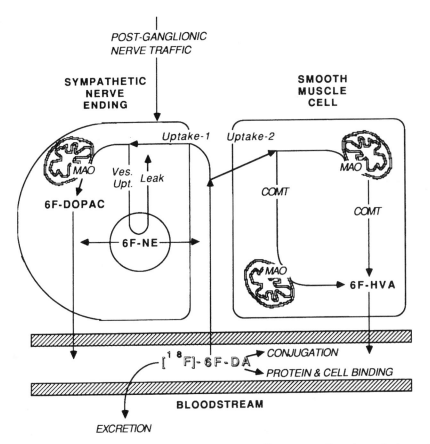

Figure 5–6. The metabolic fate of 6-[^{18}F]fluorodopamine ([^{18}F]-6F-DA). Note the analogies to the metabolic fate of endogenous catecholamines. [^{18}F]-6F-DA is removed by Uptake-1 into nerves and Uptake-2 into nonneuronal cells. In sympathetic nerves, [^{18}F]-6F-DA is metabolized to [^{18}F]-6F-DOPAC or translocated into vesicles containing dopamine-β-hydroxylase, converting the tracer to [^{18}F]-6F-NE. In extraneuronal cells, [^{18}F]-6F-DA is metabolized by monoamine oxidase and catechol-O-methyltransferase to form [^{18}F]-6F-HVA. In the bloodstream, [^{18}F]-6F-DA is sulfoconjugated to form [^{18}F]-6F-DA sulfate.

In sympathetic nerves, MAO converts [^{18}F]-6F-DA to 6F-[^{18}F]-DOPAC, with some of the [^{18}F]-6F-DOPAC entering the bloodstream and some probably converted extraneuronally to [^{18}F]-6F-HVA. Most of axoplasmic [^{18}F]-6F-DA enters storage vesicles. Vesicular [^{18}F]-6F-DA can leak back into the axoplasm, can be released during sympathetic stimulation, or can be converted slowly to [^{18}F]-6F-NE, the radioactive anlaogue of the sympathetic neurotransmitter (Chang et al., 1990). The disposition of 6F-NE is similar to that of NE itself (Chieuh et al., 1983).

Beginning virtually immediately after injection of [^{18}F]-6F-DA, the rate of disappearance of [^{18}F]-6F-DA-derived radioactivity from the bloodstream exceeds that of the radioactivity in sympathetically innervated organs (Goldstein, Chang et al., 1990;

Goldstein, Eisenhofer et al., 1993), enabling visualization of the innervated organs by PET scanning. Because of extensive neuronal uptake of catecholamines by myocardial sympathetic nerves (Goldstein, Brush et al., 1988), thoracic [^{18}F]-6F-DA PET scanning reveals striking images of the ventricular myocardium (Figure 5–7). An effective blood–brain barrier prevents exogenously administered [^{18}F]-6F-DA from entering the central nervous system. Uptake by the adrenal glands is small because of the very small proportion of the cardiac output that is distributed to the adrenal glands. Uptake by the lungs is also small, probably because of sparse sympathetic innervation. The salivary glands and spleen, which possess sympathetic innervation, concentrate [^{18}F]-6F-DA-derived radioactivity. In the urinary system, radioactivity accumulates in the renal pelvises and urinary bladder, due to excretion of [^{18}F]-6F-DA, metabolites of [^{18}F]-6F-DA, and metabolites of [^{18}F]-6F-NE. [^{18}F]-6F-DA in the liver is probably metabolized by

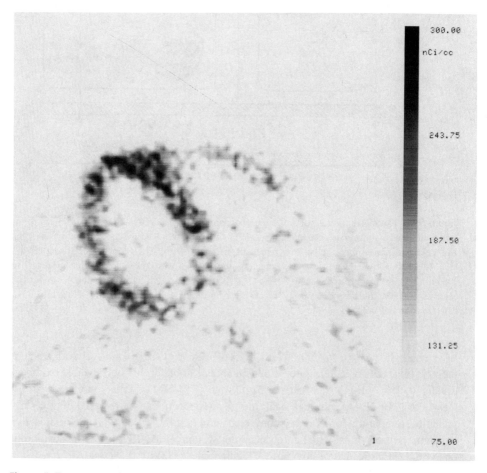

Figure 5–7. Thoracic positron emission tomographic (PET) scan after intravenous injection of 6-[^{18}F]fluorodopamine ([^{18}F]-6F-DA) into a healthy volunteer. The left ventricular free wall, the interventricular septum, and the right ventricular wall are visualized.

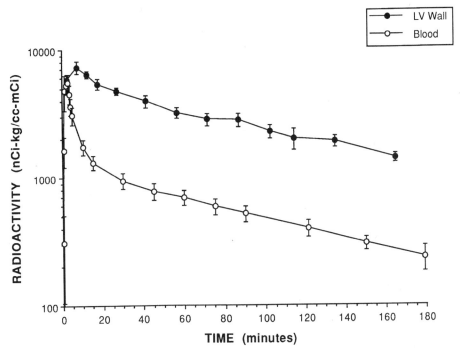

Figure 5–8. Myocardial and blood radioactivity concentrations after intravenous injection of 6-[^{18}F]fluorodopamine ([^{18}F]-6F-DA) into healthy volunteers. Within a few minutes of the injection, the myocardial radioactivity concentration exceeds that in blood by about five-fold. Myocardial radioactivity declines slowly, with a half-time of about 1.5 h.

COMT and MAO, with subsequent release of the metabolites into the bloodstream or bile.

Radiolabeling of cardiac sympathetic nerves determines PET myocardial visualization after injection of [^{18}F]-6F-DA, because chemical sympathectomy abolishes the cardiac image (Goldstein, Grossman, Tamrat et al., 1991). Specifically, radiolabeling of the storage vesicles in the nerve terminals produces the image, because pretreatment with reserpine, which blocks vesicular translocation, abolishes the cardiac image within several minutes after injection of [^{18}F]-6F-DA (Goldstein, Chang et al., 1990).

In normal volunteers, by about 10 minutes after [^{18}F]-6F-DA injection, thoracic PET scanning visualizes the left ventricular free wall, septum, right ventricular wall, and ventricular chambers. By a few minutes after the injection, the left ventricular myocardial radioactivity concentration exceeds that in whole blood by about five fold. Myocardial radioactivity subsequently declines biexponentially, with a late $t_{1/2}$ of about 1.5 hours (Figure 5–8).

Plasma levels of [^{18}F]-6F-DA and radioactivity decline extremely rapidly, with a $t_{1/2}$ of less than 2 minutes for about 10 minutes after the injection. After several minutes, the difference between the plasma total radioactivity concentration and the plasma [^{18}F]-6F-DA concentration indicates that most of the radioactivity in plasma arises from metabolites of [^{18}F]-6F-DA—including [^{18}F]-6F-HVA, [^{18}F]-6F-DA-sulfate, and [^{18}F]-6F-methoxytyramine sulfate. Urinary radioactivity excretion after [^{18}F]-6F-DA administration occurs in three phases, corresponding to sequential elimination of [^{18}F]-6F-DA, [^{18}F]-6F-HVA, and metabolites of [^{18}F]-6F-NE. Desipramine treatment attenuates similarly the accumulation of [^{18}F]-6F-DA-derived radioactivity in the myocardium (Goldstein, Chang et al., 1990; Goldstein, Eisenhofer et al., 1993) and of [^{18}F]-6F-DOPAC in the plasma (Goldstein, Eisenhofer et al., 1993).

In baboons, the rate of decline in myocardial radioactivity after administration of [^{18}F]-6F-DA exceeds the rate of decline after injection of [^{18}F]-6F-NE (Ding et al., 1993). The basis for this difference is unknown and may relate to differences in vesicular uptake and turnover of [^{18}F]-6F-DA and [^{18}F]-6F-NE.

[^{18}F]-6F-DA PET scanning can therefore visualize cardiac sympathetic innervation by PET scanning. The temporal pattern of excretion of [^{18}F]-6F-DA and its metabolites, and the results of the pharmacological treatments, imply that [^{18}F]-6F-DA is taken up into sympathetic nerves, translocated into vesicles, and converted to [^{18}F]-6F-NE, and that manipulations of Uptake-1 activity and postganglionic sympathetic nerve traffic produce predictable alterations in myocardial TACs. Thus, [^{18}F]-6F-DA PET scanning has the potential to provide unique and important information about cardiac sympathetic innervation and function noninvasively in humans. Future work in this area must focus more on elucidating the relationship between the kinetics of [^{18}F]-6F-DA-derived radioactivity in the heart and myocardial NE turnover.

Advantages and Disadvantages of Assessment Techniques

Plasma NE levels are related indirectly to sympathetically mediated exocytosis. Many factors intervene between sympathetic nerve traffic and plasma NE levels, including neuronal reuptake, presynaptic modulation of NE release, and clearance mechanisms. Moreover, during many stress responses, SNS outflows change heterogeneously in different vascular beds. One must keep in mind these factors in drawing inferences about sympathoneural outflow based on measurements of antecubital venous NE levels.

Tracer kinetic techniques based on estimates of NE spillovers into arterial and regional venous plasma have refined the neurochemical approach for measuring total body and regional NE release; however, changes not only in sympathoneural traffic but also in inhibitory modulation of NE release by adrenoceptors on sympathetic nerve endings and in Uptake-1 activity determine NE spillover. Measurements of cardiac NE kinetics require cardiac catheterization, arterial cannulation, use of radionuclides, and radioactive fraction collection. Few centers use this powerful technique.

Because of the different sources and meanings of plasma NE and DHPG levels, combined measurements of endogenous and tracer-labeled NE and DHPG can yield unique clinical information about specific aspects sympathoneural function; however, the technique is technically demanding, and the estimates are subject to extensive measurement error.

Regional spillover rates of DOPA and DOPAC seem to reflect regional TH activity, providing a means to examine the synthesis and turnover of NE in sympathetic nerves. Again, these techniques require cardiac catheterization and rather sophisticated bench laboratory support.

Sympathetic microneurography has the advantage of providing information directly about postganglionic sympathetic nerve traffic. In humans, sympathetic nerve recording is possible clinically only in skin and skeletal muscle—regions thought to participate relatively little in overall circulatory regulation under baseline conditions; however, SMSA is sensitive to stimuli affecting baroreflex-mediated changes in sympathetic out-flow. Applying the technique requires extensive training and practice, as well as access to fairly expensive monitoring equipment. Direct sympathoneural recording alone cannot assess effects of manipulations, disease states, or drugs on Uptake-1 activity, presynaptic modulation of NE release, or postsynaptic processes.

Power spectral analysis of heart rate variability is simple and inexpensive, can be automated, and requires little technical training. Whereas the high-frequency component probably does indicate cardiac parasympathetic "tone," the low-frequency component depends only partly on cardiac SNS activity. This noninvasive technique for examining cardiac SNS "tone" has not yet been validated adequately.

Radionuclide-tomographic approaches to visualize cardiac sympathetic innervation offer the unique advantage of enabling assessments of sympathetic innervation in particular regions within the heart wall, using approaches that are generally noninvasive. Radiolabeled sympathomimetic amines can image myocardial sympathetic innervation; however, since MAO and COMT do not metabolize these agents, the results cannot provide information about cardiac sympathoneural function.

Since $[^{18}F]$-6F-DA is a substrate for all the known removal and metabolic processes that affect the disposition of endogenous catecholamines, $[^{18}F]$-6F-DA PET scanning offers the potential for examining both cardiac sympathetic innervation and function. Initial findings in humans have confirmed that $[^{18}F]$-6F-DA PET scanning can visualize myocardial innervation and that manipulations altering Uptake-1 activity or postganglionic sympathoneural traffic produce predictable effects on myocardial TACs. Whether analysis of myocardial TACs after $[^{18}F]$-6F-DA administration yields valid quantitative information about cardiac sympathoneural function in humans has not been proven.

The nuclear cardiology approaches—especially those involving PET scanning—require elaborate and expensive equipment and highly trained personnel.

Summary and Conclusions

This chapter has focused on clinical methods for assessing activities of catecholaminergic systems. The SNS consists of so many facets that no single measurement tool—even direct sympathetic nerve recording—can describe adequately the events mediating sympathoneural regulation of the circulation.

Levels of each of the endogenous catechols indicate related but distinct aspects of catecholaminergic function. Simultaneous measurements of levels of catechols therefore can provide unique information about pathophysiologic mechanisms and effects of drugs in cardiology, neurology, and psychiatry.

The mainstay in the clinical neurochemical assessment of sympathoneural activity has been the measurement of plasma levels of NE. Several processes, including neuronal reuptake, heterogeneous changes in regional SNS traffic, and modulation of NE release by receptors on sympathetic nerve endings, complicate the relationship between plasma NE concentrations and sympathetically mediated exocytosis. Combinations of measurements of NE levels and responses to drugs affecting sympathoneural function, such as in yohimbine challenge and clonidine suppression testing, can aid in the identification of individuals with alterations in the sympathoneural contribution to blood pressure.

Applying tracer kinetic approaches such as simultaneous measurements of regional clearances of [^{3}H]NE and [^{3}H]isoproterenol and regional spillover rates of NE, DHPG, and O-methylated metabolites of NE can avoid many limitations of measurements of antecubital venous levels of NE. These simultaneous measurements provide a comprehensive picture of neurochemical events at sympathetic neuroeffector junctions.

The source and meaning of DA in plasma are unclear; available evidence supports the view that increments in free plasma DA levels occur only during severe stresses and may reflect release from noradrenergic nerve terminals. Virtually all of circulating DA in humans is sulfoconjugated. The source and physiological meaning of DA sulfate are unknown. The sulfoconjugation mechanism may have evolved to localize effects of DA and inactivate DA entering the circulation. Urinary excretion of DA depends importantly on renal uptake and decarboxylation of circulating DOPA.

DOPA in plasma derives substantially from sympathetic nerve endings, and regional DOPA production may therefore indicate regional catecholamine biosynthesis; however, a proportion of DOPA in plasma appears to be derived from cells that are insensitive to 6-OHDA. Plasma levels of DOPAC also probably reflect TH activity in sympathetic nerves.

SMSA can be recorded directly in humans. Since SMSA varies with alterations in baroreflex afferent activity, sympathetic microneurography can assess reflexive changes in sympathoneural postganglionic outflow. This technique cannot detect alterations in neuronal reuptake, presynaptic modulation of NE release, or postsynaptic factors determining neurogenic cardiovascular responses.

Spectral analysis of heart rate variability provides a simple, noninvasive, but probably indirect means to assess cardiac sympathetic activity; this approach has not been validated in humans.

Nuclear scanning procedures, including PET scanning, can visualize cardiac sympathetic innervation. Although manipulations of Uptake-1 activity or postganglionic sympathoneural traffic produce predictable changes in myocardial TACs after [^{18}F]-6F-DA injection, whether [^{18}F]-6F-DA PET scanning yields valid quantitative information about sympathoneural function in the heart has not yet been established.

6

Stress Response Patterns

According to Selye's stress theory, stress evokes—or is—a unitary, nonspecific, stereotyped response pattern elicited independently of the particular stressor. Cannon, who disputed Selye's doctrine of nonspecificity, asserted nevertheless that acute exposure to any of several different physiological and emotional stressors produces essentially the same neuroendocrine "emergency" response (Cannon, 1914b; Cannon 1929a). Cannon and Selye based their concepts on responses of only one effector system (sympathoadrenal or pituitary–adrenocortical) during severe and potentially overwhelming threats to homeostasis. Mason (1971, 1975a) argued that concurrent production of a distressing emotion such as anxiety could explain the resemblance of neuroendocrine responses upon exposure to the stressors Cannon and Selye used.

Life contains vastly more common and less dire stressors than encompassed in Cannon's and Selye's theories. According to the present conception, the body's stress effector systems work continuously to maintain the internal environment, based on afferent information from exteroceptors, proprioceptors, and interoceptors to the brain, cognitive simulations, and the simultaneous operation of numerous homeostats. The survival advantages afforded by relatively specific patterns fostered the evolution of those patterns, and the absence of these automatic, heterogeneous, frequently unconscious adjustments precludes normal life.

The often surprisingly large neuroendocrine and circulatory responses to purely symbolic psychosocial cues in humans testify to the power of cognitive simulations. To some extent, the occurrence of these responses in laboratory situations mitigates the deficiency of scientific understanding of distress in real-life situations, and despite sometimes substantial interspecies differences, findings in laboratory animals probably provide a glimpse at the neuroendocrine and circulatory mechanisms of distress that operate in humans.

This chapter presents patterns of effector system responses evinced by mammals upon exposure to different stressors, including physiological and metabolic stressors, such as hemorrhage, hypoglycemia, and orthostasis, and stressful emotional experiences, such as fear, anger, and grief. These patterns relate directly to putative mechanisms by which stress may contribute to cardiovascular diseases, the topic of the next and main chapter of this book.

Differences in the relative extents of activation of the AHS and SNS during different stress responses ironically provide some of the most convincing evidence for distinctive neuroendocrine stress response patterns. The reason this is ironic is that it was Cannon, so instrumental in describing and studying these components, who most forcefully propounded their combined and undifferentiated activation (Cannon, 1929a, 1939a). The two main sections of this chapter present stress response patterns where AHS or SNS activation predominates.

Much of the following discussion dwells on neuroendocrine and circulatory variables; however, as emphasized in Chapter 1, distinctions among behavioral, hormonal, and circulatory facets of stress responses largely reflect separate investigative traditions in psychology, neuroendocrinology, and cardiology, rather than intrinsically separate processes. The expression of truly adaptive stress responses requires close integration of these facets.

The evidence to be presented generally supports the following conclusions about catecholaminergic systems during stress:

1. Stressors evoking AHS activation often are distressing, in the sense of inducing a conscious, aversive experience accompanied by behavioral and autonomic signs that other members of the species instinctively recognize. Stressors perceived as posing global, metabolic challenges or threats to well-being elicit preferential adrenomedullary activation, regardless of the intensity of the stressor. Although in intact mammals distress always produces adrenomedullary activation, adrenomedullary activation does not imply the experience of distress.

2. Stresses associated with SNS activation usually include a component of skeletal muscular contraction or active movement. Patterned sympathoneural activation produces adaptive changes in the distribution of blood volume or in glandular secretion, such as in response to unloading of baroreceptors or to alterations in environmental temperature.

3. Sympathoneural responses that adequately maintain homeostasis are usually not consciously experienced. When the organism perceives that the adjustments do not or will not meet the challenge, the situation reaches consciousness, and adrenomedullary and HPA activation ensue.

4. Stress responses that include AHS activation also often include HPA activation, as indicated by circulating levels of ACTH or glucocorticoids, and increased release of endogenous opioids, as indicated by plasma levels of β-endorphin.

5. Many other systems besides the SNS, AHS, and HPA systems participate in stress responses. The brain coordinates dynamically activities of these systems using homeostats to maintain the internal environment. The patterns of AHS and SNS responses, and

their associations with other stress systems, usually make teleological sense. Dynamic aspects are especially apparent in the effector patterns elicited by hemorrhage, depending on the absence or presence of hypotension, and by exercise, as vasodilator metabolites accumulate, fatigue develops, and the anaerobic threshold is passed.

6. Distress, whether induced by physiological or psychological changes, increases the likelihood of a "giving up" or "defeat" reaction, where sympathoneural activation switches suddenly to inhibition and parasympathetic inhibition switches suddenly to activation. Combined with increased adrenomedullary secretion of EPI, hypothalamopituitary secretion of AVP, and central neural release of endogenous opioids, these changes activate a hemodynamic positive feedback loop, precipitating hypotension, bradycardia, cerebral hypoperfusion, and loss of consciousness.

Whereas one can gauge the activities of most neuroendocrine homeostatic systems chemically by measuring circulating levels of various hormones, such as EPI, ACTH, and AVP, no generally accepted chemical method measures parasympathetic activity. This is because of the very rapid metabolic breakdown of acetylcholine, the parasympathetic neurotransmitter. (Recall from the chapter about stress that the detection of the "Vagusstoff" by Loewi required the use of a bioassay preparation.) Studies have instead often used indirect chemical measures of vagal activation, such as blood levels of pancreatic polypeptide, insulin, and gastrin. One may examine cardiac sinoatrial PNS activity from power spectral analysis of heart rate variability (Randall et al., 1991), as discussed in the chapter about clinical assessment of catecholaminergic function; however, no report has compared the biochemical indices of gut parasympathetic activity with this physiological index of cardiac parasympathetic activity. For several stress responses, the vagal contribution to the neuroendocrine patterns remains obscure.

Consistent with their coordinated participation in neuroendocrine patterns, stress effector systems interact via compensatory activation and effector sharing, principles introduced in Chapter 1. For instance, depletion of endogenous glucocorticoids compensatorily enhances responses of SNS outflow during stress, explaining why adrenalectomized monkeys (treated with mineralocorticoid replacement) have normal levels of NE at rest but have exaggerated NE responses during subsequent surgical stress (Udelsman et al., 1987a). Analogously, in rats, adrenalectomy increases basal plasma NE levels and augments NE responses to ether vapor inhalation (Brown and Fisher, 1986) and to immobilization (Kvetnansky, Fukuhara et al., 1993).

The AHS, SNS, AVP system, and RAS also interact compensatorily to maintain blood pressure, as discussed in the chapter about peripheral catecholaminergic systems. The compensatory activation of other vasoactive systems after SNS destruction helps to explain why many workers, including Cannon, concluded erroneously that the SNS acts only as an emergency system.

Stresses Associated with Adrenomedullary Activation

The lucid experiments by Cannon about the physiological effects of EPI (or adrenomedullary extracts) and about the importance of EPI in the maintenance of homeostasis during emergency situations remain pertinent today. Stressors that pose immediate threats to life or that compromise distribution of essential nutrients by the cardiovascular system to body tissues evoke marked increases in adrenomedullary secretion. In contrast, in these situations SNS traffic may increase markedly, change little, or even fall.

As discussed in the chapter about stress and science, hormonal rather than neuronal responses would counter most effectively stressors requiring many compensatory adjustments throughout the body, whereas in response to less global or intense stressors, sympathoneural elicitation of patterned redistributions of blood flow or of alterations in glandular activity would suffice without distracting the organism.

Hemorrhage

Throughout mammalian evolution, traumatic hemorrhage has posed a threat to survival. Cannon (1939a) emphasized the roles of the adrenal gland and sympathetic nerves in the coordinated responses to hemorrhage. Since he reported effects of hemorrhagic hypotension only, where by definition depletion of blood volume has overwhelmed homeostatic systems maintaining blood pressure, he did not recognize the possibility of differential hormonal and neuronal responses during less severe blood loss.

The blood volume depletion during hemorrhage unloads cardiac and arterial baroreceptors, eliciting reflexive stimulation of several interacting effector systems that tend to restore cardiac and arterial filling (Figure 6–1). Increased AVP secretion during hypotensive hemorrhage produces an antidiuresis and possibly vasoconstriction; and augmented RAS activity increases AII production and aldosterone secretion, also causing vasoconstriction and an anti-natriuresis.

The pattern of neuroendocrine responses to blood loss depends on whether SNS activation to redistribute blood flow maintains blood pressure. In conscious animals, two distinct phases of neuroendocrine responses occur during acute hypovolemia (Schadt and Ludbrook, 1991). Initially, unloading of cardiac baroreceptors reflexively increases peripheral resistance via increased SNS outflows and RAS activity. These responses compensate for the fall in stroke volume and cardiac output, maintaining blood pressure. A fall in blood volume beyond a critical amount—about 30%—ushers in a second phase, characterized by sympathoneural inhibition, markedly increased EPI and AVP levels, continuing RAS activation, and relative or absolute bradycardia.

This pattern during hypotensive hemorrhage resembles that during fainting reactions, described later in this chapter. Because EPI stimulates β-adrenoceptors on skeletal smooth muscle cells, the adrenomedullary activation decreases total peripheral resistance, and in the absence of reflexive SNS stimulation in the heart and other vascular beds, blood pressure falls, evoking further adrenomedullary stimulation. The homeostatic circuit therefore includes a positive feedback loop, an inherently unstable situation.

In humans, nonhypotensive blood loss increases plasma levels of NE but not of EPI, PRA, or AVP, whereas blood loss with hypotension increases levels of all four substances (Velasquez et al., 1987). These findings agree with the view of Schadt and Ludbrook (1991) about predominantly SNS activation during nonhypotensive hemor-

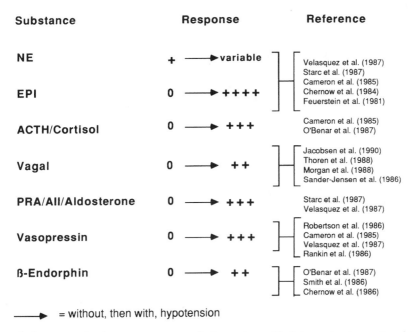

Substance	Response	Reference
NE	+ ⟶ variable	Velasquez et al. (1987) Starc et al. (1987) Cameron et al. (1985)
EPI	0 ⟶ ++++	Chernow et al. (1984) Feuerstein et al. (1981)
ACTH/Cortisol	0 ⟶ +++	Cameron et al. (1985) O'Benar et al. (1987)
Vagal	0 ⟶ ++	Jacobsen et al. (1990) Thoren et al. (1988) Morgan et al. (1988) Sander-Jensen et al. (1986)
PRA/AII/Aldosterone	0 ⟶ +++	Starc et al. (1987) Velasquez et al. (1987)
Vasopressin	0 ⟶ +++	Robertson et al. (1986) Cameron et al. (1985) Velasquez et al. (1987) Rankin et al. (1986)
ß-Endorphin	0 ⟶ ++	O'Benar et al. (1987) Smith et al. (1986) Chernow et al. (1986)

⟶ = without, then with, hypotension

Figure 6–1. Neuroendocrine response pattern in hemorrhage. Nonhypotensive hemorrhage elicits sympathoneural activation, which by redistributing blood volume counters the effects of the stressor. Hypotensive hemorrhage elicits adrenomedullary, pituitary–adrenocortical, and parasympathetic activation and increases secretion of vasopressin, whereas sympathoneural activity can increase, decrease, or remain unchanged. The organism experiences distress.

rhage and AHS activation during hypotensive hemorrhage but disagree about the effects of nonhypotensive hemorrhage on RAS activity.

Marked adrenomedullary activation in response to hypotensive hemorrhage contrasts with variable responses of plasma NE levels and renal sympathoneural activity. In rats, plasma concentrations of EPI, corticosterone, and ACTH increase markedly in this setting, with the responses related to the decreases in blood volume and mean arterial pressure, whereas plasma concentrations of NE can increase little (Graessler et al., 1989) or not at all (Brown et al., 1986). Adrenal nerve activity increases, and renal nerve activity falls (Togashi et al., 1990; Victor et al., 1989). In pigs, hemorrhage increases plasma levels of ACTH, β-endorphin, EPI, NE, and pancreatic polypeptide, with only marginal increases in AVP levels (Jacobsen et al., 1990; O'Benar et al., 1987). In conscious rabbits, hemorrhagic hypotension decreases renal sympathetic nerve activity (Morita et al., 1988). In anesthetized dogs, hemorrhagic hypotension evokes marked increases in aortic plasma levels of all the catecholamines, with especially prominent increases in EPI levels (Briand et al., 1989) and with decreased renal sympathetic nerve activity (Morita and Vatner, 1985a). In sheep, hemorrhage increases levels of β-endorphin, PRA, and EPI (R. Smith et al., 1986; Starc and Stalcup, 1987). In ketamine-anesthetized, fasting baboons, hypotensive hemorrhage evokes small increases in venous plasma NE levels but large increases in EPI levels (Chernow et al., 1984).

In dogs, temporary, bilateral, functional adrenalectomies produced by diversion of the adrenal venous effluents abolishes hemorrhage-induced increases in aortic catecholamine concentrations and augments increases in hepatic venous NE concentrations (Briand et al., 1989)—an example of compensatory activation. The combination of hepatic denervation and bilateral functional adrenalectomies abolishes the increases in hepatic venous and aortic catecholamine concentrations during hemorrhage and attenuates the hyperglycemic response by about 50%. These findings indicate that arterial catecholamine responses during hemorrhagic hypotension depend mainly on AHS activation, whereas the hyperglycemia depends on both adrenomedullary secretion and increased hepatic SNS activity.

General anesthesia blunts hemorrhage-induced increases in plasma catecholamine levels (Mayer et al., 1990). Because of the altered responsiveness to hemorrhage during general anesthesia, the neuroendocrine findings in many studies over the course of half a century—from Cannon (1939), to Briand et al., (1989)—about regulation of sympathoneural function during hemorrhage may not apply to conscious individuals.

The pattern of neuroendocrine responses to hemorrhage also depends on previous exposure to stressors. Prior hemorrhage augments ACTH responses to subsequent hemorrhage (Thrivikraman and Plotsky, 1993), whereas prior immobilization augments plasma EPI responses and attenuates ACTH responses to hemorrhage (Graessler et al., 1989). Markedly increased corticosterone levels during immobilization may feedback-inhibit central neural mechanisms determining acute changes in HPA outflow; however, exogenously administered corticosterone does not attenuate ACTH responses to hemorrhage in rats (Thrivikraman and Plotsky, 1993). Whether previous exposure to other stressors augments β-endorphin or AVP responses to hemorrhage is unknown. The occurrence of such augmentation, combined with the exaggerated adrenomedullary response, could increase the likelihood of the above-described positive feedback loop and precipitation of cardiovascular collapse.

Renal sympathoneural activity decreases during hypotensive hemorrhage in dogs (Morita and Vatner, 1985a, 1985b), rats (Togashi et al., 1990; Victor et al., 1989), and rabbits (Morita et al., 1988). The sympathoinhibition depends on cardiac vagal afferents (Gupta et al., 1987; Skoog et al., 1985; Thoren et al., 1988; Victor et al., 1989). Several mechanisms may explain the vagally mediated sympathoinhibition attending hypotensive hemorrhage. Vagal afferent activity appears to determine the large increments in circulating AVP levels in the second phase, and AVP inhibits renal nerve traffic both directly and via augmented baroreflex inhibitory control of renal nerve activity (Abboud et al., 1986; Imaizumi and Thames, 1986). Plasma β-endorphin levels also increase during hypotensive hemorrhage, and vagal afferent stimulation may inhibit renal sympathoneural outflow by a mechanism involving release of endogenous opioids (Morita et al., 1988). Others have proposed a mechanism involving serotonin (Morgan et al., 1988).

The renal sympathoinhibition in hemorrhagic hypotension contrasts with the progressive renal sympathetic stimulation in hypotension evoked by infusion of the vasodilator sodium nitroprusside (Deka-Starosta et al., 1989; Noshiro et al., 1991), indicating that the sympathoinhibition does not result from hypotension itself.

Hemorrhage-induced decreases in cardiac filling and acute increases in cardiac filling (Karim et al., 1972) both can reflexively inhibit renal sympathetic outflow. One resolution for this seeming paradox is that in different settings, the brain interprets the same afferent information differently, producing different or even opposite neuroendocrine and cardiovascular patterns. The sections about fainting in this chapter and about syncope in the chapter about cardiovascular diseases elaborate on this theme.

Because of the effects of EPI on platelet aggregability, and the tremendous increases in circulating EPI levels produced by exsanguination, decapitation to obtain blood samples can confound studies about platelet activation, as discussed in the chapter about peripheral catecholaminergic systems.

Hypoglycemia

Hypoglycemia poses a metabolic threat to all cells. In contrast with mild hemorrhage, where regionally selective increases in SNS activity to redistribute blood volume can effectively counter minor challenges to cardiovascular homeostasis, even mild hypoglycemia necessitates global—that is, hormonal—responses to counter the challenge to metabolic homeostasis. Thus, decreases in blood glucose levels too small for the individual to notice increase circulating EPI levels, with little if any concurrent SNS activation as indicated by circulating NE levels (Schwartz et al., 1987).

The selective adrenomedullary activation during hypoglycemia constitutes key evidence for the differential regulation of SNS and AHS outflows during exposure to different stressors. Ironically, it was Cannon who first demonstrated that hypoglycemia evokes adrenomedullary activation (Cannon, McIver et al., 1924). The denervated heart preparation Cannon used did not allow assessment of the effects of hypoglycemia on regional sympathoneural activity.

A central neural ''glucostat'' determines the neuroendocrine response to glucoprivation (Keller-Wood et al., 1983). Thus, intracarotid injection of glucose attenuates and ganglion blockade or spinal transection abolishes the adrenomedullary response to hypoglycemia (Goldfien, 1966; Keller-Wood et al., 1983). In contrast, responses of circulating glucagon levels during hypoglycemia do not appear to depend on central nervous connections.

Although lower brainstem centers can initiate AHS responses to hypoglycemia, the hypothalamus normally plays a critical role. Stimulation of the lateral hypothalamic area increases directly recorded adrenal nerve activity, as does icv administration of 2-deoxyglucose, which causes cellular glucoprivation. Lateral hypothalamic lesions virtually abolish the stimulatory effect of 2-deoxyglucose on adrenal nerve activity (Yoshimatsu et al., 1987), implying that the pathway by which the central nervous system senses glucoprivation and produces adrenomedullary activation includes this region. The remainder of the central neural pathways and neurotransmitters determining the drastic increases in AHS outflow during hypoglycemia are unknown.

Hypoglycemia elicits hunger, as indicated by insulin-induced eating behavior in rats (Panksepp et al., 1975). Injection of NE into the medial hypothalamus stimulates both insulin release and eating behavior (DeJong et al., 1977). The central neuronal circuitry responsible for the elicitation of hunger and eating by hypoglycemia is largely unknown. Parasympathetic stimulation to the gut appears to constitute the common final pathway for this response, since insulin-induced (Corrall and Frier, 1981; Koizumi et al., 1990; Lvgren et al., 1981) or 2-deoxyglucose-induced (Hosotani et al., 1989; Koizumi et al., 1990) glucoprivation increases circulating levels of pancreatic polypeptide. The vagal activation would then stimulate gastric production of acid and pepsin and increase intestinal motility. One may speculate that the PVN participates in hypoglycemia-induced hunger, via projections from parvocellular to vagal preganglionic neurons (Swanson, 1987).

Brown et al. (1986) reported that icv administration of a CRH antagonist attenuated responses of plasma EPI levels during insulin-induced hypoglycemia in rats, suggesting a role of central CRH release in both the HPA and AHS responses to hypoglycemia; however, Goldstein, Garty et al. (1993) failed to replicate this finding.

Hypoglycemia depletes adrenomedullary EPI selectively. The adrenomedullary EPI content decreases by about 70% three hours after insulin injection into fasted Sprague–Dawley rats, whereas the NE content remains unchanged (Vollmer et al., 1992). Electrical stimulation of particular hypothalamic sites in cats can also evoke differential release of EPI and NE (Folkow and von Euler, 1954), and vasoactive intestinal peptide (VIP), a putative adrenomedullary neurotransmitter, increases the EPI/NE concentration ratio in an isolated adrenal perfusion system (Wakade et al., 1991). Whether hypoglycemia evokes VIP release in the adrenal gland is unknown.

Glucose is so important in the body economy, and so many situations alter glucose utilization, a large number of neuroendocrine systems regulate levels of this vital fuel and react rapidly to glucoprivation. AHS activation during hypoglycemia is only part of a constellation of glucose counterregulatory adjustments (Delitala et al., 1987; Garber et al., 1976), with insulin dissipation and glucagon secretion predominating (Cryer, 1993). Glucagon deficiency increases dependence on EPI for glucose counterregulation, illustrating the principle of compensatory activation, and glucagon itself rapidly increases plasma EPI levels (Grossman, Goldstein et al., 1991), illustrating direct interactions among stress effector systems. Other hormones, such as growth hormone, cortisol, β-endorphin, AVP, renin, and prolactin (Baylis and Heath, 1977; Delitala et al., 1987; Evans et al., 1986; Higaki et al., 1984; Petraglia et al., 1986; Radosevich et al., 1988; Seckl et al., 1988; Watabe et al., 1987) play minor or as yet unknown roles (Figure 6–2).

Acute glucoprivation elicits only small and variable increases in sympathoneural activity. In humans, insulin (Anderson et al., 1991; Berne et al., 1992; Frandsen et al., 1989) or 2-deoxyglucose (Fagius and Berne, 1989) increases skeletal muscle sympathoneural activity (SMSA); however, whether these effects result from central neural glucoprivation or from reflexive sympathetic responses to systemic vasodilation and splanchnic sequestration of blood is unclear. Plasma NE levels generally increase only slightly after administration of insulin (e.g., Garber et al., 1976; Schwartz et al., 1987) or 2-deoxyglucose (Goldstein, Breier et al., 1993). The NE responses result from increased NE spillover, not from decreased NE clearance (Hilsted et al., 1985b). In

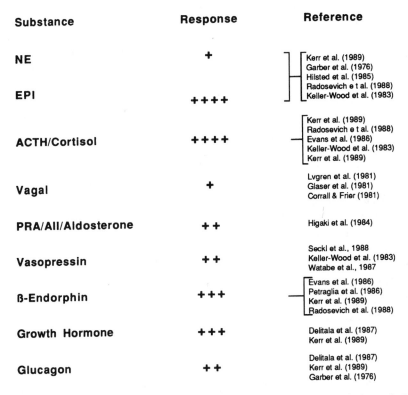

Substance	Response	Reference
NE	+	Kerr et al. (1989) Garber et al. (1976) Hilsted et al. (1985) Radosevich e t al. (1988) Keller-Wood et al. (1983)
EPI	+ + + +	
ACTH/Cortisol	+ + + +	Kerr et al. (1989) Radosevich e t al. (1988) Evans et al. (1986) Keller-Wood et al. (1983) Kerr et al. (1989)
Vagal	+	Lvgren et al. (1981) Glaser et al. (1981) Corrall & Frier (1981)
PRA/AII/Aldosterone	+ +	Higaki et al. (1984)
Vasopressin	+ +	Seckl et al., 1988 Keller-Wood et al. (1983) Watabe et al., 1987
ß-Endorphin	+ + +	Evans et al. (1986) Petraglia et al. (1986) Kerr et al. (1989) Radosevich et al. (1988)
Growth Hormone	+ + +	Delitala et al. (1987) Kerr et al. (1989)
Glucagon	+ +	Delitala et al. (1987) Kerr et al. (1989) Garber et al. (1976)

Figure 6–2. Neuroendocrine pattern in hypoglycemia. Even mild hypoglycemia elicits marked adrenomedullary and pituitary–adrenocortical activation, which contrasts with small and variable sympathoneural responses.

adrenalectomized patients, insulin-induced hypoglycemia fails to increase plasma NE concentrations (Shah et al., 1984), and studies using insulin clamp procedures, enabling assessments of effects of hyperinsulinemia independent of hypoglycemia, have disagreed about whether hyperinsulinemia of a magnitude seen in insulin-resistant humans affects plasma NE levels (Mitrakou et al., 1992; Rooney et al., 1991). During glucopenia induced by 2-deoxyglucose in healthy volunteers, plasma DHPG levels decrease rather than increase, and profound stimulation of adrenomedullary secretion, indicated by marked increases in plasma EPI levels, can account completely for the increases in plasma NE levels (Goldstein, Breier et al., 1992).

In rabbits after 2-deoxyglucose administration (Eisenhofer, Cox et al., 1990) or in rats after insulin administration (Goldstein, Garty et al., 1993), severe glucopenia increases plasma DHPG levels. In rabbits, desipramine treatment prevents the DHPG response, indicating that the response depends on augmented neuronal release and reuptake of NE. In conscious rats and rabbits, 2-deoxyglucose differentially increases adrenal nerve activity, with small or absent increases in renal nerve activity (Medvedev et al., 1988; Nijima, 1975). Tissue NE turnover remains unchanged or even decreases

(Rappaport et al., 1982; Young and Landsberg, 1979); however, as noted in the chapter about assessment of catecholaminergic function, one may question whether tissue NE turnover validly indicates sympathetic nerve traffic. In anesthetized dogs with diversion of the adrenal venous outflows, aortic NE concentrations do not increase during insulin-induced hypoglycemia (Yamaguchi et al., 1989), implying that in this preparation, increases in plasma NE levels during glucoprivic stress result exclusively from increased adrenal secretion. Severe hypoglycemia in dogs does increase pancreatic NE spillover (Havel et al., 1992). No report to date has examined comprehensively responses of regional NE spillover during hypoglycemia. In WKY rats, hyperinsulinemia increases lumbar but not renal or adrenal sympathetic nerve traffic (Morgan et al., 1993).

Neuroendocrine responses to glucoprivation, arteriolar vasodilation, and decreased cardiac filling therefore differ substantially. Mild hypoglycemia selectively stimulates AHS ouflow, but mild blood loss or vasodilation do not; severe hypoglycemia and hemorrhagic hypotension profoundly stimulate AHS outflow, with relatively small increases or with decreases in renal SNS outflow; whereas even severe vasodilator-induced hypotension evokes reflexive renal SNS stimulation (Deka-Starosta et al., 1989). Alterations in the activity of different homeostats that use the SNS and AHS effectors can explain these differences.

Asphyxiation

Asphyxiation produces the biochemical triad of hypoxemia, hypercarbia, and acute respiratory acidosis. Most research on this topic has been based on animals during general anesthesia, inadvertent asphyxiation in infants, or apneic episodes in patients with sleep-apnea syndrome. In all these settings, other factors probably influence the results.

Asphyxiation always drastically stimulates adrenomedullary secretion. Anoxia of the denervated adrenal medulla promptly releases catecholamines (Zwemer and Newton, 1928, cited in Hillarp, 1958), suggesting that adrenomedullary activation during asphyxiation occurs even without increased nerve traffic.

Which of these three stimuli actually induces the AHS response remains unclear. Hypoxia alone produces only small increases in plasma levels of catecholamines and SMSA (Leuenberger et al., 1991; Rowell, 1986; Rowell and Seals, 1990; Somers et al., 1989a, 1989b). Reflexive ventilatory stimulation probably restrains the sympathoneural response (Somers et al., 1989b), and increased NE clearance attenuates the plasma NE response (Leuenberger et al., 1991). Hypoxia does exaggerate plasma catecholamine responses to exercise (Favier et al., 1985; Rowell, 1986) and augments SMSA and plasma NE responses during application of lower-body negative pressure (LBNP; Rowell and Seals, 1990).

Hypercarbia in the presence of normal or even increased blood oxygen tension also increases directly recorded SMSA (Somers et al., 1989a, 1989b), and the increases in sympathetic activity during hyperoxic hypercapnia exceed those during isocapnic hypoxia. Acute hypoxemia and acute hypercarbic acidosis act synergistically to increase plasma levels of NE and EPI (Rose et al., 1983) and to increase directly recorded SMSA (Somers et al., 1989a, 1989b).

In healthy volunteers, mild acetazolamide-induced acidosis does not affect baseline plasma levels of catecholamines but does augment plasma catecholamine responses during bicycle ergometer exercise (Goldsmith et al., 1990). In anesthetized, artificially ventilated rats, infusion of catecholamines decreases arterial pH, possibly due to an imbalance between increased metabolism and unchanged exhalation of metabolic by-products; conversely, acidosis induced by infusion of hydrochloric acid attenuates cardiac and blood pressure responses to catecholamines (Atkinson et al., 1972).

Thus, each of the three biochemical facets of asphyxiation acts synergistically with the others to stimulate SNS and AHS outflows.

Because of the independent research interests among different groups of investigators, interrelated neurocirculatory and neurorespiratory functions have received scant research attention (Millhorn et al., 1990). The rostral ventrolateral medulla (RVLM) contains not only neurons that participate importantly in baroreflex circulatory regulation but also neurons that discharge during the inspiratory or expiratory phases of respiration (Pilowsky et al., 1990). The carotid sinus nerve carries not only baroreceptor but also chemoreceptor information to the brainstem, producing reflexive changes in SNS outflow. The vascular chemoreceptors, located especially in the carotid bodies adjacent to the carotid sinuses, respond to decreased arterial oxygen concentrations, increased arterial carbon dioxide concentrations, and decreased arterial blood pH; and chemosensitive cells near the ventral surface of the medulla respond to the same stimuli. Increased baroreceptor afferent stimulation inhibits not only circulatory parameters but also respiration, and chemoreceptor afferent stimulation augments not only respiration but also circulatory parameters.

Circulatory Collapse and Shock

Cardiac arrest profoundly and diffusely stimulates SNS and AHS outflows, as indicated by drastically increased plasma levels of NE and EPI in humans (Little et al., 1985; Wortsman et al., 1984, 1990) and in laboratory animals (Foley et al., 1987; Kern et al., 1989; Lathers et al., 1989). Cardiovascular collapse also markedly increases plasma levels of ACTH and AVP (Foley et al., 1987; Kaszaki et al., 1989).

In dogs, bilateral adrenalectomy decreases by about 70% the response of plasma NE levels during cardiac arrest, compared with values in sham-operated control dogs (Foley et al., 1987). This finding indicates that the plasma NE response arises mainly from adrenomedullary stimulation.

As discussed in the chapter about cardiovascular disorders, myocardial infarction increases plasma levels of EPI and NE, especially in patients with infarction-related ventricular fibrillation (Bertel et al., 1982a). The increases in plasma catecholamine levels correlate positively with both the extent of the infarction and with the 18-month prognosis (Karlsberg et al., 1981).

Not only circulatory but also endotoxic (Gullichsen et al., 1990; Murray et al., 1989) or anaphylactic (van der Linden et al., 1993) shock markedly increases plasma catecholamine levels. Anaphylactic shock in humans is associated with larger proportionate increments in plasma EPI than NE levels.

Pain

The experience of acute pain evokes adrenomedullary activation. Thus, in patients with suspected acute myocardial infarction, plasma EPI levels are higher in patients with chest pain than in patients without chest pain, and EPI levels are related more closely with the extent of pain than with the presence of myocardial infarction (Husebye et al., 1990). Undergoing extraction of third molars elicits about a three-fold increase in plasma EPI levels (Dionne et al., 1984; Goldstein et al., 1982). In calves, branding with a hot iron evokes larger plasma EPI responses than does sham branding or branding with a frozen iron (Lay et al., 1992).

Since pain is a subjective state, pain constitutes more than nociception, which is a neurophysiologic term referring to mechanisms of detection of noxious stimuli. In everyday situations the experience of pain draws the individual's attention to the noxious stimulus and to its bodily effects; this obviously enhances the individual's well-being and survival. In some emergency situations, however, the distraction caused by pain can more threaten than enhance survival. Strong selective pressures must have favored the evolution of systems complexly affecting the transduction of noxious stimuli by nerve endings, afferent transmission in ascending pathways in the spinal cord, and cerebrocortical interpretation of pain signals. As discussed in the chapter about central functional neuroanatomy, one such system appears to be a noradrenergic system from the LC to cells in the dorsal horn of the spinal cord. Exposure to a painful stressor evokes both adrenomedullary secretion and analgesia, consistent with concurrent activation of several pathways including the LC. Thus, for instance, during the invasion of Anzio in World War II, the majority of severely wounded soldiers denied experiencing pain and refused treatment with pain medication (Beecher, 1946).

Cardiac nociception probably involves sympathoneural and vagal afferents. Cell bodies of the sympathoneural afferents lie in the middle cervical or stellate ganglia or in the dorsal root ganglia; the afferents enter the lower cervical and upper thoracic spinal cord and terminate in dorsal horn laminae I, II, and V, synapsing on spinothalamic tract cells (Meller and Gebhart, 1992). Vagus-associated afferents transmit cardiac nociceptive information to the NTS via the aortic depressor nerve, recurrent laryngeal nerve, or vagus nerve itself, through the nodose ganglion. Thus, excision of the lower cervical and upper thoracic sympathetic ganglia can ameliorate angina pectoris. Bradykinin, serotonin, and adenosine are considered the most likely chemical mediators of cardiac pain. Local administration of bradykinin produces behavioral signs of pain and activates sympathetic afferents in laboratory animals (Felder and Thames, 1982); and serotonin and adenosine evoke chest pain when either drug is injected intravenously into humans (Hollander et al., 1957; Sylven, 1989).

Whether chronic pain stimulates adrenomedullary secretion has been unclear. Patients with functional chronic abdominal pain have if anything decreased plasma EPI levels (Jorgensen et al., 1986). In patients with neuromas, injection of EPI near the tumor evokes burning-type pain (Chabal et al., 1992), consistent with altered numbers or functions of α-adrenoceptors on nociceptor afferents (Schwartzmann, 1992). Analogously, patients with chronic limb pain due to reflex sympathetic dystrophy have evidence of α-adrenoceptor up-regulation (Arnold et al., 1993), as discussed in the chapter about cardiovascular diseases.

Emotional Distress

Difficulties in defining, measuring, and controlling the relevant independent and dependent variables in humans have impeded research about the clinical neuroendocrine and cardiovascular consequences of emotional distress—especially in those cardiovascular conditions where this information would most likely be useful. Many of the assertions presented below are highly speculative and should be viewed as attempting to provide a conceptual framework rather than summarizing an accepted body of knowledge.

Writers throughout history have associated emotions with acute cardiovascular signs, recognizing that these signs convey unerringly emotional states that verbalization cannot mask.

The Old Testament views the heart as the source of emotion: ''And he hardened Pharaoh's heart (Exodus 7:13)''; ''I caused the widow's heart to sing for joy (Job 29: 13)'' ''Let no man's heart fail because of him [Goliath] (I Samuel 17:32)''; ''My heart was hot within me; while I was musing the fire burned (Psalm 39:3)'' ''Can a man take fire in his bosom, and his clothes not be burned? (Proverbs 6:27)''; ''Hope deferred makes the heart sick (Proverbs 12:10)''; ''A merry heart makes a cheerful countenance (Proverbs 15:13).'' ''A merry heart does good like a medicine (Proverbs 17:22).''

One of the most poignant biblical stories relates Jacob's reaction to the news that his beloved son Joseph, whom he had mourned for years as dead, was not only alive but a virtual prince in Egypt:

> And they told him, saying: ''Joseph is yet alive, and he is ruler over all the land of Egypt.'' And his heart fainted, for he believed them not. And they told him all the words of Joseph, which he had said unto them; and when he saw the wagons which Joseph had sent to carry him, the spirit of Jacob their father revived. And Israel said: ''It is enough; Joseph my son is yet alive; I will go and see him before I die.'' (Genesis 45:26–28)

Jacob did not suffer a cardiac arrest or lose consciousness, and he was not resuscitated physically; rather, his initial reaction was doubt and numbness, and his uplift was spiritual. The narrative used the heart to depict the Jacob's deeply felt emotions.

William Harvey, the father of scientific medicine, recognized the link between the central nervous system, emotions, and the heart in his *De Motu Cordis*. Harvey viewed the heart not as the seat of the emotions but as a target for their expression: ''Every affection of the mind that is attended with either pain or pleasure, hope or fear, is the cause of an agitation whose influence extends to the heart'' (Harvey, 1628, cited in Eliot and Buell, 1985, p. 125).

Charles Darwin also recognized this principle when he related an anecdote about

Louis XVI, who, confronted by a murderous mob, reportedly sneered, "Am I afraid? Feel my pulse" (Darwin, 1965, p. 238).

Walter Cannon wrote that anticipatory activation of the sympathoadrenal system during "fight-or-flight" emergencies afforded survival advantages and therefore evolved (Cannon, 1945, 1929a). Physiological response patterns during emotional distress always include changes in cardiovascular function. Cannon explained the survival value of pressor responses in pain and strong emotion:

> [A] higher pressure might be required when more muscles are involved in activity, for a more widely spread dilation might then reduce the pressure to the point at which there would be insufficient circulation in active organs. Furthermore, with many muscles active, the amount of waste would be greatly augmented, and the need for abundant blood supply would thereby to a like degree be increased. For both reasons a rise of general arterial pressure would prove advantageous. The high pressure developed in excitement and pain, therefore, might be specially serviceable in the muscular activities which are likely to accompany excitement and pain. (Cannon, 1929a, p. 104)

Increased SNS vasoconstrictor and cardiac outflows usually underly the pressor response. For instance, in baboons undergoing conflict-type stress, increases in urinary NE excretion correlate positively with increases in systolic blood pressure (Turkkan, 1991), and in humans undergoing a laboratory mental stressor, increases in spillover of NE into arterial plasma correlate positively with increases in blood pressure and cardiac output (Goldstein, Eisenhofer et al., 1987). Nevertheless, as discussed below, emotional distress can also evoke vasodepressor reactions, when adrenomedullary and vagal activation coincide with sympathoinhibition.

Folkow (1982) has suggested that the physiological response pattern to psychological stress in humans resembles the "defense reaction" in animals. The hemodynamic pattern includes renal, gastrointestinal, and cutaneous vasoconstriction, skeletal muscle vasodilation, tachycardia, and predominantly systolic hypertension. Herd (1991) similarly has supported the notion of a unitary cardiovascular stress response pattern, with increased cardiac rate and contractility, skeletal muscle vasodilation, venoconstriction, and renal, splanchnic, and cutaneous vasoconstriction. Although one may surmise that sympathetic noradrenergic inhibition underlies the skeletal muscle vasodilation of the defense reaction, microneurographic evidence has indicated if anything increased SMSA, especially in the legs, during exposure to laboratory psychological stressors in humans (Anderson et al., 1987; Hjemdahl et al., 1989). One may speculate that a combination of increased circulating EPI levels, accumulation of vasodilator metabolites, and cholinergic vasodilation determines the skeletal vasodilation attending the defense reaction.

In contrast with the views of Folkow (1987, 1988) and Herd (1991), who have argued that the organism evinces a defense reaction during even slight alerting or mental engagement, with psychological stress and distress differing only in intensity, the present discussion distinguishes between simple problem-solving or mental challenge and emotional distress. Evidence presented below suggests that emotional distress evokes predominantly AHS activation, whereas performance of attention-requiring but non-distressing tasks elicits predominantly SNS activation. Just as no unitary neurocirculatory or neuroendocrine response pattern occurs during different forms of physiological stress, such as hemorrhagic hypotension and hypoglycemia, no unitary neurocirculatory or neuroendocrine response pattern may occur during different forms of emotional distress. In particular, the following discussion develops the theme that the neurocirculatory and neuroendocrine patterns during "fight" differ from those during "flight" and from those during "defeat," although all three contain an element of distress.

The abundance of laboratory stressors that elicit anxiety compared with other emotional experiences such as anger may help to explain the failure to recognize this differentiation in clinical studies. Because of the lack of relevant information from studies of humans and laboratory animals, the following discussion introduces several ideas with scanty experimental support.

For several dimensions of psychological stressors, available evidence provides support for patterning of neuroendocrine or neurocirculatory responses. These dimensions, which overlap, include aggression vs. fear; activity vs. passivity; novelty vs. habituation; perceived ability to cope vs. perceived inability to cope; perceived control or dominance vs. perceived lack of control or submissiveness; low vs. high intensity; and positive vs. negative emotions.

Aggression (Anger/Rage/Frenzy) vs. Fear (Anxiety/Terror/Panic)

Cannon (1914b, 1929a), Selye (1956), Folkow (1982), and Herd (1991) all theorized that "fight-or-flight" situations elicit essentially the same autonomic changes. Observations dating back at least to the time of Darwin, however, disagree with this conceptualization.

Terror does share several features with rage, including tremor, hyperventilation, tachycardia, diaphoresis, and piloerection. Despite these similarities, behaviors obviously distinguish fear and aggression, and the behavioral differences require appropriate neuroendocrine and circulatory support. From the concepts introduced in Chapter 1, one may hypothesize that the behaviors, neuroendocrine changes, and circulatory adjustments probably evolved together.

Darwin recognized all the main signs distinguishing extreme fear (terror) from extreme anger (rage). Writers and playwrights since antiquity have recognized and exploited these signs. The following discussion considers four such differences: the state of effective skeletal muscular tension (trembling and weakness vs. concerted tonic contraction); skin color (pallor vs. flushing); defecation; and salivation. All these differences depend on differences in autonomic effector patterns, and the autonomic effector patterns in turn depend to at least some extent on differential SNS and AHS activation (Table 6–1).

Writers about the psychology of emotion have not considered these distinctions. In neither Buck's *Human Motivation and Emotion* (1988) nor Lazarus's *Emotion and Adaptation* (1991) do the indices list trembling, pallor, defecation, or salivation.

The trembling associated with fear represents a peculiar form of ineffective skeletal muscle contraction, contrasting with the more obviously purposeful, concerted, and yet

Table 6–1. Neuroendocrine and Physiological Factors Distinguishing Fear from Anger.

	Anger	Fear
Skeletal muscle	Locomotion, clenching, erect posture	Immobility, prominent trembling
Skin	Flushing	Pallor
Gastrointestinal		Defecation, "butterflies"
Salivation	Increased	Decreased
Δ Catecholamine levels	Δ NE > Δ EPI	Δ EPI > Δ NE
Defeat reaction	Unlikely	Likely

Note: Although extreme fear (terror) and extreme anger (rage) share several characteristics, such as sweating, piloerection, shaking, and increased metabolic activity, they also differ in some ways. In fear, skeletal muscle contraction seems disorganized and ineffectual; cutaneous vasoconstriction produces pallor; gastrointestinal motility increases, possibly due to concurrent vagal parasympathetic activation; salivary glandular secretion decreases; plasma epinephrine levels increase more than plasma norepinephrine levels; and there is an increased tendency to evince a "giving up" or "defeat" reaction, characterized by sudden sympathoinhibition, high circulating levels of epinephrine, vasopressin, and β-endorphin, and vagal bradycardia, resulting in a neurocirculatory positive feedback loop leading to hypotension and loss of consciousness.

largely involuntary skeletal muscle contraction that produces the clenched fists, grimacing, and upright or advancing posture associated with anger. Of course, humans shake during either terror or rage. Thus, the words "agitate," "quiver," and "quake" imply both shaking and a state of emotional upset, without necessarily indicating fear or anger. One may speculate that trembling has provided an evolutionary advantage as a form of skeletal muscle "idling" prior "flight-or-flight" behavior. Trembling also communicates extreme emotional intensity.

In the absence of signs of purposeful skeletal muscle contraction, and in the presence of other signs discussed below, trembling probably mainly indicates intense fear, explaining the most common use of trembling by classical writers:

And among these nations shalt thou have no repose, and there shall be no rest for the sole of thy foot; but the Lord shall give thee there a trembling heart, and failing of eyes, and languishing of soul. And thy life shall hang in doubt before thee; and thou shalt fear night and day, and shalt have no assurance of thy life. (*Deuteronomy* 28:65–66)

Then the king's countenance was changed, and his thoughts troubled him, so that the joints of his loins were loosed, and his knees smote one against another. . . . (*Daniel* 5:26)

I shudder at the word. (Virgil, *The Aeneid* II, 204)

Right as an aspes leef she gan to quake. (Chaucer, *Troilus and Criseyde* III, 656)

Less than a drop of blood remains in me that does not tremble; I recognize the signals of the ancient flame. (Dante, *Purgatorio* XXX, 46)

How all the other passions fleet to air,
As doubtful thoughts, and rash-embrac'd despair
And suddering fear, and green-ey'd jealousy.
(Shakespeare, *The Merchant of Venice,* III, ii 100)

Distilled
Almost to jelly with the act of fear. (Shakespeare, *Hamlet* I, ii, 204)

What man dare, I dare:
Approach thou like the rugged Russian bear,
The arm'd rhinoceros, or the Hyrcan tiger,
Take any shape but that, and my firm nerves
Shall never tremble. (Shakespeare, *Macbeth* III, iv, 99)

Darwin associated terror with muscular weakness, in contrast with the association between rage and contraction of skeletal muscle:

We may . . . infer that fear was expressed from an extremely remote period, in almost the same manner as it now is by man; namely, by trembling, the erection of the hair, cold perspiration, pallor, widely opened eyes, the relaxation of most of the muscles, and by the whole body cowering downwards or held motionless. . . .

Rage will have been expressed at a very early period by threatening or frantic gestures, by the reddening of the skin, and by glaring eyes, but not by frowning . . . (Darwin, 1965, pp. 360–361)

The excited brain gives strength to the muscles, and at the same time energy to the will. The body is commonly held erect ready for instant action, but sometimes it is bent forward towards the offending person, with the limbs more or less rigid. The mouth is generally closed with firmness, showing fixed determination, and the teeth are clenched or ground together. Such gestures as the raising of the arms, with the fists clenched, as if to strike the offender, are common. Few men in a great passion, and telling some one to begone, can resist acting as if they intended to strike or push the man violently away. (Darwin, 1965, p. 239)

Both injected EPI (Cameron et al., 1990) and endogenously released NE (Grossman, Rea et al., 1991) elicit trembling in humans.

The state of contraction of cutaneous vascular smooth muscle—that is, pale or red skin color—also differentiates terror from rage. In many animal species, including humans, the color red signals aggressive feeling and intent (Lorenz, 1952, 1963).

Human cultural evolution has extended the meanings of the colors red and white. When enraged, we "see red" and our "blood boils," whereas when we surrender we wave a white flag. The English adjectives "pale," "wan," and "pallid," denote not only whiteness but feebleness or weakness, whereas "sanguine" denotes not only bloodiness but confidence, and "ruddy" denotes not only redness but vigor.

The Queen turned crimson with fury, and after glaring at her for a moment like a wild beast, began screaming, "Off with her head!" (Carroll, *Alice in Wonderland,* Chapter 8)

We "seethe" with anger but "freeze" and turn "pale as a ghost" with fright.

These associations are not peculiar to English. For instance, in the Old Testament (Genesis 25:24), Esau was born ruddy, and commentators have interpreted Esau's ruddiness as a premonition of his love for hunting and therefore bloodshed (Hertz, 1985). His father Isaac predicted that Esau would live "by the sword" (Genesis 27:40).

These considerations help to explain why the expression of fear in humans decreases skin temperature, whereas expression of anger increases skin temperature (Ekman et al., 1983). In the study of Ekman et al. (1983), professional actors produced "facial prototypes" of different emotions and relived past emotional experiences; the results incidentally demonstrate that people can learn to evince autonomic changes that would not be expected to be under direct voluntary control.

During rage reactions, cholinergic stimulation may contribute to the flushing, whereas during fear, cholinergic inhibition combined with SNS and AHS stimulation may contribute to the pallor (Arnold, 1967). In cats, increases in blood flow in the trained limb accompany aversive, classically conditioned leg flexion, and methylatropine blocks the responses, whereas blood flow decreases in the untrained limb (Ellison and Zanchetti, 1971). Cholinergic dilation may therefore partly explain the association between increased skeletal muscle blood flow and movement during agonistic behavior, and the absence of such dilation may partly explain the association between skeletal muscle vasoconstriction and immobile expectation, as during fear without flight (Mancia et al., 1972).

The state of contraction of gastrointestinal smooth muscle constitutes a third physiological basis for distinguishing terror from rage.

The Old Testament contains only one example of "trial by ordeal" (Numbers 5:27–28), to test a woman accused of adultery. Failure to digest a type of potion, the "water of bitterness," would produce abdominal distention, indicating guilt. Since adrenomedullary activation and cholinergic inhibition during intense fear can cause a form of ileus, the biblical test may have had a rational basis.

The 23d Psalm includes: "He sets a table for me in the presence of my enemies," which may refer to fear interfering with digestion, since the ability to eat in the presence of one's enemies would require a sense of calm confidence. Shakespeare similarly recognized the effects of emotional distress on the gastrointestinal system when he wrote, "Unquiet meals make ill digestions" (*The Comedy of Errors,* V, i, 73).

In the film, *Shoah,* Franz Suchomel, the former SS Unterscharfuhrer at the Treblinka death camp, recalls with sardonic detachedness the "death panic" of Jews in the tunnel to the gas chambers:

> In the "funnel" the women had to wait. They heard the motors of the gas chambers. Maybe they also heard people screaming and imploring. As they waited, "death panic" overwhelmed them. "Death panic" makes people let go. They empty themselves, from the front or the rear. So often, where the women stood, there were five or six rows of excrement. . . .
>
> When this "death panic sets in, one lets go. It's well known that when someone's terrified, and knows he's about to die. . . ." (Lanzmann, 1985, p. 118)

The above biblical quotation about King Belshazzar's reaction to the handwriting on the wall—"the joints of his loins were loosed"—may refer to the same sort of gastrointestinal "letting go" evoked by terror. Whether adrenomedullary activation plays a role in the defecation attending extreme fear is unknown. Maudsley "stress-susceptible" rats, inbred based on defecation during emotional distress, have decreased, not increased, basal plasma levels of catecholamines (Blizard et al., 1980). Gastrointestinal "letting go" may mainly reflect intense vagal stimulation as part of a "giving up" reaction, discussed below.

The state of contraction of myoepithelial cells in glands—for example, the state of salivary secretion—provides a fourth physiological difference between terror and rage. Darwin wrote that during terror,

> [t]he salivary glands act imperfectly; the mouth becomes dry, and is often opened . . . One of the best-marked symptoms is the trembling of all the muscles of the body; and this is often first seen in the lips. From this cause, and from the dryness of the mouth, the voice becomes husky or indistinct, or may altogether fail. "Obstupui, steteruntque comae, et vox faucibus haesit." (Darwin, 1965, p. 291)

Anxiety-provoking situations generally inhibit salivary secretion (Morse et al., 1983). This inhibition explains a component of stage fright in musicians:

> In one case a promising French horn player got dry in the mouth at every audition. "You can't play the French horn if you haven't got spit," a music school official pointed out. (Rubin and McNeil, 1987, p. 261)

In contrast, increased drooling during rage recalls anticipatory salivation before predatory attack. To "spit in another's face" signals aggression in cats and humans. Yohimbine tends to increase salivation (Linden et al., 1985). Whether provoked anger increases salivation has not been tested.

Most germane to the concepts of this book, the pattern of AHS and SNS activation may provide a fifth distinction between manifestations of terror and rage. Based on effects of injections of NE and EPI, Ax (1953) and Funkenstein (1956) linked EPI with fear or anxiety and NE with anger or aggression. Subsequent research discarded these views, because EPI secretion was found to increase in a variety of emotional states, administration of NE did not evoke rage or any other particular emotion (Frankenhaeuser et al., 1961), increased catecholamine output was found to occur during pleasant, not merely unpleasant, emotions (Levi, 1965), and EPI administration was found to intensify different emotional experiences, with the type of emotion depending on the subject's cognitions (Schachter and Singer, 1962).

Ironically, clinical findings involving plasma levels of endogenous NE and EPI have tended to support the suggestions of Ax and Funkenstein. In general, situations producing panic or anxiety increase plasma EPI levels proportionately more than they increase plasma NE levels (Bolm-Audorff et al., 1986; Dimsdale and Moss, 1980; Dionne et al., 1984; Ekeberg et al., 1990; Fell et al., 1985; Grossman et al., 1989; Hjemdahl et al., 1984; Horikoshi et al., 1985; Jorgensen et al., 1985; Perini et al., 1990a, 1990b). Indeed, arterial plasma NE concentrations may not increase at all during some laboratory mental stress tests (Jorgensen et al., 1985). In subjects with acute flight phobia, actual flying increases heart rate, blood pressure, perceived anxiety, and plasma EPI levels, whereas plasma NE levels remain unchanged (Ekeberg et al., 1990). In patients undergoing induction of general anesthesia, plasma EPI levels, but not NE levels, correlate positively with self-reported anxiety as assessed using linear analog scales (Fell, 1985). In professional hockey players and in neuropsychiatric patients, selective increases in NE excretion accompany aggressive, active emotional displays; whereas selective increases in urinary EPI excretion accompany tense and anxious, but passive emotional behaviors (Elmadjian et al., 1965).

At least three potential problems limit inferences from clinical studies using antecubital venous plasma levels of catecholamines to indicate AHS and SBS activation during exposure to psychological stressors. Stressors that alter forearm and total body blood flows can distort relationships among antecubital venous levels of NE, arterial levels of NE, and spillover of NE into arterial plasma (Chang et al., 1989; Grossman, Chang et al., 1991b) and lead to underestimation by antecubital venous NE of the extent of sympathoneural recruitment. Studies that have taken these hemodynamic and kinetic factors into account have indicated that exposure to mentally challenging laboratory tests increases both AHS and overall SNS outflows. Thus, undergoing the Stroop color–word conflict test increases arterial levels of both NE and EPI (Hjemdahl et al., 1989; Tidgren and Hjemdahl, 1989). Goldstein, Eisenhofer et al. (1987) reported increases in arterial EPI levels and in spillover of NE into arterial plasma in subjects playing a video game, with the increases in arterial NE spillover correlated significantly positively with the increases in mean arterial pressure and cardiac output. Ushiyama et al. (1991) did note a positive correlation between changes in antecubital venous plasma NE concentrations and increments in systolic blood pressure in healthy volunteers performing mental arithmetic; however, Goldstein, Eisenhofer et al. (1987) found no relationship between changes in antecubital venous NE and increments in blood pressure or cardiac output in healthy volunteers playing a video game.

Second, studies of responses of humans during laboratory mental challenge often have not considered adequately the effects of associated locomotor activity on neuroendocrine outflows, nor the relationship between the locomotor–neuroendocrine response and the type of emotional experience. For instance, during aggressive behavior, physical activity, not the experience of anger, may produce a relatively large sympathoneural response. Consistent with this view, passive avoidance elicits larger plasma EPI and corticosterone responses and smaller plasma NE responses than does active avoidance (de Boer et al., 1990).

Third, studies that have used public speaking as a naturalistic model of an anxiety-provoking situation (e.g., Bolm-Audorff et al., 1986) often have neither monitored nor controlled for alterations in dietary intake that may affect plasma catecholamine levels at baseline or during stress.

Despite these theoretical limitations, the above studies of humans support an association between fear or anxiety and AHS activation and between aggressive behavior or anger and SNS activation. Studies of laboratory animals confirm these associations. In dogs exposed to a food-access confrontation protocol, animals exhibiting anger have prominent increases in plasma NE levels, whereas those exhibiting fear (indicated by cowering posture and trembling) have prominent increases in plasma EPI levels (Verrier and Dickerson, 1991). In cats, defensive behavior associated with exposure to a dog elicits predominantly adrenomedullary activation, whereas exposure to another cat elicits both sympathoneural and adrenomedullary activation (Stoddard et al., 1986a, 1986b). In rats, passive avoidance is associated with larger responses in plasma EPI levels than in NE levels (de Boer et al., 1990).

Adrenomedullary activation during anxiety may intensify but probably does not cause emotional experiences. Patients with pheochromocytomas, with high circulating catecholamine levels due to release by the tumor, do not have excessive anxiety (Starkman et al., 1990); and EPI when administered exogenously amplifies emotional experiences (Schachter and Singer, 1962) but does not elicit any specific emotion. Moreover, plasma EPI levels required for healthy people to discriminate between infusions of EPI or saline exceed those typically noted in situations eliciting emotional distress (Cameron et al., 1990).

Several studies have supported a closer link between AHS and HPA responses than between AHS and SNS responses during distress. Public speaking markedly increases plasma levels and urinary excretion of EPI and cortisol, with only small changes in NE levels (Bolm-Audorff et al., 1986). In humans playing a video game, responses of arterial ACTH levels correlate positively with responses of EPI levels but not NE levels (Goldstein, Eisenhofer et al., 1987). In rats, electroconvulsive shock increases jugular venous plasma concentrations of ACTH, β-endorphin, and EPI, whereas plasma concentrations of NE remain unchanged (Thiagarajan et al., 1989); and passive avoidance elicits large plasma EPI and corticosterone responses but small plasma NE responses (de Boer et al., 1990).

The central neuroanatomy of "fight-or-flight" behaviors includes pathways from the limbic system to the hypothalamus and lower brainstem, as discussed in Chapter 4. Determinants of the interactions among the centers these pathways connect remain poorly understood. In 1892, Goltz reported that decortication in dogs exaggerates attack behavior. Cannon and Britton (1925) later confirmed this finding, naming the phenomenon "sham rage." Bard (1928) identified the posterior hypothalamus as the most rostral portion of the neuraxis required for elicitation of sham rage. Electrical stimulation along a pathway including the amygdala, BNST, perifornical lateral hypothalamus, and periaquaductal gray region evokes defensive behavior (Fernandez de Molina and Hunsperger, 1962), and this pathway appears to extend caudally in the dorsomedial pons and medulla (Coote et al., 1973).

The immediate early gene *c-fos* is expressed in neurons that produce biogenic amines such as NE and 5-HT or neuropeptides such as CRH and endogenous opiates. In rats exposed acutely to pain or immobilization, both of which would be expected to elicit distress and attempts to escape, *c-fos* expression increases similarly in several brainstem catecholaminergic or serotonergic nuclei (Senba et al., 1993). On the basis of *c-fos* expression during pain or immobilization and on the basis of projection to the intermediolateral columns of the spinal cord, brainstem catecholaminergic cells can be divided into three groups: catecholaminergic cells in the A7 and RVLM regions that project to the intermediolateral cord but do not express *c-fos*; catecholaminergic cells in the A1, NTS, and LC, and RVLM regions that express *c-fos* but do not project to the intermediolateral cord; and catecholaminergic cells in the A5 and ventral A6 (subceruleus) regions that both express *c-fos* and project to the intermediolateral cord. Non-catecholaminergic (presumably serotonergic) raphe cells, especially in the raphe pallidus, both express *c-fos* during pain or immobilization and project to the intermediolateral cord. Whereas neurons in the dorsomedial parvocellular PVN express *c-fos* during pain or immobilization, spatially distinct neurons in the dorsal and ventro-medial parvocellular PVN project to the intermediolateral columns.

These findings, while confirming the sources of descending projections to spinal preganglionic neurons (SPNs) discussed in Chapter 4, suggest that exposure to acute pain or immobilization can activate *c-fos* in clusters of cells that differ from those projecting directly to the SPNs. For instance, whereas pain or immobilization markedly increases *c-fos* expression in parvocellular PVN cells, the activated cells are localized differently from the parvocellular cells that project directly to the SPN's; and whereas these stressors also markedly increase *c-fos* expression in the LC, the LC activation probably does not directly increase sympathoadrenal outflows. The sources and mean-ings of increased *c-fos* expression in the PVN and LC during exposure to these and other stressors therefore remain to be established. The report of Senba et al. (1993) did not consider interoceptor input via the NTS, separate pathways to adrenomedullary and sympathoneural effectors, stressors that do not elicit distress, relationships between *c-fos* expression and actual neurotransmitter release, other immediate early genes besides *c-fos,* or effects of chronic as opposed to acute stress. Nevertheless, the approach using *c-fos* expression enables identifying at least some of the brain centers activated during exposure to stressors. Future research should apply this technique to delineate pathways linking regional metabolic activation, central neurotransmitter release and synthesis, and alterations in autonomic outflows during exposure to different stressors.

Stoddard (1991) summarized several studies about plasma catecholamine responses during hypothalamically elicited defense reactions in cats. The largest increases in fem-oral venous plasma NE and EPI levels occurred during electrical stimulation of the ventromedial nucleus, perifornical area, and MFB. As discussed in the chapter about central neuroanatomy, Smith et al. (1990) have proposed that cells in the perifornical "HACER" region determine alterations in neurocirculatory function during the defense reaction.

The role of higher cortical and limbic system structures in the central neuroanatomy of distress remains a mystery. Consistent with cortical inhibition of defensive attack behavior, prefrontal cortical electrical stimulation in cats suppresses hypothalamically mediated defensive behavior (Siegel et al., 1974, 1975). In psychiatric patients, how-ever, prefrontal lobe destruction ameliorates aggressive behavior (Fulton, 1951); and until the introduction of the major tranquilizers, lobotomy was an accepted neurosur-gical method for controlling intractable patients. Although portions of the limbic system may trigger or otherwise influence "defensive attack" by natural stimuli, limbic struc-tures are not necessary, whereas the posterior hypothalamus is. Swanson (1987) has opined:

[T]he closest one can come to a neural model of affect or emotion at the present time is the platitude that the limbic system (including the hypothalamus) is involved. The term limbic system is now so vague . . . that it has no real meaning, and in effect there is today no viable model based on neuroanatomical circuitry for the elaboration of affective experience. (Swanson, 1987, p. 100)

Central pathways mediating defensive attack behavior differ from those mediating predatory behavior. Whereas exposure of a cat to a dog or to an aggressive cat evokes marked increases in LC firing, heart rate (Levine et al., 1990), and plasma NE levels, exposure of a cat to rats does not elicit these responses in the cat, despite behavioral evidence of "activation" (Abercrombie and Jacobs, 1987b; Jacobs, 1990). Predatory attack may not be associated with the experience of distress, in contrast with defensive attack; purely aggressive behavior can even be associated with decreased adrenomedullary secretion of EPI (Stoddard et al., 1987). Swanson (1987) has suggested that descending pathways for defensive attack behavior traverse the central gray and those for predatory behavior traverse the ventral tegmental area, following the two main portions of the MFB.

In summary, patterns of skeletal and smooth muscle responses associated with terror and rage differ, probably due at least partly to differential AHS and SNS activation. Emotional distress due to fear or anxiety is linked with HPA and AHS activation. The latter may amplify the emotional experience but does not produce it. Except for purely predatory situations, antagonistic encounters involve some fear, and therefore, adrenomedullary activation can accompany intraspecific fighting. SMSA and NE spillover into arterial plasma increase in situations involving heightened vigilance and active responding (Table 6–2), consistent with a role for the SNS in rapid circulatory adjustments supporting brain blood flow and skeletal muscle contraction. Combining *c-fos* expression, immunocytochemistry, and neurochemistry offers the potential to delineate the central neural pathways of distress; however, these approaches have not yet been used to test whether different stressors elicit different patterns of skeletal and smooth muscle responses.

Activity vs. Passivity

As the intensity of a "fight-or-flight" emotion increases, the tendency to evince locomotor activity increases. Thus, the continuum of fear ranges from boredom to unex-

Table 6–2. Psychological Dimensions and
Neuroendocrine Correlates

Engagement	↑ NE > ↑ ACTH ↑ EPI
Locomotion	↑ NE > ↑ EPI
Anxiety/Distress	↑ EPI ↑ ACTH > ↑ NE
Fear vs. Anger	↑ EPI ↑ X > ↑ NE
Novelty	↑ ACTH
Hopelessness	↑ ACTH ↑ X
Defeat/Giving Up	↑ EPI ↑ ACTH ↑ X ↑ AVP ↑ Opioids

Note: This table summarizes suggestions about adrenomedullary (EPN), sympathoneural (NE), pituitary–adrenocortical (ACTH), vagal (X), vasopressin (AVP), and endogenous opioid responses as a function of several dimensions of psychological stressors. Because of the lack of literature involving simultaneous assessments of activities of neuroendocrine systems, the listings are speculative.

pressed but experienced anxiety to visible, trembling terror to uncontrollable panic and head-long flight; and the continuum of anger ranges from boredom to unexpressed anger to visible rage to uncontrollable frenzy. The circulatory and neuroendocrine patterns accompanying fear or anger probably depend importantly on the extent of expression of locomotor behaviors—that is, the amount of activity or passivity, and therefore on the intensity of the emotional experience, independent of the quality of the emotion itself.

Little is known about the neuroendocrine and circulatory patterns associated with active and passive fear. As noted above, passive avoidance is associated with larger plasma EPI and smaller plasma NE responses than is active avoidance (de Boer et al., 1990). Adams et al. (1969) used a model where cats were exposed to other cats that had undergone implantation of hypothalamic electrodes; hypothalamic stimulation evoked defense responses in the cats with the implants. The test cats also displayed defensive behaviors. Different cardiovascular patterns occurred during immobile confrontation, "nonsupportive fighting," involving defensive movements of the forelimbs to ward off the aggressor; and "supportive fighting," where all four limbs were used to attack. In contrast with defense reactions elicited by hypothalamic stimulation, naturally occurring defense was not accompanied by large increases in blood pressure, because during immobile confrontation, bradycardia and decreased cardiac output countered renal and splanchnic vasoconstriction. During actual fighting, marked skeletal vasodilation occurred. Whether immobile confrontation differs from actual fighting in terms of SNS activity or plasma catecholamine levels has not been determined.

As the intensity of fear increases, any of several reaction patterns can occur: The organism may tremble but otherwise remain attentive and motionless (the "freezing reaction"; Folkow, 1987); it may attack defensively (the "defense reaction"; Folkow, 1982); it may suddenly attempt to flee; or it may suddenly lose consciousness in a "playing dead" or "defeat" reaction (Folkow, 1987). Species vary in their tendencies for these behaviors. The triggers and mechanisms causing abrupt shifts among these reaction patterns are unknown.

Fainting, Defeat, and Giving Up

Darwin recognized that extreme fear can evoke sudden loss of consciousness in lower animals and in humans:

> A terrified canary-bird has been seen not only to tremble and to turn white about the base of the bill, but to faint; and I once caught a robin in a room, which fainted so completely, that for a time I thought it dead. (Darwin, 1965, p. 77)

Psychological theorists have viewed fainting as an expression of helpless defeat, when the individual perceives the futility of either fighting or fleeing in an emotionally distressing situation (Engel, 1978), and the central nervous system directs a physiological response pattern resembling primitive "freezing" or "playing dead" reactions (Engel, 1978; Goldstein, Spanarkel et al., 1982). Many situations in modern-day life, such as undergoing blood sampling at the doctor's office, receiving an injection of dental anesthetic, witnessing a traumatic automobile accident, or receiving tragic news in public, cause distress without the possibility of fighting or fleeing as coping options. Standing for a long period, warm external temperature, and delayed ingestion of food increase the likelihood of developing vasodepressor syncope, possibly because they tend to decrease effective arterial filling and therefore require sympathoneural activation to maintain venous return to the heart.

Physiologically, vasodepressor syncope occurs when a failure of orthostatic sympathetic reflexes combines with vagal bradycardia to decrease cerebral perfusion, despite (or perhaps due to) large increases in circulating levels of AVP (Jensen et al., 1986) and EPI (Robertson, Johnson et al., 1979). The pattern of neuroendocrine responses in this setting therefore includes AHS, PNS, and vasopressinergic activation but with SNS inhibition (Figure 6–3). Directly recorded SMSA decreases markedly during vasovagal responses in humans (Wallin and Sundlof, 1982). Plasma NE levels either do not increase or increase inappropriately, considering the fall in mean arterial pressure (Esler, Jennings et al., 1990; Goldstein, Spanarkel et al., 1982; Jensen et al., 1986; Robertson, Johnson et al., 1979; Ziegler et al., 1986). Estimated NE spillover rates into arterial and into cardiac and renal venous plasma all decrease markedly (Esler et al., 1990; Tidgren et al., 1990).

Substantial literature about neurophysiological and hemodynamic correlates of vasodepressor reactions contrasts with a lack of information about the neurophysiological trigger. Two different triggering mechanisms, peripheral and central, have been proposed (van Lieshout et al., 1991).

Several investigators have suggested that in volume-depleted subjects, enhanced cardiac contraction with a near-empty ventricular chamber can paradoxically stimulate inhibitory ventricular myocardial receptors, evoking a depressor reflex (Barcroft and Edholm, 1945; Oberg and Thoren, 1972; Sharpey-Schaefer, 1956). For instance, in anesthetized cats, rapid hemorrhage can increase activity in left ventricular non-myelinated vagal afferents (Thoren et al., 1988). This mechanism, although widely accepted, has never actually been demonstrated as a cause of vasovagal syncope (Hainsworth, 1991). On the contrary, since infusion of a vasodilator has been reported to evoke vasodepressor syncope in a heart-transplant recipient lacking cardiac innervation (Scherrer et al., 1990a), the reaction does not appear to require altered neuronal afferent input from ventricular baroreceptors. Analogously, in conscious dogs, surgical cardiac denervation does not prevent sympathoinhibition during hemorrhagic hypotension (Morita and Vatner, 1985a).

Alternatively, sudden activation of a central neuroendocrine pattern may evoke vasovagal syncope. Koizumi and Kollai (1981) elicited vagal bradycardia, sympathoinhibition, and hypotension by stimulating hypothalamic sites close to those eliciting the pattern of the defense reaction.

Endogenous opioids decrease LC firing, participate in sedation and anti-nociception, and, as discussed above, contribute to the sudden sympathoinhibition attending hypotensive hemorrhage (Morita et al., 1988). Morphine has long been known to exert a vagal stimulatory effect (Eyster and Meek, 1912), possibly by enhancing baroreflex–cardiac sensitivity (Saini et al., 1988), and the opioid anesthetic fentanyl produces both

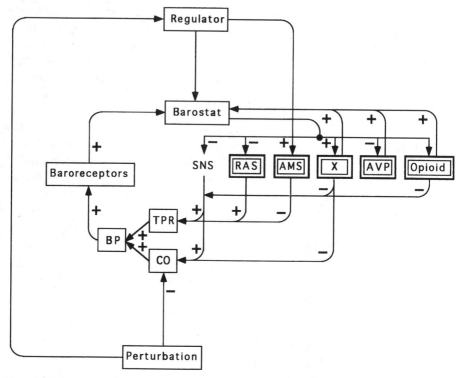

Figure 6–3. The "defeat" or "giving up" reaction and vasodepressor syncope. Normally, perturbations decreasing cardiac filling reflexively increase sympathoneural outflow to skeletal muscle and the heart, and noradrenergic vasoconstriction and increased cardiac rate and contractility tend to restore cardiac filling and blood pressure. In vasodepressor reactions, elaboration of a centrally determined neuroendocrine pattern abruptly increases baroreflex–sympathoneural gain, possibly via increased occupation of receptors for vasopressin (AVP) or an endogenous opioid. This decreases sympathoneural outflow and disrupts homeostatic regulation of blood pressure. Concurrently increased circulating epinephrine (EPI) levels cause skeletal muscle vasodilation, and increased vagal cholinergic outflow (X) decreases cardiac rate and contractility and interferes with sympathetically mediated release of norepinephrine (NE). Since these processes block the noradrenergically mediated vasoconstriction and increased cardiac rate and contractility, blood pressure and cardiac output fall, further increasing release of vasopressin and epinephrine. The hemodynamic derangements decrease cerebral perfusion, and so the situation reaches consciousness and evokes distress, which further increases secretion of vasopressin, epinephrine, and endogenous opioids, and increases vagal cholinergic outflow. The multiple positive feedback loops produce precipitous declines in blood pressure, cerebral perfusion, and consciousness.

a central vagotonic and sympatholytic effect (Faden and Holaday, 1979). Endogenous opioids inhibit cardiac sympathoneural reactivity to interoceptive input to the brain (Weinstock et al., 1984), and the opioid antagonist naloxone can reverse hypovolemic shock (Faden and Holaday, 1979). These findings suggest that sudden activation of an endogenous opioid pathway during distress may contribute to sympathoinhibition and vagal stimulation, increasing the likelihood of a neurocirculatory positive feedback loop that eventuates in profound hypotension and fainting.

Decreased cardiac filling increases release of AVP from the posterior pituitary. Since AVP increases baroreflex–sympathoneural gain (e.g., Hasser et al., 1988), and high circulating AVP levels inhibit reflexive increases in sympathoneural outflow during hemorrhage (Abboud et al., 1986; Imaizumi and Thames, 1986), increased occupation of AVP receptors in the brain during orthostasis could act synergistically with endogenous opioids to prevent sympathoneural responses during unloading of cardiac baroreceptors. This would further enhance AVP release, again increasing the likelihood of a neurocirculatory positive-feedback loop.

Increased circulating EPI levels may also decrease the threshold for triggering vasodepressor syncope during emotional distress. Physiological increases in plasma EPI levels stimulate vascular β_2-adrenoceptors, dilating skeletal muscle beds. EPI administration reflexively increases sympathoneural outflow and regional NE spillover (Persson et al., 1989), countering the tendency to decrease total peripheral resistance. Resetting of the baroreceptor-sympathoneural reflex, perhaps owing to endogenous opiates or AVP, could prevent sympathetically mediated vasoconstriction, leaving EPI-induced vasodilation unopposed. The resulting cerebral hypoperfusion could exacerbate the sense of distress—again increasing the likelihood of a positive feedback loop. Thus, distress-associated increases in circulating EPI levels, in the setting of an orthostatic decrease in cardiac filling, may combine with AVP and endogenous opioids to evoke sudden hypotension and syncope. Consistent with this view, β-adrenoceptor blockade can successfully be used to treat patients with recurrent vasodepressor syncope (Perry and Garson, 1991).

Despite the common occurrence of vagal bradycardia in vasodepressor syncope, atropinization often does not prevent the hypotension. Increased vagal outflow probably nevertheless contributes to the triggering mechanism, since vagal cholinergic stimulation not only slows the heart but also inhibits release of NE from regional sympathetic nerves (Levy and Blattberg, 1976) and may decrease cardiac contractility (DeGeest et al., 1965). Hypoglycemia or hypotensive hemorrhage increases vagal outflow; and a delay in the normal routine of food intake or the sight of blood is commonly associated with vasodepressor reactions. From the principle of accentuated antagonism (Levy, 1971, 1984), discussed in Chapter 2, situations increasing cardiac sympathoneural outflow would be expected to increase concurrently the extent of cholinergic antagonism during vagal stimulation.

PNS stimulation during extreme terror would also be expected to increase gut motility and thereby contribute to gastrointestinal ''letting go.''

In sum, a neuroendocrine pattern including SNS inhibition, AHS and PNS stimulation, and release of endogenous opioids and AVP, may trigger vasodepressor syncope via activation of neurocirculatory positive feedback loops.

One may ask what survival advantage a ''giving up'' or defeat reaction would have provided in evolution. Predators may instinctively avoid eating an animal they have not killed, since eating any discovered carcasses would pose an infectious or toxic threat. Thus, when attacked, an opossum enters a deathlike trance; the predator may shake the animal but eventually loses interest in the prey that looks and feels already dead. Within a species, including humans, combat usually ends abruptly when one of the combatants displays a defeat reaction (Lorenz, 1963). This would allow the "underdog" to survive. A defeat reaction may arouse altruistic behavior in others. Finally, "giving up" may sacrifice consciousness to allay pain and suffering.

Henry et al. (1986) proposed that chronic exposure to situations eliciting defense reactions leads eventually to passive, immobile, helplessness, with vagal and pituitary–adrenocortical system activation causing ulceration, immunosuppression, and hypertension without tachycardia. Frankenhaeuser (1983) suggested that increased release of catecholamines accompanies effort without distress; elevations in cortisol and catecholamines accompany effort with distress; and elevations in cortisol alone accompany distress without effort (i.e., giving up, helplessness). Henry and Grim (1990) elaborated further on the theory that during the defense reaction, increases in NE, gonadotropin, and testosterone levels reflect "control," and increases in EPI, β-endorphin, PRA, prolactin, and glycogenolysis reflect "striving"; whereas during the "defeat reaction," increases in levels of ACTH and pepsin, decreases in levels of gonadotropins and testosterone, and no changes in plasma catecholamines reflect "loss of control." They hypothesized further that a threat to control evokes arousal and fight-or-flight behavior via the amygdala, whereas loss of control evokes depression via the hippocampus–septal system.

Studies involving simultaneous measurements of activities of several effector systems can test these hypotheses by determining if neuroendocrine responses "cluster" as predicted. In contrast to predictions from the hypothesis of Henry and Grim (1990), Prince and Anisman (1990) reported that stressor controllability did not affect the magnitude of the glucocorticoid response to footshock in rats; and Contrada et al. (1982) found in humans that control over a laboratory psychological stressor enhances responses of plasma EPI levels. In rats, chronic repetition of exposure to distressing, inescapable stimuli, such as immobilization and electroconvulsive shock, does not lead to recrudescent pituitary–adrenocortical activation and does not attenuate acute responses of plasma catecholamines (e.g., Kvetnansky and Mikulaj, 1970; Kvetnansky, Nemeth et al., 1984). The findings in rats do not support the development of "defeat reactions" (in Henry and Grim's terms), or the "stage of exhaustion" (in Selye's terms) after repeated exposure to a stressor.

The present conception views chronic "defeat" or "giving up" reactions somewhat differently. Applying the same hypothesized mechanisms triggering vasodepressor syncope during acute distress to a chronic "giving up" reaction during chronic distress, "giving up" would be characterized experientially by depression and resignation; behaviorally by inaction, inattentiveness, and blunted affect; neuroendocrinologically by increased vagal outflow, sympathoinhibition, increased secretion of EPI, ACTH, β-endorphin, AVP, and pancreatic polypeptide; and hemodynamically by intolerance to exercise or orthostasis. According to this view, the long-term consequence of "giving up" would not be hypertension but, if anything, hypotension. In 1942, Cannon described "voodoo death," which may exemplify an extreme defeat reaction, with depression, failure to care, bradycardia, and eventual vagal cardiac arrest (Engel, 1971).

The interplay of parasympathetic, endogenous opioid, pituitary–adrenocortical, and catecholaminergic systems in this phenomenon is unknown.

Novelty vs. Predictability

HPA activation seems especially prominent in distressing situations perceived as novel. Brady (1975) reported that when no coping behavior was possible, novel, threatening or distressing conditions were associated with both HPA and AHS activation (Brady, 1975). Thiagarajan et al. (1989) confirmed this in naive rats exposed to electroconvulsive shock, since following the tenth exposure, responses of ACTH and corticosterone were significantly attenuated, whereas responses of plasma catecholamine levels were augmented. Levine et al. (1989) reported a positive correlation between the extent of novelty and of glucocorticoid secretion. de Boer et al. (1989) exposed rats to repeated predictable or unpredictable noise and found that plasma corticosterone levels decreased with repeated regular, but not irregular, presentations of the stimulus, plasma EPI responses were abolished regardless of the irregularity of the presentations, and plasma NE responses were attenuated partially after repeated irregular presentations. Weiss (1970, 1971) found that rats receiving unpredictable shock had higher plasma corticosteroid levels and more extensive gastric ulcers than did rats receiving predictable shock. Prince and Anisman (1990) reported that glucocorticoid responses to an aversive stressor (swimming in rats) depended on stressor controllability when the animals were highly prepared to escape but not when they were unprepared; that is, controllability and preparedness both appeared to influence the pituitary–adrenocortical response.

Early clinical studies about HPA activation in stressful situations such as surgery did not take into account separately the factors of novelty, predictability, and controllability. Voigt et al. (1990) reported that during repetition of exhausting bicycle exercise, physiological and performance measures were reproducible, whereas responses of ACTH, cortisol, and AVP levels diminished with increasing experience. Mason et al. (1976) concluded that threatening situations, such as free shock avoidance, ambiguous signals, and first episodes of bleeding, increase excretion of NE, EPI, and 17-hydroxycorticosteroids. Unpleasant but anticipated stimuli were associated with increases in cortisol and NE but not with increases in EPI levels. The finding of Mason et al. (1976) that uncertainty or unpredictability was not associated with increased 17-hydroxycorticosteroid excretion disagrees with the above results about HPA activation in novel distressing situations; however, as indicated above, most evidence supports the view that repeated exposure to distressing stimuli attenuates responses of ACTH and corticosterone levels, with generally maintained responses of plasma levels of catecholamines (Graessler et al., 1989; Natelson et al., 1987; Thiagarajan et al., 1989).

Chronic, repeated exposure to a distressing stimulus augments plasma catecholamine responses to a novel distressing stimulus (Graessler et al., 1989; Kvetnansky et al., 1984)—a phenomenon called "stressor shift hyperresponsiveness" or "dishabituation" (McCarty et al., 1992). Thus, rats subjected to repeated immobilization have augmented AHS responses to subsequent hemorrhage (Graessler et al., 1989). The response to either a physiological or psychological stimulus evoking distress therefore depends importantly on the previous experiences of the organism.

Dominance vs. Submissiveness

Subordinate baboons in the wild have higher basal plasma concentrations of cortisol than do dominant animals. The chronic hypercortisolemia in subordinate animals has been proposed to produce resistance to suppression of the HPA axis by exogenous glucocorticoids such as dexamethasone. Actual position in the dominance hierarchy appears to be not as important a determinant of basal cortisol levels as aspects of the individual's personality, including social skillfulness, outlets for frustration, affiliations, and the correctness of perceptions about predictability and control in confrontational situations (Sapolsky, 1990). Farabollini (1987) reported increased ACTH and cortico-sterone levels in subordinate rabbits.

Intensity

Frankenhaeuser (1975) proposed a higher threshold for NE responses than for EPI responses during psychosocial stimulation. As discussed above, the higher NE threshold may reflect the greater amount of skeletal muscle contraction associated with more intense emotional experiences.

In summary, the character and intensity of neuroendocrine and circulatory patterns during emotional distress depend importantly on the perceptions of the organism, both about the stressor and about the available repertoire of coping responses. HPA and AHS activation accompanies unanticipated distress. At least three patterns of experiential, behavioral, neuroendocrine, and physiological responses can occur during emotional distress: (1) anger, which can develop into rage and fighting; (2) fear, which can develop into terror and flight; and (3) immobile passivity, which can develop into vasodepression and syncope. Physiological distinctions between fear and anger reflect differential changes in contraction of skeletal muscle, cutaneous vascular and gastrointestinal smooth muscle, and glandular myoepithelium. The extent of skeletal muscle contraction and of recruitment of SNS activation to redistribute blood flows appropriately, generally vary with the intensity of the emotional experience, helping to explain why AHS acti-vation accompanies fear and SNS activation anger. When the organism perceives a failure to gain control or cope, a combination of vagal PNS stimulation, high plasma EPI, AVP, and β-endorphin levels, and SNS inhibition can trigger neurocirculatory positive feedback loops precipitating cerebral hypoperfusion and loss of consciousness.

Stresses Associated with Regional Sympathoneural Activation

The stress responses described above have in common the elicitation of AHS activation. Other stressors elicit mainly patterned responses of regional SNS outflows, redistrib-uting blood volume or altering glandular secretion.

Orthostasis

When a person stands up, dependent pooling of blood rapidly decreases cardiac filling, stroke volume, and delivery of blood from the heart into the aorta. Low-pressure baroreceptors in the heart and high-pressure baroreceptors in the carotid arteries and aorta virtually immediately sense the perturbation. Proprioceptive and vestibular system inputs about the change in body position also rapidly reach the central nervous system. Reflexive adjustments both in behavior and in the distribution of blood volume normally soon follow. Orthostasis decreases cardiac filling and stroke volume, because reflexive decreases in splanchnic capacity do not offset completely the effects of hydrostatic pooling of blood in the legs.

The main behavioral response to orthostasis is leg muscle pumping, which enhances venous return to the heart. Skeletal muscle veins possess little or no sympathetic innervation, and so muscle pumping during orthostasis determines the venous capacity. In the practice of *crurifragium* ancient Romans may have recognized the role of leg muscle pumping in maintaining blood pressure during orthostasis. They found that smashing the shinbones of crucified victims would precipitate collapse and death (Keller, 1980). Muscle pumping probably also prevents orthostatic hypotension in climbing snakes. Water snakes, which appear to lack this capacity, develop orthostatic hypotension when tilted in a tube, but climbing snakes do not (Lillywhite, 1988).

The main effector systems mediating reflexive adjustments of blood volume distribution during orthostasis are the SNS and RAS (Figure 6–4). At least four homeostats regulate the effectors in this setting: the arterial barostat, the cardiac "volustat," homeostats monitoring proprioception and vestibular variables, and homeostats monitoring input from "ergoreceptors" activated by changes in skeletal muscle tension.

Skeletal SNS activity increases virtually instantaneously in response to orthostasis in humans (Delius et al., 1972b), and plasma levels of NE double within a few minutes (Lake et al., 1976). The results of activation of the SNS effector during orthostasis include vasoconstriction, increased total peripheral resistance, and increased heart rate, maintaining mean arterial pressure. The neurogenic vasoconstriction during orthostasis occurs by at least three mechanisms: (1) supraspinal arterial baroreflexes affecting skeletal muscle sympathetic vasomotor tone; (2) spinal reflexes elicited by altered cardiopulmonary baroreceptor activity, affecting subcutaneous blood flow; and (3) a local venoarteriolar axon reflex elicited by venous distention (Henriksen and Skagen, 1986).

The central neural pathways involved in determining the sympathetic adjustments during orthostasis appear to involve brainstem interconnections between the fastigial nucleus of the cerebellum and several brainstem cell clusters (Luft et al., 1986; Miura and Reis, 1970). The fastigial nucleus receives input from the vestibular apparatus, and the NTS receives afferent input from carotid and aortic baroreceptors. Brainstem pathways beyond the NTS synapse are discussed in the chapter about central functional neuroanatomy.

Orthostasis does not elicit distress. Adrenomedullary secretion increases relatively little during orthostasis (Jensen et al., 1986; Robertson, Johnson et al., 1979), whereas traffic in sympathetic nerves supplying skeletal muscle in the legs normally increases markedly (e.g., Burke et al., 1977). Although virtually completely imperceptible, the adaptive neural responses are absolutely required for maintaining cerebral perfusion and consciousness during orthostasis. Activation of the RAS during orthostasis plays a

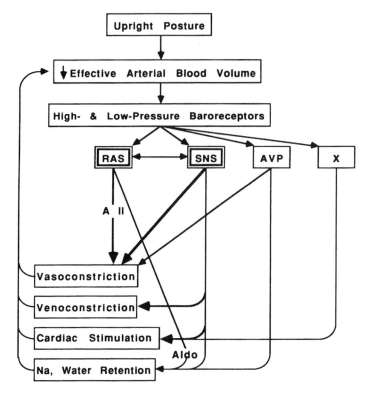

Figure 6–4. Neuroendocrine responses to orthostasis. The sympathoneural and renin–angiotensin–aldosterone systems predominate in the neuroendocrine response pattern evoked by assuming the upright posture.

minor role in the vasoconstrictor response (Jensen et al., 1986; Johnson et al., 1977; Mueller et al., 1974); administration of an ACE inhibitor produces orthostatic hypotension in salt-depleted but not salt-replete subjects (Oparil et al., 1970). Levels of aldosterone and AVP change relatively little during orthostasis, unless hypotension occurs (Jensen et al., 1986; Mueller et al., 1974; Robertson, Johnson et al., 1979).

Lower body negative pressure (LBNP) applies controllable intensities of orthostatic stress. LBNP at low intensities (less than about −15 mm Hg) is thought to unload cardiac "low pressure" mechanoreceptors, although one may question the specificity of the stimulus (Hainsworth, 1991). In humans, LBNP increases radial and peroneal SMSA reflexively (e.g., Rea and Hamden, 1990; Rea and Wallin, 1989; Rowell and Deals, 1990; Sanders et al., 1989b; Seals, 1991; Sundlof and Wallin, 1978b; Vissing et al., 1989), vasoconstricts the extremities, and increases renal NE spillover and renal vascular resistance (Tidgren et al., 1990).

As during orthostasis, during LBNP plasma NE levels increase within a few minutes (Giannattasio et al., 1993; Rea et al., 1990). Baily et al. (1990) reported that LBNP increased directly recorded SMSA without increasing estimated spillover of NE into arterial plasma. The difference between responses of NE spillover to LBNP and to orthostasis has not been explained.

Since heart transplant patients exposed to LBNP have not only blunted responses of plasma NE levels but also absent responses of PRA and AVP levels (Giannattasio et al., 1993), neuroendocrine responses to decreased cardiac filling depend importantly on alterations in afferent neural information to the brain.

Systemic administration of nitroprusside to produce mild hypotension in humans unloads cardiac and arterial baroreceptors and evokes larger increases in plasma NE than EPI levels (Grossman, Chang et al., 1991a; Shepherd and Irvine, 1986), indicating selective stimulation of sympathoneural outflow. Directly recorded SMSA also increases in this setting (Rea et al., 1990).

Exercise

Many homeostatic systems contribute to maintaining appropriate delivery of metabolic fuels and removing waste during exercise. These include chemoreceptor systems, responding rapidly to changes in arterial concentrations of oxygen, carbon dioxide, and hydrogen ions; low- and high-pressure baroreceptor systems; proprioceptor systems; and glucostatic, osmostatic, and thermostatic systems. The neuroendocrine, physiological, and experiential aspects of exercise are therefore very complex and dynamic, with alterations in SNS outflows during exercise resulting partly from "central command" by the cerebral cortex, partly from reflexive effects of hemodynamic changes, and partly by stimulation of chemical receptors in the exercising muscle.

Increased cardiac output is the hemodynamic hallmark of isotonic exercise. Rhythmic contraction of skeletal muscle during isotonic exercise acts as a pump, increasing venous return to the heart. Products of skeletal muscle metabolism act locally to dilate blood vessels, redistributing blood flow to the exercising muscle. This dilatory response may result not only from direct effects of cellular metabolites on vascular smooth muscle cells but also indirectly from presynaptic modulation of NE release. Parasympathetic inhibition combines with sympathetic stimulation to increase heart rate during exercise. As exercise continues, body temperature tends to increase, and temperature-sensitive cells in the anterior hypothalamus activate cholinergic fibers to sweat glands and inhibit sympathetic cutaneous vasoconstriction. The resulting flushing and sweating limit further increases in core temperature. The tendency for skeletal vasodilation to decrease filling pressures and total peripheral resistance releases SNS outflows from inhibition by low- and high-pressure baroreceptors, increasing renal, arterial, and especially cardiac spillovers of NE (Esler, Jennings et al., 1990). During severe exercise, adrenomedullary secretion of EPI augments cardiac rate and contractility as well as venous and renal vasoconstriction.

Regional changes in SNS outflows therefore contribute importantly to the redistribution of blood volume to skeletal muscle during exercise. As vasodilator metabolites accumulate and oxygen debt increases during prolonged exercise, the neuroendocrine pattern changes, in order to balance the increased skeletal muscle flow against the tendency to decrease blood pressure. Beyond an "anaerobic threshold," accumulation of lactate probably leads to further SNS enhancement by recruiting a chemoreceptor homeostatic system that uses the SNS effector.

Isotonic exercise increases plasma NE and EPI levels (Banister and Griffiths, 1972). The plasma NE response exceeds the EPI response (Haggendal et al., 1970; Kotchen et al., 1971; Ludwig et al., 1988) and varies with the workload or oxygen consumption (Haggendal et al., 1970), whereas the requirement for supplying glucose to exercising muscle appears to determine the EPI response. Thus, infusion of glucose during exercise attenuates the plasma EPI response without greatly affecting the plasma NE response (Christensen et al., 1979). This finding confirms the importance of glucose metabolism in regulation of the AHS during exercise.

In rats swimming against a counter-current for 15 minutes, plasma levels of EPI, NE, and corticosterone all increase (Scheurink et al., 1990). Infusion of the nonselective α-adrenoceptor antagonist phentolamine into the lateral hypothalamic area enhances selectively the plasma NE response, and infusion of the β-adrenoceptor antagonist timolol enhances selectively the plasma EPI response. Neither adrenoceptor antagonist affects the corticosterone response. These results suggest separate central neural mechanisms of HPA, SNS, and AHS responses during severe distress-associated exercise.

Isometric handgrip exercise increases SMSA in nonexercising muscle (Sanders et al., 1989a; Seals, 1991) and produces relatively small, delayed increases in plasma NE levels, compared with the rapid, often large hemodynamic changes (Jorgensen et al., 1985; Wallin et al., 1987). During isometric handgrip exercise, plasma NE and EPI levels and total peripheral resistance increase (Grossman et al., 1989). At the initiation of isometric handgrip exercise, cholinergically mediated vasodilation occurs in the nonexercising forearm (Sanders et al., 1989).

Responses of ACTH and PRA are not prominent during exercise except at severe intensities (Kotchen et al., 1971; Luger et al., 1987). AVP levels increase in an intensity-dependent manner during exercise; the physiological role of increased AVP levels in this setting is unknown (Wade, 1984).

Postprandial State

After a large meal, increased vagal PNS activity contributes to the "cephalic" phase of digestion, augmenting release of gastrin and insulin and increasing gut motility. Whereas vagal outflow to the gut increases after a meal, cardiac parasympathetic activity appears to change relatively little (Heseltine et al., 1990), possibly because hemodynamic changes produce counterbalancing reflexive PNS inhibition.

Increased PNS activity in the cephalic phase results in postprandial increases in insulin levels before the increases in blood glucose levels (Steffens et al., 1986). Afferent information relayed from the gut to the NTS and then to the PVN leads to the stimulation of vagal efferent activity to the pancreas (Swanson, 1987).

SNS outflows to most vascular beds also increase after a meal, for at least three reasons. First, splanchnic pooling of blood decreases cardiac filling and stimulates sympathoneural outflows reflexively. Second, increased vagal outflow and postprandial hyperglycemia stimulate insulin secretion, and insulin increases sympathoneural outflows (Mark, 1990), possibly by acting at receptors in the ventromedial hypothalamus (Christensen et al., 1984; Rowe et al., 1981) or by inducing vasodilation. Third, sympathetic outflow may increase on a central basis, since in cats, the act of eating itself increases renal sympathetic nerve activity and plasma levels of NE but not of EPI (Matsukawa et al., 1989). The postprandial state therefore represents a situation where SNS outflow to several regions increases concurrently with increased PNS outflow.

Because the liver removes most of the catecholamines in portal venous blood, plasma catecholamines in the systemic circulation reflect only distantly changes in splanchnic sympathetic outflow. Postprandial increases in plasma NE levels therefore probably indicate sympathetically mediated vasoconstriction in other vascular beds. Effects of eating on splanchnic NE spillover are unknown.

In young people, ingestion of a high-carbohydrate meal, but not a high-fat meal, increases plasma NE levels and pulse rate. The basis for the difference between the effects of the diets is unclear (Heseltine et al., 1990).

Postprandial redistribution of blood flow to the gut can contribute to postprandial angina pectoris in patients with coronary artery disease and postprandial orthostatic hypotension in elderly people, as discussed in the chapter about cardiovascular diseases.

Altered Temperature

Without an intact SNS, mammals cannot survive either cold or hot environments; conversely, an intact SNS endows mammals including humans with a most remarkable ability to maintain internal temperature.

On January 23, 1774, five men entered a room that was heated with dry air to the temperature of boiling water. In this room, where an egg roasted solid in 20 minutes, the almost incredible ability of the human body to maintain its internal temperature by perspiration and evaporative heat loss was demonstrated for the first time (Fulton, 1930). Dr. Charles Blagden, 26 years old at the time, reported his novel observations to the Royal Society of London three weeks later "[T]he most striking effects proceeded from our power of preserving our natural temperature. . . . Whenever we breathed on a thermometer the quicksilver sank several degrees . . ." (Blagden, 1775).

Cutaneous sympathetic activity responds markedly to changes in environmental temperature (Delius et al., 1972a). Sympathetic noradrenergic stimulation of apocrine glands causes axillary sweating, whereas eccrine glands, which receive both sympathetic noradrenergic and sympathetic cholinergic innervation, are responsible for thermoregulatory sweating.

Alterations in sympathetic nervous activity effectively counter mild thermal stressors by shifting blood volume distribution and altering glandular activity. When these responses prove inadequate, AHS outflow increases. Thus, hyperthermic cancer therapy to a core temperature of 39.5°C in humans increases arterial levels of NE but not EPI (Kim et al., 1979), with the increases in NE levels directly related to the increases in cardiac output. At 41.5°C, increases in both plasma NE and EPI occur, possibly because the sympathoneurally mediated changes no longer prevent metabolic derangements. This situation would be expected to evoke anxiety, as Blagden noted in 1775:

[At 260°] I sweated, but not very profusely. For seven minutes my breathing continued perfectly good; but after that time I began to feel an oppression in my lungs, attended with a sense of anxiety; which gradually increasing for the space of a minute, I thought it most prudent to put an end to the experiment, and immediately left the room. My pulse, counted as soon as I came into the cool air, was found to beat at the rate of 144 pulsations in a minute, which is more than double its ordinary quickness. . . . (Blagden, 1775)

As with other homeostatic systems of the body, the mammalian thermoregulatory system is organized hierarchically, with the hypothalamus regulating coordinated changes in SNS outflows during exposure to altered environmental temperature (Swanson, 1987). Two hypothalamic mechanisms seem to carry out this vital function: (1) a heat-dissipating mechanism in the anterior hypothalamus (medial preoptic nucelus), involving sensation of blood temperature and eliciting sweating and cutaneous vasodilation; and (2) a heat-producing mechanism in the posterior hypothalamus, eliciting cutaneous vasoconstriction, cessation of sweating, and shivering. Anteromedial hypothalamic neurons respond briskly to alterations in local or skin temperature, and medial preoptic lesions appear to render mammals into ectotherms, with behavioral but without visceral means to control temperature (Satinoff and Rutstein, 1970). Anterior hypothalamic damage can cause hyperpyrexia, whereas posterior hypothalamic lesions usually produce a condition in which body temperature approaches that of the environment (poikilothermia).

The neuropeptide bombesin seems to interfere with the hypothalamic thermostat; when given icv, the drug decreases body temperature in cold-exposed rats, increases temperature in heat-exposed rats, and produces no change in temperature in rats exposed to a thermoneutral environment (Tache et al., 1980). The central site of action of bombesin is in the anterior hypothalamic–preoptic area.

Cold

In response to decreases in environmental temperature, activation of the hypothalamic thermostat elicits cutaneous vasoconstriction, shivering, and piloerection—all mediated importantly by the SNS—and by behavioral responses seeking warmer conditions. Cold exposure stimulates sympathetic activity in the skin, skeletal muscle (Fagius and Kay, 1991; Victor et al., 1987), spleen, and heart, with little effect on sympathetic activity in the kidney or gut. This pattern redistributes blood away from the extremities and increases cardiac filling and output. Cutaneous vasoconstriction during cold exposure shunts blood to vital organs and decreases evaporative heat loss, and shivering tends to generate metabolic heat.

Cannon, Querido et al. (1927) used the denervated heart preparation to show for the first time that exposure to cold increases adrenomedullary secretion. Since physiological increases in circulating EPI levels increase metabolic activity in humans (Staten et al., 1987), this adrenomedullary response is homeostatic. As noted above, exposure to decreased environmental temperature stimulates SNS outflows relatively selectively, with AHS activation occurring only when alterations in cutaneous vascular resistance fail to prevent hypothermia. Thus, exposure to cold air increases plasma NE but not EPI levels in humans (Graham et al., 1991).

In the cold pressor test, the subject voluntarily immerses a hand in ice-cold water for 1–3 minutes. This rapidly increases blood pressure. The stimuli and responses involve not only cold but also pain, novelty, and numbness. The mechanisms of the rapid regional and systemic hemodynamic changes probably change dynamically. During the cold pressor test, SMSA increases in nonimmersed limbs (Matsukawa et al., 1991a; Victor et al., 1987). The increases in sympathoneural outflow proportionately exceed the accompanying increases in plasma NE levels (Matsukawa et al., 1991a), perhaps because the short time period of immersion, and regional vasoconstriction, may not allow plasma NE levels to reach plateau concentrations. Nevertheless, antecubital venous levels of NE usually increase during the test (Matsukawa et al., 1991a; Robertson, Johnson et al., 1979; Ward et al., 1983). Plasma EPI levels tend to increase during the cold pressor test but to a proportionately much smaller extent than do plasma NE levels (LeBlanc et al., 1979; Robertson, Johnson et al., 1979; Ward et al., 1983).

Exposure of the face to cold water produces cutaneous vasoconstriction and vagally mediated bradycardia. Two reflexes determine the response pattern. Stimulation of trigeminal nerve endings in this setting evokes reflexive apnea; vagal bradycardia; splanchnic, skeletal muscle, renal, and cutaneous vasoconstriction; constriction of venous capacitance vessels; and coronary vasodilation. Hypoxemia and hypercarbia rapidly follow, stimulating chemoreceptors, which augment the reflexive vasoconstriction and bradycardia. The decreased metabolic activity, absence of ventilation, decreased cerebral metabolism during unconsciousness, decreased cardiac metabolism, and redistribution of blood flow toward the heart and brain can enable humans to survive prolonged immersion in ice-cold water, such as in near-drownings in partially frozen lakes. The current world record for the longest survival of out-of-hospital cardiac arrest—four hours—belongs to a 41-year-old man who fell overboard into icy water near Bergen, Norway in 1987 (McFarlan, 1992).

Mental Challenge or Active Attention

Active attention and coping behavior, such as during playing a video game, increase overall sympathoneural activity, as reflected by the spillover of NE into arterial plasma (Goldstein, Eisenhofer et al., 1987). This and other laboratory mental stressors, such as the Stroop color–word conflict test and forced arithmetic, involve a complex interplay of novelty, emotional distress related to harassment, and verbalization, in addition to simple problem-solving. These laboratory stressors generally increase plasma EPI levels proportionately more than plasma NE levels (Grossman et al., 1989; Hjemdahl et al., 1984, 1989; LeBlanc et al., 1979; Matsukawa et al., 1991a; Perini et al., 1990a, 1990b; Robertson, Johnson et al., 1979; Ushiyama et al., 1991; Ward et al., 1983) but nevertheless increase directly recorded SMSA, especially in the legs (Anderson et al., 1987).

Most studies using these stressors have involved antecubital venous blood sampling, and as noted above, this can underestimate responses of NE spillover into arterial plasma. Esler, Jennings, et al. (1989b) found that during performance of mental arithmetic by untreated hypertensive patients, increases in antecubital venous concentrations of NE were negligibly small, whereas arterial NE levels and estimated spillover rates of NE into arterial plasma increased significantly. Mental arithmetic also markedly increased cardiac NE spillover. Playing a video game or undergoing the Stroop color–word conflict test increases arterial NE levels but not antecubital venous NE levels in healthy volunteers (Goldstein, Eisenhofer et al., 1987; Hjemdahl et al., 1989).

Dietary Salt Intake

The main neuroendocrine change during dietary salt restriction is RAS activation (Figure 6–5). Homeostats monitoring cardiac filling, renal perfusion, and the amount of sodium filtered by the kidney all use the RAS effector, and sodium deprivation affects all three variables monitored by these homeostats. The prominence of this system during

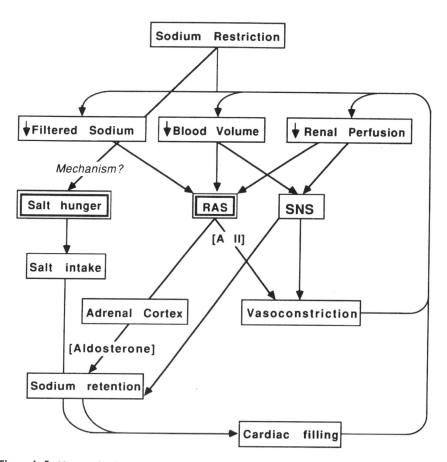

Figure 6–5. Neuroendocrine responses to dietary salt restriction. The renin–angiotensin–aldosterone system (RAS) predominates in the neuroendocrine response pattern evoked by salt restriction.

salt restriction fits with aldosterone being the foremost salt-retaining hormone of the body. By stimulating exchange of Na^+ for K^+ in the kidneys, aldosterone counters the perturbation of all the monitored variables. Salt deprivation also leads to salt-seeking behavior and a preference for salty food, and aldosterone can act in the brain to increase salt appetite (McEwen et al., 1986; Schulkin, 1991). Central neural pathways mediating salt hunger involve the anterior NTS and medial parabrachial region, since lesions in either region virtually abolish salt deprivation-induced increases in NaCl intake in rats (Shulkin, 1991).

Consistent with the view that deprivation of salt, without deprivation of water, does not stimulate the osmolar homeostat, AVP levels change relatively little in this situation (Os et al., 1986). Conversely, whereas increased cardiopulmonary filling decreases AVP levels (Seckl et al., 1986), dietary salt loading augments the osmolar stimulus to AVP release, and the competition between the volustat and osmostat results in no net effect of chronic dietary salt loading on plasma AVP levels (Krieger et al., 1990).

SMSA increases slightly during dietary salt restriction (Anderson et al., 1989). Plasma NE levels also tend to increase. The increases in plasma NE levels during dietary salt restriction do not result from increased release of NE into the extravascular compartment but from a decreased volume of distribution of plasma NE (Linares et al., 1988; Supiano et al., 1990). Salt restriction increases renal NE spillover without affecting total body or cardiac NE spillover (Friberg et al., 1990).

Dietary salt loading markedly suppresses RAS activity, with large falls in levels of PRA, AII, and aldosterone (e.g., Krieger et al., 1990). Plasma NE levels tend to decrease slightly (Dimsdale et al., 1990a, 1990b; Gill et al., 1988, 1991; Luft et al., 1979; Zimlichman, Goldstein, Stull et al., 1987), and plasma EPI levels remain unchanged (Dimsdale et al., 1990a, 1990b). Probably because of increased cardiac filling, dietary salt loading increases plasma levels of ANP (Sagnella et al., 1986).

Dietary salt loading also increases urinary excretion of DA (Alexander et al., 1974; Goldstein, Stull et al., 1989; Oates et al., 1979) and DOPA (Gill et al., 1991; Goldstein, Stull et al., 1989), as discussed in the chapter about peripheral catecholaminergic systems. In humans, increased DOPA spillover does not explain the increased excretion of DOPA and DA during salt loading (Wolfovitz et al., 1993), suggesting that ingestion of a high-salt diet may enhance basolateral membrane uptake of circulating DOPA by proximal tubular cells. In the adrenal cortex, where circulating DOPA also seems to provide the main source of local DA production (Buu and Lussier, 1990), DA tends to inhibit aldosterone secretion.

Increased Cardiac Filling

Application of lower-body positive pressure, assumption of the head-down (Trendelenburg) position, head-out water immersion, weightlessness during space flight, autotransfusion, and rapid intravenous administration of saline all increase cardiac filling. Stimulation of cardiopulmonary mechanoreceptors in these situations reflexively decreases renal sympathetic outflow, decreases secretion of AVP, inhibits RAS activity, and increases cardiac secretion of ANP, in turn increasing leg vein distensibility, decreasing total peripheral vascular resistance, evoking a diuresis and natriuresis, and increasing pulse rate—responses that buffer the effects of the initial perturbation.

Renal sympathoinhibition contributes importantly to the diuresis and natriuresis evoked by increased cardiac filling (Karim et al., 1972; Morita and Vatner, 1985b). Sreeharan et al. (1981) stimulated left atrial receptors by inflating balloons at the pulmonary vein–left atrial junctions or in the left atrium. Surgically denervated kidneys had attenuated natriuretic responses to stimulation of the atrial receptors. Residual natriuretic responses in the denervated kidney were thought to be mediated by humoral mechanisms.

The cardiac sympathoneural response to alterations in cardiac filling appears to be U-shaped: Both severe cardiac underfilling and overfilling increase cardiac SNS outflow, whereas mild increases in filling decrease cardiac SNS outflow. The pattern of autonomic activation attending congestive heart failure, discussed in the chapter about cardiovascular diseases, exemplifies responses to cardiac overfilling in humans.

Mildly increased cardiac filling induced by blood transfusion in humans produces small effects on central blood volume, cardiac output, and left ventricular stroke work; however, transfusion in the setting of ganglion blockade markedly increases values for all these parameters, indicating that during acute, mild central hypervolemia in healthy humans, reflexive vasodilation and decreased myocardial contractility buffer the changes in circulatory dynamics (Frye and Braunwald, 1960).

Head-out water immersion redistributes blood volume to the chest and evokes a prompt, marked diuresis and natriuresis. Immersion increases plasma levels of ANP, tends to decrease AVP levels, increases urinary excretion of prostaglandins, and decreases PRA (Epstein et al., 1983, 1989; Grossman, Goldstein et al., 1992; Norsk and Epstein, 1988). Although Epstein et al. (1983) found no changes in plasma NE or EPI levels during head-out water immersion, a more recent study revealed decreases in plasma NE levels and in urinary NE excretion (Grossman, Goldstein et al., 1992). In conscious dogs, immersion decreases renal sympathetic nerve activity and produces a natriuresis, and dogs with renal denervation fail to evince renal sympathoinhibition or natriuresis in this setting (Miki et al., 1989), indicating that renal sympathoinhibition produces the natriuresis attending immersion. Increased ANP secretion can act directly in the kidney to induce natriuresis or indirectly via vagal afferents or in the central nervous system to augment the reflexive renal sympathoinhibition (Gammage et al., 1987; Kaneko et al., 1987; Thoren et al., 1986).

Saline infusion evokes a natriuresis by several mechanisms, including renal vasodilation due to sympathoinhibition, shutdown of the RAS, increased release of ANP, and stimulation of the renal DOPA–dopamine system. Most studies have failed to distinguish DA responses to intravascular volume loading from responses to an increased filtered load of Na$^+$. Faucheux et al. (1977) found in dogs that saline infusion more potently stimulated increases in urinary DA excretion than did albumin infusion, suggesting that an increased filtered load of sodium contributes to the activation of the renal DOPA–DA system in this setting. Blockade of DA receptors or of the enzymatic conversion of DOPA to dopamine in the kidneys usually interferes with acute natriuretic responses to infused saline (Ball and Lee, 1977; Bennett et al., 1982; Krishna et al., 1985; Sowers et al., 1984; Williams et al., 1986); however, the literature on this point is not entirely consistent (Bradley et al., 1986).

The body's responses to the weightlessness of space flight demonstrate by contrast the actions of reflexive adjustments that evolved to counter the effects of gravity during upright posture (e.g., Davydova et al., 1989; Kvetnansky, Davydova et al., 1978; Kvetnansky et al., 1988). During zero-gravity conditions, astronauts commonly note periorbital fullness, nasal congestion, and distended neck veins, reflecting redistribution of blood from the legs to the upper body. The increase in cardiac filling evokes a natriuresis and diuresis, which decrease blood volume. Prolonged weightlessness dissociates blood volume from cardiac filling. The "volustat," which uses cardiopulmonary stretching as the monitored variable in the regulation of blood volume as the controlled variable, seems to reset, so that indices of sympathoneural outflows normalize despite persistent hypovolemia (Davydova et al., 1989). Upon return to earth's gravity after prolonged space flight, cardiac filling pressures and stroke volume suddenly decrease, resulting in poor tolerance of orthostasis.

The actions of at least three types of homeostats determine the neuroendocrine and behavioral responses to water deprivation. An osmostat, probably located in the hypothalamus, senses the osmolality of the plasma; barostats integrate afferent information from "low pressure" baroreceptors in the heart and "high pressure" baroreceptors in the carotid arteries and aorta; and a third homeostat interprets oropharyngeal afferent information (dry throat and mouth) via the glossopharyngeal and vagus nerves (Swanson, 1987). Water deprivation increases plasma osmolality and decreases effective circulating blood volume, both stimuli synergistically increasing AVP release, and so AVP dominates in the neuroendocrine response pattern (Figure 1–9). This fits with AVP being the foremost hormone to retain "free water."

Although AII and AVP both participate in central neural mechanisms eliciting thirst and water intake, the exact central neural mechanisms relating increased serum osmolality and decreased cardiac filling to water intake are poorly understood. Water deprivation without hypotension does not stimulate sympathoneural activity (Trapani et al., 1988), and increased AVP levels and RAS activity maintain blood pressure in this setting (Ryan et al., 1989).

Summary and Conclusions

Patterns of neuroendocrine stress responses depend importantly on the character and intensity of the stressor, on the organism's perceived ability to cope with it, and on the history of the organism with respect to the stressor and other stressors.

The neuroendocrine response patterns described above reflect different relative contributions of many effector systems during different forms of stress. The effector systems include the AHS and SNS, the HPA system, the PNS, the RAS, and neuropeptidergic systems involving ANP, AVP, and opioids. During manipulations of glucose availability, responses of insulin, glucagon, and adrenomedullary secretion predominate, with concurrent increases in HPA system activity and levels of other glucostatic hormones. During orthostasis, SNS activation predominates; however, during fainting, a rapid switch occurs from orthostatically increased SNS activity to SNS shutdown, associated with PNS and AHS activation and increased levels of AVP and endogenous opioids. During manipulations of dietary salt intake, RAS responses predominate, and during manipulations of water availability, AVP responses predominate. These patterns have a degree of primitive specificity that one can comprehend in terms of the evolution of adaptively advantageous adjustments, as discussed in Chapter 1.

One basis for classifying neuroendocrine stress response patterns is in terms of the relative extent of activation of the AHS and SNS. Stresses associated with AHS activation usually elicit distress. Conversely, stressors that pose global, metabolic challenges or are perceived as threats to well-being elicit AHS activation, even when the intensity of the stressor is mild. AHS activation is prominent in hemorrhage, hypoglycemia, shock, emotional distress, and pain. Stresses eliciting AHS activation typically also elicit HPA activation, as indicated by circulating levels of ACTH or glucocorticoids, and increase release of endogenous opioids, as indicated by plasma levels of β-endorphin, even when SNS activity declines.

Stresses associated with SNS activation often include a component of skeletal muscle contraction. Patterned SNS activation during stress produces adaptive shifts in the distribution of blood volume or in glandular secretion. When these changes suffice to maintain homeostasis, they are not consciously experienced, but when the responses do not mitigate effects of the stressor, the situation can reach consciousness, and AHS activation ensues. SNS activation is prominent in orthostasis, mild-to-moderate exercise, thermoregulation, and the postprandial state.

Neuroendocrine responses during emotional distress can be distinguished behaviorally, neuroendocrinologically, and physiologically in at least three patterns: fear/terror, anger/rage, and submission/giving up. In particular, fear and anger involve different extents of concerted skeletal muscle contraction, cutaneous vasoconstriction, gastrointestinal motility, glandular secretion, and SNS activation. Novel, distressing situations appear to evoke prominent HPA system activation, which habituates as exposure to the stressor is repeated. After repeated exposure to a stressor, the habituated organism has excessive responses to novel stressors: dishabituation. Mechanisms of dishabituation are currently unknown.

Defeat reactions can develop suddenly in situations involving increased SNS outflow. In these reactions, vagal PNS stimulation, increased AVP secretion, release of endogenous opioids, and AHS activation combine with sudden SNS inhibition to produce neurocirculatory positive feedback loops, resulting in hypotension, cerebral hypoperfusion, and syncope.

As researchers assess further the activities of several stress systems concurrently, clearer depictions of primitively specific patterns should emerge, enabling identification of central neural mechanisms determining the elaboration of those patterns and ultimately of genetic bases for stressor-specificity of neuroendocrine responses.

7

Stress and Catecholaminergic Function in Cardiovascular Diseases

Physicians and writers throughout history have appreciated the associations between the experience of distress and changes in cardiovascular function; however, the idea that stress, by way of various neuroendocrine responses, can itself cause disease was not proposed until relatively recently (Willis, 1681, cited in Wolf, 1985) and has remained controversial to this day.

Selye attributed the existence of a wide variety of common disorders to maladaptive stress responses. Among these disorders he included high blood pressure, other cardiovascular diseases, gastrointestinal ulceration, eclampsia, rheumatoid arthritis, inflammatory disorders of the skin and eyes, infections, allergic and hypersensitivity diseases, nervous and mental diseases, cancer, and diseases of resistance in general (Selye, 1956). He emphasized that the development of a disease process requires not only an inciting stimulus but also an ineffective or inappropriate bodily response.

Continuing the tradition of Selye, a tenet of modern psychosomatic medicine holds that whereas activation of homeostatic systems can counter perturbations of the external and internal environments, maladaptive responses contribute to tissue damage or disease. In patients with underlying cardiovascular disease, acute SNS or AHS activation can produce obvious and immediate threats to health; however, the etiologic relationship between repeated activation and the long-term development of cardiovascular disease remains in dispute.

The present conception about the role of the sympathetic nervous system in cardiovascular diseases adopts the view expressed by Peters: "The disorders encountered in disease may be regarded as normal physiologic responses to unusual conditions produced by pathologic processes" (Peters, 1948, p. 353).

Because of the crucial and ubiquitous role of catecholaminergic systems in maintaining circulatory homeostasis, virtually every cardiovascular disease state and every medication used in clinical cardiology affects catecholaminergic function directly or indirectly. Compensatory recruitment of the SNS and AHS effector systems hinders identifying disorders where increased activity of these systems plays a truly etiologic role.

According to the concepts introduced in Chapter 1, several homeostats share the SNS and AHS effectors, the effectors acting in concert with many others in maintaining cardiovascular performance (Figure 7–1). Therefore, the occurrence of abnormal

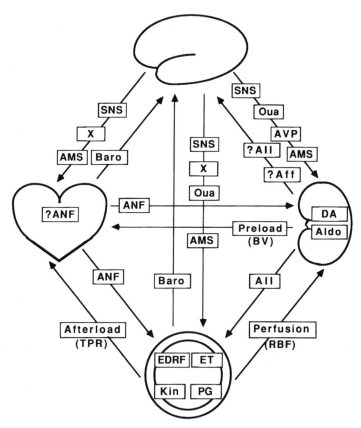

Figure 7–1. Vertical integration of the circulation. A tremendous array of neuronal, endocrine, autocrine/paracrine, and intracellular systems in the brain, heart, kidneys, and blood vessels interact to regulate cardiovascular performance and blood pressure. Neuronal systems include the sympathoneural (SNS) and vagal cholinergic (X) efferent systems and possibly SNS and renal afferents (Aff); endocrine systems include the adrenomedullary (AMS), vasopressin (AVP), atrial natriuretic factor (ANF), endogenous ouabainlike (Oua), and renin–angiotensin–aldosterone (AII, Aldo) systems. Autocrine/paracrine systems include those involving renal production of dopamine (DA) from DOPA, endothelium-derived relaxing factor (EDRF), endothelin (ET), prostaglandins (PG), kinins (K), and possibly ANF. The complexity of interactions among these systems suggests that no single abnormality can explain the occurrence of clinical hypertension.

SNS activity must relate only indirectly to abnormal regulation of any single monitored variable. For instance, although increased SNS activity or reactivity probably occurs early in the development of hypertension, the determination of both blood pressure and SNS outflow by multiple homeostats implies a complex and indirect relationship between SNS activity, however measured, and blood pressure.

The structures of the multiple homeostatic systems regulating blood pressure suggest that, at least in some individuals, interference with inhibitory feedback can produce hypertension. Disinhibition of sympathetically mediated NE release could reflect interruption of reflex arcs at any of several levels, as discussed in the section about baroreflexes in Chapter 2. Alternatively, abnormal neurocirculatory regulation could reflect inappropriate elicitation of neuroendocrine stress response patterns that include resetting of barostats. Inability to separate cause from effect has frustrated efforts to elucidate the relationship between baroreflex function and sympathoneural outflow in patients with hypertension.

Moreover, evidence discussed below about pathophysiological mechanisms in spontaneously hypertensive rats (SHRs) indicates that inbreeding animals based only on high blood pressure, the value for a single physiological variable, selects alterations at several genetic loci. Theoretically, inbreeding for a sufficient number of generations should affect the expression of *all* genes related to the determination of blood pressure, even if only remotely so. This suggests that no matter how intense the study of laboratory animals inbred for high blood pressure alone, no single detected genetic abnormality will explain fully the mechanism of hypertension.

One may ask why modern treatments in clinical cardiology offset, rather than assist, the activation of neuroendocrine systems ''designed'' to foster homeostasis. Harris (1983, 1985) has considered this apparent paradox in a discussion of cardiac edema and offers an appealingly straightforward answer, based on the likely determinants of the evolution of stress responses:

> Cardiac failure is, in nature, a rare event and not likely to have had a perceptible influence on the survival of the species. The mechanisms which are set in motion in cardiac oedema are more likely to have evolved to deal with circumstances vital to preservation which are far more commonplace. In which case it may be that, rather by accident, disease of the heart calls up these mechanisms by somehow simulating the circumstances for which they had properly been developed. . . .

> When the output of the diseased heart becomes diminished, the body responds in exactly the way it has been programmed to function in shock or physical stress. But the programming was designed to service the body during a few hours of physical stress or a few days of traumatic shock. Now it is maintained in action over months of years and an over-retention of saline ensues. (Harris, 1985, pp. 328–329)

One can offer an identical argument for the occurrence of hypertension or any other chronic disorder in modern cardiology. These conditions have been irrelevant throughout human evolution, in contrast with life-preserving neurocirculatory reflexes. Chronic disorders such as hypertension and congestive heart failure may plague the elderly today, but natural selection has favored the evolution of acute mechanisms of self-preservation in the young. According to Harris's concept, the occurrence of chronic cardiovascular disorders in modern civilization has resulted partly from powerful but inappropriate activation of neuroendocrine systems.

The above considerations explain why alterations in SNS or AHS activity accompany so many clinical physiological (Table 7–1) and pathophysiological (Table 7–2) situations, several of which receive extensive attention in this chapter. In addition, commonly used drugs in cardiovascular pharmacotherapy, listed in Table 7–3, act in the nervous system to alter NE concentrations or noradrenergic effects at cardiac or vascular sympathetic neuroeffector junctions.

Hypertension

Many neuronal, endocrine, paracrine, autocrine, and intracellular systems, affecting hemodynamic conditions in several vascular beds, regulate blood pressure (Figure 7–1). The activities of virtually all these systems, including the SNS, AHS, PNS, HPA system, AVP system, and RAS, vary during exposure to different stressors, as discussed in Chapter 6.

The chapters about stress and stress response patterns emphasized the preservation of the internal environment at rest and during stress as putative ''goals'' of alterations in activities of the effectors; and that as homeostatic systems evolved, so did controls over them, resulting in the potential for homeostat resetting in rapid response to or in anticipation of exposure to distressing stimuli. If one accepts these points, then hypertension may represent not so much the consequence of abnormal function of a single effector system as the consequence of dyscoordination of mutually compensating effector systems; and if so, then the real issue in assessing the role of the SNS system in essential hypertension would not be whether the activity of the effector system is excessive, but why the brain does not regulate activity of the SNS, along with activities of other systems, in a manner determining ''normal'' blood pressure—why the brain seems

Table 7–1. Some Factors Affecting Sympathoneural or Adrenomedullary Outflows

Cardiovascular	Neuropsychiatric
Vasodilation/ vasoconstriction	Fear
	Anger
Hemorrhage	Anxiety
Shock	Pain
Tilt	Mental challenge
Exercise	Consciousness
Cardiac pacing	
	Other
Metabolic	
	Time of day
Hypoglycemia	Posture
Hypoxemia/asphyxiation	Normal aging
Hyperthermia/hypothermia	
Sodium homeostasis	
Caloric intake	

Table 7-2. Disorders with Altered Catecholaminergic Function

Cardiovascular	Neurologic
Myocardial infarction	Dysautonomias
Shock	Neurogenic orthostatic hypotension
Hypertension	Shy-Drager syndrome
Early essential hypertension	Pure autonomic failure
Neurogenic hypertension	Reflex sympathetic dystrophy
Post-bypass hypertension	Pure autonomic failure
Post-coarct repair hypertension	Intracranial bleeding
Heart failure	Hypothermia
Low output	Hyperthermia
High output	Seizures (autonomic, grand mal)
Cardiomyopathy	Psychiatric
Hypertrophic	Depression
Dilated	Panic/anxiety
Neurocirculatory	Anorexia/bulemia
Hyperdynamic circulation syndrome	Alcohol or opiate withdrawal
Symptomatic mitral valve prolapse	Genetic
syndrome	DHPR deficiency
Neurocirculatory asthenia	DDC deficiency
Baroreflex failure	DBH deficiency
Neurocardiogenic syncope	Norrie disease
Ventricular arrhythmias	MAO_A deficiency
	Menkes' disease
Endocrinologic	
	Other
Pheochromocytoma	
Hyper/hypothyroidism	Parenchymal failure of liver, lungs, kidneys
Hypocorticotropic hypopituitarism	
Hypercortisolemia	
Diabetic autonomic neuropathy	

to "seek" a higher operating pressure (Julius, 1990). In terms of Dawkins's "selfish gene" theory, discussed in Chapter 1, why and how do the genes of hypertensives direct algorithms for cardiovascular performance that include high blood pressure? As Folkow (1982) has stated, "The more it is realized that unitary explanations do not suffice and therefore a multifactorial background must be considered, the more urgent it becomes to formulate some type of principal interaction scheme for participating mechanisms. Such a scheme would not only aid the search for individual predisposing elements but also provide a more realistic evaluation of how they may exert their triggering influences."

Spontaneously Hypertensive Rats

Young spontaneously hypertensive rats of the Okamoto strain (SHRs) have elevated systemic blood pressure mainly due to increased cardiac output (Lundin and Hallback-Nordlander, 1982). As they mature, the hemodynamic determinant switches to increased total peripheral resistance. This trend resembles that in humans with essential hypertension (Lund-Johansen, 1986), providing one reason many investigators have viewed the SHR as a model of clinical primary hypertension.

Table 7-3. Drugs That Affect Catecholaminergic Function

Cardiovascular

Blockers and stimulators of ganglionic neurotransmission (e.g., trimethaphan, bethanidine; nicotine)
Drugs that deplete catecholamine stores
    Drugs interfering with catecholamine biosynthesis (e.g., α-methyl-*para*-tyrosine, forskolin)
    Other (e.g., reserpine, guanethidine)
Drugs affecting norepinephrine release
    Sympathomimetic amines (e.g., tyramine, amphetamine, aramine)
    Other (e.g., bretylium)
Drugs affecting norepinephrine reuptake
    Digitalis glycosides
Adrenoceptor agonists and antagonists (e.g., norepinephrine, epinephrine, dopamine, dobutamine, isoproterenol,
    methoxamine, yohimbine, propranolol, atenolol, prazosin, salbutamol, clonidine, guanabenz, phenylephrine)
Drugs affecting intracellular messenger function in vascular smooth muscle cells
    Caffeine
    Theophyllines
Anti-hypertensive medications
    Vasoactive drugs producing reflexive effects (e.g., nitroprusside, hydralazine, diuretics)
    Other (e.g., calcium channel blockers, ACE inhibitors)

Neurologic

MPTP
DOPA
Carbidopa
Atropine
Deoxyphenylserine (DOPS)
Bromocriptine

Psychiatric

MAO inhibitors (e.g., debrisoquin, clorgyline, deprenyl)
Anti-depressants (e.g., desipramine)
Sedatives (e.g., benzodiazepines)
Cocaine
Alcohol

Other

Cyclosporine
Barbiturate anesthesia

Multiple Loci of Abnormalities

During the development of hypertension in SHRs, catecholaminergic abnormalities occur at many levels of the sympathetic neuraxis (Figure 7–2). All the abnormalities tend to increase occupation of cardiovascular adrenoceptors by catecholamines or enhance vascular smooth muscle responses to adrenoceptor occupation.

SHRs have increased rates of directly recorded sympathetic activity (Iriuchijima, 1973; Judy et al., 1976; Kumagai et al., 1992; Lundin et al., 1983, 1984; Okamoto et al., 1967). Even after spinal cord transection, SHRs have more sympathetic nerve traffic than do Wistar–Kyoto (WKY) control rats (Schramm and Chornoboy, 1982).

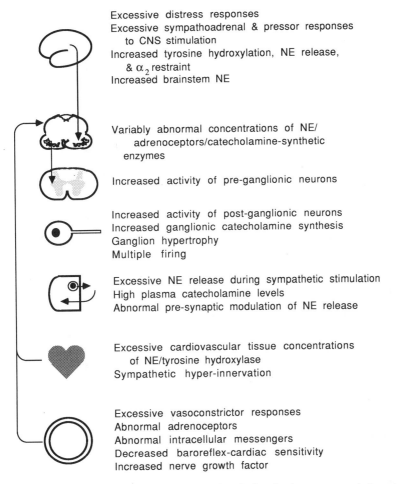

Excessive distress responses
Excessive sympathoadrenal & pressor responses
    to CNS stimulation
Increased tyrosine hydroxylation, NE release,
    & α_2 restraint
Increased brainstem NE

Variably abnormal concentrations of NE/
    adrenoceptors/catecholamine-synthetic
    enzymes

Increased activity of pre-ganglionic neurons

Increased activity of post-ganglionic neurons
Increased ganglionic catecholamine synthesis
Ganglion hypertrophy
Multiple firing

Excessive NE release during sympathetic stimulation
High plasma catecholamine levels
Abnormal pre-synaptic modulation of NE release

Excessive cardiovascular tissue concentrations
    of NE/tyrosine hydroxylase
Sympathetic hyper-innervation

Excessive vasoconstrictor responses
Abnormal adrenoceptors
Abnormal intracellular messengers
Decreased baroreflex-cardiac sensitivity
Increased nerve growth factor

Figure 7–2. Multiple loci of alterations in catecholaminergic function in spontaneously hypertensive rats of the Okamoto strain (SHRs).

Several studies, using a variety of immunohistochemical, histofluorescence, and neurochemical techniques, have reported hyper-innervation of the vasculature and increased NE concentrations in vascular tissue of SHRs (Adams et al., 1989; Burnstock, 1990; Cassis et al., 1985; Scott and Pang, 1983). Scott and Pang (1983) noted jejunal arterial hyper-innervation in SHRs from two weeks of age onwards, suggesting that the hyper-innervation does not result from hypertension or medial hypertrophy. Adams et al. (1989) reported increased tissue NE concentrations in the forelimb muscles, kidney, and left ventricle and septum at most ages in SHRs, and increased NE turnover (as indicated by fractional rate constants of tissue NE concentrations after inhibition of catecholamine synthesis) in these tissues (especially in the heart) in juvenile SHRs.

Monofluoromethyldopa, an irreversible DDC inhibitor, produces a much larger decrease in blood pressure in SHRs than in WKY control rats (Fozard et al., 1980;

1981). Depletion of NE in the heart and portal vein and attenuated cardiovascular responses to stimulation of SNS outflow accompany the hypotensive responses. Assuming that these changes result from blockade of decarboxylation of DOPA, they also support increased NE turnover and an increased SNS contribution to hypertension in SHRs.

Many reports have described exaggerated release of NE during regional sympathetic stimulation of vascular tissue in SHRs (Ekas et al., 1982, 1983; Cassis et al., 1985; Collis et al., 1979; Galloway and Westfall, 1982; Kowasaki et al., 1982; Scott and Pang, 1983; Tsuda et al., 1984a, 1984b, 1986, 1987a, 1987b; Westfall et al., 1987), the phenomenon again most apparent in juvenile animals.

Juvenile SHRs have increased plasma levels of NE, compared with values in normotensive WKY rats (Grobecker et al., 1975; Nakamura and Nakamura, 1978; Pak, 1981; Palermo et al., 1981; Roizen et al., 1975; Szemeredi, Bagdy et al., 1988b). In adults, the strain difference is less apparent or absent. One report indicated increased plasma levels of metabolites of NE and normal plasma levels of NE itself (Vlachakis and Alexander, 1981). Juvenile SHRs also have augmented plasma EPI responses to icv CRH (Brown, Hauger et al., 1988).

Stroke-prone SHRs have particularly high plasma EPI concentrations (Howe et al., 1986). Even after ganglion blockade with pentolinium, stroke-prone SHRs have higher basal plasma catecholamine levels than do normotensive control rats, suggesting that increased preganglionic sympathetic nerve traffic underlies the adrenomedullary hypersecretion. In response to hydralazine-induced hypotension, SHRs have markedly excessive increases in plasma EPI levels, indicating augmented reflexive release of EPI.

The excessive NE release in juvenile SHRs depends partly on abnormal peripheral presynaptic modulation of NE release, by α_2-adrenoceptors (Ekas et al., 1982, 1983; Masuyama et al., 1986; Tsuda et al., 1987b), AII receptors (Kowasaki et al., 1982), prostaglandins (Tsuda et al., 1987a), or ANP (Tsuda et al., 1986). Regarding α_2-adrenoceptors, juvenile SHRs have markedly augmented responses of plasma levels of NE, EPI, and DHPG after systemic administration of yohimbine (Szemeredi, Bagdy et al., 1988b), indicating enhanced α_2-adrenoceptor-mediated restraint of catecholamine release; however, Westfall et al. (1987) reported no differences between juvenile SHRs and WKY control rats in the amount of yohimbine-induced enhancement of NE release during field stimulation of isolated caudal arteries.

Since adrenal tissue from fetal SHRs has increased TH activity (Teitelman et al., 1981), accelerated adrenomedullary catecholamine biosynthesis appears to occur early in the ontogenesis of SHRs. Grobecker et al. (1982), however, reported significantly decreased activities of TH, DBH, and PNMT in juvenile SHRs. No studies have compared the expression of mRNAs for catecholamine-synthesizing enzymes in adrenals of juvenile SHRs and WKY control rats.

Juvenile SHRs have increased concentrations of autoradiographic grains in superior cervical and stellate ganglia after incubation of the tissues with [^{3}H]DOPA (Kondo, 1987), implying increased ganglionic synthesis of NE. Newborn animals have the most prominent increases in [^{3}H]DOPA incorporation. Dissociated superior ganglion cells from SHRs have characteristic multiple action potentials in response to intracellular, long-duration, depolarization pulses. This multiple firing results from lack of stimulation of Ca^{2+}-activated K^+ conductance (Jubelin and Kannan, 1990).

Central neural pathways, including noradrenergic centers, contribute to the augmented sympathoneural and pressor responses of SHRs. Posterior hypothalamic ablation immediately decreases blood pressure of SHRs (Bunag and Eferakeya, 1976), and posterior hypothalamic stimulation evokes excessive pressor responses in SHRs (Kawasaki et al., 1991), with normal responses to infused NE or AII. Juvenile SHRs have increased NE concentrations in the posterior hypothalamus, LC, and medullary A1 area (Winternitz et al., 1984). Tsai and Lin (1987) reported higher rates of turnover of catecholamines in the hypothalamus and brainstem of SHRs than in normotensive WKY control rats; Nakamura and Nakamura (1978) found increased DBH in the LC, A2 region of the brainstem, and intermediolateral columns of the spinal cord, suggesting increased NE turnover; Qualy and Westfall (1988) noted increased NE release, measured using a push-pull cannula, in the PVN in SHRs; Koulu et al. (1986) reported increased rates of catecholamine synthesis in the LC of young SHRs; and Kawasaki et al. (1991) reported enhanced posterior hypothalamic NE release during chemical stimulation of the LC in SHRs. Hypothalamic synaptosomes from juvenile (7-week-old) SHRs have increased release of endogenous NE during electric field stimulation and have increased uptake of [^{3}H]NE, compared with findings in WKY control rats, with no strain differences in adult (13-week old) animals (Hano et al., 1989).

Eilam et al. (1991) provided probably the most spectacular evidence for a role of the hypothalamus in the pathogenesis of hypertension in SHRs. Grafting hypothalamic neurons from embryonic SHRs into the hypothalamus of adult normotensive rats increased blood pressure of the recipient rats by 31%, compared with values in a group receiving grafts from embryonic WKY control rats.

Other studies have disagreed with the notion of globally increased central noradrenergic function in SHRs, instead supporting deficient ascending inhibition by medullary noradrenergic centers. Fujino (1984) reported decreased NE concentrations and decreased rates of catecholamine synthesis in the NTS of young SHRs, and Nomura et al. (1985) found decreased medullary NE levels. Smith and Barron (1990a, 1990b, 1990c) proposed, based on results of local microinjections of bicuculline to block GABA-ergic activity and glutamate to stimulate cellular activity, that SHRs have a deficiency of tonic sympathoinhibition by the CVLM.

Several reports have noted augmented central α_2-adrenoceptor-mediated responses in SHRs, including mydriatic responses (Yarbrough et al., 1983) and responses of growth hormone levels (Eriksson et al., 1986) to clonidine. Clonidine also abolishes the exaggerated sympathoneural response to shaker stress in SHRs (Takeda et al., 1990). Recent findings using microdialysis have indicated increased α_2-adrenoceptor-mediated restraint of NE release and of in vivo catecholamine biosynthesis in the posterolateral hypothalamus of juvenile SHRs (Pacak, Yadid et al., 1993), and Luque et al. (1991) reported increased α_2-adrenoceptor binding in the LC of SHRs. Nomura et al. (1985) and Gulati (1991), however, reported decreased medullary α_2-adrenoceptor numbers in

SHRs. One explanation for these disparate findings is that SHRs may have decreased post-synaptic α_2-adrenoceptors in the medulla and increased presynaptic α_2-adrenoceptors at sites higher in the brainstem.

Augmented central neural catecholamine biosynthesis in SHRs does not necessarily imply augmented central NE synthesis. Pituitary gland concentrations of DOPAC, a deaminated metabolite of DA, in SHRs exceed by about six fold values in WKY control rats (Sim and Hsu, 1990), suggesting excessive DA turnover in the tuberoinfundibular tract or adenohypophysis of SHRs; and increased DOPAC levels in posterior hypothalamic microdialysate (Pacak, Yadid et al., 1993) may result from increased NE or DA synthesis, or both. Van den Buuse and co-workers (van den Buuse, De Kloet et al., 1984; van den Buuse, Versteeg et al., 1984; van den Buuse et al., 1986) have focused on the possible pathophysiological role of increased central neural dopaminergic function in SHRs.

SHRs have markedly excessive sympathoneural responses to a variety of stressors (Chieuh and McCarty, 1981; Koepke and DiBona, 1985a, 1985b, 1986; Lundin and Thoren, 1982; Lundin et al., 1983, 1984; McCarty and Kopin, 1978; Takeda et al., 1990; Yamamoto et al., 1985, 1987). Chiueh and McCarty (1981) reported not only excessive plasma catecholamine responses but also excessive corticosterone responses to footshock in SHRs, consistent with excessive elicitation of a patterned distress response, rather than isolated dysregulation of SNS outflow. After systemic administration of yohimbine, however, juvenile SHRs have exaggerated responses of plasma levels of catechols without exaggerated responses of plasma ACTH levels (Szemeredi, Bagdy et al., 1988b, 1993).

The role of augmented stress responses in the development of hypertension in SHRs remains unclear. In contrast with SHRs of the Okamoto strain, New Zealand SHRs do not have excessive plasma catecholamine responses during aversive classical conditioning (McCarty, 1981). F1 hybrids of SHRs, presumably genetically susceptible to develop hypertension, fail to develop elevated blood pressure in response to aggregation or isolation, despite increased plasma NE levels, adrenal hypertrophy, and gastric erosions (Harrap et al., 1984). In contrast, Hubbard et al. (1986a, 1986b) reported that similar hybrid offspring of hypertensive rats (female SHRs mated with male WKY normotensive rats) developed stress-induced hypertension, with excessive blood pressure and catecholamine responses during classical aversive conditioning. Hendley et al. (1988) obtained evidence from different substrains derived from the Okamoto WKY rats that behavioral hyperreactivity could be separated from blood pressure dysregulation in adult animals. Hyperactive inbred adults had excessive plasma catecholamine responses to footshock, whereas hypertensives did not. Whether this is the case before hypertension develops is unclear. Peruzzi et al. (1991) noted hypertrophy of stellate ganglion cells in the hypertensive but not in the hyperactive substrain. Thus, evidence to date is inadequate to determine whether the exaggerated behavioral and catecholaminergic responses of SHRs of the Okamoto strain actually are related causally to the development of hypertension.

Several reports by Koepke and coworkers (Koepke and DiBona, 1985a, 1985b, 1986;

Koepke et al., 1986, 1987) have indicated participation of central neural α_2- and β_2-adrenoceptors in the excessive anti-natriuretic and sympathoneural responses of SHRs to stress. Koepke et al. (1987) obtained evidence that α_2-adrenoceptors in the amygdala participate in the excessive renal sympathoneural responses to air-puff stress in SHRs, and Folkow et al. (1982) reported attenuation of hypertension development in SHRs with amygdala lesions.

As noted in Chapter 2, emotional stress or hypothalamic stimulation resets the arterial baroreflex—especially the cardiac vagal component. Knuepfer et al. (1991) noted decreased baroreflex–cardiac gain in SHRs and greater suppression of baroreflex–cardiac gain by electrical stimulation of the amygdala in SHRs than in WKY rats. Lundin et al. (1983, 1984) reported excessive renal sympathoneural responsiveness to stress in SHRs and altered baroreflex–cardiac sensitivity, without baroreflex–sympathoneural resetting. Morrison and Whitehorn (1982), and Luft, Demmert et al. (1986) reported diminished baroreflex–cardiac gain and normal or even accentuated baroreflex–sympathoneural gain in SHRs. Kumagai et al. (1992) reported both blunted arterial baroreflex–heart rate and baroreflex–renal sympathoneural gain in SHRs. Taken together, these observations suggest altered central integration of baroreflex responses in SHRs of the Okamoto strain; however, whether SHRs have both decreased baroreflex–vagal and baroreflex–SNS responsiveness has not been established. Abolition of baroreflexes does not normalize excessive sympathoneural activity in SHRs (Morrison and Whitehorn, 1982; Schramm and Chornoboy, 1982).

The massive literature about SNS and AHS abnormalities in SHRs justifies a few conclusions. First, young SHRs have increased SNS and AHS outflows at rest, compared with outflows in age-matched WKY rats, and distress augments the strain differences. Insufficient evidence about responses of other stress systems in SHRs prevents conclusions about whether SHRs have abnormal expression of stress response patterns in general that may cause or contribute to development of hypertension. Second, SHRs have abnormalities of catecholaminergic function at all levels of the sympathetic neuraxis, including the brain, spinal cord, postganglionic nerves, and nerve terminals. This multiplicity of abnormalities leads to the suggestion that SHRs possess an abnormal genetic "algorithm" that directs abnormal development of sympathetic neuroeffector mechanisms. Third, juvenile SHRs have enhanced α_2-adrenoceptor-mediated restraint of hypothalamic NE release and catecholamine biosynthesis. These changes may result from decreased release of NE as an inhibitory transmitter in ascending pathways from the lower brainstem, or from compensatory up-regulation in response to increased local NE release.

What the "algorithm" consists of remains a mystery. One possibility is that SHRs have augmented growth of catecholamine-synthesizing neurons in the periphery and in the central nervous system. The mesenteric arteries, aorta, and spleen of juvenile but not adult SHRs have higher concentrations of nerve growth factor (NGF) than do age-matched WKY control rats (Donohue et al., 1989; Ueyama et al., 1992). SHRs also have enhanced tissue expression of mRNA for NGF in mesenteric arteries from 2-, 10-, and 43-day old animals (Falckh et al., 1992).

Prevention of Hypertension and Cardiovascular Hypertrophy

The finding of catecholaminergic abnormalities in juvenile SHRs does not imply that these abnormalities actually contribute to the development of the hypertension. Evidence from studies of effects of sympatholytic procedures in neonatal or juvenile animals has generally supported such a contribution.

Sympathetic activity exerts a trophic effect on the development of blood vessels. In neonatal SHRs, administration of antiserum to NGF, combined with guanethidine, completely prevents the development of hypertension (Lee et al., 1987). Cutilletta et al. (1977) reported that peripheral sympathectomy with NGF antiserum alone prevented the development of hypertension in male SHRs. The combination of NGF antiserum, guanethidine, and prazosin prevents not only the development of hypertension but also the development of cardiovascular hypertrophy in SHRs (Korner et al., 1993). Systemic administration of 6-OHDA, a neurotoxin at noradrenergic and dopaminergic terminals, in neonatal SHRs attenuates by at least one-half increments in mean arterial pressure measured later in life (Provoost and De Jong, 1978; Rascher et al., 1983). These results imply that the development of the hypertension requires an intact sympathoneural system.

Renal sympathectomy inhibits development of hypertension in SHRs (Liard, 1977; Saynavalammi et al., 1982), and since SHRs have excessive renal neural responses during aversive conditions, as described above, augmented neurogenic sodium retention in SHRs may provide a mechanism whereby excessive neurogenic pressor responses eventually lead to fixed hypertension. PVN lesions retard the hypertension (Ciriello et al., 1984), as does adrenal demedullation or β_2-adrenoceptor blockade (Borkowski and Quinn, 1985), the latter findings consistent with the "epinephrine hypothesis."

The development of cardiovascular hypertrophy in SHRs also appears to depend at least partly on catecholaminergic mechanisms. Administration of sympatholytic agents to SHRs prevents hyperplastic changes in small resistance vessels (Lee et al., 1987). β-Adrenoceptor antagonists or central sympatholytics such as α-methylDOPA attenuate the development of cardiac hypertrophy in SHRs, and blockade of NE formation by DBH inhibition decreases heart weights of SHRs (Ohlstein et al., 1987). Superior cervical ganglionectomy prevents the development of cerebrovascular hypertrophy in young SHRs (Sadoshima et al., 1986). As noted above, the combination of NGF antiseum, guanethidine, and prazosin prevents both the vascular and myocardial hypertrophy (Korner et al., 1993).

SHRs have an excessive rate of protein synthesis in venous tissue (Greenberg and Wilborn, 1982a), and propranolol or clonidine treatment normalizes the protein synthetic rate, independently of the anti-hypertensive actions of these drugs (Greenberg, 1981; Greenberg and Wilborn, 1982b). Similar findings have been noted in myocardial tissue (Greenberg and Wilborn, 1982c) and in posterior cerebral arteries of SHRs (Nakada et al., 1986).

The structural cardiovascular changes in SHRs probably do not simply reflect consequences of increased pressure, since detectable structural vascular changes in small arteries and arterioles of SHRs appear as early as 15 days after birth, when blood pressure is normal or only slightly increased (Folkow and Karlstrom, 1984; Nordborg and Johannson, 1982); and even neonatal SHRs can have enlarged left ventricles (Hallback-Nordlander, 1980). Moreover, peripheral sympathectomy with NGF antiserum can prevent the development of hypertension without preventing left ventricular hypertrophy in SHRs (Cutilleta et al., 1977).

Instead, catecholamines appear to foster pressure-independent cardiovascular hypertrophy (Alicandri et al., 1982; Egan and Julius, 1985; Kanbe et al., 1983). In vivo as well as in vitro studies have shown that NE directly stimulates medial hypertrophy and polyploidization of aortic smooth muscle cells (Yamori et al., 1980, 1981) and increases the growth rate of smooth muscle cells in secondary culture (Blaes and Bloissel, 1983). In rats, long-term treatment with low doses of catecholamines or with tyramine to release endogenous amines produces myocardial hypertrophy and increased collagen synthesis (as indicated by ventricular concentrations of hydroxyproline), without affecting blood pressure or heart rate (Genovese et al., 1984; Newling et al. (1989).

Treatment with prazosin or metoprolol alone attenuates but does not prevent NE-induced ventricular hypertrophy, as indicated by left ventricular weight and RNA content, whereas the combination of these agents prevents the NE-induced alterations (Zierhut and Zimmer, 1989). Cardiac hypertrophy due to systemic NE administration therefore appears to depend on agonistic occupation of both α_1- and β_1-adrenoceptors. Whether adrenoceptors mediate cardiac hypertrophy due to increased release of endogenous amines, such as by tyramine, is unknown.

Human Essential Hypertension

Abnormalities of sympathoneural activity, catecholamine uptake or metabolism, and cardiovascular smooth muscle responses to endogenous NE have long been suspected to contribute to the pathogenesis of clinical primary hypertension. Decades before epidemiologic studies showed that even moderate hypertension shortens life-span and increases cardiovascular morbidity, surgical sympathectomy successfully ameliorated severe hypertension in a substantial proportion of patients (Allen and Adson, 1938). After pharmacotherapy superseded neurosurgery in the treatment of hypertension, many effective antihypertensive agents were found to work by interfering with sympathetic neurotransmission, blocking cardiac or vascular adrenoceptors, or stimulating central neural adrenoceptors, implicating adrenergic mechanisms in the hypertensive process.

According to the model proposed by Shepherd (1990), four factors produce increased sympathetic outflow and increased total peripheral resistance in clinical primary hypertension: baroreflex resetting, genetic constitution, stress, and RAS activity in the brain and periphery. Alterations in circulating levels of humoral factors such as an endogenous digoxin-like substance (Blaustein and Hamlyn, 1991), ANP (Ferrari et al., 1990; Ganau et al., 1989; Taylor et al., 1989), steroids, and EPI; structural adaptive changes in vascular walls (Folkow, 1982); endothelium-derived relaxing and contracting factors; membrane and intracellular mechanisms such as adrenoceptor numbers and types, second messengers, ion channels, and protein phosphorylation all would interact with the increased sympathoneural outflow, leading to an abnormal renal function curve, the long-term determinant of high blood pressure (Guyton, 1991).

The important issue in considering this sort of model is not the individual tiles in a complex mosaic (since they change continually with the discovery of additional vaso-active substances) but, rather the goal-directedness of the entire mosaic. What homeostats regulate them, and how and why do the homeostats reset? As in SHRs, patients with essential hypertension can have abnormalities of catecholaminergic function at virtually all levels of the sympathetic neuraxis (Figure 7–3); and as in SHRs, these abnormalities are more apparent or are detectable only in relatively young patients, suggesting a role in the development of the hypertension.

Overall, patients with established essential hypertension do not appear to have increased directly recorded skeletal muscle sympathetic activity (SMSA) at rest (Morlin et al, 1983; Sundlof and Wallin, 1978a; Wallin et al., 1987) or during isometric handgrip exercise (Wallin et al., 1987). A proportion of patients with borderline or mild hypertension, however, do have excessive peroneal SMSA at baseline (Anderson et al., 1989; Mark, 1990; Matsukawa et al., 1991a, 1991b), during the cold pressor test (Matsukawa et al., 1987, 1991b), during unloading of cardiopulmonary ''low pressure'' baroreceptors (Rea and Hamdan, 1990), or during stimulation of arterial baroreceptors (Matsukawa et al., 1991a).

Yamada et al. (1989) reported higher SMSA in hypertensives than normotensives, regardless of the age of the compared groups. The findings of Yamada et al. (1989) and Matsukawa et al. (1991a, 1991b), which disagree with those of Sundlof and Wallin (1978a), Wallin et al. (1987), and Morlin et al. (1983), corroborate an impression from the literature about plasma NE levels (Fujita et al., 1984; Horikoshi et al., 1985; Iimura et al., 1984; Kawano et al., 1982; Masuo et al., 1984; Masuyama, 1982; Matsukawa et al., 1991a, 1991b; Ogawa et al., 1981; Saito et al., 1984) that Japanese hypertensives are more likely to have evidence for increased SNS outflow than are hypertensives from other ethnic groups.

The findings of Rea and Hamdan (1990) suggest increased gain of the cardiac baroreceptor–sympathoneural reflex in borderline hypertensives, in contrast with the common finding of decreased gain of the arterial baroreceptor–cardiac reflex (Bristow et al., 1969; Goldstein, 1983a; Mark, 1990).

Plasma Norepinephrine and the Autonomic Contribution to Hypertension

Given the large number of factors regulating blood pressure, and the likely heterogeneity of clinical hypertension, the contribution of increased autonomic activity to essential hypertension must vary widely across individual patients. Doyle and Smirk (1955) used a pharmacologic method to estimate the neurogenic component, based on the fall in blood pressure during ganglionic blockade. Applying an analogous method, Korner et al. (1973) found an increased autonomic contribution to total peripheral resistance in hypertensives, but with 60% to 80% of the observed difference from that in normotensives due to nonautonomic factors. As discussed previously, compensatory activation of other pressure-regulatory systems would lead to underestimation of the contribution of the autonomic component. Compensatory activation acutely, and

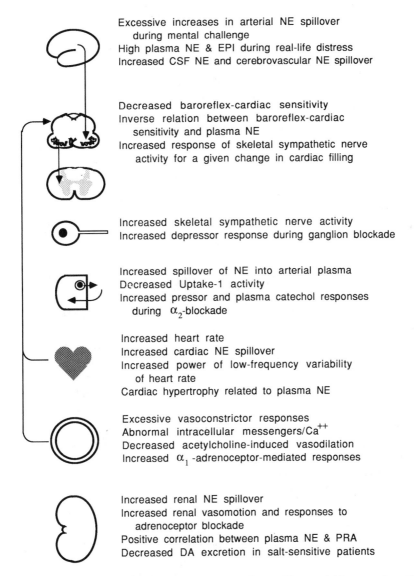

Excessive increases in arterial NE spillover
    during mental challenge
High plasma NE & EPI during real-life distress
Increased CSF NE and cerebrovascular NE spillover

Decreased baroreflex-cardiac sensitivity
Inverse relation between baroreflex-cardiac
    sensitivity and plasma NE
Increased response of skeletal sympathetic nerve
    activity for a given change in cardiac filling

Increased skeletal sympathetic nerve activity
Increased depressor response during ganglion blockade

Increased spillover of NE into arterial plasma
Decreased Uptake-1 activity
Increased pressor and plasma catechol responses
    during α_2-blockade

Increased heart rate
Increased cardiac NE spillover
Increased power of low-frequency variability
    of heart rate
Cardiac hypertrophy related to plasma NE

Excessive vasoconstrictor responses
Abnormal intracellular messengers/Ca^{++}
Decreased acetylcholine-induced vasodilation
Increased α_1-adrenoceptor-mediated responses

Increased renal NE spillover
Increased renal vasomotion and responses to
    adrenoceptor blockade
Positive correlation between plasma NE & PRA
Decreased DA excretion in salt-sensitive patients

Figure 7–3. Some catecholaminergic abnormalities in patients with essential hypertension. All the findings are more apparent or only detected in relatively young patients (less than about 40 years old). The multiplicity of loci of abnormalities resembles that in SHRs, probably because of heterogeneity in hypertensive mechanisms in the clinical hypertensive population. For all these abnormalities, extensive overlap exists with findings in normotensives.

hypertrophic processes that produce "amplifier" effects chronically (Korner, 1982), compromise inferences from depressor or vasodilator responses during autonomic blockade in the estimation of autonomic cardiovascular "tone" in hypertension. Moreover, evidence summarized by De Champlain (1990) has supported the view that as hypertension becomes established, postsynaptic α_1-adrenoceptor-mediated responses become enhanced and β-adrenoceptor-mediated responses attenuated. These limitations have led to abandonment of the use of ganglionic or adrenoceptor blockers to estimate autonomic tone from effects on blood pressure or peripheral resistance.

Both cardiac parasympathetic inhibition and sympathoneural activation contribute to the elevated mean heart rate in young hypertensives (Julius et al., 1971; Julius and Esler, 1975). Borderline hypertensives have decreased salivary flow, consistent with decreased PNS activity (Henquet et al., 1982). Antecubital venous plasma NE levels tend to correlate positively with pulse rate and negatively with baroreflex–cardiac sensitivity among hypertensive patients (Goldstein, 1983a; Goldstein, Levinson et al., 1985).

Analytical reviews have summarized the voluminous literature about plasma NE levels in clinical hypertension (Goldstein, 1981a, 1983b). Distributions of antecubital venous plasma NE levels in hypertensive patients are wider and shifted significantly toward higher values than distributions in normotensive control subjects, but with substantial overlap between the distributions (Goldstein, Lake et al., 1983; Goldstein, Levinson et al, 1985), indicating the absence of a discrete hypernoradrenergic subgroup. Other reports have noted increased plasma levels of NE metabolites in hypertensives (Ludwig et al., 1991; Vlachakis et al., 1981), with normal levels of NE itself.

After taking into account several possibly confounding factors, including body-mass index, individual maximum physical work capacity, urinary sodium excretion, and anxiety scores, relatively young patients with borderline hypertension have increased antecubital venous plasma NE concentrations compared to values in age-matched normotensive subjects (Matsukawa et al., 1991a, 1991b; Perini et al., 1990a, 1990b). Plasma EPI levels at baseline may be normal (Perini et al., 1990a, 1990b) or increased (Matsukawa et al., 1991a, 1991b).

Combined assessments of neurohormonal factors and hemodynamic responses to adrenergic drugs can improve the accuracy of identifying patients with an augmented sympathoneural contribution to blood pressure. For instance, hypernoradrenergic patients have larger depressor responses to clonidine and larger pressor responses to yohimbine than do pressure-matched patients with normal plasma NE levels (Goldstein, Grossman, Listwak et al., 1991; Goldstein, Levinson et al., 1985; Grossman et al., 1993). Hypernoradrenergic hypertensives have augmented depressor responses during treatment with atenolol (Myers and De Champlain, 1983), and depressor responses during acute α- and β-adrenoceptor blockade vary directly with baseline plasma NE levels (Agabiti-Rosei et al., 1982), but depressor responses to hydrochlorothiazide do not (Myers and De Champlain, 1983). Hypernoradrenergic hypertensives tend to have increased PRA (Esler, Jennings et al., 1986; Goldstein, 1985), and whereas most patients with both high plasma NE levels and increased PRA respond well to treatment with a β-adrenoceptor blocker or a combined α- and β-adrenoceptor blocker, few respond to a diuretic (Esler et al., 1977; Masuyama, 1982). The combination of high baseline levels of NE and PRA, a large depressor response to clonidine, and a large pressor response to yohimbine may therefore identify patients with an increased sympathoneural contribution to blood pressure better than does any of these measures in isolation. The value of this profiling, both in therapeutic decision-making and in predicting cardiovascular morbidity, is unknown.

Hypertensive patients with elevated plasma NE concentrations also appear to respond well to relaxation therapy for hypertension (Lee et al., 1989). McGrady and Higgins (1989) have suggested that a "hypertensive predictor profile," based on evidence of autonomic overactivity (e.g., cool hands, fast pulse rate, high anxiety scores), can predict responses to biofeedback-assisted relaxation in patients with essential hypertension.

A small proportion of hypertensive patients have a hyperkinetic syndrome characterized by increased heart rate and cardiac output, labile hypertension with prominent increases in systolic blood pressure, diaphoresis, tremor, sensitivity to isoproterenol, and amelioration of all of these manifestations by propranolol treatment (Frohlich, 1977; Frohlich et al., 1969). In a detailed study of one such patient, Goldstein and Keiser (1985) found excessive increments in plasma catecholamines during administration of isoproterenol or yohimbine and poor baroreflex–cardiac sensitivity that improved after acute sedation with intravenous diazepam. Some of these findings resemble those in juvenile SHRs. Increased heart rate and cardiac output may be early findings in the development of essential hypertension; in young, borderline hypertensives, these abnormalities seem to be neurogenic, resulting from a combination of increased cardiac sympathetic and decreased vagal outflow (Julius et al, 1971; Widimsky et al, 1957). The hyperdynamic circulation syndrome is discussed later in this chapter.

The Age Factor

Since cardiac output decreases and total peripheral resistance increases in hypertensive patients followed longitudinally (Lund-Johansen, 1986, 1989), the hemodynamic mechanism of essential hypertension shifts, but the hypertension persists. Julius (1990) has proposed that the central nervous system "seeks" to maintain a higher blood pressure, with increasing vascular responsiveness due at least partly to structural cardiovascular adaptation (Folkow, 1982) and with less sympathetic drive to maintain the hypertension over time. The bulk of available evidence about plasma NE levels and aging supports the view that at least in some patients with primary hypertension, a transition occurs from a neurogenic to a nonneurogenic basis for the high blood pressure.

Plasma NE concentrations increase with increasing subject age (e.g., Ziegler et al., 1976; Goldstein, 1983b; Goldstein, Lake et al., 1983). Directly recorded SMSA also increases with subject age in hypertensive as well as normotensive groups (Morlin et al., 1983; Sundlof and Wallin, 1978; Yamada et al., 1989). Groups of hypertensives often do not have age-related increases in plasma NE levels, because a proportion of young patients have elevated plasma NE levels (Barnes et al., 1982; Dominiak and Grobecker, 1982; Esler, Lambert et al., 1990; Esler et al., 1986; Fujita et al., 1984; Goldstein, Lake et al., 1984; Iimura et al., 1984; Izzo et al., 1987; Kawano et al., 1982; Masuo et al., 1984; Matsukawa et al., 1991a, 1991b; Ogawa et al., 1981; Premel-Cabic et al., 1987; Saito et al., 1984; Sowers et al., 1987; Tuck et al., 1985). Nevertheless, even young patients with borderline hypertension do not consistently have increased plasma NE levels at baseline (Goldstein, Eisenhofer et al., 1989; Saito et al., 1984). Izzo et al. (1987) reported that among white men with essential hypertension, plasma NE levels correlated positively with mean arterial pressure, after correction for age.

Esler et al. (1986) and Esler, Lambert et al. (1990) found that the magnitude of increase in total body spillover of NE in hypertensive patients varied inversely with age. Findings about NE kinetics are summarized later in this chapter.

Whereas plasma NE levels tend to increase with age among normotensive people, plasma EPI levels do not. Elderly subjects can have larger plasma NE responses to experimental ''mental stress'' than do younger subjects; plasma EPI responses do not appear to change with aging (Barnes et al., 1982).

Norepinephrine Kinetics in Hypertension

Relatively young patients with essential hypertension have increased spillover of NE into antecubital venous or arterial plasma (Esler, Jackman et al., 1981; Esler, Jennings et al., 1984a, 1986, 1989a; Goldstein, Horwitz et al., 1983), with normal plasma NE clearance (Esler, Hasking et al., 1985; Goldstein, Horwitz et al., 1983). Since normotensive subjects with a family history of hypertension have higher rates of NE spillover into arterial plasma than do normotensives without a family history of hypertension (Ferrier et al., 1993), increased sympathetically mediated NE release may either contribute to or provide a marker for the later development of hypertension in humans.

Increased sympathetic outflow or decreased Uptake-1 activity increases estimated NE spillover (Esler, Jackman et al., 1981; Goldstein, Horwitz et al., 1983; Ohashi et al, 1985), and no study has clearly differentiated these factors in patients with essential hypertension. Esler, Jackman et al. (1981) and Goldstein, Horwitz et al. (1983), reported indirect evidence for decreased Uptake-1 activity in some patients; and elevated circulating levels of chromogranin A (O'Connor et al., 1984) and of SMSA have suggested increased sympathetically mediated exocytosis.

Since measurements of spillover rates of endogenous NE into arterial plasma can fail to detect abnormalities of regional NE spillover in particular vascular beds, recent research has emphasized assessments of regional NE kinetics. Hypertensive patients have increased cardiac and renal spillover of NE (Esler, Hasking et al., 1985; Esler, Jennings et al., 1986, 1989a), the hypertensive–normotensive differences again most apparent in young subject groups. Since hypertensive patients do not have reduced regional fractional extractions of [^{3}H]-labeled NE in the heart and kidneys, decreased Uptake-1 activity alone cannot explain the increased spillover of NE in these beds (Esler, Lambert et al., 1990). Preliminary results have indicated increased spillover of NE into internal jugular venous plasma in some hypertensive patients, consistent with but by no means proving increased NE spillover in the central nervous system (Esler, Ferrier et al., 1991). In contrast with the positive findings in the heart and kidneys, hypertensives do not have increased NE spillover in the forearm, lungs, or hepatosplanchnic complex (Esler, Jennings et al., 1989a; Goldstein, Eisenhofer et al., 1989).

Studies using power spectral analysis of heart rate variability have reported evidence consistent with increased cardiac sympathetic and decreased cardiac parasympathetic activity (Guzzetti et al., 1988; Malliani et al., 1991) in hypertensives; however, as noted in the chapter about assessment techniques, power spectral analysis for measuring cardiac SNS activity has not yet been validated adequately.

Stress Responses

Brod and coworkers (Brod et al., 1959) were the first to measure regional hemodynamic responses to psychological stress (forced mental arithmetic) in patients with hypertension. Performance of forced mental arithmetic evoked renal vasoconstriction, decreased forearm skin temperature, increased forearm blood flow, and increased blood pressure in hypertensive and normotensive groups. Whereas in control subjects the increases in blood pressure resulted from increases in cardiac output, in hypertensive patients the increases in blood pressure resulted from increases in total peripheral resistance. Analogously, during playing a video game, young patients with hypertension increase their total peripheral resistance, whereas normotensive control subjects of similar age increase their cardiac output (Goldstein, Eisenhofer et al., 1989).

Many studies since then have reported excessive catecholaminergic, pressor, or vasoconstrictor responses to a variety of stressors in young patients with borderline or mild hypertension (Eliasson et al., 1983; Falkner et al., 1979, 1981; Goldstein, Eisenhofer et al., 1989; Horikoshi et al., 1985; Lenders et al., 1989a; Matsukawa et al., 1991b). Goldstein, Eisenhofer et al. (1989) found that during playing a video game, hypertensives aged 40 years old or younger had larger responses of arterial levels of EPI and of spillover of NE into arterial blood than did age-matched normotensive control subjects. The cardiac output and blood pressure responses in this setting correlated positively with changes in spillover of NE into arterial plasma. Goldstein, Grossman, Listwak et al. (1991) reported similar findings when yohimbine was used to increase sympathetic outflow pharmacologically. Falkner et al. (1979, 1981) reported that in borderline hypertensive adolescents, those with excessive physiologic responses to mental challenge had enhanced plasma catecholamine responses, as well as a higher risk for subsequent progression to established hypertension during a 41-month follow-up period.

Young Japanese subjects with borderline hypertension have been reported to have increased directly recorded SMSA, as well as increased plasma EPI and NE levels, compared to values in age-matched normotensive control subjects (Matsukawa et al., 1991a, 1991b). The hypertensives in the study of Matsukawa et al. (1991b) also had augmented SMSA and plasma NE responses during the cold pressor test, and whereas the controls had decreased SMSA during performance of mental arithmetic, the hypertensives did not. The pressor, plasma NE, and plasma EPI responses to mental arithmetic all were larger in the hypertensive than in the normotensive group.

Low et al. (1986) reported one of the few studies about catecholamine responses of hypertensives to other than laboratory stressors. During laryngoscopy prior to elective vascular surgery, hypertensives had markedly larger increases in plasma NE levels than did normotensive patients, and plasma EPI levels increased only in the hypertensive group.

Analogous to the findings described above in SHRs, excessive renal vasoconstrictor responses during emotional stress in hypertensives would be expected to contribute to a tendency to retain sodium. Brod (Brod, 1963; Brod et al., 1959) noted that some hypertensive patients responded to mental arithmetic with severe, prolonged renal vaso-constriction as well as excessive cutaneous and splanchnic vasoconstriction. Hollenberg et al. (1978) reported increased renovascular tone in the majority of young patients with uncomplicated hypertension, and Hollenberg and Sandor (1984) and Hollenberg et al. (1981) found excessive decreases in renal blood flow during emotional provocation in hypertensives. These investigators also noted emotion-related, exaggerated increases in renal oscillatory vasomotion in hypertensives.

Pressure-induced natriuresis can offset the antinatriuretic effect of renal vaso-constriction, complicating inferences about the pathophysiological significance of stress-related sodium retention in hypertensive patients. In men with borderline hypertension or a positive family history as a predisposition to develop hypertension, Light et al. (1983) reported increased renal sodium retention during a laboratory mental stress. In the high-risk group, the magnitude of urinary sodium retention cor-related positively with the magnitude of the heart rate response, suggesting common mediation by the SNS.

Folkow (1982) has hypothesized that individuals undergo many defense reactions daily, without the actual physical fight-or-flight behavior that would amplify skeletal vasodilation; and that chronic repetition of pressor episodes could cause long-lasting structural adaptation of arterioles, biasing toward the development of sustained hyper-tension. Studies of chronically repeated pressor episodes elicited by instrumental car-diovascular conditioning in nonhuman primates, however, have not consistently noted persistent hypertension after removal of the reinforcement contingencies (Turkkan et al., 1984). Chronic exposure of nonhuman primates to conflict-type stress also produces only small increases in blood pressure, although stress coupled with high dietary salt intake does produce moderate hypertension (Turkkan, 1991; Turkkan and Goldstein, 1991a, 1991b). Taken together, the results suggest that the defense reaction hypothesis may explain the development of hypertension only in individuals with underlying, as yet unidentified, susceptibilities. Consistent with this view, social disruption induces chronic hypertension in some normotensive inbred rat strains but not others (Henry et al., 1993).

Diagnostic labeling appears to increase plasma catecholamine levels at baseline and augment catecholamine and hemodynamic responses during exposure to a laboratory mental stressor in young hypertensives (Rostrup et al., 1991). Whether these effects occur specifically in hypertensives is unknown.

Personality

The possible existence and constituents of a "hypertensive personality" have incited debate for many years. Sommers-Flanagan and Greenberg (1989) concluded from a review of 48 studies that personality factors do characterize hypertensives. Researchers have failed to agree about the exact components of such a personality; most have implicated restrained aggressive impulses. Alexander (1939) suggested that hyperten-sives have an instability of vasomotor control, coupled with inhibited rage. Saul (1939) concluded that some hypertensives have chronic, unexpressed rage. Saslow et al. (1950)

reported an association between hypertension and obsessive-compulsive or subnormal assertiveness traits. Perini et al. (1990b) noted less externalized aggression, more internalized aggression, and more submissiveness in borderline hypertensives than in normotensive control subjects, with somewhat similar although less marked findings in offspring of hypertensive parents. Cottier et al. (1987) analyzed literature about suppressed hostility, the Type A behavior pattern, a constellation of neuroticism, anxiety and depression, inability to deal with life stresses, and ''alexithymia,'' referring to inappropriate affect, difficulty in verbal description of feelings, absence of fantasies, and acting on impulse. They concluded that although personality factors may characterize certain subgroups of patients, there is no convincing evidence that any of these factors actually relates causally to the development of hypertension. Markovitz et al. (1991) reported that Framingham Tension scores (a measure of anxiety) at baseline predicted increments in systolic blood pressure at a three-year followup examination in middle-aged women.

If there is a hypertensive personality, the patients who have it may also have increased sympathoneural outflows. Young patients with mild neurogenic hypertension (characterized by high plasma levels of catecholamines or PRA and sensitivity of blood pressure to autonomic blockade) tend to have anger or suppressed hostility (Esler, Julius et al., 1977; Sullivan et al., 1981a, 1981b). Starkman et al. (1990) found that in hypertensives with elevated plasma catecholamine levels, plasma NE levels were significantly positively correlated with self-rated anxiety scores. Goldstein, Grossman, Listwak et al. (1991) reported that in a subgroup of hypertensives with excessive pressor and catechol responses to yohimbine, virtually all the patients reported a history of anxiety, panic, depression, or antisocial behavior. Perini et al. (1991) conducted a prospective study of personality factors as predictors of hypertension development in young (18–24 year old) normotensive and borderline hypertensive subjects. Stress-induced pressor responses, indices of sympathoneural activity, and psychological factors predicted only weakly blood pressure classification at a mean of 30 months of follow-up. The largest pressure increases in pressure, however, occurred in subjects with suppressed aggression.

CSF Norepinephrine and Hypertension

Most studies about CSF NE in primary hypertension have reported increased levels in hypertensive patients (Cubeddu et al., 1984; DeQuattro et al., 1984; Eide et al., 1979; Kawano et al, 1982; Lake, Polinsky et al., 1980; Lake et al., 1981; Ziegler et al., 1982), leading to the inference that hypertensives have increased brain ''noradrenergic activity.'' Because the source of NE in CSF is unclear, as discussed in the chapter about assessment of catecholaminergic function, the extent to which CSF NE provides a ''window on the brain'' in clinical hypertension is also unclear.

As noted above, hypertensives have a higher mean rate of estimated NE spillover into the internal jugular veins than do normotensive control subjects (Esler, Jennings, and Lambert, 1988), consistent with increased NE spillover in the central nervous system. Whether patients with increased cerebrovascular NE spillover also have increased CSF NE levels has not been determined.

The Epinephrine Hypothesis

According to the "epinephrine hypothesis" for the development of essential hypertension (Floras, 1992; Majewski et al., 1981, 1982; Rand and Majewski, 1984), high circulating EPI levels in hypertensive patients increase neuronal uptake of EPI, and subsequent sympathetic stimulation coreleases neuronal EPI with NE, the released EPI activating presynaptic β-adrenoceptors and augmenting further NE release. The hypothesis therefore views EPI as an amplifier of sympathetically mediated pressor responses.

The role of this mechanism in the pathophysiology of clinical hypertension has received substantial attention; however, direct confirmatory evidence remains lacking. The chapter about peripheral catecholaminergic systems cites studies refuting key elements of the EPI hypothesis in laboratory animals. Several clinical studies have reported increased plasma EPI concentrations at baseline in patients with essential hypertension (for review see Goldstein, 1983b), but many other studies have not. Exogenously administered EPI may enhance neurogenic vasoconstriction (e.g., Floras et al., 1988a, 1990) in humans, but exactly how remains unknown. Amann et al. (1981) reported a positive correlation between plasma EPI levels and decrements in forearm vascular resistance during α_1-adrenoceptor blockade in hypertensives; however, the study did not determine whether EPI directly or indirectly augmented α_1-adrenoceptor-mediated responses. Finally, the EPI hypothesis cannot account easily for the generally poor correlations between plasma NE and EPI levels among individual patients (Goldstein and Lake, 1984).

Salt Sensitivity

Several groups have studied possible pathophysiologic mechanisms of salt-sensitive hypertension, generally referring to hypertensive patients in whom blood pressure increases by more than 3 to 10 mm Hg between a low- and high-salt diet. The research has emphasized the role of the RAS and catecholamines.

Williams, Hollenberg, and coworkers have reported that a substantial proportion of patients with hypertension fail to exhibit the usual enhancement of aldosterone responses and responses of renal blood flow to administered AII during sodium restriction (Williams and Hollenberg, 1985). This group of patients, designated "nonmodulators," also have a reduced ability to excrete a sodium load and delayed suppression of renin release after sodium loading (Tuck et al., 1976). The exact relationship between these findings and salt-sensitivity remains undefined, because a substantial minority of nonmodulators fail to increase their blood pressure on a high-salt diet.

In healthy people and in experimental animals, salt deprivation tends to increase and salt loading tends to decrease plasma NE levels (Brosnihan et al., 1981; Lake and Ziegler, 1978; Luft et al., 1979). Several reports have noted a failure to suppress plasma NE levels normally during dietary salt loading in salt-sensitive hypertensives (Campese et al., 1982; Dimsdale et al., 1990a; Fujita et al., 1980, 1984; Koolen et al., 1983). Other reports have indicated higher plasma NE levels in salt-sensitive than in salt-resistant hypertensives or normotensive control subjects even during normal salt intake (Masuo et al., 1984; Koolen et al., 1983, 1984). These findings are consistent with the suggestion that enhanced sympathoneural responsiveness contributes to salt sensitivity (Skrabal et al., 1983). Anderson et al. (1989) reported that hypertensives suppressed directly recorded SMSA normally during dietary salt loading; however, the investigators did not consider separately responses in salt-sensitive and salt-resistant hypertensives.

These studies have not considered the possibility that the failure of salt loading to suppress plasma NE levels in salt-sensitive patients may result from production of subclinical heart failure and compensatory recruitment of sympathoneural activity to maintain cardiac performance.

Several groups have hypothesized that an imbalance between the antinatriuretic catecholamine, NE, and the natriuretic catecholamine, DA, causes or contributes to salt sensitivity. Gill et al. (1988) reported an association between deficient responses of urinary DA excretion and deficient suppression of plasma NE levels dietary salt loading in salt-sensitive hypertensives. Weinberger et al. (1982) analogously reported lower values for a ''natriuretic index,'' the ratio of urinary DOPAC to urinary NE, in hypertensive than normotensive men during rapid administration or depletion of sodium; the investigators did not analyze results separately for salt-sensitive and salt-resistant subjects. Kuchel et al. (1979) reported decreased urinary DA excretion in patients with essential hypertension. In normotensive subjects with genetic risk of hypertension, Saito et al. (1984) reported the absence of the usual relationship between urinary DA and urinary sodium, and in salt-sensitive hypertensives, Harvey et al. (1984) and Shikuma et al. (1986) reported a failure to increase urinary DA excretion during dietary salt loading. Aoki et al. (1989) found that low-renin hypertensives, who would be expected to be salt-sensitive, had decreased urinary DA excretion for a given amount of estimated delivery of DOPA to the kidney. Iimura et al. (1990) reported similar findings in normotensive subjects with a family history of hypertension. Gill et al. (1991) studied responses of urinary DOPA and DA excretion during dietary salt restriction and loading in salt-sensitive and salt-resistant hypertensive inpatients. Salt-sensitive patients had a higher mean rate of DOPA excretion and a lower urinary DA/DOPA ratio than salt-resistant patients, regardless of dietary salt intake, suggesting deficient renal uptake or decarboxylation of DOPA in salt-sensitive patients.

Pressor Responsiveness and Baroreflexes

Patients with established hypertension often have exaggerated increments in blood pressure or total peripheral resistance after administration of any of a variety of vasoactive drugs, including NE. Excessive pressor responsiveness in hypertensives probably results from a complex combination of presynaptic and postsynaptic factors (Amman et al., 1981; Bianchetti et al., 1984; Bristow et al., 1969; De Champlain, 1990; Erne et al., 1984; Esler et al., 1981; Floras et al., 1988b; Folkow, 1982; Goldstein, 1983a; Matsukawa et al., 1991a, 1991b; Ohashi et al., 1985; Rea and Hamdan, 1990; Urabe et al., 1990; Weidmann et al., 1979; Figure 7–4). Mechanisms of presynaptic hyperresponsiveness include increased sympathoneural outflow, abnormal processing of baroreflex afferent information, or overexpression of centrally determined emotional or behavioral reactions. Mechanisms of postsynaptic hyperresponsiveness include altered vascular

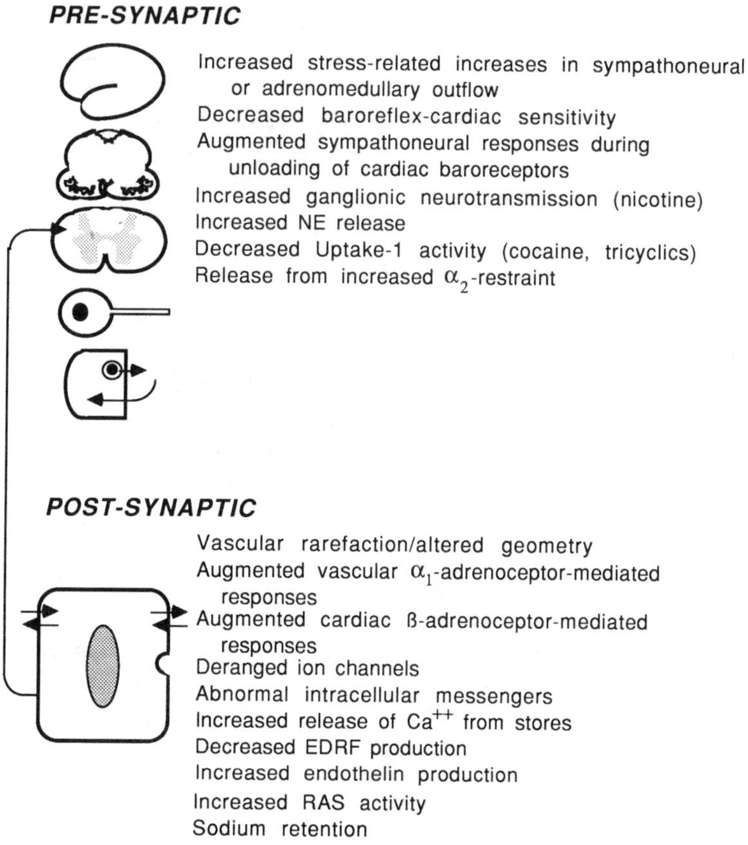

PRE-SYNAPTIC

Increased stress-related increases in sympathoneural
    or adrenomedullary outflow
Decreased baroreflex-cardiac sensitivity
Augmented sympathoneural responses during
    unloading of cardiac baroreceptors
Increased ganglionic neurotransmission (nicotine)
Increased NE release
Decreased Uptake-1 activity (cocaine, tricyclics)
Release from increased α_2-restraint

POST-SYNAPTIC

Vascular rarefaction/altered geometry
Augmented vascular α_1-adrenoceptor-mediated
    responses
Augmented cardiac ß-adrenoceptor-mediated
    responses
Deranged ion channels
Abnormal intracellular messengers
Increased release of Ca^{++} from stores
Decreased EDRF production
Increased endothelin production
Increased RAS activity
Sodium retention

Figure 7–4. Some potential mechanisms of excessive pressor responses in hypertensives. The many processes can be classified in terms of presynaptic and postsynaptic locations.

geometry, microvascular rarefaction, altered vascular smooth muscle excitation–contraction mechanisms, deranged local generation of vascular relaxant or stimulant factors, and altered adrenoceptor numbers or function.

Most studies have not assessed simultaneously more than one of these processes. Goldstein, Grossman, Listwak et al. (1991) provided a step in this direction, using a "yohimbine challenge test." Among young patients with borderline or mild hypertension, some had normal pressor responses and normal responses of arterial NE levels during yohimbine infusion; some had excessive pressor responses for a normal increment in plasma NE; and some had excessive increments in plasma NE levels, with pressor responses appropriate for the increases in NE levels. Thus, the yohimbine challenge test may distinguish patients with pressor hyperresponsiveness due to increased sympathetically mediated NE release from patients with pressor hyperresponsiveness due to increased postsynaptic responsiveness for a given amount of NE release.

Patients with essential hypertension do not appear to have overall increased responsiveness of isolated arteriolar smooth muscle to NE. Most studies have found normal or even decreased responsiveness, after exclusion of geometric factors such as wall thickness/lumen ratios (Aalkjaer et al., 1987a, 1987b; Horwitz et al., 1974). Egan et al. (1987) studied mechanisms of augmented vasoconstrictor responses to α-adrenoceptor agonists in patients with essential hypertension. Young men with mild hypertension had significantly higher arterial plasma NE levels than did normotensive control subjects. Although forearm vascular responses to intra-arterially infused NE were normal, α-adrenoceptor blockade by phentolamine produced larger decreases in forearm vascular resistance in hypertensives than in control subjects, suggesting that the increased α-adrenergic "tone" in hypertensives resulted from increased sympathetically mediated NE release.

Patients with essential hypertension have decreased baroreflex–cardiac gain (Bristow et al., 1969; Goldstein, 1983a). Atropinization, which markedly decreases baroreflex–cardiac sensitivity in humans, accentuates pressor responses (Goldstein and Keiser, 1984). Subjects with decreased baroreflex–cardiac sensitivity have increased spontaneous systolic pressures and pressure variability (Conway et al., 1984), and hypertensives with relatively low baroreflex–cardiac sensitivity have augmented pressor responses during bicycle exercise (Floras et al., 1988b).

Because resetting of the cardiac limb of the arterial baroreflex accompanies virtually all forms of experimental hypertension, it is unclear whether alterations in baroreflex function in essential hypertension constitute a primary or secondary phenomenon. Goldstein (1983a) reported an inverse relationship between arterial baroreflex sensitivity and arterial plasma NE concentrations. Although several explanations can potentially apply to this relationship, one is that hypertensives with increased sympathoneural activity also have decreased arterial baroreflex–cardiac gain. Chadwick et al. (1986) reported an association between increased arterial NE levels and decreased modulation of the brachial arterial dicrotic wave after injection of nitroglycerin in relatively young hypertensives, interpreted as evidence for a sympathoneural contribution to both the increased arterial stiffness and augmented pressor responsiveness in early hypertension. Parmer et al. (1992) reported lower mean arterial baroreflex–cardiac gain in normotensives with a family history of hypertension than in those without a family history of hypertension, suggesting that low arterial baroreflex sensitivity can indicate a risk for the development of hypertension rather than simply result from hypertension. Mark (1990) has proposed that increases in SMSA in mild hypertension do not result from impaired arterial baroreflexes but from increased central sympathetic outflow.

Whether patients with essential hypertension have alterations in arterial baroreflex–vascular or arterial baroreflex–sympathoneural gain has been less clear. Goldstein (1983a) obtained evidence for baroreflex–cardiac resetting in young hypertensives, without evidence for baroreflex–vascular resetting. Duprez et al. (1987) similarly observed no large differences between hypertensives and normotensives in vascular responsiveness to carotid baroreceptor stimulation or inhibition. Matsukawa et al. (1991b) reported decreased arterial baroreflex-mediated inhibition of SMSA after phenylephrine administration, with normal reflexive stimulation of sympathoneural activity after injection of nitroglycerine, an asymmetry that would tend to elevate blood pressure. Borderline hypertensives have changes in SMSA that are similar to those in normotensive control subjects when arterial baroreceptors are stimulated or inhibited by infusions of nitroprusside or phenylephrine while LBNP is used to hold central venous pressure (CVP) constant (Rea and Hamdan, 1990).

Patients with mild or borderline essential hypertension appear to have, if anything, increased cardiopulmonary baroreceptor reflex gain, in contrast with blunted barore-flex–cardiac gain. Unloading cardiopulmonary baroreceptors, by application of non-hypotensive LBNP, reduces CVP similarly in hypertensive and normotensive subjects, and heart rate and blood pressure remain unchanged; however, for any given decrease in CVP, hypertensives have larger increments in forearm vascular resistance (Mark and Kerber, 1982) and directly recorded SMSA (Rea and Hamdan, 1990). These results support the view that borderline hypertensives have increased gain of the low-pressure baroreceptor–sympathetic reflex. Since this augmented gain would tonically restrain sympathetic outflow, increased cardiopulmonary baroreflex gain could offset a central neural abnormality in regulation of sympathetic vascular tone, and LBNP would expose the abnormality. In established hypertension, or hypertension associated with myocardial hypertrophy and increased stiffness, the restraining influence of the cardiopulmonary baroreceptors could decline (Zanchetti and Mancia, 1991). This would help to explain the failure to detect augmented SMSA to LBNP in patients with chronic hypertension, as well as positive correlations between plasma NE levels and the severity of left ventricular hypertrophy, as discussed below.

Cardiovascular Stiffness and Hypertrophy

Cardiovascular hypertrophy in clinical hypertension does not appear to relate as directly to blood pressure as one might expect. One explanation for this discrepancy is that sympathetic activity can contribute to cardiac and vascular hypertrophy even in the absence of alterations in blood pressure (e.g., Alicandri et al., 1982; Borkowski and Quinn, 1985; Chadwick et al., 1986; Corea et al., 1982, 1983; Egan and Julius, 1985; Ganguly and Anderson, 1989; Genovese et al., 1984; Greenberg, 1981; Greenberg and Wilborn, 1982a, 1982b, 1982c; King et al., 1987; Newling et al., 1989; Ostman-Smith, 1981; Pauletto and Pessina, 1991; Sadoshima et al., 1986; Saynavalammi et al., 1982; Simpson et al., 1982; Zierhut and Zimmer, 1989). Among borderline hypertensives, baseline plasma NE levels correlate positively with minimum forearm vascular resistance (Egan and Julius, 1985), consistent with the view that increased sympathoneural activity contributes to the development of vascular hypertrophy. Corea and coworkers (Corea et al., 1982, 1983, 1984) reported positive correlations between plasma NE levels and severity of left ventricular hypertrophy in hypertensives. In young hypertensives, arterial plasma NE levels correlate positively with the extent of limitation in arteriolar dilation and arterial distensibility (Chadwick et al., 1986). Mental stress or systemic administration of EPI in humans increases plasma levels of a vascular growth factor, as indicated by the fraction of [³H]thymidine-positive nuclei assessed autoradiographically in cultured rat aortic smooth muscle cells (Larsson et al., 1989). Mechanisms by which catecholamines stimulate cardiovascular cell growth constitute an important subject matter for future applications of molecular biological techniques.

Chronic subcutaneous infusion of NE in dogs does not produce hypertension but does produce biventricular cardiac hypertrophy (King et al., 1987). Chronic repetition of neurogenic pressor episodes in dogs also elicits cardiac hypertrophy without hypertension (Julius et al., 1989). In borderline hypertensives, echocardiographically determined interventricular septal thickness correlates positively with plasma NE levels (Corea et al., 1982, 1983). No study has determined whether cardiac hypertrophy in hypertensives correlates with cardiac NE spillover.

Although associations between plasma NE levels and cardiac hypertrophy are consistent with a sympathoneural contribution to cardiovascular hypertrophy in hypertension, another explanation for these relationships is that impaired cardiac function resulting from ventricular hypertrophy may recruit sympathetic outflow compensatorily to maintain hemodynamic homeostasis. Thus, the association between SNS activation and cardiovascular hypertrophy in clinical hypertension may be causal, via effects of catecholamines on cardiovascular cell growth, or indirect and not causal, via compensatory activation of SNS outflows. The discussion below about the role of the SNS in congestive heart failure returns to this theme.

Long-term follow-up studies of patients with essential hypertension have confirmed that the extent of alterations in left ventricular mass and geometry markedly influences prognosis (Koren et al., 1991). Patients with essential hypertension uncomplicated by left ventricular structural alterations have such an excellent prognosis, one may question whether hypertension without cardiovascular hypertrophy or coronary atherosclerosis actually constitutes a disease. No study has considered the possible prognostic implications of high plasma NE levels in patients with hypertension-associated left ventricular hypertrophy. Mechanisms relating SNS activity to left ventricular hypertrophy and to prognosis seem important topics for future research.

Secondary Hypertension

Neurogenic Hypertension

Increased sympathoneural outflow contributes to the hypertension attending various neurologic syndromes, including baroreceptor deafferentation (Koch and Mies, 1929), hyperdynamic circulation associated with autonomic epilepsy (Metz et al., 1978), the Guillain–Barre syndrome (Ventura et al., 1986; Yao et al., 1985; Ahmad et al., 1985), bladder stimulation in tetraplegics (Mathias et al., 1976), generalized seizures (Simon, 1985), and intracranial bleeding (Myers et al., 1981, 1982; Shigeno, 1982). Cardiac and catecholaminergic effects of intracranial bleeding are discussed below in the section about stroke and the heart.

As noted in the chapter about functional neuroanatomy, lesions of the A1 region of the CVLM (Minson et al., 1986; Sved and Reis, 1985), of the NTS (Doba and Reis, 1973), or of the rostral hypothalamus (Nathan and Reis, 1981) can cause severe hypertension mediated by several interacting vasoactive systems. Hypothalamic stimulation increases blood pressure and sympathoneural activity acutely, but it is unclear whether chronic hypothalamic stimulation produces sustained hypertension (Bunag and Riley, 1979; Folkow and Rubinstein, 1966).

Koch and Mies (1929) probably were the first to describe hypertension related to section of the buffer nerves, a phenomenon confirmed later by many investigators (e.g., Thomas, 1944). Subsequent studies by Cowley and coworkers (1973) led to the conclusion that baroreceptor deafferentiation increases the lability of blood pressure, including exaggerated pressor responses to various environmental stimuli, without necessarily increasing the mean level of pressure in individuals at rest. More recent work has questioned this conclusion. Some animals become clearly hypertensive and others hypotensive, and individual differences may result from concurrent sympathetic afferent or efferent denervation (Sleight, 1986). Sino-aortic deafferentiation increases blood pressure and plasma levels of NE and EPI in rats (Dominiak et al., 1986). In nonhuman primates, sino-aortic denervation also produces chronic elevations in blood pressure and plasma NE levels (Shade et al., 1990), whereas carotid sinus denervation alone elicits only transient hypertension.

In cats, bilateral NTS destruction elicits labile hypertension, sustained tachycardia, and exaggerated pressor responsiveness to conditioned and unconditioned stimuli (Nathan et al., 1978; Nathan and Reis, 1977). In rats, bilateral NTS ablation produces fulminant, usually fatal hypertension (Doba and Reis, 1973). Intravenous administration of clonidine ameliorates both the hypertension and the elevated levels of AVP resulting from bilateral NTS lesions in rats (Sved and Reis, 1985; Sved et al., 1985), consistent with a role of central neural adrenoceptors in regulating AVP release in this setting.

Whereas adrenalectomy does not affect the hypertension produced by bilateral NTS lesions, adrenalectomy prevents the hypertension (as well as the tachycardia, hyperthermia, and increased motor activity) resulting from bilateral lesions of the rostral hypothalamus, suggesting the participation of increased circulating EPI levels in the latter form of neurogenic hypertension (Nathan and Reis, 1981); however, plasma catecholamine levels appear not to have been assessed in this model.

In rats, destruction of the A1 region of the CVLM also produces severe hypertension, via increased SNS vasoconstrictor outflows and to a lesser extent from increased circulating EPI levels, with little influence by the associated increases in circulating AVP (Minson et al., 1986).

Immunosuppressive therapy with cyclosporine often causes hypertension. Hypertensive patients on cyclosporine have increased SMSA without increased plasma NE levels (Scherrer et al., 1990b). The basis for the discrepancy is unknown.

Patients with arterial baroreflex failure have extremely labile blood pressures, headache, diaphoresis, emotional instability, and hypertensive paroxysms during distress, anxiety, or pain (Robertson et al., 1993). Associated pathologic states include paraganglioma, neck irradiation, bilateral NTS lesions, or glossopharyngeal nerve section. Clonidine treatment can ameliorate the hypertensive and tachycardic paroxysms. The symptoms and signs mimic those in pheochromocytoma; however, unlike most patients with pheochromocytoma, patients with arterial baroreflex failure have normal clonidine-induced suppression of plasma NE levels.

Pheochromocytoma

Pheochromocytoma, a rare cause of clinical hypertension, is a tumor of chromaffin cells. Pheochromocytomas occur most commonly in the adrenal gland or along pathways of embryological development from the neural crest, i.e., along the aorta to the organ of Zuckerkandl at the aortic bifurcation. The tumor presents clinically as sustained or paroxysmal hypertension, pallor, sweating, headache, anxiety, palpitations, orthostatic hypotension, and hyperglycemia. The absence of sweating, headache, palpitations, or hypertension casts doubt on the diagnosis.

Pheochromocytomas are often benign, thus surgical removal is curative. The associated severe hypertensive paroxysms or catecholamine-induced cardiomyopathy can be life-threatening. These consequences justify efforts to diagnose pheochromocytoma in patients with suggestive signs or symptoms, despite the rarity of the tumor.

Screening tests to detect release of catecholamines by the tumor, such as measurements of urinary excretion of "metanephrines" (NMN and MN) and of VMA, are sensitive and specific. Patients with pheochromocytoma usually have high plasma levels of NE, EPI, or both—most commonly of NE. The relative usefulness of urinary and plasma measurements has been controversial (Bravo et al., 1981).

Some hypertensive patients can have high plasma catecholamine levels due to anxiety. Clonidine suppression testing decreases the frequency of false-positive results (Bravo et al., 1981). In this test, blood pressure is measured and antecubital venous blood sampled before and three hours after oral clonidine administration. Clonidine normally substantially decreases plasma NE levels; patients with pheochromocytoma have a failure of clonidine suppression of plasma NE. The failure to suppress plasma NE levels therefore constitutes a positive clonidine suppression test. One can also conduct analogous suppression testing using the ganglion blocker, pentolinium (Brown, Allison et al., 1981).

The occurrence of false-negative results using screening biochemical tests for pheochromocytoma presents a more difficult problem. Provocative tests have included administration of tyramine, calcium with pentagastrin, or glucagon (Bravo and Gifford, 1984; Lawrence, 1967). Because these agents can evoke hypertensive crises in pheochromocytoma patients, and since many patients with suspected pheochromocytoma undergo treatment with α-adrenoceptor blockers, clinicians have largely abandoned testing based on the magnitude of pressor responses to drugs. Grossman, Goldstein et al. (1991) introduced a schema using plasma levels of catechols for diagnostic testing of hypertensive patients with suspected pheochromocytoma. Positive results include high baseline levels of NE, EPI, or DOPA; excessive increases in plasma NE levels after administration of glucagon; and a failure to suppress plasma NE levels after administration of clonidine. This approach yields conclusive results in about 80% of hypertensive patients with suspected pheochromocytoma. The testing protocol has the advantage of applicability to patients treated with phenoxybenzamine, which blocks or attenuates pressor responses to glucagon but leaves intact responses of plasma levels of catecholamines (Zweifler et al., 1983). Since glucagon administration normally increases plasma EPI levels, the neurochemical diagnosis does not depend on EPI responses.

Consistent with the intraneuronal source of DHPG, as discussed in the chapter about assessment methods, patients with pheochromocytoma usually have high plasma NE/DHPG ratios (Brown, 1984). Use of this ratio for diagnostic purposes does not improve diagnostic accuracy, because patients with pheochromocytoma can have high plasma levels or urinary excretion of DHPG (Duncan et al., 1988; Lenders et al., 1992). Thus, a normal NE/DHPG ratio does not exclude the diagnosis of pheochromocytoma. Because pheochromocytomas secrete directly into the bloodstream, patients with these tumors usually have high plasma NMN levels (Lenders et al., 1993), and measurement of plasma levels of metanephrines provides a very sensitive screening test (Lenders et al., unpublished observations).

In patients with pheochromocytoma, the occurrence of metastases, not the pathological appearance of the tumor, defines malignancy. Patients with malignant pheochromocytoma may not have hypertension, and the tumors can occur in unusual locations. About 60% of patients with malignant pheochromocytoma have high plasma levels of the catecholamine precursor, DOPA (Goldstein, Stull et al., 1986), whereas patients with benign pheochromocytoma have normal plasma DOPA levels. This may result from the fact that malignant pheochromocytomas are less well differentiated than are benign pheochromocytomas.

High NE levels in patients with pheochromocytoma can cause cardiomyopathy, as discussed later in this chapter; excision of the tumor can reverse the cardiomyopathy (Imperato-McGinley et al., 1987).

Case reports have indicated that adrenomedullary hyperfunction can cause hypertension and high plasma catecholamine levels without pheochromocytomas. Streeten et al. (1990) reported five cases of spontaneous hyperepinephrinemia. One patient had suspected adrenal medullary hyperplasia, based on a family history of multiple endocrine neoplasia type IIa. Two others had adrenal cysts, with amelioration of symptoms after surgical removal of the cysts. The two others had relief of symptoms during administration of propranolol or atenolol, consistent with the hyperdynamic circulation syndrome. In a case reported by Letizia and Scavo (1990), a 30-year-old man with paroxysmal hypertension, high plasma catecholamine levels, and MIBG scanning results suggesting an adrenal pheochromocytoma, computed tomography did not reveal a tumor, and after surgical adrenalectomy, histopathologic examination showed only hyperplastic medullary tissue. The hypercatecholaminergic syndrome recurred in the other adrenal after one year. Kuchel and co-workers (Kuchel et al., 1979, 1981, 1987) have suggested that deficient catecholamine conjugation can produce a syndrome that resembles pheochromocytoma clinically: "pseudopheochromocytoma."

Renovascular Hypertension

Increased SNS outflows accompany the development of renovascular hypertension in animal models (Suzuki et al., 1983). Sympatholytic procedures attenuate the development of the hypertension, and AV3V lesions prevent it (Brody and Johnson, 1980; Brody et al., 1991). Once established, the hypertension persists despite these procedures.

Patients with renovascular hypertension have normal plasma NE levels and large depressor responses to clonidine (Lake et al., 1984; Mathias, 1991).

Adrenal Corticosteroid-Related Hypertension

Uninephrectomized rats with deoxycorticosterone (DOCA)–salt hypertension, have increased SNS activity (De Champlain, 1990), as evidenced by high tissue turnover of NE (Reid et al., 1975), high plasma levels of catecholamines (Bouvier and De Champlain, 1986), increased spillover of NE into plasma (Bouvier and De Champlain, 1985), and large depressor responses to ganglion blockade (Chen et al., 1985). DOCA–salt hypertensive rats also have larger hemorrhage-induced increases in NE levels than do normotensive rats, and since the group differences persist following Uptake-1 blockade, decreased neuronal reuptake of the neurotransmitter does not cause the increased NE levels in this setting (Drolet et al., 1989).

Intact baboons with DOCA–salt hypertension, however, have normal plasma NE levels, and whereas treatment with β-adrenoceptor blockade or clonidine fails to ameliorate the hypertension, treatment with a diuretic combination causes the animals rapidly to become normotensive (Turkkan and Goldstein, 1987). These results cast doubt on the hypothesis that increased SNS outflows contribute to this low-renin form of hypertension in primates. Analogously, patients with hypertension related to adrenocortical hyperfunction typically have normal or decreased plasma NE levels, with little or no depressor response to β-adrenoceptor blockade or to combined α- and β-adrenoceptor blockade (Bravo et al., 1985).

High circulating levels of glucocorticoids suppress SNS and AHS outflows (e.g., Szemeredi, Bagdy et al., 1988a; Brown and Fisher, 1986). In healthy volunteers, hypercortisolemia for one week does not affect NE spillover into plasma but does increase blood pressure, cardiac output, and regional vascular responsiveness to exogenous NE (Sudhir et al., 1989). Clinical reports have not described indices of SNS outflows in patients with Cushing's syndrome.

Rats with moderate hypertension produced by chronic hypercortisolemia have normal pressor responses to phenylephrine, normal baroreflex–cardiac and baroreflex–sympathoneural sensitivity, and augmented tachycardic responses to isoproterenol (Szemeredi et al., 1989). Patients with Cushing's disease and hypertension also have increased tachycardia responses to isoproterenol, apparently without increased β-adrenoceptor density (Ritchie et al., 1990).

Postoperative Hypertension

Severe postoperative hypertension often occurs in coronary bypass patients; the afferent signal triggering this hypertension has not been identified. Wallach et al. (1980) reported that 54% of patients studied prospectively after saphenous vein bypass grafting developed new hypertension within 1 hour after surgery. Some investigators have postulated that destruction of the left coronary glomus activates a hypertensive chemoreflex (James, 1983; Wallach et al., 1980), eliciting increases in plasma NE and EPI concentrations (Wallach et al., 1980). Rossi (1988) described a case of a patient with post-bypass hypertension and painless ischemia who died during a silent ischemic attack about three months postoperatively. In the field of operative trauma, marked neuronal degeneration and lymphocytic periendoneuritis of the left coronary artery nerve plexus were observed.

Hypertension also occurs frequently after carotid endarterectomy. Consistent with disruption of carotid baroreflexes, patients with post–carotid endarterectomy hypertension have increased CSF and plasma NE levels (Ahn et al., 1989). Bilateral lidocaine blockade of the glossopharyngeal and vagus nerves also produces marked acute hypertension (Guz et al., 1966), and Pickering and Sleight (1977) cited anecdotal evidence that carotid sinus denervation in humans produces sustained hypertension. Aksamit et al. (1987) described a case of episodes of paroxysmal hypertension, without sustained hypertension, in a patient with a remote history of neck and mediastinal radiation who underwent bilateral carotid bypass surgery.

In hypertension after repair of coarctation of the aorta, reports have indicated either increased or normal levels of plasma NE, with excessive pressor responsiveness to exogenous NE (Gidding et al., 1985).

Coronary Heart Disease

Catecholamines contribute to values for every known risk factor and epidemiological feature of coronary heart disease—hyperlipidemia, hypertension, nicotinic effects of cigarette smoking, obesity, the Type A behavior pattern, and insulin resistance (Lee, cited in Antaloczy, 1984)—and catecholamines can precipitate acute events in coronary patients. Nevertheless, despite suggestive evidence from studies of laboratory animals, the role of chronically repeated episodes of stress in the development of clinical coronary heart disease remains controversial; a catecholaminergic link, while rational, remains unproven.

Atherosclerosis Development

Ethical and practical limitations have prevented rigorous scientific testing of the hypothesis that chronic emotional distress contributes to the development of coronary heart disease in humans. This notion remains one of the major unproven ideas in psychosomatic medicine.

SNS or AHS activation can accelerate the development of atherosclerosis via hemodynamic changes that increase peak blood flow velocity and heart rate, both of which increase the likelihood of turbulence and therefore increase endothelial cell turnover and arterial wall damage (Pauletto et al., 1991). Catecholamines also affect processes related to the disposition of cholesterol, as discussed in the chapter about peripheral catecholaminergic systems. By mobilizing free fatty acids, EPI theoretically can indirectly inhibit production of high density lipoproteins, by transformation of excess free fatty acids to triglycerides in the liver and inhibition of lipoprotein lipase by high triglyceride levels (Pauletto et al., 1991). Catecholamines can also activate acyl-cholesterol-acyl-transferase, which catalyzes production of cholesterol esters in arterial walls (Sacks and Dzau, 1986). In rabbits on a normal diet (Helin et al., 1970), and monkeys on a high-cholesterol diet (Kukreja et al., 1981) injections of NE or EPI produce aortic sudanophilic lesions.

Emotional distress seems to increase serum cholesterol levels subacutely or chronically, in humans and laboratory animals (Cathey et al., 1962; Grundy and Griffin, 1959; Taggart and Carruthers, 1971; Wertlake et al., 1958; Wolf et al., 1962). Wolf (1985) reported that exposure to a "stress interview" increased serum cholesterol concentrations within one hour; however, the acute psychological stress induced by undergoing third molar extractions does not alter cholesterol or lipoprotein levels (Goldstein, Dionne et al., 1982). In tax accountants, serum cholesterol levels have been reported to peak about April 15 (Friedman et al., 1958). In a longitudinal study of Johns Hopkins medical students, the stress of examinations was associated with increased cholesterol levels (Thomas and Murphy, 1958). Although long-term emotional distress probably does bias toward increased circulating lipid levels, the magnitude, time course, mechanisms, and interindividual consistency of this effect in humans remain incompletely understood.

In laboratory monkeys on a high cholesterol diet, social instability and dominance interact to accelerate atherosclerosis (Clarkson et al., 1986; Kaplan et al., 1982, 1983). Manuck et al. (1983) reported that in cynomolgus monkeys subjected to psychosocial stress (the threat of capture and physical handling by the investigator while the animals were in their social groups), animals with relatively large heart rate responses had more extensive coronary atherosclerosis than those with small heart rate responses. In zoo animals, crowding and social perturbation increase the frequency of atherosclerosis (Ratcliffe et al., 1958).

Hypertension and high catecholamine levels interact in the development of atherosclerosis in broad-breasted white turkeys (Pauletto et al., 1991). The animals have marked age-related increases in blood pressure and high plasma levels of catecholamines—especially of NE—and they develop aortic atherosclerosis despite high serum α-lipoprotein levels. Treatment with the β-adrenoceptor blocker oxprenolol decreases the extent of plaque formation.

The Type A Behavior Pattern and Related Theories

According to the theory of the "Type A coronary prone behavior pattern," the Type A individual's style of reaction to stress constitutes an independent coronary risk factor. The theory therefore shifts emphasis from stressors that may accelerate development of atherosclerosis to aspects of the individual's personality that increase coronary risk. Although Friedman and Rosenman introduced and popularized the Type A theory, William Osler presaged it in his characterization of the typical coronary patient as "not the delicate neurotic but the robust, the vigorous in mind and body, the keen ambitious man, the indicator of whose engine is always full speed ahead" (Osler, 1910).

The Type A behavior pattern includes time urgency, competitiveness, and aggressiveness. Results of the Western Collaborative Group Study (WCGS) of 3524 men followed prospectively for 8½ years provided convincing evidence for the existence and pathophysiological significance of this pattern (Rosenman et al., 1975). After taking into account all other known major risk factors, Type A subjects had a twofold greater risk of developing overt ischemic heart disease than did subjects without Type A behavior. Findings of the Framingham study tended to confirm the WCGS results (Haynes et al., 1978).

Several studies subsequently failed to support the Type A theory. These studies usually stratified patients in terms of the existence of the Type A pattern and then tested the association with the extent of angiographically demonstrable coronary atherosclerosis (Matthews and Haynes, 1986). The results of the Multiple Risk Factor Intervention Trial (MRFIT) were also very damaging, since this prospective study of 3000 healthy men failed to reveal increased susceptibility to develop coronary disease in Type A subjects (Shekelle et al., 1983, 1985).

If only a portion of the Type A pattern actually were related to coronary risk, this would help to explain the inconsistent findings. Whereas Friedman, Rosenman, and coworkers (Rosenman et al., 1964, 1975) dwelled on the constellation of aggressiveness, time urgency, and competitiveness, Williams and coworkers (Barefoot et al., 1983; Williams et al., 1980; Williams, 1989) and others (Dembroski and Costa, 1988; Shekelle et al., 1983) have concentrated on the specific component of anger or hostility. Reanalysis of the structured interview data from the MRFIT trial indicated that, whereas the global Type A pattern failed to predict the development of coronary artery disease, the component of hostility did (Dembroski and Costa, 1988). A 30-year longitudinal study, however, did not find that hostility scores predicted coronary disease or mortality (Hearn et al., 1989). Williams (1989) suggested that because the subjects had studied at the University of Minnesota and had lived in the upper Midwest during the follow-up period, they were in a ''low-stress environment,'' insufficiently activating the pathogenic process in those who were coronary-prone due to hostility. A 25-year follow-up study of law students found that the score on the hostility scale component of the Minnesota Multphasic Personality Inventory did predict mortality during the follow-up period (Barefoot et al., 1989). Statistical reanalysis of the original WCGS data of Friedman and Rosenman confirmed that when responses in the structured interview by 250 subjects who subsequently suffered heart attacks were compared with responses by 500 subjects who remained healthy, hostility ratings predicted overt coronary heart disease, whereas after exclusion of the hostility component, no other component of the coronary prone behavior pattern was predictive (Hecker et al, 1988).

Syme (1985) suggested that the relationship between the Type A personality and coronary risk may depend on the extent of social support. In a study of Japanese men in California, a subpopulation of immigrants who became ''acculturated'' had coronary heart disease rates 2.5 to 5 times that of the subpopulation retaining a Japanese lifestyle (Berkman and Syme, 1979; Marmot and Syme, 1976). Wolf (1985) obtained analogous results in a study of Roseto, an Italian-American town in eastern Pennsylvania. Residents of this community, who retained their European culture from the time of immigration in 1882 until the 1960s, had fewer heart attacks than did inhabitants of nearby towns, despite similar consumption of animal fats and similar prevalence of smoking, sedentary life-style, hypertension, and diabetes.

Wolf (1960) emphasized a different personality characteristic that could typify Type A individuals: joyless striving, also termed the ''Sisyphus reaction,'' after the mythical

King of Corinth who was condemned to Hades and forced to push a rock endlessly up the side of a mountain (Wolf, 1985).

Whether hostility, lack of social support, or joyless striving are "toxic" components of the Type A pattern has not yet been resolved.

Eliot, Buell, and coworkers have suggested that patterns of hemodynamic response during emotional stress, rather than the Type A pattern itself, explain the association between cardiovascular morbidity and stress (Eliot and Buell, 1985). These investigators have categorized patients as "hot reactors" or "cold reactors," based on the occurrence of excessive hemodynamic responses to a panel of tests, including mathematical problems, competitive video games, and the cold pressor test. The authors have related anecdotes where myocardial infarction patients with abnormal hemodynamic responses underwent reinfarction within two years, and patients with large increases in total peripheral resistance subsequently suffered cardiovascular catastrophes; however, the report did not test scientifically the predictive value of the "hot reactor" categorization.

A related view holds that stress-related coronary risk results from excessive catecholaminergic responses that elicit pathologic hemodynamic patterns. Since the "hypertensive personality" and the Type A pattern seem to share a component of hostility, and since there is an association between this personality characteristic and elevated NE and PRA levels in hypertensives, one may hypothesize that catecholamines mediate increased coronary risk in hostile, Type A hypertensives. Williams et al. (1982) reported that Type A men had exaggerated responses of muscle blood flow and circulating blood levels of NE, EPI, and cortisol during mental arithmetic. The combination of hostility and harassment was associated with especially large changes in diastolic blood pressure and forearm blood flow during a mental task (Suarez and Williams, 1989). Glass et al. (1980) reported that Type A individuals responded with excessive increases of plasma catecholamine levels and blood pressure during challenges perceived as personally threatening. Other studies involving challenge, competition, or harassment have supported the view that Type A men have excessive increases in levels of NE, EPI, and cortisol, compared with responses in Type B men (Krantz et al., 1984; Williams et al., 1982). DeQuattro et al. (1985) summarized results from 33 experiments and concluded that Type A individuals have about threefold larger plasma NE responses and about fourfold larger EPI responses during exposure to various laboratory and clinical stressors than do Type B individuals.

Although the neuroendocrine mediator hypothesis can explain increased coronary risk in hypertensives with the hostile Type A pattern, the pathophysiologic meaning of excessive catecholamine responses in the long-term development of coronary disease is unknown.

Myocardial Infarction

Changes in sympathoneural function associated with myocardial infarction can be primary, with augmented cardiac or extracardiac NE release increasing myocardial oxygen consumption and exacerbating ischemia, or can be secondary, with recruitment of cardiac and extracardiac SNS outflows maintaining cardiovascular performance.

Separating pathologic from beneficial increases in sympathetic activity in patients with myocardial infarction has proven very difficult.

Ethical limitations obviate scientifically meaningful testing of the role of distress-induced catecholaminergic activation as a precipitant of acute myocardial infarction in humans. Miminoshvili et al. and Lapin and Cherkovitch (cited in OA Smith et al., 1986) provided experimental support for such a role in primates. Dominant baboons were separated physically from their harems but were allowed to have visual and auditory contact with the colony. Subdominant males were given first choice of food and snacks and were allowed to copulate with females of the harem, evoking evident hostility and frustration in the previously dominant baboons. About ¼ of the previously dominant animals became hypertensive, and about ¹⁄₁₀ suffered myocardial infarctions—conditions virtually nonexistent in the normal baboon population.

The frequency of myocardial infarction varies during the day, with the peak incidence early in the morning (Muller et al., 1985; Willich et al., 1989). Since plasma catecholamine levels also peak at this time (Tofler et al., 1987), one may speculate that increased SNS or AHS outflow in the morning contributes to the circadian variation in the frequency of myocardial infarction. Consistent with this hypothesis, patients treated with β-adrenergic blockers do not have an increased morning incidence of myocardial infarction (Willich et al., 1989).

Effects of Coronary Occlusion on Sympathoneural Function

It is generally accepted that cardiac sympathetic outflow increases in response to clinical myocardial infarction. Coronary occlusion rapidly and markedly impedes ventricular function, and atrial distention due to decreased ventricular compliance would be expected to increase cardiac efferent SNS traffic (Karim et al., 1972) and therefore cardiac NE spillover (Hasking et al., 1985). Malliani et al. (1969) and Gillis (1971) reported increased sympathetic efferent activity during coronary occlusion in laboratory animals.

Whether these increases reflect compensatory activation to maintain cardiac performance or responses to coronary occlusion or myocardial anoxia is unknown. In patients with myocardial infarction, plasma catecholamine levels increase with the severity of cardiac damage, as assessed by creatine phosphokinase (Bertel et al, 1982a; Nadeau and De Champlain, 1979; Steiger and McCann, 1982) and the extent of pump dysfunction (Seino et al., 1989). These results do not distinguish sympathetic recruitment to maintain cardiac performance from a primary pathological role of increased myocardial catecholamines.

Schwartz, Malliani, and coworkers have proposed that acute myocardial ischemia elicits vagal depressor and sympathetic excitatory reflexes by stimulation of vagal and sympathetic afferent fibers (Malliani et al., 1969, 1986). The sympathetic excitatory cardio-cardiac reflex (Felder and Thames, 1981; Malliani et al., 1969, 1986; Minisi and Thames, 1991) would increase the likelihood of a neurocardiac positive feedback loop, which could play a role in the mechanism of sudden death soon after the onset of myocardial ischemia.

During myocardial ischemia, cardiac release of NE, as reflected by the cardiac venous

NE concentration, generally does not increase (McGrath et al., 1981). As noted below, patients with stable angina pectoris have normal cardiac NE spillover during cardiac catheterization.

Local anoxia or ischemia can increase cardiac release of NE in laboratory animals, even in the absence of increased postganglionic sympathoneural activity (Wollenberger and Shahab, 1965), possibly via reverse transport through the Uptake-1 carrier (Carlsson et al., 1986; Malliani et al., 1986; Schomig, 1988; Staszewska-Barczak, 1971). The increased release by this process is associated with increased net leakage of NE from storage vesicles into the axonal cytoplasm (Schomig et al., 1987; Schomig, 1988). NE washout increases markedly after release of coronary occlusion (Abrahamsson et al., 1984), suggesting that decreased coronary blood flow augments accumulation of NE in the heart.

Cardiac nerves and muscle differ in their susceptibility to ischemia (Rossi, 1988). Nerve fibers tend to have lower oxygen requirements than myocardial cells, and whereas the local blood supply provides the sole source of fuel and waste removal for myocardial cells, local blood supply and perfusion of the cell bodies in sympathetic ganglia may both contribute to these processes for sympathetic nerve terminals. Myocardial sympathetic nerves therefore would be expected to be less susceptible to damage resulting from coronary occlusion than would myocardial smooth muscle cells. Acute ligation of the left anterior descending coronary artery in rats produces little change in the accumulation of radiolabeled NE in the ischemic zone; in nonischemic regions, the accumulation is enhanced (Antaloczy, 1984). At 3 and 14 days after the ligation, however, accumulation of radiolabeled NE declines. This dysfunction may result from inflammatory infiltration at the site of myocardial necrosis, with proteoloysis caused by granulocytic enzymes. Clinical researchers have generally ignored perineuritis associated with this inflammatory response in considering mechanisms of pain, arrhythmias, and disordered regional hemodynamics after acute myocardial infarction (Rossi, 1988).

Transmural myocardial infarction of the anterior left ventricle interferes with sympathetic and parasympathetic neurotransmission in the infarcted region as well as apical to the infarct (Barber et al., 1983; Minardo et al., 1988; Zipes and Inoue, 1988). Myocardial concentrations of NE and NE histofluorescence decrease in the noninfarcted areas, with physiological evidence of denervation. In contrast, subendocardial infarction appears to spare sympathetic transmission apical to the infarct, since the sympathetic fibers travel in the subepicardium (Inoue and Zipes, 1987), and only regional sympathetic denervation seems to occur. Scintigraphic assessment of sympathetic cardiac innervation using [^{123}I]MIBG or thallium imaging in dogs with transmural or nontransmural myocardial infarctions has revealed that after transmural infarction, the zone of reduced MIBG-derived radioactivity exceeds in size the zone of reduced thallium uptake, indicating viable but dysfunctional or denervated myocardium distal to the infarct (Dae et al., 1991).

Schwaiger et al. (1990a) found that reperfusion after 30 minutes of occlusion of the left anterior descending artery in dogs was associated with decreased regional [^{18}F]fluorometaraminol-derived myocardial radioactivity and NE concentrations, indicating residual failure to retain amines in sympathetic terminals. Thus, decreased MIBG-derived radioactivity in a perfused region after myocardial infarction may indicate either sympathoneural denervation or dysfunction.

There is no clinical evidence about whether denervated myocardium related to myocardial infarction can undergo reinnervation.

Differential loss of sympathetic nerve terminals and myocardial cells after myocardial infarction probably predisposes to the development of arrhythmias, as discussed below.

Autonomic Nerves and Arrhythmogenesis

Myocardial ischemia or infarction decreases thresholds for lethal ventricular arrhythmias. About ½ of patients with myocardial infarction die from this complication (Packer, 1985). Proposed mechanisms of ventricular arrhythmias in the setting of acute myocardial infarction include localized conduction defects due to necrosis and fibrosis, electrolyte abnormalities such as hypokalemia, side effects of drugs, myocyte damage, sympathoneural activation, and NE accumulation at sites of denervation supersensitivity.

Skinner (1985) has emphasized that myocardial ischemia alone may not explain sudden cardiac death and that superimposed activation of autonomic outflow is required. Many studies of laboratory animals have shown that SNS or AHS activation contributes to arrhythmogenesis in the setting of acute myocardial infarction (e.g., Corr and Gillis, 1978). This activation exaggerates the spatial dispersion of action potential durations in infarcted hearts, increasing the probability of developing reentry-type ventricular arrhythmias, and enlarges delayed afterdepolarizations, increasing the probability of developing ectopic arrhythmias. In addition, EPI produces hypokalemia (Struthers et al., 1983; Vincent et al., 1984), which may add to the hypokalemic effects of diuretics and increase the probability of digitalis toxicity. Moreover, since ventricular extrasystoles, by momentarily decreasing systemic blood pressure, almost immediately evoke reflexive increases in cardiac preganglionic sympathetic activity (Lombardi et al., 1988), and since cardiac NE release increases ventricular automaticity, a neurocardiologic positive feedback loop may lead to rapid degeneration of cardiac rhythm in patients with myocardial infarction. These mechanisms may explain why signs of sympathetic activation often precede ventricular fibrillation in myocardial infarction patients (Adgey et al., 1982).

In 1931, Leriche and coworkers reported that excision of the upper thoracic sympathetic ganglia decreased the frequency of occurrence of ventricular fibrillation associated with sudden coronary occlusion. Manning et al. (1939) and Ebert et al. (1967) confirmed and extended these findings. Verrier and Lown (1981) reported that sympathetic blockade increased the threshold for ventricular arrhythmias in dogs with acute coronary ligation. In anesthetized dogs, maximal increases in sympathetic neural activity and in vulnerability to ventricular fibrillation occur concurrently during brief occlusion of the left anterior descending artery; and bilateral stellectomy attenuates the increased susceptibility to ventricular fibrillation in this preparation (Lombardi et al., 1983, 1988). Saini et al. (1988) obtained evidence indicating that a sympatholytic effect mediated the antifibrillatory action of fentanyl.

Chronic, bilateral stellate ganglionectomy, administration of the noradrenergic neurotoxin, 6-OHDA, or total cardiac denervation decreases the likelihood of ventricular fibrillation induced by acute coronary occlusion (Ebert et al., 1970; Fowlis et al., 1974; Harris et al., 1951; Leriche et al., 1931; Schaal et al., 1969; Sheridan et al., 1980). These findings imply that the arrhythmogenic effect of cardiac sympathetic activation during coronary occlusion depends on release of NE from sympathetic nerves. According to the theory of Schwartz, stimulation specifically of the left stellate ganglion is arrhythmogenic in the ischemic heart, and left stellate blockade is anti-arrhythmogenic (Pandey et al., 1979; Schwartz et al., 1976). Possibly because of offsetting influences of the right and left ganglia, acute bilateral stellate ganglionectomy does not consistently affect the frequency of ventricular fibrillation during coronary occlusion (Gillis, 1971; Schwartz et al., 1976).

Abundant evidence indicates that emotional distress in the setting of myocardial infarction increases the likelihood of ventricular arrhythmias and that sympatholytic procedures or adrenoceptor blockade prevents this tendency. In conscious animals, coronary ligation does not produce ventricular fibrillation if either psychological stress is minimized by behavioral adaptation or, in the presence of psychological stress, a central neural pathway from the frontal cortex to brainstem nuclei is blocked or the amygdala frozen (Skinner, 1985; Skinner et al., 1975; Skinner and Reed, 1981). Conversely, Lown and Verrier (1976) reported that emotional stress markedly reduced the threshold for ventricular arrhythmias in animals with coronary ligation. In pigs, Carpeggiani and Skinner (1991) studied arrhythmic consequences of a psychological stressor—presentation of food to a fasting but restrained animal. When ''food deprivation stress'' was applied in intact animals, there were no ischemic or arrhythmic effects; when left anterior descending coronary occlusion was performed without application of the stressor, 1 of the 5 subjects developed ventricular fibrillation; but when the stress was applied in animals with coronary occlusion in the presence of the stressor, all the animals developed ventricular fibrillation.

In pigs with snare occlusion of the left anterior descending artery 1 week before acute testing, arousal induced by being lifted in a sling or by bringing a stall mate into the room increases the inducibility and rate of ventricular tachycardia and increases plasma NE and EPI levels; β_1-adrenoceptor blockade normalizes the increased inducibility of ventricular tachycardia (Kirby et al., 1991). Intracerebral injection of as little as 0.01 mg/kg of the nonselective β-blocker propranolol also prevents ventricular fibrillation after occlusion of the left anterior descending artery in psychologically stressed pigs (Skinner, 1985).

In dogs with acute coronary ischemia, exposure to a classically conditioned aversive stimulus does not precipitate ventricular arrhythmias (Billman et al., 1990). In the setting of acute anterior myocardial infarction, however, coronary ischemia can interact with the classically conditioned stimulus to precipitate ventricular arrhythmias. During subsequent exercise or coronary occlusion, only a proportion of ''susceptible'' animals develop worsening of ventricular arrhythmias when exposed to the conditioned stimulus, suggesting that at least in dogs, classically conditioned aversive stimuli do not consistently increase susceptibility to ventricular arrhythmias during coronary ischemia, even in the setting of a previous anterior myocardial infarction.

A dog will become obviously enraged when another dog challenges its access to food. In dogs with circumflex coronary stenosis produced using an adjustable occluder, exposure to this situation increases coronary flow, but within 2–4 minutes after the episode, coronary flow proximal to the occluder decreases, and coronary vascular resistance increases markedly (Verrier et al., 1987), accompanied by electrocardiographic evidence of ischemia. The coronary vasoconstriction is neurogenic, since stellate ganglion ablation prevents the post-anger ischemic changes. During agonistic behavior, sympathetically mediated increases in systemic blood pressure may increase the distending force in coronary vessels; after the behavior ends, blood pressure may fall abruptly, leaving the artery susceptible to local sympathetic vasoconstriction. The canine data lead to the suggestion that patients with moderately severe coronary disease who are prone to coronary vasoconstriction during anger reactions may be predisposed to develop acute coronary ischemic events.

Attenuation of vagal reflexive bradycardia, as indicated by low baroreflex–cardiac gain, is a major risk factor for the development of ischemia-related ventricular fibrillation in dogs that previously have undergone anterior myocardial infarction (Billman et al., 1982; Vanoli et al., 1987). Myocardial infarction itself produces reversible decreases in baroreflex gain (Schwartz and Stramba-Badiale, 1988). Schwartz and Stramba-Badiale (1988) have therefore suggested that low baroreflex sensitivity in post-myocardial infarction patients may be associated with an increased risk of mortality in the follow-up period. According to Skinner (1985), emotional stressors trigger a frontocortical–brainstem noradrenergic pathway ("process-P"), eliciting dual autonomic activation that increases myocardial vulnerability to ventricular fibrillation. Behavioral adaptation, blockade of the pathway between frontal cortex and the brainstem, or intracerebral injection of propranolol would prevent the lethal arrhythmogenesis. The hypothalamus is a major intervening station in this pathway, and hypothalamic stimulation interferes with baroreceptor–cardiac reflexes, as discussed in Chapter 2. This central neural mechanism may explain the positive correlation between inhibition of baroreflexes and increased vulnerability to ventricular fibrillation during myocardial ischemia (Billman et al., 1982).

Since vagal stimulation during acute myocardial ischemia generally increases electrical stability (Kent et al., 1973), and intravenous injection of atropine can evoke ventricular fibrillation in bradycardic subjects (Massumi et al., 1972), increased PNS outflow probably decreases susceptibility to ventricular fibrillation during myocardial ischemia; however, in patients with a neuroendocrine "giving up" response pattern, the increased PNS outflow could occur simultaneously with adrenomedullary secretion of EPI, which would decrease arrhythmia thresholds. Lombardi et al. (1988) have hypothesized that during severe left ventricular ischemia, ventricular dilatation activates ventricular vagal afferents, leading to depressor reflexes, whereas lesser amounts of ischemia may result in sympathetic stimulation, producing circulatory excitation. An alternative explanation for the pattern during severe ischemia is central neural elicitation of a "giving up" reaction.

Cellular electrophysiologic effects of catecholamines resulting in arrhythmogenesis have been ascribed to β- and α_1-adrenoceptors (Sheridan et al., 1980; Surawicz, 1971). By several mechanisms, stimulation of myocardial β-adrenoceptors during myocardial ischemia increases susceptibility to ventricular fibrillation. As noted above, ischemia produces heterogeneity of refractory periods, and concurrent β-adrenoceptor stimulation would exaggerate the temporal dispersion of refractory periods. Tachycardia produces a functional conduction delay in the ischemic region. Increases in the size of delayed after-depolarizations may increase the likelihood of triggered rhythms. β-Adrenoceptor stimulation also increases the already accelerated rate of depolarization of ischemic tissue. Superimposed on all these changes, β-adrenoceptor stimulation increases myocardial oxygen consumption, worsening the ischemic state.

Administration of β-adrenoceptor blockers such as propranolol therefore decreases the occurrence of ventricular arrhythmias during acute myocardial ischemia (Khan et al., 1972; Matta et al., 1976; Pentecost and Austen, 1966). Whether acute treatment with β-adrenoceptor blockers affects the short-term prognosis of patients with acute myocardial infarction has been controversial (Frishman et al., 1984); long-term treatment with these agents reduces the incidence of sudden death in survivors of myocardial infarction (May et al., 1982).

The role of α-adrenoceptors in the susceptibility to ventricular arrhythmias during myocardial ischemia is incompletely understood. NE prolongs effective refractory periods, apparently via stimulation of α-adrenoceptors (Govier, 1967). Although the number of β-adrenoceptors on myocyte cell membranes remains unchanged in the setting of myocardial ischemia, the number of α_1-adrenoceptors increases rapidly in the ischemic region (Corr et al., 1981). In canine myocytes, increases in surface α_1-adrenoceptor density occur within 10 minutes of cellular hypoxia; reoxygenation reverses these increases (Heathers et al., 1988). Thus, whereas under normal conditions stimulation of β-adrenoceptors mediates the cardiac effects of catecholamines, during myocardial ischemia α_1-adrenoceptors may play an increased role. Calcium channel blockade with nifedipine or α_1-adrenoceptor blockade with prazosin prevents coronary vasoconstriction after cessation of stellate ganglion stimulation in anesthetized dogs with coronary stenosis (Hagestad and Verrier, 1988). Whereas β-adrenoceptor blockade does not prevent reperfusion-induced arrhythmias in experimental animals, α_1-adrenoceptor blockers do (Heathers et al., 1988).

Although it is commonly thought that left ventricular inferior wall myocardial infarction results in vagal hyperactivity and anterolateral infarction results in sympathetic hyperactivity, clinical evidence for this distinction has been indirect, based mainly on electrocardiographic and hemodynamic findings. Increased discharge of both parasympathetic and sympathetic nerves can occur simultaneously in patients with myocardial infarction—for example, in inferior wall myocardial infarction with reflexive sympathetic stimulation in response to hypotension (Webb et al., 1972). In this setting, vagal effects may predominate at the sinus node or atrioventricular node and noradrenergic effects in the ventricles (Zipes and Inoue, 1988).

As noted above, coronary occlusion produces sympathetic denervation in and apical to the infarcted area. In a patient with a noninfarcted region apical to a myocardial infarction, the denervated region could become supersensitive to circulating catechol-amines, leading to a predisposition to the development of ventricular arrhythmias. Dogs with chronic myocardial infarction or denervation have supersensitivity, as indicated by exaggerated shortening of electrocardiographic refractory periods in response to intracoronary infusions of NE or isoproterenol (Vatner et al., 1985; Zipes and Inoue, 1988).

Prognosis

High plasma levels of NE and EPI indicate a poor 18-month prognosis in patients with myocardial infarction (Karlsberg et al., 1981). Whether the worse prognosis results from decreased thresholds for ventricular arrhythmias, sympathetic stimulation superimposed on denervation supersensitivity, or more compensatory sympathoneural activation due to more extensive infarction, is unknown.

Angina Pectoris

In patients with coronary heart disease, emotional distress can provoke attacks of angina pectoris. One of the earliest, best-documented, and ironic illustrations of this phenom-enon was the case of Dr. John Hunter (Kligfield, 1980). Hunter, a renowned eighteenth-century surgeon, was by all accounts an extraordinarily hard worker, customarily arising before dawn. He was also notoriously prone to defensive argument, irrational outbursts, obstinateness, and impatience—epitomizing a hostile "Type A" individual. In 1785, he began to experience angina pectoris, a syndrome that his friend, William Heberden, had only recently described. Despite having conducted the dissection of one of Heber-den's cases, Hunter never admitted his own condition for what it was and thought that rheumatism or dyspepsia caused it. He did recognize, however, the relationship between emotional upset and his symptoms, and because argumentation frequently brought them on, he claimed, "My life is at the mercy of any rogue who chooses to provoke me" (Kobler, 1960).

This proved to be one of the most ironic statements in the history of medicine. On October 16, 1793, Hunter became incensed at critical, insolent remarks against him at a meeting of the board of governors of St. George's Hospital. He left the room, col-lapsed, and dropped dead. His brother-in-law and colleague, Everard Home, published Hunter's *A Treatise on the Blood, Inflammation, and Gun-Shot Wounds;* as a preface, Home described Hunter's condition and death. This description is a classic of cardiology (Willius and Keys, 1941):

> [T]he first attack of these complaints was produced by an affection of the mind, and every future return of any consequence arose from the same cause; and although bodily exercise, or distention of the stomach, brought on slighter affections, it still required the mind to be affected to render them severe; and as his mind was irritated by trifles, these produced the most violent effects on the disease. His coachman being beyond his times, or a servant not attending to his directions, brought on the spasms, while a real misfortune produced no effect. . . .

On October 16, 1793, when in his usual state of health, he went to St. George's Hospital, and meeting with some things which irritated his mind, and not being perfectly master of the circumstances, he withheld his sentiments, in which state of restraint he went into the next room, and turning around to Dr. Robertson, one of the physicians of the hospital, he gave a deep groan and dropt down dead.

Laboratory mental challenges such as performance of forced mental arithmetic frequently can evoke myocardial ischemia in patients with coronary artery disease (L'Abatte et al., 1985). During emotionally arousing self-descriptions, coronary patients often have left ventricular wall motion abnormalities and decreased ejection fraction, as indicated by radionuclide ventriculography, even without anginal pain (Rozanski et al., 1988). Electrocardiographic indices usually do not detect the silent ischemia attending mental stress in patients with coronary disease (Rozanski et al., 1991). Mental challenge can reveal ischemic segments that are not evident during exercise (Giubbini et al., 1991). The role of the cardiac sympathetics in mental stress-induced silent ischemia is unknown.

Laboratory mental stressors can elicit myocardial ischemia in coronary patients not only by catecholamine-induced increases in cardiac myocardial oxygen consumption but also by activation of platelets. Brief (10-minute) periods of mental stress increase serum EPI and NE levels, heart rate, blood pressure, the heart rate × systolic pressure product (a measure of myocardial oxygen consumption) and platelet aggregability concurrently; these responses, which cessation of the stress rapidly reverses, are more prominent in coronary patients than in age-matched control subjects (Grignani et al., 1991).

Patients undergoing cardiac catheterization for stable angina pectoris have approximately normal arterial plasma levels of NE and normal NE spillover into arterial plasma (McCance and Forfar, 1990), in contrast with patients with unstable angina, recent acute myocardial infarction, or heart failure, who have increased values for these parameters (McCance and Forfar, 1989a, 1989b). Coronary patients have apparently selectively enhanced increases in cardiac NE spillover during exercise-induced angina (McCance and Forfar, 1989a).

Coronary Spasm

Typical angina pectoris results from an excess of myocardial oxygen consumption over supply provided by coronary arteries that have limited flow reserve. Coronary artery spasm, which occurs usually in areas of underlying coronary atherosclerosis, can evoke angina pectoris even in the absence of increased myocardial oxygen consumption.

Over a century ago, Huchard (cited in Wolf, 1985) wrote that angina pectoris can result when emotions produce coronary spasm and thereby myocardial ischemia. Leriche continued this idea:

From tonus to vasoconstriction, that is to physiological hypertonia, from vasoconstriction to spasm, there is no borderline. One passes from one state to the other without transition, and it is the effects rather than the thing itself which makes for differentiations. Between physiology and pathology there is no threshold. Even with perfect conservation of the arterial structure the spasm, at a distance, has grave pathological effects. It causes pain, produces fragmented or diffuse necroses; last but not least it gives rise to capillary and arterial obliteration at the periphery of the system. (Leriche, 1932, cited in Wolf, 1985)

Osler (1910) also recognized that coronary arteries can undergo spasm, evoking angina pectoris and myocardial infarction. In 1959, Prinzmetal described 32 patients with an atypical form of angina (Prinzmetal et al., 1959) characterized by chest pain at rest or with mild exertion and by transiently elevated electrocardiographic ST segments. It was thought at first that this syndrome was rare, until studies of patients during coronary angiography revealed the common occurrence of spasm in coronary arteries already narrowed by atherosclerosis. This has led to a revival of interest in coronary spasm as a cause of or contributor to ischemic heart disease (Maseri et al., 1978, 1982).

Of the many postulated mechanisms of coronary spasm, several impute abnormalities at the level of the coronary sympathetic neuroeffector junctions (Ricci et al., 1979; Sewell et al., 1955). Coronary vascular smooth muscle cells possess α- and β-adrenoceptors, and since β-blockade unmasks coronary vasoconstrictor responses to NE (Beamish and Dhalla, 1985), desensitization of β-adrenoceptor-mediated processes due to chronic increases in local concentrations of endogenous NE or EPI could intensify α-adrenoceptor-mediated coronary vasoconstriction. Adrenochrome, a product of catecholamine auto-oxidation, constricts coronary arteries (Karmazyn et al., 1981; Singal, Dhillon et al., 1982). Oxidative deamination of catecholamines produces free radicals, implicated in coronary spasm as well as arrhythmias, cellular pathology, and cardiac dysfunction (Singal, Kapur et al., 1982). High circulating levels of catecholamines produce functional hypoxia, due to the marked increases in heart rate and contractility, and prolonged hypoxia elicits coronary vasoconstriction (Karmazyn et al., 1984).

Some patients without fixed coronary narrowing or coronary arterial spasm have pacing-induced angina and limited coronary vasodilator reserve (Cannon et al., 1992). There is no consensus yet whether "microvascular angina," or "Syndrome X," constitutes a distinct clinical pathophysiological entity and if so whether coronary sympathoneural or adrenoceptor function plays a pathophysiological role. In cardiomyopathic hamsters, liquid silicone rubber perfusion of the heart has revealed microvascular spasm (Factor et al., 1982). Calcium channel or α_1-adrenoceptor blockade prevents the spasm and cardiomyopathy.

Heart Failure

Generalized and Cardiac Sympathoneural Activation

Activation of the sympathetic nervous system plays an important role in maintaining cardiovascular performance in "compensated" heart failure. Thus, administration of reserpine (Chidsey et al., 1963) or guanethidine (Gaffney and Braunwald, 1963) causes marked clinical deterioration in patients with heart failure. Consistent with the view that recruited sympathoneural outflow maintains cardiovascular performance in clinical heart failure, beneficial treatments such as diuretics and vasodilators decrease or do not change plasma NE levels, whereas the same drugs increase plasma NE levels in healthy subjects (Bertel et al., 1982b; Creager et al., 1982; Kluger et al., 1982; Levine and Cohn, 1982; Levine et al., 1986a; Olivari et al., 1983). In dogs with chronic mitral regurgitation, acute β-adrenoceptor blockade decreases the mass-corrected slope of the end-ejection stress-volume relation (Nagatsu et al., 1994), indicating that adrenergic support masks contractile depression in this preparation.

Patients with heart failure usually have high NE concentrations in systemic venous plasma. The antecubital venous NE concentration varies directly with the severity of heart failure, as indicated by New York Heart Association functional class (Thomas and Marks, 1978). Although low cardiac output would be expected to prolong NE clearance, elevated plasma NE concentrations in heart failure patients result from increased NE spillover (Abraham et al., 1990; Hasking et al., 1986).

Clinical congestive heart failure has been proposed to develop in three stages (Abboud and Schmid, 1978). First, decreased arterial filling would elicit compensatory neurohumoral activation, with vasoconstriction and sodium retention, a phenomenon called ''forward'' failure. As myocardial dysfunction progressed, cardiac filling pressures would increase, and the hypervolemia would exert a counterbalancing effect on the neurohumoral activation. Eventually, perhaps due to loss of restraint by dysfunctional cardiac baroreceptors, high levels of PRA, AII, aldosterone, AVP, and SNS activity would ensue. These factors would expand extracellular fluid volume severely and further increase cardiac filling pressures, producing ''backwards'' failure, with renal and splanchnic blood shunted preferentially to the heart and brain via the lungs, causing pulmonary edema.

Judging from plasma NE levels, one may question whether the second stage, where SNS activity normalizes due to hypervolemia, actually occurs. Plasma NE concentrations increase inversely with declining functional status in patients with congestive heart failure (Cody et al, 1982; Kluger et al., 1982; Thomas and Marks, 1978). In patients with left ventricular dysfunction but without clinically overt heart failure, plasma levels of NE, ANP, and AVP already are increased (Francis et al., 1990). The neuroendocrine values increase further, accompanied by high PRA levels, as overt heart failure develops. Sympathoneural activity therefore does not normalize, despite hypervolemia, in patients with heart failure, possibly because of activation of several homeostats that use the sympathoneural effector.

Patients with compensated heart failure do not have elevated EPI levels (Abraham et al., 1990), but distress, hypoxemia, and acidosis related to pulmonary edema would be expected to evoke AHS activation. Since β-adrenoceptors in the kidney contribute to renin secretion, combined AHS and renal SNS (Hasking et al., 1986) activation in symptomatic heart failure may help to explain the late increase in RAS activity.

Patients with congestive heart failure have markedly increased cardiac spillover of NE (Hasking et al., 1986). As discussed in the chapter about assessment of catecholaminergic function, measurements of myocardial NE spillover using steady-state systemic intravenous infusions of [³H]NE cannot distinguish increased cardiac sympathetically mediated NE release from decreased neuronal reuptake; the relative importance of these mechanisms in heart failure has been disputed. Rose et al. (1985) interpreted tracer NE kinetic evidence using a bolus-injection technique as indicating reduced cardiac NE release as well as reduced uptake in heart failure patients. In contrast, recent findings by Esler and coworkers, based on simultaneous measurements of spillovers of NE and DHPG, have indicated markedly increased cardiac NE spillover—about 10-fold—in heart failure patients, which the relatively small concurrent decreases in cardiac Uptake-1 activity cannot explain (G. Eisenhofer, personal communication).

Patients with heart failure who have high plasma NE concentrations have poor long-term survival (Cohn et al., 1984; Keogh et al., 1990; Rector et al., 1987; Swedberg et al., 1990). For instance, in the study of Rector et al. (1987), in patients with plasma NE levels more than 600 pg/ml, mortality at four years of follow-up averaged about eight times that in patients with levels less than 600 pg/ml. Heart failure patients with poor prognoses not only have high plasma catecholamine levels but also increased levels of AII, aldosterone, and ANP (Swedberg et al., 1990), indicating concurrent compensatory activation of other circulatory homeostatic effectors. Cardiac transplantation rapidly decreases plasma NE concentrations in patients with severe heart failure (Levine et al., 1986).

These findings have led to reconsideration of whether sympathetic activation in heart failure is beneficial or deleterious (Cohn, 1990; Daly and Sole, 1990; Francis and Cohn, 1986; Packer, 1990). As noted at the beginning of this chapter, even a homeostatic system can produce deleterious effects in the setting of an underlying pathologic process. Generalized increases in sympathetic outflow would be expected acutely to increase myocardial oxygen consumption and cardiac afterload due to increased blood pressure and vasoconstriction. As noted in Chapter 2, both cardiac underfilling and overfilling increase cardiac sympathoneural traffic. In patients with cardiac overfilling due to heart failure, increases in cardiac SNS outflow may fail to augment cardiac output adequately, compared to the amount of increase in myocardial oxygen consumption. This would exacerbate the myocardial dysfunction and produce further overfilling. In addition, chronic cardiac SNS activation could accelerate the pathologic process by accelerating cardiac hypertrophy, thereby decreasing myocardial compliance and diminishing cardiac baroreceptor restraint of SNS outflows. The combined operation of these factors therefore would increase the likelihood of positive feedback loops. This would help to explain the susceptibility of heart failure patients to develop life-threatening pulmonary edema rapidly after apparently trivially small amounts of volume loading due to dietary salt.

Cautious β-blockade seems beneficial in patients with heart failure related to dilated cardiomyopathy (Swedberg et al., 1979; Waagstein et al., 1975). Attempts to improve clinical status or survival in heart failure patients by blocking catecholamine synthesis using α-MT (Franciosa and Schwartz, 1989), sympathetic outflow using clonidine (Hermiller et al., 1983), or α_1-adrenoceptors using prazosin (Cohn et al., 1986) have been disappointing (Cohn, 1990; Leier et al., 1990).

Myocardial Norepinephrine Depletion

In animal models of congestive heart failure, as well as in humans with heart failure, myocardial NE stores decrease (Spann et al., 1964; Vogel et al., 1969). The NE depletion may be clinically significant, because reduced availability of releasable NE stores can impair homeostatic increases of myocardial contractility during stress. For instance, dogs with reserpine-induced depletion of myocardial NE stores have attenuated responses of ventricular max dp/dt and left ventricular end-systolic pressure–segment length slope (indices of left ventricular myocardial contractility) during sympathetic stimulation (Ikeda et al., 1991).

Several explanations have been proposed for the mechanism of depletion of NE stores in congestive heart failure. The most obvious is that the increased rate of synthesis of NE does not keep pace with the markedly increased NE turnover. Pool et al. (1967), Schmid et al. (1982), and Sassa (1971) provided evidence for decreased, rather than increased, myocardial TH activity in heart failure; however, the myocardial content of TH activity is not decreased in the myocardium of laboratory animals with preterminal idiopathic dilated cardiomyopathy (Pierpont et al., 1983). Sole et al. (1982) reported that hamsters with heart failure had increased myocardial concentrations of DA, suggesting a deficiency not of tyrosine hydroxylation but of the vesicular uptake or β-hydroxylation of DA. Pierpont et al. (1983) reported similar findings in animals with dilated cardiomyopathy.

According to another hypothesis, in sodium-retaining states such as heart failure, elaboration of a circulating inhibitor of Na/K-ATPase decreases the extracellular–intracellular gradient of sodium ion, partly inhibiting Uptake-1. Cardiac NE stores would then decline as a consequence of inadequate recycling of the released NE. As noted above, Rose et al. (1985) reported decreased cardiac Uptake-1 activity in heart failure patients; and Liang et al. (1989) reported that in dogs with isolated right heart failure produced by tricuspid avulsion and progressive pulmonary artery constriction, right ventricular myocardial uptake of NE was decreased by about ½; and Sassa (1971) reported that rabbits with cardiac hypertrophy and failure due to supravalvular aortic constriction had decreased left ventricular myocardial uptake of exogenous NE. A combination of increased cardiac sympathetic activity and decreased reuptake would increase the requirement for accelerated synthesis of NE, in order to maintain normal NE stores.

Another hypothesis proposes attenuation of metabolic processes that normally maintain the steep gradient of amine concentrations between the interior of vesicles and the axoplasm. These processes depend on ATP, which may be depleted in heart failure. Somewhat consistent with this view, patients with hypertrophic cardiomyopathy have decreased cardiac spillover of DHPG per unit of mass of myocardium, compared with patients with chest pain and normal coronary arteries (Brush et al., 1989). Although this also may reflect decreased Uptake-1 activity, recent evidence has indicated that most of cardiac DHPG production in humans derives not from reuptake of endogenously released NE but from net leakage of NE from the vesicles into the cytoplasm (Eisenhofer, Esler et al., 1992). Decreased DHPG production in cardiomyopathy patients therefore could result from decreased NE synthesis, due to deficient vesicular uptake of axoplasmic DA and NE. This defect would also explain the buildup of tissue DA. Rats with cardiac hypertrophy due to aortic constriction have decreased myocardial concentrations of [^{3}H]NE after injection of the tracer (Fischer et al., 1965). The results do not distinguish whether the increased NE turnover arises from decreased uptake, increased release, or decreased retention of the tracer.

Patients with heart failure have down-regulation of cardiac β_1-adrenoceptors (Bristow et al., 1982, 1986; Liang et al., 1989), possibly in response to increased concentrations of neuronally released NE or of circulating EPI at neuroeffector junctions in the heart. Myocardial failure may also be associated with abnormalities in the function of G-proteins that link β-receptors to cellular contraction mechanisms (Bristow et al., 1990; Horn and Bilezikian, 1990), although no abnormality has been identified definitively.

Patchy depletion of myocardial NE stores in heart failure (Daly and Sole, 1990; Sole, 1988; Vogel et al., 1969) may predispose to the development mechanical or electrical cardiac dysfunction. Consistent with the notion that regional sympathetic denervation decreases thresholds for ventricular arrhythmias, Wichter et al. (1994) reported that most patients with arrhythmogenic right ventricular cardiomyopathy had localized decreases in ^{123}I-MIBG-derived radioactivity in left ventricular myocardium. Because of the poor spatial resolution of ^{123}I-MIBG scanning, the right ventricular myocardium was not visualized in the patients or controls.

Ventricular Arrhythmias and Sudden Death

Literature since antiquity has noted an association between acute distress and sudden cardiovascular collapse. In the New Testament, in the Acts of the Apostles, Ananias and his wife Sapphira "fell down and gave up the ghost" after being chastised by Peter. Josephus wrote about the circumstances of the death of the murderous king Aristobulus:

> But Aristobulus instantly repented the slaughter of his brother. Guilt aggravated a disease and so disturbed his mind that his entrails were wracked by intolerable pain and he vomited blood. Once, a servant carrying away this blood slipped and shed some of it—by divine providence, as I cannot but think—at the very spot where stains of Antigonus' blood still remained . . . he shed many tears and gave a deep groan: "I am not, I see, to escape God's detection of the impious and hideous crimes I have been guilty of. Unforeseen punishment threatens me for shedding the blood of my kin. And now, most impudent body of mine, how long will you retain a soul that, to appease the ghosts of my brother and my mother, ought to die? . . . With these words he died. . . . (Glatzer, 1960, pp. 58–59)

Hypotheses about external triggers precipitating sudden death often center on sympathoneural activation (Willich et al., 1993), providing a straightforward link between distress and sudden cardiac death. Modern medical reports generally have confirmed an association between acute emotional distress and sudden cardiac death. Engel

(1971) reviewed 170 cases of sudden death during psychological stress, noting that "people are described as dying suddenly while in the throes of fear, rage, grief, humiliation, joy . . . as far back as written records exist . . . intense emotional distress may induce sudden death." Greene et al. (1972) suggested that in more than half of patients with sudden death, social or psychological factors are evident at the time of death. Wolf (1969) also described patients in whom emotional crisis preceded a lethal arrhythmia.

Supplementing this body of largely anecdotal literature, a study cited by Wehrmacher and Randall (1984) included 45,000 workers for the Eastman Kodak Company. Among 22 patients who died suddenly, death occurred in "a setting of acute arousal engendered by increased work activity or circumstances precipitating reactions of anxiety or anger." Compared with an unselected population studied over a similar time frame, people undergoing unusually emotionally disturbing events have an increased frequency of sudden cardiac death (Reich et al., 1981). Other epidemiological evidence has confirmed the view that presumed psychosocial stressors, such as the recent death of a spouse, increase the likelihood of subsequent sudden death (Cannon, 1942; Jenkins, 1976, 1982; Rees and Lutkins, 1976; Rissanen et al., 1978; Wolf, 1969).

The following discussion considers four types of conditions where emotional distress or catecholaminergic activation can produce sudden arrhythmic death: vasovagal circulatory collapse, such as associated with severe hemorrhage (the case of Aristobulus may be an early example); ventricular arrhythmias due to sympathetic activation during myocardial ischemia; the long QT syndrome; and catecholamine-induced myocardial necrosis.

Vasovagal circulatory collapse represents a situation where markedly increased PNS outflow occurs concurrently with withdrawal of SNS vasoconstrictor tone, as discussed in the chapter about stress response patterns. This reaction develops rapidly, often in a setting where the individual senses a failure to cope despite activation of homeostatic systems. Intense SNS stimulation gives way abruptly to sympathoinhibition, increased AHS and PNS outflows, bradycardia, and hypotension. Vasovagal reactions can include potentially lethal heart block and ventricular arrhythmias; if the individual is held upright, cerebral hypoperfusion occurs. Tilt-table testing in the diagnostic evaluation of unexplained syncope detects "malignant vasovagal syncope" (abrupt onset of hypotension and bradycardia and loss of consciousness) in about 20% of patients (Hiner, 1992). Whereas neither atropinization nor permanent cardiac pacing prevents hypotension during vasodepressor episodes, measures to counteract dependent pooling of blood (e.g., elastic stockings) or increase blood volume (e.g., mineralocorticoid combined with dietary salt loading, head-up tilt at night), isometric exercise training of leg muscles, and β-adrenoceptor blockade can be effective treatments (Perry et al., 1991; van Lieshout et al., 1991).

Hypotension due to carotid sinus hypersensitivity can be viewed as a form of vasovagal response. As in vasovagal reactions, carotid sinus hypersensitivity revealed by effects of carotid massage can be primarily cardioinhibitory or primarily vasodepressor. Profound sympathoinhibition can occur during carotid sinus massage in either syndrome (Smith et al., 1992); however, whether carotid sinus massage-induced sympathoinhibition characterizes all patients with carotid sinus hypersensitivity and whether the sympathoinhibition causes the hypotension have not yet been established.

In the presence of normal coronary arteries, emotional distress rarely induces life-threatening arrhythmias in animals (Billman et al., 1990; Carpeggiani and Skinner, 1991) or in humans (Amsterdam, 1990). In contrast, substantial clinical and laboratory animal evidence supports the view that stress can evoke lethal ventricular arrhythmias in the setting of coronary ischemia, as discussed in the section about acute myocardial infarction. In laboratory animals, electrical stimulation of the frontal cortex, hypothalamus, and brainstem reticular formation can produce ventricular arrhythmias, even in the absence of coronary ischemia (Delgado, 1960; Garvey and Melville, 1969; Hall et al., 1977; Hockman et al., 1966; Manning and Cotten, 1962; Mauck et al., 1964; Melville et al., 1963; Weinberg and Fuster, 1960). Corley et al. (1975, 1977) reported myocardial damage and cardiac arrest in squirrel monkeys undergoing 24-hour sessions of avoidance conditioning, with negative reinforcement being mild electric shocks.

Patients with sustained ventricular arrhythmias have increased cardiac NE spillover (Meredith et al., 1991). Although this is consistent with a pathophysiologic role for increased cardiac sympathoneural release of NE, in the study of Meredith et al. (1991) most of the patients had coronary artery disease, and those patients with high cardiac NE spillover had reduced left ventricular ejection fractions. Myocardial dysfunction therefore could have elicited compensatory increases in cardiac SNS outflow in these patients.

Patients with the idiopathic long QT syndrome have increased susceptibility to develop life-threatening ventricular arrhythmias during exposure to physical or emotional stressors, including fear, exercise during emotional distress, swimming, and being awakened by a loud noise. In some patients with prolonged electrocardiographic QT intervals, left stellate ganglionitis or inflammation of ganglia within the sinoatrial node has been identified pathologically (Rossi, 1988). β-Adrenergic blockade is the treatment of choice, and left cardiac sympathetic denervation can be effective (Schwartz et al., 1991). In conscious cats with right stellate ganglion ablation, emotional distress prolongs the QT interval and can precipitate ventricular arrhythmias. Schwartz and coworkers have suggested that increased cardiac sympathetic activity derived from the left stellate ganglion results in an increased risk of ventricular arrhythmias (Schwartz, 1985; Schwartz et al., 1991). This is the basis of the ''sympathetic imbalance'' hypothesis.

The occurrence of afferent and efferent cardiac nerves in the same trunks complicates inferences from the effects of electrical stimulation or surgical sectioning. Another complicating feature is that stimulation of efferent sympathetic neurons from a variety of intrathoracic sites can produce substantial localized changes in repolarization that are not detected by total electrocardiographic QT intervals (Savard et al., 1991).

LeNoble et al. (1985) introduced the use of renal intra-arterial injections of 6-OHDA to produce selective renal efferent sympathectomy. This approach could be used in the heart to evaluate the relationship between regional sympathetic denervation and thresholds for ventricular arrhythmias, with or without coronary ischemia.

Cardiac Necrosis and Cardiomyopathy

There are two main forms of cardiac necrosis: coagulation necrosis and necrosis with contraction bands (Ferrans et al., 1969; Ferrans and Van Vleet, 1985). The former typically occurs in areas of myocardial infarction (i.e., areas of myocardial cell death due to ischemia without reflow). In coagulative necrosis due to myocardial infarction, the cells die in a relaxed state; the pathologic changes are not detectable for many hours or even days, when there is a polymorphonuclear infiltrate; and calcification occurs late.

In contrast, myofibrillar degeneration (also called myocytolysis, coagulative myocytolysis, or contraction band necrosis) occurs within seconds or minutes. Contraction bands reflect the hypercontracted, rather than relaxed, state of the cells. If there is an infiltrate, it is mononuclear; and calcification occurs rapidly. On the light microscopic level, mildly affected areas have increased eosinophilic staining of the cytoplasm with preserved striations; more severely affected cases have transformation of the entire cytoplasm, with dense eosinophilic bands (''contraction bands'') between areas of granularity (''myofibrillar degeneration''). Electron microscopy reveals hypercontraction, tearing, and dislocation of cellular myofibrils. Other pathological findings include mitochondrial deposits of calcium, loss of cellular glycogen, margination of nuclear chromatin, and nonspecific changes of cell death. In less severely affected regions, the finding of small bulges in the cells on either side of the intercalated disk has led to the designation, ''paradiscal'' lesion (Todd, 1984). In more severely affected regions, the entire cell contains coagulated contractile proteins, with clumped mitochondria—a ''holocytic'' contraction band lesion.

Contraction band necrosis appears to arise when large amounts of calcium enter living myocardial cells through damaged membranes (Ferrans and Van Vleet, 1985; Fleckenstein et al., 1969; Milei et al., 1979; Todd, 1984). The lesions occur in the outer regions of myocardial infarcts and subendocardially.

Infusion of catecholamines, stimulation of the central nervous system, the combination of stress and steroids, myocardial reperfusion, the ''stone heart'' syndrome after heart surgery, and pheochromocytoma all can produce contraction band necrosis, which is also observed in the majority of cases of sudden cardiac death (Baroldi et al., 1979; Samuels, 1985; Todd, 1984). The combination of subendocardial damage and arrhythmogenic actions of catecholamines may explain the high frequency of sudden death in patients with stroke, epilepsy (Jay and Leestma, 1981), head trauma (Evans et al., 1976), intracranial hypertension (Smith and Ray, 1972), and severe emotional distress (Corbalan et al., 1974).

Stress Cardiomyopathy

In 1907, Josue (cited in Samuels, 1985) demonstrated cardiac necrosis after infusions of EPI. The pathologic picture resembles that in patients suffering extreme stress (Eliot et al., 1977), sudden death (Baroldi et al., 1979), intracranial bleeding, or pheochromocytoma. Sixty minutes after administration of isoproterenol at 100 ng/kg/min, paradiscal contraction band lesions begin to accumulate (Todd, 1984). This dose would be expected to result in a circulating isoproterenol level of about 1500 pg/ml (Goldstein, Zimlichman et al., 1986a) and would correspond to levels of EPI observed only during maximal AHS responses such as evoked by severe hypoglycemia or cardiac arrest. A 10-fold larger dose of isoproterenol produces holocytic contraction band lesions. By about 1–2 weeks after production of contraction band lesions in rats, the lesions have disappeared. Remnants of myocardial cells become condensed fragments, and necrotic areas fibrose. The histopathological nonspecificity of the chronic lesions makes it difficult or impossible to identify catecholamine-induced myocardial damage by a few weeks after the injury.

Injection of large amounts of NE also produces myocardial necrosis, in rats (Lee and Sponenberg, 1984) and monkeys (Wahi et al., 1984). Pretreatment with the α_1-adrenoceptor blocker prazosin or a calcium channel blocker ameliorates NE-induced necrosis (Lee and Sponenberg, 1984). Activation of α_1-adrenoceptors by NE, with consequently increased cytoplasmic Ca^{2+} concentrations, therefore appears to be the mechanism of NE-induced cardiomyopathy (Downing and Lee, 1983). α_1-Adrenoceptor stimulation probably also contributes to Ca^{2+} accumulation in myocardium during reperfusion injury (Sharma et al., 1983); and α_1-blockers ameliorate reperfusion-related arrhythmias (Stewart et al., 1980). Auto-oxidation of catecholamines increases the production of free radicals that peroxidate lipids and disrupt cellular structure (Singal, Kapur et al., 1982; Singal et al., 1983). The auto-oxidation hypothesis may apply to cardiac necrosis from reperfusion injury, since, as noted above, acute coronary occlusion and myocardial anoxia markedly increases the efflux of NE from sympathetic nerve terminals.

Hans Selye showed that injection of large doses of adrenal corticosteroids or analogues increases the frequency of cardiac necrosis after exposure to any of several stressors (e.g., immobilization, bacteremia, surgery, toxins, and vagotomy; Selye, 1958). Treatment with corticosteroids also exacerbates cardiac necrosis produced by injections of catecholamines (Eliot, 1988, 1989). Exactly how adrenocortical hormones render the myocardium vulnerable to catecholamine-induced necrosis is unknown. One explanation is that glucocorticoids upregulate cardiac β-adrenoceptors.

Contraction bands have been observed in about 80% of all victims of sudden death (Baroldi et al., 1979). Cebelin and Hirsch (1980), analyzed autopsy results in victims of homicidal assault who died despite the lack of sufficient evidence of internal or external injury. Contraction band necrosis—"stress cardiomyopathy"—was observed in 11 of the 15 cases, without evidence of myocardial infarction. Ryan and Fallon (1986) described the case of a 44-year-old woman who, after learning that her son had just committed suicide, developed substernal chest pain and pulmonary edema. Endomyocardial biopsy showed findings consistent with "a stress-induced myocarditis caused by high circulating levels of catecholamines."

In 1968, Topel et al. introduced the term "porcine stress syndrome" to describe rapid shock and death in pigs during handling, transportation, exposure to hot, humid conditions, and physical or emotional excitement. This susceptibility is inherited as a single recessive gene with high penetrance. The mechanism of cardiopathy in the porcine stress syndrome is unknown (Johansson et al., 1974).

Cardiac necrosis has also been reported in rats subjected to immobilization (Sharma and Barar, 1966), overcrowding (Fani et al., 1977), restraint and water immersion (Tanaka, 1981), repeated, small electric shocks (Lauria et al., 1972), and laboratory emotional stressors (Lawler et al., 1981; Raab, 1966; Raab et al., 1964).

In laboratory animals, electrical stimulation of central neural regions such as the hypothalamus, limbic cortex, and midbrain reticular formation, can produce myofibrillar degeneration, ventricular arrhythmias, or subendocardial necrosis (Garvey et al., 1969; Greenhoot and Reichenbach, 1969; Hall et al., 1974; Melville et al., 1963, 1969). Cervical spinal transection or stellate ganglionectomy prevents the electrocardiographic and pressor effects, but vagotomy does not, indicating a sympathoneural mechanism (Samuels, 1985).

In patients with pheochromocytoma, persistently high circulating catecholamine levels can induce cardiac hypertrophy and cardiomyopathy. The cardiomyopathy can progress to a dilated form, producing congestive heart failure. Even at this late stage, however, curative surgical removal of the tumor can reverse the cardiomyopathy (Imperato-McGinley et al., 1987).

Other Forms of Cardiomyopathy

Hypertrophic cardiomyopathy is an unusual disease characterized by massive overgrowth of the muscular interventricular septum, variable amounts of obstruction of ventricular outflow, a hypercontractile myocardium, and impaired diastolic filling of the left ventricle. About 50% of the patients die suddenly. Pathologically, there is cellular disarray, with patchy areas of necrosis and fibrosis. Catecholamines, by increasing the force and rate of cardiac contraction, worsen the outflow obstruction and decrease the threshold for ventricular arrhythmias in response to several types of stressors.

Hypotheses about the pathogenesis of hypertrophic cardiomyopathy have imputed abnormalities of cardiac sympathoneural function. In utero, the developing myocardium may not handle catecholamines normally (Goodwin, 1980). Correct alignment of myofibrils may require appropriate modulation of catecholamines during embryogenesis (Perloff, 1981). Repeated administration of subpressor doses of catecholamines including NE (King et al., 1987; Laks et al., 1973) or of NGF (Witzke and Kaye, 1976) produces left ventricular hypertrophy. Ostman-Smith (1981) proposed that cardiac sympathetic nerves, via release of endogenous NE, constitute the final common pathway in adaptive cardiac hypertrophic responses.

Although an early study indicated excessive NE concentrations in the septum of patients with hypertrophic cardiomyopathy (Pearse, 1964), this has not been confirmed. Patients with hypertrophic cardiomyopathy have a few abnormalities of cardiac NE kinetics, compared with findings in patients with chest pain and normal coronary arteries (Brush et al., 1989). The left ventricular extraction percent of circulating NE is decreased, whereas the extraction percent of isoproterenol is not, consistent with decreased neuronal uptake of circulating catecholamines per unit of mass of tissue. The cardiac arteriovenous increment in plasma DHPG levels is also significantly decreased.

Most of the findings could be explained if the hypertrophic myocardium were relatively denervated, with increased traffic in the remaining sympathetic nerves.

The cardiomyopathic Syrian hamster represents an animal model of inherited, congestive cardiomyopathy. The cardiomyopathy appears to result from repeated episodes of microvascular spasm, followed by reperfusion injury, resulting in regions of patchy necrosis. According to Sole and Factor (1984), the cardiomyopathy depends on genetic transmission of hypersensitivity, both of cardiac and vascular smooth muscle, to catecholamines. Juvenile cardiomyopathic hamsters have increased rates of urinary NE excretion and cardiac NE turnover (Jasmin et al., 1979; Sole et al., 1975). Treatment with the calcium channel blocker verapamil or with the α_1-adrenoceptor blocker prazosin prevents the cardiomyopathy, whereas treatment with the β-blocker propranolol does not. As cycles of spasm and reperfusion injury lead to myocardial necrosis and cell loss, sympathetic outflow increases compensatorily (Ostmann-Smith, 1981). Eventually, there is loss of sympathetic nerve terminals apposed to myocardial cells and sprouting of terminals in connective tissue. The heterogeneity of sympathetic innervation then would predispose to sudden death. Kagiya et al. (1991) confirmed that in the prehypertrophic stage in cardiomyopathic Syrian hamsters, myocardial NE content and densities of α_1-adrenoceptors and β-adrenoceptors were increased, and blockade of α_1-adrenoceptors by bunazosin reduced the myocardial hypertrophy and focal myocardial necrosis.

Chagas' disease represents a unique form of cardiomyopathy, where abnormalities of cardiac SNS function develop in stages (Iosa et al., 1989, 1990). Early in the disease, decreased numbers of α-adrenoceptors and cholinergic receptors produce orthostatic hypotension. The adrenergic receptor pathology advances, and nerve and muscle impairment become prominent, with fatigue, dizziness, failure of orthostatic reflexes, and palpitations. High plasma NE levels reflect an ineffectual compensatory mechanism in this stage. In the last stage, denervation is superimposed on receptor malfunction. Unlike other forms of heart failure, in heart failure due to Chagas' disease there is no increase in plasma NE levels. The patients have bradycardia, absence of sweating, and weakness. The high frequency of sudden death may result from denervation supersensitivity.

Orthostatic Hypotension

Physical manipulation of the region of the carotid sinus in the neck has long been thought to evoke circulatory abnormalities such as arrhythmias, hypotension, and syncope (Leatham, 1982). Surprisingly little is known about the mechanism of clinical carotid sinus syncope. Some patients continue to have bradycardic syncope even after surgical bilateral removal of the carotid glomus, and the removed tissue can be histologically normal (Rossi, 1988).

Decreased cardiac filling, such as occurs clinically in hemorrhage or dehydration, would be expected to enhance orthostatic responses of sympathoneural traffic and plasma NE levels, since orthostatic hypotension in this setting occurs despite compensatory increases in SNS outflows and is associated with tachycardia.

Orthostatic hypotension as part of autonomic neuropathy occurs in several disorders, most notably diabetes mellitus. This form of hypotension is associated with relatively constant heart rate and decreased basal and reflexive increases in plasma NE during standing.

Three types of primary neurogenic orthostatic hypotension have been described: pure autonomic failure (PAF), multiple system atrophy (MSA), and DBH deficiency. PAF reflects degenerative loss of peripheral sympathetic nerve endings. MSA involves concurrent neurogenic orthostatic hypotension and central neural degeneration, such as parkinsonism or cerebellar–pontine atrophy. DBH-deficient patients have a congenital absence of DBH.

Whether PAF and MSA constitute distinct syndromes or extremes along a continuous pathophysiologic spectrum has not been resolved. Thus, patients with clinical evidence of MSA can have markedly decreased levels of catecholamine-synthesizing enzymes in the LC as well as in sympathetic ganglia (Black and Petito, 1976). Patients with evidence of central neural degeneration have a shorter median duration of illness until disability and death.

Patients with primary neurogenic orthostatic hypotension usually have a failure to increase plasma NE levels normally during standing (Ziegler et al., 1977a). Orthostatic blood pooling, which decreases NE clearance, can result in orthostatic increases in plasma NE levels in autonomic failure patients—a false-negative test. Assessments of [³H]NE kinetics can reveal decreased or absent orthostatic increases in NE spillover in these patients (Meredith et al., 1992).

Patients with autonomic failure have markedly decreased total, cardiac, and renal spillover of NE, as well as very low cardiac spillovers of DOPA and DHPG (Meredith et al., 1991).

In supine subjects, patterns of plasma levels of catechols can help to distinguish among the diagnostic subgroups (Goldstein, Polinsky et al., 1989). PAF patients usually have very low levels of NE, often also with low levels of DHPG, DOPA, and DOPAC, consistent with decreased populations of NE-synthesizing terminals. MSA patients usually have normal levels of all catechols, and DBH-deficient patients have a virtual absence of NE and DHPG and high levels of DA, DOPA, and DOPAC.

Within the group of PAF patients, some have normal plasma levels of DHPG and DOPA, suggesting an abnormality in the exocytotic process rather than a simple loss of sympathetic nerve terminals. Nanda et al. (1977) reported a case of idiopathic orthostatic hypotension with failure of NE release despite fluorescence microscopic evidence of vascular innervation.

Consistent with abnormal central pathways mediating baroreflexes, patients with MSA often have a failure to increase plasma AVP levels during tilt-induced hypotension (Kaufmann et al., 1992). MSA patients also have an absence of clonidine-induced increases in growth hormone levels, unlike PAF patients or patients with Parkinson's disease (Thomaides et al., 1992).

The etiology of MSA may be autoimmune, since CSF of MSA patients contains an antibody that reacts with rat LC tissue in vitro (Polinsky et al., 1991). Patients with other neurological diagnoses associated with clinical signs and symptoms of sympathetic failure (diabetic polyneuropathy, Parkinson's disease, or idiopathic autonomic failure) often have circulating immunoglobulins that recognize proteins in extracts of rat sympathetic neurons (Murphy et al., 1993). In rats, injection of a monocloncal antibody against the low-affinity receptor for nerve growth factor (NGF) destroys post-ganglionic sympathetic nerves (Wiley, 1993). These findings justify further research into the possibility of autoimmune bases for autonomic failure and the development of treatments involving neurotrophic agents.

Treatment with dihydroxyphenylserine (DOPS) can effectively reverse orthostatic hypotension due to DBH deficiency (Biaggioni et al., 1990). Decarboxylation of the drug generates NE, bypassing the enzymatic defect. In patients with PAF and very low plasma NE levels, treatment with clonidine increases blood pressure via stimulation of α_2-adrenoceptors on vascular smooth muscle cells (Robertson et al., 1983).

Stroke and the Heart

Physicians have long known that cardiac disorders can cause stroke; however, the recognition that strokes can produce cardiac abnormalities is much more recent. Beginning with the observations of Byer, Ashman, and Toth (Byer et al., 1947), many studies have reported electrocardiographic abnormalities in patients with acute stroke. Burch et al. (1954) considered the triad of prolonged electrocardiographic QT interval, abnormal T waves, and U waves to be pathognomonic of acute stroke. Hammermeister and Reichenbach (1969) associated electrocardiographic QRS changes, myocardial necrosis, and neurogenic pulmonary edema in patients with subarachnoid hemorrhage.

Since most patients with acute stroke have associated atherosclerotic coronary heart disease, it is important to know which electrocardiographic changes actually are new at the time of the stroke. In a study of 150 patients with acute stroke, over 90% had electrocardiographic abnormalities (Goldstein, 1979). Of these, the most common abnormalities were also changes from previous tracings: QT prolongation, ischemic changes, U waves, tachycardia, and arrhythmias. Patients with embolic strokes had a high frequency of atrial fibrillation, and patients with subarachnoid hemorrhage had a high frequency of QT prolongation and sinus arrhythmia. Stroke patients also had a higher frequency of pathologic Q waves and left ventricular hypertrophy than did age- and sex-matched control inpatients, but these findings were not new at the time of the stroke. Patients with either extremely low or extremely high blood pressure on admission had an increased frequency of QT prolongation and ischemic changes that were unrelated to mortality. The findings were consistent with the view that QT prolongation in acute stroke results from cardiac sympathetic activation, which, in turn, can be a compensatory mechanism or reflect a primary neurocardiologic process.

Strokes due to intracranial bleeding are often associated with acute hypertension, arrhythmias, electrocardiographic changes suggesting myocardial ischemia, and increased levels of cardiac isozymes (Norris et al., 1979). In the study of Goldstein (1979), 61% of patients with acute stroke had elevated CPK levels, and of patients who had CPK isozymes measured, 40% had elevated levels. Twenty-six percent of the patients who had LDH isozymes measured also had elevated levels. Most remarkably, all patients with intracranial bleeding had elevated CPK levels. The time course of development of focal myocardial damage is about 6 hours after the acute neurological event. Cardiac lesions are not evident after 2 weeks, implying that they are reversible (Kolin and Norris, 1984).

In cases of subarachnoid hemorrhage associated with myocardial necrosis, Greenhoot and Reichenbach (1969) reported that intramyocardial nerves, identified by external laminae, microtubules, neurofibrils, and axoplasmic vesicles, occasionally were adjacent to the involved myocardial cells, with the extent of myocardial cell pathology inversely related to the distance from the nerves and with structurally intact cells appearing by 2–4 μm from the nerves. These findings suggest that high local concentrations of NE, released during marked cardiac sympathoneural stimulation, cause contraction band necrosis in patients with intracranial bleeding (Reichenbach and Benditt, 1970). Several groups have confirmed the occurrence of stroke-induced, autonomically mediated cardiac necrosis, especially in hemorrhagic stroke (Burch et al., 1969).

Stroke-induced myocardial necrosis is associated with generalized increases in SNS outflows, since the rate of occurrence of cardiac arrhythmias and the extent of increase in cardiac-specific enzymes correlate with plasma levels of catecholamines in stroke patients (Myers et al., 1981, 1982). Vasospasm evoked by intracerebral bleeding is associated with large increases in both CSF and plasma NE levels (Shigeno, 1982). Analogously, plasma NE levels in stroke-prone SHRs are higher in animals with actual cerebral bleeding than in those without bleeding (Minami et al., 1984). The occurrence of high plasma catecholamine levels is a sign of poor prognosis in patients with aneurysmal subarachnoid hemorrhage (Dilraj et al., 1992).

Intracranial bleeding would be expected to increase intracranial pressure. In dogs, progressive intracranial hypertension produced by an epidural balloon elicits marked increases in plasma catecholamine levels, with mean increases of 286-fold for EPI and 78-fold for NE (van Loon et al., 1993); and in chronically catheterized fetal sheep, lateral ventricular injection of artificial CSF to increase intracranial pressure increases arterial plasma levels of NE, EPI, and AVP by almost two orders of magnitude (Harris et al., 1989). Extremely high catecholamine levels due to intracranial hypertension therefore may produce the hemodynamic changes occurring in the Cushing response and in fetal head compression during labor.

High levels of catecholamines in the heart probably contribute importantly to the cardiac necrosis attending acute stroke. β-Adrenoceptor blockade ameliorates the electrocardiographic changes in patients with subarachnoid hemorrhage (Cruickshank and Dwyer, 1974), and adrenoceptor blockade (Hunt and Gore, 1972; Neil-Dwyer et al., 1978) or depletion of catecholamine stores by reserpine (McNair et al., 1971) can prevent myocardial necrosis produced by intracranial bleeding.

These findings support the view that cardiac necrosis and electrocardiographic changes in patients with acute stroke result at least partly from high myocardial concentrations of catecholamines.

Functional Cardiorespiratory Syndromes

Patients with signs or symptoms of combined cardiovascular and psychiatric disorders represent a large proportion of any internist's medical practice. These patients often pose a diagnostic, therapeutic, and management challenge, especially when angiography or noninvasive tests document coincident coronary ischemia, when Holter monitoring reveals arrhythmias, or when ambulatory blood pressure monitoring records pressor episodes.

Many different diagnostic appellations have been proposed for functional cardiorespiratory syndromes: hyperdynamic circulation syndrome, hyperkinetic heart syndrome, vasoregulatory asthenia, hypernoradrenergic hypertension, mitral valve prolapse syndrome, chronic fatigue syndrome, neurocirculatory asthenia, soldier's heart, effort syndrome, hyperventilation syndrome, Da Costa's syndrome, somatization psychogenic cardiovascular reaction, psychophysiologic cardiovascular disorder, nervous heart complaint, psychogenic cardiac nondisease, panic disorder, and psychogenic autonomic dysfunction (Bass, 1990). The length of this list probably indicates not so much the variety of psychocardiologic conditions as ignorance about their pathophysiologic mechanisms.

The most common complaints of patients with functional cardiorespiratory disorders are breathlessness, palpitations, fatigue, sweating, and chest pain (Bass, 1990). There also can be paresthesias, faintness, sighs, nervousness, and syncope.

The following discussion explores separately neurocirculatory asthenia, hyperdynamic circulation syndrome, hypertension with SNS hyperresponsiveness, mitral valve prolapse syndrome, and anxiety-related chest pain. These may not constitute distinct nosologic entities and may instead reflect different emphases by clinical observers.

''Neurasthenia,'' a term introduced by Beard in 1867, refers to a syndrome initially described by Da Costa in Civil War soldiers and used subsequently by Osler, MacKenzie, and Paul Dudley White (Rosenman, 1990). Others have called the same condition neurocirculatory asthenia, Da Costa's syndrome, effort syndrome, soldier's heart, irritable heart, shell shock, combat fatigue, vasomotor instability, vasomotor neurosis, autonomic imbalance, somatization psychogenic cardiovascular reaction, and posttraumatic stress disorder (Caranasos, 1974). The syndrome consists of a large number of symptoms, including breathlessness, palpitations, precordial chest pain, fatigue, dizziness, exertional dyspnea and fatigue, excessive sweating, trembling, flushing, dry mouth, paresthesias, irritability, and exercise intolerance (Friedman, 1945). Family members often have a similar syndrome.

The multiplicity of symptoms in these patients contrasts with the dearth of signs of disease, which all are nonspecific: relative tachycardia and tachypnea, facial and neck flushing, slight tremor, excessive palmar sweating, a functional heart murmur, and hyperactive deep tendon reflexes, with generally normal resting blood pressure. There are no characteristic laboratory or electrocardiographic findings.

Injections of EPI may (Wearn and Sturgis, 1919) or may not (Friedman, 1945) evoke these symptoms. β-Blockade often normalizes the cardiovascular and somatic findings without affecting the emotional symptoms. Drugs such as caffeine and benzadrine can produce tachycardia, tachypnea, tremor, and diaphoresis in patients with neurocirculatory asthenia. These drugs are thought to increase sympathetic outflow by actions in the brain, whereas exogenous EPI produces tachycardia directly.

Caranasos (1974) has hypothesized that excessive central stimulation of sympathetic outflow, rather than augmented responsiveness to adrenoceptor agonists, produces the symptoms in patients with neurocirculatory asthenia. Rosenman (1990) has suggested that patients with neurocirculatory asthenia have a biological anxiety disorder associated with mitral valve prolapse, as discussed below.

Most modern research about neurocirculatory asthenia has been conducted in Russia. Meerson et al. (1990) reported increased baseline EPI excretion, normal baseline NE excretion, and excessive NE responses to stress in patients with neurocirculatory asthenia. More than ½ of the patients were reported to develop arrhythmias during adrenergic stress responses but not during exercise.

Western cardiovascular researchers have evinced little interest in this topic. The diagnosis is rarely made in modern medical practice, probably because of vague nosology and medical benignity. Patients with neurocirculatory asthenia do not appear to have an increased risk of organic heart disease or other medical illnesses.

In the hyperdynamic circulation syndrome, resting tachycardia, labile, predominantly systolic hypertension, and increased heart rate responsiveness to isoproterenol are associated with increased catecholamine levels at rest and during provocative maneuvers (Frohlich, 1977; Frohlich et al., 1969; Goldstein and Keiser, 1985). β-Adrenoceptor blockers or benzodiazepines ameliorate the syndrome. It is unclear whether patients with this syndrome have an increased frequency of subsequent development of established hypertension.

In a case of hyperdynamic circulation syndrome studied in detail, Goldstein and Keiser (1985) reported markedly decreased baroreflex–cardiac sensitivity that normalized during sedation induced by intravenous diazepam. Episodes of tachycardia and systolic hypertension were associated with remarkable blotchy flushing of the face, nape, and upper chest. Emotional facial flushing appears to depend on active sympathetic vasodilation (Drummond and Lance, 1987). Kuchel et al. (1987) reported a similar case of a patient followed for 30 years with emotion-induced severe hypertensive paroxysms. The attacks were associated with increased cardiac output, flushing, decreased reflexive bradycardia, and variably increased plasma levels of catecholamines.

Anxiety or panic can be associated with chest pain that mimics angina pectoris due to coronary heart disease. An example may have been the attack that Mickey Mantle suffered in April 1987 (*New York Times,* April 14, I, 26:2; April 15, II p:1):

> Mickey Mantle, the former Yankee star, was released from the hospital in good condition today after tests that showed chest pains he suffered probably stemmed from stress syndrome, a hospital spokesman said.
>
> "Mr. Mantle has had no previous history of heart problems," said Dr. Michael Rothkopf, medical director of Irving Heart Institute. "He does have evidence of bronchitis and has had physical symptoms suggesting stress syndrome—chest pains, shortness of breath and

dizziness.'' Rothkopf said Mantle's heart appeared normal and his condition was probably caused by ''too many pressing social engagements.'' (*New York Times*, April 15, 1987)

Anxiety and panic attacks often include important catecholaminergic components, with systolic hypertension, tachycardia, palpitations, and patterned changes in cutaneous blood flow (Winters et al., 1990). Munjack et al. (1990) reported that patients with generalized anxiety disorder had approximately normal plasma levels of catecholamines and metabolites under resting conditions. Panic patients can have increased plasma EPI levels related to anxiety ratings (Villacres et al., 1987). Gale and Edwards (1986) have severely criticized psychophysiological research in this area, noting that most of the studies ''merely select an 'off-the-rack' self-report measure of trait anxiety, choose an equally 'off the rack' physiological index, and subject the experimental population to an 'off-the-rack' and ecologically meaningless laboratory test'' (p. 468).

Even during panic attacks, catecholaminergic activation may not occur. Cameron et al. (1987) followed neuroendocrine and cardiovascular changes during 36-hour periods of bed rest in patients with panic attacks and in normal control subjects. Panic attacks were not associated with increased plasma levels of NE, EPI, or MHPG, suggesting a dissociation between neuroendocrine responses and experiential reports in panic patients.

The benzodiazepines have proven to be effective in the treatment of several types of anxiety disorder. Benzodiazepines are thought to augment modulatory actions of GABA at $GABA_a$ receptors regulating Cl^- channels in the brain (Paul et al., 1986). Administration of the benzodiazepine antagonist β-carboline-3-carboxylic acid ethyl ester (β-CCE) produces behavioral and physiological effects in rhesus monkeys that are analogous to those during natural conditions eliciting anxiety. Neurochemical effects of β-CCE include increased plasma levels of catecholamines, cortisol, and ACTH (Crawley et al., 1985; Ninan et al., 1982). Treatment with diazepam blocks the behavioral, cardiovascular, and autonomic responses to β-CCE. Administration of benzodiazepines decreases SNS and AHS outflows and reactivity in laboratory animals (Antonaccio and Halley, 1975; Chai and Wang, 1966; Morpurgo, 1968; Sigg, 1975; Sigg et al., 1971) and in humans (Goldstein et al., 1982; Hossmann et al., 1980; Marty et al., 1986; Stratton and Halter, 1985). Alprazolam treatment has been found to be effective in the management of panic patients with chest pain and normal coronary arteries (Beitman et al., 1988).

Intravenous administration of yohimbine can evoke attacks in patients with panic/anxiety disorder. Symptom ratings after yohimbine administration correlate positively with peak changes in plasma levels of MHPG in patients with panic disorder (Gurguis and Uhde, 1990). Treatment with alprazolam or tricyclic antidepressants attenuates MHPG responses to yohimbine (Edlund et al., 1987). These results are consistent with the view that in the brain, α_2-adrenoceptors on noradrenergic terminals restrain SNS outflows, and in patients with panic/anxiety, interference with this restraining influence releases the sympathetic nervous system from inhibition, concurrently precipitating the psychopathologic emotional experience.

There is no convincing evidence from prospective studies that anxiety or panic disorder increases the risk for developing coronary heart disease (Byrne and Byrne, 1990). Thus, Army veterans with disability separations for psychoneurosis had normal 25-year mortality rates from arteriosclerotic cardiovascular disease, degenerative cardiac disease, diseases of arteries or veins, and hypertension (Keehn et al., 1974).

Patients with depression associated with anxiety have increased plasma NE levels, due to increased NE spillover (Esler, Jennings et al., 1988, 1990). Despite these findings, blood pressure is not elevated. Apparently, for hypertension to be expressed, other compensatory systems must also fail.

Patients with mitral valve prolapse can complain of chest pain or pressure, exertional dyspnea, palpitations, orthostatic faintness, fatigue, poor exercise tolerance, pallor, sweating, anxiety, and panic (Rosenman, 1990). This constellation of symptoms suggests autonomic imbalance, and a proportion of patients with mitral valve prolapse have high venous plasma levels of NE (Paddu et al, 1983; Pasternac et al., 1982). Patients with mitral valve prolapse have an increased incidence of anxiety disorders, although it remains unclear whether the prolapse and the adrenergically associated anxiety are merely coincidental. Chesler et al. (1985) failed to confirm both the psychiatric and biochemical associations. Taylor et al. (1989) reported increased heart rate and plasma NE levels and exaggerated tachycardic responses to isoproterenol in patients complaining of dysautonomic symptoms, regardless of the presence of mitral valve prolapse. Lenders et al. (1986) found no differences in plasma catecholamine levels among groups of mitral valve prolapse patients with or without symptoms and healthy control subjects, at rest, during head-up tilt, or during isometric exercise. Boudoulas and Reynolds (1983) reported that patients with high baseline plasma levels of catecholamines had increased responsiveness to β-adrenoceptor agonists.

Rosenman (1990) has suggested that some of the excessive ''sympathicotonic'' responsiveness of symptomatic patients with mitral valve prolapse syndrome results from abnormal processing of baroreceptor information or from hypovolemia, which would augment sympathoneural responses to orthostasis. According to Rosenman's hypothesis, functional mitral valve prolapse results from decreased ventricular volume compared to the size of the mitral orifice. The decreased ventricular volume may in turn result from deficient blood volume produced by an abnormality of sodium homeostasis; this would stimulate SNS outflows compensatorily. Alternatively, since patients with mitral valve prolapse syndrome tend to be thin for their height, with a narrow anterior–posterior chest diameter, and occasionally have pectus excavatum, they may on a constitutional basis have decreased ventricular volume compared to mitral annulus area. Regardless, hyperadrenergic activity would be associated with mitral valve prolapse not because of a neurocirculatory disorder or because of anxiety but because of a specific hemodynamic abnormality eliciting appropriate autonomic responses.

Among hypertensives, pressor and plasma catecholamine responses to yohimbine are distinctly bimodal (Goldstein, Grossman, Listwak et al., 1991). An identifiable subgroup have both large pressor responses to yohimbine and large responses of arterial plasma NE levels. Patients in this subgroup typically report yohimbine-elicited anxiety, panic, or emotional feelings similar to those experienced at some time in the past. In this series, the patient with the largest pressor and catecholamine responses had a chronic anxiety disorder. The patient exhibited marked labile systolic hypertension, with extreme blood pressure elevations during exposure to minor psychological stressors, and with clinic blood pressure readings invariably much higher than home readings. The patient was tall and thin, with cool, sweaty palms but without evidence of blotchy flushing of the face or neck. In this patient, treatment with alprazolam markedly attenuated the physiological, neuroendocrine, and experiential effects of yohimbine, and chronic alprazolam treatment prophylactically, combined with a long-acting calcium channel blocker, effectively controlled his blood pressure at baseline and limited pressor responses during emotionally stressful conditions. The patient did not have the hyperdynamic circulation syndrome, since his tachycardic and psychiatric responses to intravenously infused isoproterenol were normal. In two other patients with combined hypertension and excessive pressor and catecholamine responses to yohimbine, clinical symptoms and signs included exertion- and emotion-related chest pain and palpitations, excessive sweating, breathlessness, frequent clearing of the throat, hyperglycemia, and a rapid style of speaking, so that the patients often seemed to be tripping over their words. Another patient with this combination had a chronic somatization disorder. Another had a history of sensitivity to caffeine, palpitations, and frequent atrial premature contractions, and had had severe panic and tachycardia at the time of childbirth, necessitating hospitalization for this reaction. Another, discussed previously in the section about the hyperdynamic circulation syndrome, had stress-, isoproterenol-, lactate- and yohimbine-induced blotchy flushing of the face, neck, and upper back and chest, thin body habitus, resting tachycardia, and a history of paroxysmal hypertension triggered by seemingly trivial emotional stressors.

Interrelationships among these psychiatric, autonomic, and cardiovascular abnormalities obviously pose a challenge to researchers interested in the role of stress and catecholaminergic reactivity in clinical cardiovascular diseases.

Other Conditions

Quadriplegia due to spinal cord section is usually associated with decreased plasma NE levels and with adrenoceptor supersensitivity (Mathias and Frankel, 1983).

Acute increases in blood pressure and pulse rate commonly accompany seizures. NE levels in CSF and plasma increase (Devinsky et al., 1992). Patients with "autonomic epilepsy" have increased plasma NE during seizure activity (Metz et al., 1978).

Guillain–Barre syndrome occasionally is associated with neurogenic hypertension or supraventricular tachycardia, possibly as a consequence of impaired baroreflexes (Yao et al., 1985). The tachycardia and hypertension are correlated with plasma levels of NE and with urinary VMA excretion (Ahmad et al., 1985).

Simonovsky, a student of the Russian physician S. Botkin, taught that prolonged stimulation of sensory nerves in the arm can result in structural damage in myocardium (Zavodskaya et al., 1980). Simonovsky coined the term "reflex sympathetic dystrophy" (RSD) to describe this phenomenon, since he considered the mechanism to be an abnormal sympathetic reflex. The term has been expanded to include severe limb pain that develops after seemingly minor trauma such as surgery.

The diagnosis of RSD depends on the clinical presentation (burning pain, allodynia, skin temperature or color changes, edema, and hair, skin, and nail growth changes) and on results of clinical tests (thermography, bone X-ray, bone scan, sweat test, sensory testing, and responsiveness to sympathetic blockade). Clinical staging into acute, dystrophic, and atrophic forms is based on trophic changes, decreased blood flow and skin temperature, cyanosis, and absence of sweating (Raj et al., 1992).

Whether RSD as encountered clinically results from abnormal reflexes or abnormal SNS activity is unknown. Patients with RSD have decreased, rather than increased, plasma NE levels in the venous drainage of the affected limb (Drummond et al., 1991). Research attention therefore has begun to focus on possible abnormalities of adrenoceptors (Arnold et al., 1993), including adrenoceptors on nociceptor afferents (Raja, 1992; Schwartzmann, 1992).

Summary and Conclusions

The main role of the SNS in cardiovascular function is homeostatic. Sympathoneural activation can be pathologic in effect because of worsening of a largely independent cardiac pathologic state. Only in relatively rare conditions, such as PAF, pheochromocytoma, and cardiac necrosis attending intracranial bleeding, does abnormal catecholaminergic function play an incontrovertibly etiologic role.

SHRs of the Okamoto strain have increased sympathoneural activity and reactivity that is most prominent in young animals. Because of the many loci of catecholaminergic abnormalities in this strain, an abnormal "algorithm" for development of catecholaminergic systems in the brain and periphery, or for the development of neuroendocrine stress responses, seems more likely than an isolated biochemical or genetic abnormality. Nevertheless, researchers studying SHRs continue to focus on single effector systems.

Clinical essential hypertension is a heterogeneous disorder; however, as with studies of SHRs, most experimental approaches to the pathophysiology of clinical primary hypertension have been monolithic. Relatively young patients with borderline hypertension often have increased cardiac, renal, and skeletal muscle sympathoneural activity and augmented reactivity during stimuli that increase SNS outflows reflexively, pharmacologically, or psychologically. Yohimbine challenge testing can identify patients with hypertension and sympathetically mediated pressor hyperresponsiveness.

NE is a hypertrophogenic factor in the heart and vascular system, acting independently of increases in blood pressure.

Pheochromocytoma, a tumor that secretes catecholamines into the bloodstream, is a rare but curable cause of secondary hypertension. Diagnostic approaches include measurements of plasma levels of catechols during glucagon stimulation and clonidine suppression testing. Patients with pheochromocytoma can have a catecholamine-induced cardiomyopathy that is reversible upon excision of the tumor.

Myocardial infarction and congestive heart failure are associated with marked cardiac sympathoneural activation that probably decreases thresholds for the occurrence of malignant ventricular arrhythmias. The extent of recruitment of sympathetic outflow appears to provide a prognostic index in both myocardial infarction and heart failure.

Whether this association results from deleterious effects of high local concentrations of catecholamines or compensatory sympathoneural recruitment remains unclear. Heart failure depletes NE stores, possibly contributing to exercise intolerance. The mechanism of this depletion is incompletely understood.

Catecholaminergic activation during acute emotional distress, superimposed on a substrate of coronary insufficiency, can precipitate myocardial infarction, cardiac necrosis, or sudden death. Whether chronic emotional stress accelerates the development of hypertension, coronary disease, or any cardiovascular disorder in otherwise healthy people is unknown.

Patients with different types of neurogenic orthostatic hypotension have distinctive patterns of plasma levels of catechols. In rare cases of DBH deficiency, treatment with DOPS can provide NE and cure the hypotension.

Intracranial bleeding can evoke SNS and AHS activation, producing characteristic electrocardiographic changes and cardiac necrosis.

Clinical diagnostic attempts to date have failed to provide objective means to evaluate patients with functional cardiorespiratory syndromes pathophysiologically.

Hypotheses that particular personality characteristics, such as the "Type A coronary prone behavior pattern," hostility, and the "Sisyphus reaction," accelerate the development of coronary heart disease have aroused persistent controversy. The next chapter examines further several prevalent opinions about personality and environmental factors that may mediate relationships among stress, catecholamines, and cardiovascular disease.

8

Current Opinions and
Future Directions

Substantial interest within the medical community and among lay people about the long-term health consequences of stress contrasts with an inadequate fund of clinically relevant, valid research information about whether and how chronic stress affects cardiovascular performance and risk.

Previous chapters discussed how acute emotional distress increases heart rate and blood pressure by mechanisms where catecholamines dominate. As exemplified in the classic case of the death of Dr. John Hunter in 1793 (Kligfield, 1980), described in Chapter 7, acute emotional distress in an individual with underlying coronary heart disease can precipitate myocardial ischemia or sudden death. Much more controversial are the views that chronically repeated episodes of emotional distress can produce hypertension that persists after the stress ends, and that chronic emotional stress constitutes an independent risk factor for the development of coronary heart disease.

These views derive mainly from evidence about responses during acute stresses, from Selye's notions about "diseases of adaptation," from psychosomatic concepts about "reactivity," and from literature about the relationship between aspects of personality and cardiovascular risk.

This chapter attempts to separate facts from opinions about these ideas and presents a homeostatic model for the relationship between exposure to a distressing stimulus and the occurrence of cardiovascular pathology. The chapter and book close with predictions about future trends in the area of stress, catecholamines, and cardiovascular diseases.

Beyond Selye

Many researchers continue to accept Selye's view of stress as a stereotyped response pattern with characteristic neuroendocrine changes—in particular, increased HPA activity (Kalin, 1993). An alternative view, presented in Chapters 1, 2, and 6 of this book, posits that different stressors elicit primitively specific patterns of responses, involving many effector systems.

Differential responses of SNS and AHS outflows provide persuasive evidence for this patterning. For instance, hypoglycemia selectively increases adrenomedullary secretion; unloading of cardiopulmonary baroreceptors selectively increases skeletal sympathoneural outflow; and hemorrhagic hypotension produces adrenomedullary activation with renal sympathoinhibition. One may hypothesize that patterning of central neurochemical responses underlies the stressor specificity of peripheral autonomic responses.

Neuroendocrine patterning may also occur during different forms of psychological stress, depending on the quality of the emotion, the occurrence of locomotion, the novelty or predictability of the stressor, and the individual's perception of coping options. Whereas Selye considered ''distress'' in a rather vague and circular manner, the present theory proposes several distinguishing and defining characteristics of distress: consciousness, aversiveness, external signs, and homeostat resetting, leading to HPA and AHS activation.

The homeostatic model in Figure 8–1 depicts how distress can contribute to cardiovascular pathology. According to the model, exposure to a distressing stimulus, such as an agonistic confrontation at work, contributes only indirectly to cardiovascular pathology. Inputs from receptors to the brain; regulation of psychological homeostats based on factors such as instinct, learning, and simulation; activities of effector systems; alterations in levels of monitored variables; and concurrent risk factors such as drugs (e.g., nicotine, caffeine, alcohol, cocaine, medications) and coexisting cardiovascular pathologic states (e.g., coronary artery disease, cerebrovascular disease, valvular heart disease, myocardial dysfunction, and degenerative cardiovascular changes) intervene between the stressor and the cardiovascular pathologic consequences.

The model suggests that assessments of interactions among risk factors, monitored variables, and activities of neuroendocrine effector systems may predict cardiovascular pathologic events better than assessments of elements of stressors.

Do Life Changes Accelerate Heart Disease?

Until the late 1960s, scientific support for a causal link between stress and the development of chronic cardiovascular disease depended mainly on collections of case reports (Wolf et al., 1968). In 1967, Holmes and Rahe published a ''Schedule of Recent Experience'' to quantify major life changes and their relationship to illness in general. The authors proposed that the sum of the life changes requiring adjustment would predict subsequent illness. In the inventory, subjects reviewed a checklist of positive and negative life experiences, such as marriage, divorce, birth or death of a close family

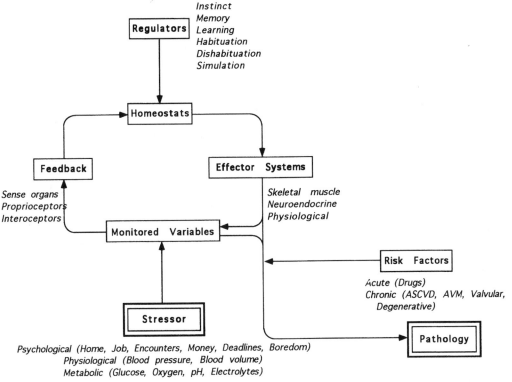

Figure 8–1. Homeostatic model of distress-related cardiovascular pathology. According to the model, exposure to a stressor, such as an agonistic confrontation at work, is related only indirectly to cardiovascular pathology. Intervening are levels of monitored variables; inputs from receptors to the brain; regulation of homeostats based on factors such as instinct, learning, and simulation; activities of effector systems, including the sympathoneural and adrenomedullary systems; and concurrent risk factors such as drugs (e.g., nicotine, caffeine, alcohol, cocaine, medications) and coexisting cardiovascular pathological states (e.g., coronary artery disease, cerebrovascular disease, valvular heart disease, myocardial dysfunction, and degenerative cardiovascular changes). The model assumes no direct link between any of the other components and the risk factors, since research literature on this topic is very controversial; and the model suggests that assessments of interactions among levels of monitored variables, risk factors and activities of neuroendocrine effector systems predict cardiovascular pathological events better than assessments of more distant factors such as elements of stressors.

member, loss of employment, and relocation. The 43 life events were ranked numerically, with death of a spouse rated 100, divorce 73, marital separation 65, a jail term 63, death of a close family member 63, loss of employment 47, and so forth. The subjects were asked to think back over a specific time interval and report events during that interval. The total score was compared with health outcomes, such as visits to a doctor. Studies using this approach generally found that recalled life changes preceded the recalled onset of illness (Rahe et al., 1970, 1974).

The approach using life change rating scales accepts Selye's notions that stress can contribute to any of a wide variety of diseases, depending on ''conditioning factors'' operating in the individual and the extent and appropriateness of the stress response; and that stress is the sum of all the ''wear and tear'' in an individual. This approach has proven very popular, and an abundance of lay literature purports to instruct the reader about how to tote stress to predict risk (e.g., Tanner, 1976). Stress management organizations and writers have claimed that a score over 300 raises substantially the chances of serious illness of some kind during the subsequent year (Hanson, 1985).

The low predictability of morbid events or mortality has led to reliance on retrospective or case-control analyses in testing the validity of rating scale results. The retrospective approach allows the possibility of biases, both intentional and unintentional, to influence or even determine the results. For example, subjects stricken with serious illness probably try to identify preceding factors in their lives that could have caused their disease. Case-control approaches have well-known and inescapable limitations. One is that they provide no information about the actual increase in risk due to the event, since this would require a comparison between the incidence of death after the event and the incidence of death in the absence of the event—that is, a predictive study design. Rosengren et al. (1993) recently reported that among 752 middle-aged Swedish men, the self-report of three or more life events (illness or concern about death of a family member, divorce or separation, being forced to move one's household or change jobs, job insecurity or unemployment, financial problems, and prosecution) during the year before the baseline examination was associated with more than a three-fold increase in mortality. The association remained statistically significant after adjustment for smoking, emotional support, and self-perceived health.

A major problem with the rating scale approach is that the same events may have different psychological impacts in different people. This could be especially relevant in studies of people with the ''Type A'' pattern, where the stressor itself is not so important as the patient's interpretation of and response to the stressor. A more appropriate life experience inventory would take into account the impact of the events on the individual (Beamish et al., 1991; Byrne and Byrne, 1990). Lazarus (1966) has theorized that no life events are inherently stressful, and the experience and reactions to stress require interpretations in terms of cognitive and personal frameworks—especially about the ability to cope. To date, no prospective study has determined whether taking into account both events and their personal impact improves the predictability of life change scores in terms of cardiovascular risk.

Some of the listed life changes can themselves indicate underlying disease. In the rating scale of Holmes and Rahe, the occurrence of personal injury or illness receives a score of 53, change in living conditions 25, change in work conditions or hours 20, and change in sleeping habits 16. In myocardial infarction patients, these associations alone can explain a relationship between self-reported life changes and health outcomes.

Finally, the literature is inconsistent about whether life change inventory scores predict any specific cardiovascular morbid events (Byrne and Byrne, 1990).

After major life crises, such as the death of a spouse, mortality does transiently increase (Clayton, 1974; Cottingham and Matthews, 1980; Jacobs and Ostfeld, 1977; Parkes and Brown, 1972; Parkes et al., 1969; Rahe et al., 1970; Spilken and Jacobs,

1971). Upon review of nine studies, Clayton and Darvish (1979) concluded that mortality following bereavement did not result from coronary heart disease. The mechanism of increased mortality in this setting therefore remains obscure. Loss of a long-term companion would be expected to depress the survivor, increasing the likelihood of self-neglect—including failure to take prescribed medications—and suicide. The loss would also eliminate a source of warning and assistance in the event of a fall or acute, progressive disease process. Moreover, bereaved people increase their consumption of alcohol and tobacco (Parkes and Brown, 1972). All these factors could complicate the relationship between the stress itself and the occurrence of overt coronary events.

Episodes of emotional distress exacerbate hypertension acutely (e.g., Reiser et al., 1951), but the long-term consequences in humans are unclear. An oft-quoted report by Graham (1945) noted a high frequency of hypertension in soldiers after a year or more of desert warfare. With two months of rest, however, blood pressure normalized in virtually all the subjects. Whether chronic neurotic illness incited by wartime stress causes or contributes to chronic cardiovascular disease remains unsettled and controversial. When an Administrative Appeals Tribunal decided to grant war pensions for ischemic heart disease arising out of military service in World War II, the decision incited severe criticism (Boman, 1982; Tennant, 1982). Keehn et al. (1974) reported that Army veterans with disability separation for psychoneurosis in 1944 did not have increased 24-year mortality from hypertension or atherosclerotic or degenerative cardiovascular diseases.

All modern wars have been associated with temporarily increased cardiovascular morbidity or mortality in the civilians. When London was bombed by the Germans, there was an increase in heart attacks (Boman, 1982). When the Israeli citizenry underwent Iraqi "Scud" missile attacks in 1990, the only reported deaths resulted from cardiac causes in elderly people, and the frequency of myocardial infarction and sudden death suddenly increased (Meisel et al., 1991). Survivors of internment in concentration camps or of imprisonment during war have suffered few if any long-term sequelae in terms of cardiovascular risk, although psychiatric problems often persist (Eaton et al., 1982; Gill, 1983; Levav and Abrahamson, 1984). These studies of course included only the survivors.

Trevisan et al. (1986) obtained screening data from groups of people a few weeks before and a few weeks after an earthquake. Both groups had had baseline examinations five years previously. Pulse rates were higher in the group after the disaster, whereas blood pressures did not differ. During the first three days after the Athens earthquake of 1981, fatal cardiac events increased by 50% and deaths from atherosclerotic heart disease by about a 100%, compared with corresponding periods in 1980 and 1982 (Trichopoulos et al., 1983).

Does Job Stress Contribute to Heart Disease?

Literature about occupational stress and cardiovascular disease has suggested that job settings involving both large demands and little autonomy (i.e., little latitude in decisionmaking) are associated with increased cardiovascular risk (Karasek et al., 1981,

1982; Langosch et al., 1983). Beamish et al. (1991) have listed excessive overtime, monotonous assembly line labor, unrealistic time schedules, more than one job at a time, too little (or too much) responsibility, and conflicts with supervisors or fellow employees as relevant job-related stressors affecting cardiovascular health. This would fit with the view that emotional stress contributes to heart disease when there is a sense of lack of control or inability to cope.

Studies in this area have mainly used either cross-sectional or retrospective designs and have assessed patients with already clinically overt hypertension or coronary heart disease. Several articles contain little more than intuitive opinions.

In Japan, "karoshi," death from overwork, refers not to the fatal consequences of emotionally exhausting office work. The Japanese Government has funded a study about the pathophysiologic significance, if any, of job stress. The results have not been published as of this writing.

Byrne and Byrne (1990) reviewed studies about the relationship between the amount of "inherent" stress of occupations and risk of coronary heart disease. Reports have suggested increased coronary risk in general medical practitioners as opposed to specialists (Russek, 1960); sea officers (Mundal et al., 1982); blue-collar workers as opposed to white-collar workers (Bolm-Audorff and Siegrist, 1983); police officers (Ely and Mostardi, 1986); and self-employed individuals as opposed to employees (Magnus et al., 1983). It also has been proposed that increased work demand (Liljefors and Rahe, 1970), job dissatisfaction (Sales and House, 1971), and lack of control (Alfredson et al., 1982) increase coronary risk. Syme (1985) has hypothesized that job elements related to increased cardiovascular risk include tight scheduling with an impossibility of meeting time requirements, social isolation, and interpersonal provocation producing anger and impatience. For instance, Japanese who acculturated after they immigrated to the San Francisco Bay area had higher rates of coronary heart disease than those who did not acculturate (Marmot and Syme, 1976).

For most of these studies, the effects of self-selection and of behavioral factors such as cigarette smoking, intake of alcohol, fat, salt, and caffeine, obesity, and sedentariness probably complicated the results. In a recent cross-sectional study of urban bus drivers (Albright et al., 1992), after controlling for 12 confounding variables, no relationship was detected between hypertension and job strain, demands, or decision latitude.

Occasionally, studies have appeared by their titles to use a longitudinal design, whereas the design actually has been cross-sectional. Bartone (1989) reported "predictors" of stress-related illness in city bus drivers. What was predicted was not the future development of illness but concurrently obtained questionnaire results. The truly prospective study of Siegrist et al. (1992) did note that among blue-collar male workers, multivariate logistic regression analysis revealed that status inconsistency (low reward at work) and "immersion" (high intrinsic effort at work) constituted independent factors predicting cardiovascular events. Other identified risk factors included hypertension, left ventricular hypertrophy, and hyperlipidemia.

Another problem in this line of research is the assessment of the amount of distress experienced by individuals who self-select their employment. The study of Cobb and Rose (1973) exemplifies this problem. Air traffic controllers had excessive rates of hypertension, diabetes, and other risk factors that would be expected to contribute to the development of coronary heart disease. The union of air traffic controllers, PATCO, struck at least partly because of the position that the controllers should be compensated for the increased risk due to the stress inherent in their job. Relatively few people, however, become air traffic controllers. In a free society, perhaps individuals who feel a thrill holding for a few minutes the lives of hundreds of people in their hands, or who smoke cigarettes and drink coffee, or who prefer a sedentary job, tend to become air traffic controllers; for them the job may not be distressing but stimulating.

An additional limitation applies to use of case-control studies to uncover relationships between job stress and heart disease. Schnall et al. (1990) screened blood pressure in 2,556 male employees at 7 work sites; 87 cases of hypertension and a random sample of 128 controls were studied further. After adjusting for age, race, body-mass index, type A behavior, alcohol intake, smoking, sodium excretion, education, the work site, and the physical demand of the job, job strain—defined as high psychological demand and low decision latitude on the job—was associated with hypertension and increased left ventricular mass index. The case-control method is cross-sectional in design, rendering interpretations in terms of cause and effect most difficult and risky, as pointed out in an editorial by Williams (1990) and a summary of the literature by Pickering (1990). For instance, the results of Schnall et al. (1990) did not exclude the possibility that patients with elevated blood pressure—perhaps in response to publicity about the topic—tended to report more stress on their jobs. Brody and Natelson (1987) have concluded that there is no compelling evidence that chronic stress alone, in an otherwise healthy individual, causes hypertension that is sustained after removal of the stressor.

Reynolds (1974) and Warheit (1974) studied groups of workers at the Kennedy Space Center who either were or were not directly responsible for aspects of an upcoming rocket launch to the moon. The former group were considered to be under occupational stress. As the launch date approached, neither group had changes in serum total cholesterol levels or blood pressure. Electrocardiographic abnormalities were more frequent in the stressed group; however, the types of abnormalities (e.g., right bundle branch block and changes consistent with an old myocardial infarction) probably indicated underlying coronary heart disease that was not induced by the stress of the job itself.

The inadequate number of prospective studies prevents drawing firm conclusions about the role of chronic job-related emotional stress in the development of heart disease. Nevertheless, physicians are often asked to provide opinions about occupational stress and heart disease in individual patients. The following seem reasonable if largely intuitive criteria in forming such opinions: (1) The situation's rarity or severity render the individual unprepared to face it, inciting a perceived inability to cope. (2) The situation actually allows few if any coping options. (3) The situation involves confrontation, challenging the individual's integrity, with evident anger, fear, or humiliation. (4) No other precipitant, such as nicotine inhalation, caffeine ingestion, self-medication, or physical or emotional stress outside the job setting, could have elicited the catecholaminergic activation. (5) The event would not have occurred but for the experience of emotional distress; that is, the event could not have resulted from the continued operation of established pathogenic factors. And, (6) the individual complains of symptoms referable to catecholaminergic activation (such as palpitations or a feeling of impending doom), or evinces signs of such activation (such as tachycardia, paroxysmal hypertension, sweating, pallor, piloerection, and hyperventilation) after the stressful experience and before the acute morbid event.

Stress Management

Stress management programs currently are in vogue. These programs may improve worker morale, productivity, and mental outlook; their effects on the development of cardiovascular disease have been unclear. Many studies have examined whether application of stress management techniques decreases blood pressure or decreases medication requirements in patients with hypertension (Johnston, 1991). Reductions in blood pressure after stress management for 2 or 3 months average about 9 mm systolic and 6 diastolic, compared with 3 and 3 mm Hg in control subjects. Whether these beneficial effects persist is unknown. Although it is widely assumed that the mechanism of blood pressure reduction is neurohumoral, data about catecholamine levels have been inconsistent. Stress management usually is applied as a package that includes dietary changes and decreases in nicotine and alcohol consumption. One may therefore hypothesize that if stress management programs do help to prevent heart disease, they do so because of amelioration of established cardiovascular risk factors rather than because of ''stress reduction'' itself.

The Reactivity Hypothesis

Coronary Atherosclerosis

Studies about job stress and cardiovascular disease often have relied on biochemical or acute physiological responses (''reactivity'') to draw conclusions about risk. These approaches are fraught with interpretational difficulties. Two main problems involve an emphasis on acute rather than chronic outcomes and also on largely unknown relevance of responses in laboratory settings to responses in real life (Pickering, 1990).

In a frequently cited study, Friedman et al. (1958) reported serum cholesterol levels of tax accountants biweekly between January and June. The cholesterol levels peaked early in April, exactly when the subjects would have been expected to experience the most emotional stress. In this study, caffeine intake, cigarette smoking, alcohol intake, and dietary fat ingestion were not controlled, and there was no comparison group where the subjects would not be expected to experience stress early in April. Instead, data about dietary intake were obtained from diary information for two 1-week periods, April 2–9 and May 14–21. The absence of a control group means that other temporal factors were not excluded. The same limitations could apply in the studies of Thomas and Murphy (1958) and Grundy and Griffin (1959) about cholesterol levels in medical students undergoing academic examinations.

Wolf et al. (1962) reported changes in serum concentrations of cholesterol in subjects on a metabolic ward during several months of constant diet and exercise. Periods separately judged to be emotionally stressful were associated with increased cholesterol levels. Dimsdale and Herd (1982) summarized many studies about plasma lipids during emotional arousal and concluded that whereas free fatty acid levels almost invariably increase in this setting, results about cholesterol have been more inconsistent; the majority of studies have reported increased cholesterol levels. Again, the rigor of control of dietary intake varied widely among the studies.

In the above-cited study of Trevisan et al. (1986), screening cholesterol data had been obtained from the subject groups a few weeks before and a few weeks after an earthquake. Both groups had previously had baseline examinations five years previously. Cholesterol, triglyceride, and heart rate levels were higher in the group after the disaster, whereas blood pressures did not differ. Although the results are suggestive, the study failed to control for possible differences in several behaviors in the exposed group after the acute stress.

Eliot and co-workers (Eliot, 1988, 1989; Eliot and Buell, 1985) have developed a "SHAPE" (Stress, Health, and Physical Examination) program to diagnose and treat "hot reactors" and "cold reactors" during stress. The testing, "Life Stress Simulation," includes hemodynamic assessments during tilting, playing a video game, performing mental arithmetic, hyperventilation, Valsalva maneuver, handgrip exercise, and the cold pressor test. "Hot reactors" have increased peripheral resistance and decreased cardiac output (measured using impedance cardiography) during stress—a presumably high-risk situation. Treatment is then tailored based on the hemodynamic pattern—for example, β-blockade for "output reactors" and a vasodilator for "vasoconstrictive reactors." No convincing evidence in peer-reviewed journals has supported the validity or clinical significance of this reactivity testing procedure.

Hypertension

As a pathophysiologic explanation for the development of hypertension, the reactivity hypothesis contains two elements, both of which are controversial (Freeeman, 1990). The first is that people destined to develop hypertension have excessive pressor reactivity during a standard challenge. The second is that repeated neurogenic pressor episodes produce structural cardiovascular adaptation, resulting in a long-lasting tendency to excessive vasoconstriction.

Since the initial suggestions of Hines and Brown (1936) and Keys (Keys, 1966; Keys et al., 1971), whether an excessive increase in blood pressure during the cold pressor test predicts the future development of sustained hypertension has aroused persistent controversy. Several prospective studies, summarized by Pickering and Gerin (1990), have failed to confirm this idea. For instance, Thomas and Duszynski (1982) found little predictive power of the cold pressor test in a longitudinal study of Johns Hopkins medical students. Coresh et al. (1992) confirmed this in an updated analysis of the Johns Hopkins database. In a longitudinal study of residents of Tecumseh, Michigan, blood pressure reactivity occurred independently of the development of hypertension (Julius et al., 1991). Pickering (1990) has concluded that there is little or no evidence that acute stress-related pressor responses have any pathologic relevance, except for a possible relationship to the development of left ventricular hypertrophy.

Falkner and co-workers (Falkner, Kushner et al., 1981; Falkner, Onesti et al., 1981) reported that in adolescents with borderline hypertension, strongly positive family history, tachycardia at rest, and a large cardiovascular response to mental stress characterized patients who developed sustained essential hypertension after several years. Perini et al. (1991) conducted a prospective study about personality factors as predictors of hypertension development in young normotensive and borderline hypertensive humans. Stress-induced pressure responses, indices of sympathoneural activity, and psychological factors all predicted, albeit weakly, blood pressure classification at a mean of 30 months of follow-up. The largest pressure increases occurred in subjects with suppressed aggression.

Folkow (1982) has suggested that repetition of acute pressor episodes leads to structural cardiovascular adaptation, where arteriolar wall/lumen ratios increase. This would amplify increases in resistance to blood flow for a given amount of smooth muscle contraction. Korner and co-workers (Adams et al., 1989; Korner, 1982; Korner et al., 1989) have analogously hypothesized that cardiovascular amplifiers contribute to the development and maintenance of elevated blood pressures in hypertensive subjects. In dogs (Julius et al., 1989) and baboons (Turkkan et al., 1984), chronic repetition of neurogenic pressor episodes does not consistently produce sustained hypertension.

Benschop et al. (1994) recently assessed whether self-reported chronic stress affected immunologic or cardiovascular responsiveness to an acute psychological stressor in male high school teachers. The groups of subjects reporting extremely high or low frequencies of daily stress differed in terms of natural killer and T-cell responses to the stressor but did not differ in terms of heart rate or blood pressure responses.

Julius and Brandt (1988) and Julius et al. (1989) reported that repeated neurogenic pressor episodes do not produce sustained hypertension but do produce left ventricular hypertrophy; and the cold pressor test can elicit coronary spasm (Raizner et al., 1980). Thus, the reactivity hypothesis may live on, to explain other pathophysiologic states besides hypertension or coronary atherosclerosis.

Acute vs. Chronic Stress

Whereas much literature describes neuroendocrine responses during acute emotional distress, long-term effects of repeated episodes have received relatively little attention.

Kvetnansky and co-workers have used chronic or repeated immobilization to examine chronic effects of distress on neuroendocrine parameters in rats. Rats exposed repeatedly to immobilization have increased tissue concentrations of catecholamine-synthesizing enzymes (Kvetnansky et al., 1970, 1971; Kvetnansky and Mikulaj, 1970). In the heart, concentrations of NE decrease and of EPI increase after a single period of immobilization, whereas after repeated immobilization, myocardial NE concentrations return to about baseline, and high EPI concentrations persist (Kvetnansky and Torda, 1984). The return of NE concentrations to control levels is associated with increased activities of TH and DBH. Kvetnansky and Torda (1984) attributed the depletion of myocardial

NE in repeatedly immobilized animals to enhanced release that was not balanced by increases in NE synthesis and storage.

Chronic repetition of exposure to stressors often results in habituation of responses to the same stressor and exaggerated acute responses to a novel one—the phenomenon of dishabituation (Kvetnansky and Mikulaj, 1970; McCarty et al., 1992; Nisenbaum et al., 1991). Repeated restraint of rats decreases the response of cAMP concentrations to catecholamines in brain slices (Stone et al., 1985), consistent with decreased β-adrenoceptor sensitivity. Repeated exposure to a variety of other stressors, including cold, forced exercise, intraperitoneal injection of saline, and electroconvulsive shock, increases brain NE stores and TH activity and decreases α_2-adrenoceptor numbers (Birch et al., 1986; Ostman-Smith, 1980; Stanford and Nutt, 1982). Smith et al. (1991) reported increased expression of TH mRNA in the LC after acute but not after chronically repeated restraint stress in rats. How these changes relate to behavioral habituation or dishabituation is unknown.

Future Directions

Each chapter of this book represents a field of interest related to stress, catecholamines, and cardiovascular disease. This section provides viewpoints about directions in which these fields may develop and poses questions for future research.

Stress Theory

Despite a wealth of literature about neuroendocrine, behavioral, and physiological responses to stress, the lack of an agreed-on definition has retarded acceptance of stress as a legitimate object of medical scientific research. Experimental results have refuted key elements of Selye's theory—especially the doctrine of nonspecificity—but researchers have not agreed on an alternative theory explaining those findings. This book presents a homeostatic theory of stress, including a doctrine of ''primitive specificity''—where adaptive advantages in natural selection are viewed to have led to the evolution of distinguishable neuroendocrine response patterns.

The task now is to derive hypotheses to test the homeostat theory. The proposed organizational principles for interactions among stress systems seem amenable to experimental testing and computer modeling. These principles include negative feedback regulation; multiple effectors for the same homeostat, allowing neuroendocrine patterning and compensatory activation; effector sharing, obscuring relationships between activity of a single effector system and values for a parameter regulated by a homeostat; resetting; and increased variability and drift of the regulated parameter after homeostatic disruption.

Concerning stress as a scientific concept, what is the basis for the coordination of behavioral, neuroendocrine, and cardiovascular responses during stress? Are patterns of stress responses inherited? What and where are psychological homeostats? What are the bases for compensatory interaction among stress systems, and for dishabituation? How do homeostats reset?

Peripheral Catecholaminergic Systems

The application of molecular biologic techniques has enhanced our knowledge about catecholaminergic systems in several ways. Recent advances include the identification of the structures of adrenoceptor subtypes and sub-subtypes; elucidation of intracellular mechanisms relating receptor occupation to cellular activity; description of molecular bases of desensitization; identification of genes regulating the expression of catechol-amine-synthesizing enzymes; identification of the structures of catecholamine transporters; and adaptive changes in expression of catecholamine-synthesizing enzymes and adrenoceptors during acute and chronic stress.

The development of neurochemical assays, microdialysis, nuclear scanning, and other techniques affords an opportunity to study in detail aspects of sympathoneural function in vivo in laboratory animals and in humans. Combining molecular biologic approaches with these in vivo techniques seems to hold particular promise for enhancing our understanding of the role of peripheral catecholaminergic systems in stress and disease.

The DOPA–DA system may constitute a third type of peripheral catecholaminergic system, besides the classical sympathetic neural and adrenomedullary hormonal systems. The third system would be autocrine/paracrine, with conjugation the main means for terminating and localizing the actions of the amine.

Despite the long and rich history of catecholamine research, several questions remain inadequately answered: What exactly is the basis for exocytosis? What determines the balance between catecholamine synthesis, turnover, and release? How do presynaptic receptors modulate release of transmitters? What, if anything, regulates neuronal reuptake? Do endogenous substances coreleased with NE play any physiological role in the sympathetic neuroeffector junction? Can adrenoceptors on sympathetic nerve endings up- and down-regulate? If there is an autocrine/paracrine endogenous catecholaminergic system, what regulates it, and what are its functions?

Brain Pathways

The length of the chapter about the central functional neuroanatomy reflects a large body of still inadequately conceptualized information. Data about pathways and localization of putative transmitters abound, but organizational principles and functional relevance seem lacking. What exactly does NE do in the brain? How do catecholaminergic brain pathways participate in regulation of SNS outflows? What is the central neural basis for differential SNS and AHS responses during different forms of stress? What is the meaning of the colocalization of catecholamines and neuropeptides; is there a central neurochemical ''code''?

Technological Improvements

The past several years have seen the introduction of new tools to assess sympathetic and catecholaminergic function clinically and in laboratory animals. Techniques using infusions of tracer-labeled catecholamines have become more and more sophisticated.

Regional sampling now allows estimates of cardiac, renal, cranial, and limb spillovers of NE in humans. Since regional spillover rates of DOPA and DOPAC appear to reflect the regional rate of catecholamine biosynthesis, combined assessments of DOPA, DOPAC, DHPG, and NE kinetics, coupled with pharmacological manipulations, allow comprehensive examinations of exocytosis, vesicular transformation, and leakage from storage vesicles in sympathetically innervated organs in humans and delineation of pathophysiologic mechanisms and responses to treatments.

Combined assessments of directly recorded SMSA and regional NE spillover can examine presynaptic actions of various drugs and effects of various physiological manipulations on the presynaptic modulation of neurotransmitter release in humans. PET scanning after injection of positron-emitting analogues of catecholamines or sympathomimetic amines can examine cardiac sympathetic innervation and possibly function in humans.

Microdialysis offers a new tool for measuring changes in extracellular fluid concentrations of a large number of low-molecular-weight substances in the brain. This technique lends itself especially well to measuring simultaneously release of catecholamines and catecholamine metabolites in specific brain areas, while delivering drugs in the same region via the microdialysis probe (Itoh et al., 1990) or an attached cannula (Yadid et al., 1993). This technique may enable answers to difficult questions about the patterns of release of different central neurotransmitters.

Concerning assessment techniques, can combined assessments of spillovers of NE and its metabolites enable estimation of the regional rate of exocytosis? What are the source and meaning of NE in CSF? From where does plasma DOPA emanate? Does spectral analysis of heart rate variability validly measure cardiac SNS activity? Can PET scanning detect regional abnormalities of cardiac sympathetic function?

Patterning of Stress Responses

Simultaneous measurements of several neuroendocrine substances have revealed complex neuroendocrine patterns of responses to different stressors. Questions for future research in this area include the following: Do different patterns of neurotransmitter release in the brain explain different patterns of activation of effector systems during stress? Which homeostats determine which patterns? Are patterns inherited or learned? What are the dimensions for patterning of responses during psychological stress?

Neurocardiology as a New Discipline in Medicine

Neurocardiology seems to be evolving as a new discipline in clinical medicine (Johnson et al., 1984; Kulburtus and Franck, 1988; Natelson, 1985; Williams, 1989). Tables 8–1 and 8–2 list diagnostic entities and clinical assessment tools of this discipline.

Regarding the nervous system and hypertension, is hypertension a disease of dysregulation by the brain—that is, a neurological disease? What is the basis for the association between SNS or AHS hyperreactivity in juvenile SHRs and the development of hypertension? What causes the behavioral hyperreactivity of SHRs, and is this hyper-

Table 8-1. Neurocardiology: Diagnostic Entities

Neurogenic Abnormalities of the Heart: Altered Rate/Rhythm

Tachycardia

Reflexive
  Increased/decreased cardiac filling
  Decreased arterial filling
  Decreased BP or pulse pressure
    Shock
  Orthostatic tachycardia
Emotional/Psychiatric
  Distress
  Neurocirculatory asthenia
  Hyperkinetic heart syndrome
Drugs
  Alcohol
  β-Adrenoceptor agonists
  Vasodilators
  Anticholinergics
  Ganglion blockers
  Desipramine
Metabolic
  Fever
  Diabetes
  Thyrotoxicosis
Neurologic
  Guillain–Barre syndrome
  Porphyria
  Tetanus

Bradycardia

Drugs
  β-Adrenoceptor blockers
  Clonidine
  Parasympathomimetics
Vagal reactions
  Fainting
  Cold exposure
  Diving reflex
  Apnea
  "Voodoo death"
Anorexia
Myxedema
Fetal/neonatal (Sudden infant death syndrome)

Neurogenic Abnormalities of the Heart: Altered Function

Neurologic Diseases

Stroke
  Cardiac myocytolysis
  Electrocardiographic changes
Spinal cord injury
Guillain–Barre syndrome
Basilar artery migraine
Cluster headache
Friedrich's ataxia
Epilepsy
Narcolepsy
Chagas' disease
Tumors of neural crest origin
  Pheochromocytoma
Diagnostic procedures

Psychiatric disorders

Neurocirculatory asthenia
Mitral valve prolapse syndrome

Stress-related

Acute
  Hypertension
  Angina pectoris
  Silent ischemia
  Myocardial infarction
  Arthythmias
  Sudden death
Chronic
  Type A behavior pattern
  Hypertrophy

Drugs

Cocaine
Catecholamines

Table 8-1. (continued)

Neurogenic Hypertension	

Drugs

Alcohol
Nicotine
Caffeine
Cocaine
Yohimbine
Desipramine
MAO inhibitors

Central nervous system disease

Intracranial hypertension
Seizures
   Autonomic epilepsy
Stroke (especially intracranial bleeding)
Tetanus
Familial dysautonomia (Riley–Day syndrome)
Brainstem lesions/altered vascular supply
Poliomyelitis

Primary hypertension

Hypernoradrenergic
Orthostatic hypertension

Postoperative

Carotid endarterectomy
Aortic coarctation repair
Coronary bypass

Neuropathy

Guillain–Barre syndrome
Acute autonomic neuropathy
Acute intermittent porphyria
Diabetes mellitus

Baroreflex disorders

Baroreceptor denervation
Baroreflex failure

Tumors of neural crest origin

Pheochromocytoma
Carotid body

Neurogenic Orthostatic Hypotension	

Acute neurological disorders

Acute spinal cord lesion/injury
Post-dialysis
Guillain–Barre syndrome
Pure autonomic polyneuropathy

Chronic neurological disorders

Parkinson's disease
Pure autonomic failure
Multiple system atrophy (Shy–Drager syndrome)
Dopamine-β-hydroxylase deficiency
Diabetes mellitus
Brainstem/spinal cord lesions
Familial orthostatic hypotension
Familial dysautonomia (Riley–Day syndrome)
Anorexia nervosa
Adie's syndrome
Pophyria
Amyloidosis
Pernicious anemia
Renal failure
Mitral valve prolapse
Tabes dorsalis
Tetanus
Pheochromocytoma

Drugs

Alcohol
Desipramine

Miscellaneous

Old age
Heart failure

continued

Table 8-1. Neurocardiology: Diagnostic Entities (continued)

Noncardiac Syncope

Acute depletion of blood volume

Gastrointestinal bleeding
Trauma

Emotional

Common faint
Breath holding

Reflexive

Carotid sinus hypersensitivity
Airway stimulation
Gastrointestinal stimulation
Meniere's disease
Eyeball pressure
Micturition

Raised intrathoracic pressure

Self-induced
Occupational
Cough/sneeze

Seizures

Epilepsy
Febrile

Migraine

Miscellaneous
Pulmonary embolism

Cardiac Syncope

Arrhythmias

Supraventricular tachycardia
Ventricular tachycardia
   Torsade de pointes
   Long QT syndrome
Sick sinus syndrome

Heart block

Stokes–Adams syndrome
Pacemaker failure

Obstruction

Aortic stenosis
Mitral stenosis
Atrial myxoma

Heart muscle disease

Hypertrophic cardiomyopathy
Dilated cardiomyopathy

Cardiac arrest

Other Neurovascular Disorders

Headache

Migraine
   Basilar artery
   Ophthalmoplegic
   Retinal
   Hemiplegic
Cluster

Reflex sympathetic dystrophy

Vascular dementia

Disorders of vascular supply to the spinal cord

Anterior spinal artery thrombosis
Posterior spinal artery thrombosis
Venous infarction
Embolism
Vascular malformation
Intermittent claudication
Post-cordotomy

Collagen vascular diseases

Polyarteritis nodosa
Systemic lupus erythematosis
Giant cell arteritis
Thromboangiitis obliterans
Takayashu's arteritis

Raynaud's disease

Peripheral neuropathy

Diabetes
Amyloidosis
Charcot–Marie Tooth disease

Miscellaneous

Muscular dystrophies
Multiple sclerosis
Post-sympathectomy

Table 8–2. Clinical Assessment Tools in Neurocardiology

General	Specialized continued
Medical history and physical examination	Reflexes
Orthostatic pulse rate and blood pressure	Arterial baroreflex gain
Electrocardiogram	Lower body negative pressure
Respiratory sinus arrhythmia	Valsalva maneuver
QTc	Responses to vasoactive drugs
Valsalva	Tilt
Echocardiogram	Sweating and vasodilation
Valvular lesions	Acetylcholine axon reflex
Hypertrophy	Neurochemical analyses
Ejection fraction	Plasma catechols and metabolites
	CSF
Specialized	Soft probe microdialysis
Related to underlying diagnosis	Receptors
Ambulatory monitoring	Direct sympathetic nerve recording
Heart rate and rhythm	Skin
Blood pressure	Skeletal muscle
Blood flow	Tracer norepinephrine kinetics
Laser–Doppler skin flow	Total body
Cold pressor test	Regional
Forearm vascular resistance	Heart
	Linb
	PET scanning

reactivity relevant to the development of hypertension or cardiovascular hypertrophy? Does epidemiologic, physiological, or biochemical profiling rationalize antihypertensive treatment, and does this rationalization matter? Is cardiac hypertrophy, whether neurogenic or not, an independent cardiovascular risk factor, and after taking hypertrophy into account, is hypertension a disease?

Regarding coronary disease, is the Type A behavior pattern, or a component of the pattern, an independent risk factor for the development of coronary heart disease? Does the coronary risk of the Type A individual depend on neuroendocrine activation?

Regarding heart failure, do increased plasma NE levels indicate early cardiac decompensation? What is the mechanism of depletion of cardiac NE in heart failure, and what are the pathologic consequences, if any? Does increased release of endogenous NE in the heart contribute to the development of cardiac hypertrophy?

Regarding functional cardiorespiratory syndromes, should hyperreactive patients receive treatment with sedatives? Are there objective neurochemical abnormalities in hyperdynamic circulation syndrome, neurocirculatory asthenia, and symptomatic mitral valve prolapse syndrome? What causes reflex sympathetic dystrophy? What causes chest pain in patients with normal coronary arteries (or diseased coronaries, for that matter)?

Conclusions

In this book I have attempted to expand on concepts introduced by Bernard, Cannon, Darwin, and Selye, in conveying the roles of catecholaminergic systems in the maintenance of homeostasis in stress and heart disease. The theories these giants of scientific medicine propounded cannot be true or untrue, only useful or not useful, in the sense of generating hypotheses that observation and experience can test.

The present theory distinguishes between stress and distress. Stress is not a stimulus, as Cannon would argue, or a stereotyped response pattern independent of the stressor, as Selye would argue, but a form of intervening variable, a condition where expectations—whether genetically programmed, established by prior learning, or deduced from circumstances—do not match the current or anticipated perceptions of the internal or external environment, and this discrepancy, sensed by comparator homeostats, between the observed and the expected elicits patterned, largely inherited, compensatory responses. Distress is a conscious, aversive experience that elicits instinctive behavioral and autonomic signs and resets homeostats, resulting in HPA and AHS activation. The theory does not assume that distress is pathologic.

By means of a hierarchical meshwork of central neural clusters, higher centers such as in the hypothalamus modulate the operations of homeostatic systems. That is, the brain constantly redefines homeostasis by resetting homeostats.

As homeostatic systems evolved, so did mechanisms to regulate them. Advantageousness in natural selection led to the evolution of primitively specific stress response patterns. The patterns include experiential, behavioral, neuroendocrine, and physiological components.

Two of the most potent and rapidly acting of neuroendocrine effectors are the SNS and AHS. AHS activity is closely tied with HPA system activity and to the experience of emotional distress, whereas the SNS functions largely unconsciously to regulate the distribution of blood volume and the secretory actions of sweat, salivary, and other glands.

The main role of the SNS in cardiovascular disease is compensatory—to maintain circulatory homeostasis. In heart patients this role can actually worsen rather than help the condition of the patient. Dysregulation of these systems may cause or contribute to the development of hypertension, cardiovascular hypertrophy, or arrhythmias.

Acute emotional distress, superimposed on underlying cardiovascular disease, can elicit SNS and AHS activation, and this activation can be deleterious or even fatal; however, the role of chronic stress and chronic catecholaminergic activation in the development of cardiovascular disease remains poorly understood.

Abel first deduced the chemical structure of a hormone: EPI. Elliott's hypothesis about the neuronal release of an EPI-like substance foreshadowed the theory of chemical neurotransmission. The discovery of cAMP, the first identified intracellular messenger, and of cellular activation by phosphorylation, depended on hormonal effects of EPI. Ahlquist's explanation for the different effects of catecholamines, and Iversen's and Axelrod's findings about the disposition of catecholamines, led to the identification of the molecular structures of adrenoceptors and catecholamine transporters and to a cascade of discovery of pharmacologic agents now widely used in cardiology, neurology, and psychiatry. The discovery of NGF, the first identified neurotrophic factor, was based on in vitro studies of sympathetic and sensory ganglia. Thus, for a century, the study of catecholaminergic systems has proven a most fruitful endeavor. One may predict that our knowledge of cardiovascular physiology and pathophysiology will advance further when we understand in a comprehensive way the factors regulating concentrations of catecholamines and sympathoneural cotransmitters at cardiovascular receptors; the numbers, types, functions, and regulation of membrane adrenoceptors and catecholamine transporters; intracellular mechanisms of catecholamine action, recycling, and degradation; and the roles of catecholamines in the transmission of afferent information to the brain and in how the brain acts on this information. If a goal of physiological research is to identify the strategies the body uses to maintain the internal environment, the means to achieve this goal may be the elucidation of mechanisms by which homeostats operate during stress and reset during distress. Medical history predicts that catecholamine research will spearhead this quest.

References

Aalkjaer C, Heagerty AM, Mulvaney MJ. In vitro characteristics of vessels from patients with essential hypertension. *J Clin Hypertens* 1987a;3:317–322.

Aalkjaer C, Heagerty AM, Petersen KK, Swales JD, Mulvany MJ. Studies of resistance vessels from offspring of essential hypertensive patients. *Hypertension* 1987b; 9 (Suppl III): III155–III158.

Aars H, Akre S. Effect of angiotensin on sympathetic nerve activity. *Acta Physiol Scand* 1968; 74:134–141.

Aars H. Aortic baroreceptor activity in normal and hypertensive rabbits. *Acta Physiol Scand* 1968;72:298–309.

Abboud FM, Aylward PE, Floras JS, Gupta BN. Sensitization of aortic and cardiac baroreceptors by arginine vasopressin in mammals. *J Physiol (Lond)* 1986;377:251–265.

Abboud FM, Eckberg DL, Johannson UJ, Mark AL. Carotid and cardiopulmonary baroreceptor control of splanchnic and forearm vascular resistance during venous pooling in man. *J Physiol (Lond)* 1979;286:173–184.

Abboud FM, Heistad DD, Mark AL, Schmid PG. Reflex control of the peripheral circulation. *Prog Cardiovasc Dis* 1976;18:371–403.

Abboud FM, Schmid PG. Circulatory adjustments to heart failure. In Fishman AP (Ed) *Heart Failure*. Washington, DC: Hemisphere, 1978, pp 249–260.

Abel JJ, Crawford AC. On the blood-pressure-raising constituent of the suprarenal capsule. *Bull Johns Hopkins Hosp* 1897;8:151–157.

Abel JJ. On a simple method of preparing epinephrin and its compounds. *Bull Johns Hopkins Hosp* 1902;13:29–36.

Abercrombie ED, Jacobs BL. Microinjected clonidine inhibits noradrenergic neurons of the locus coeruleus in freely moving rats. *Neurosci Lett* 1987a;76:203–208.

Abercrombie ED, Jacobs BL. Single unit response of noradrenergic neurons in the locus coeruleus of freely moving cats. I. Acutely presented stressful and non-stressful stimuli. *J Neurosci* 1987b;7:2837–2843.

Abercrombie ED, Jacobs BL. Single unit response of noradrenergic neurons in the locus coeruleus of freely moving cats. II. Adaptation to chronically presented stressful stimuli. *J Neurosci* 1987c;7:2844–2848.

413

Abercrombie ED, Jacobs BL. Systemic naloxone administration potentiates locus coeruleus noradrenergic neuronal activity under stressful but not non-stressful conditions. *Brain Res* 1988;441:362–366.

Abercrombie ED, Keefe KA, DiFrischia DS, Zigmond MJ. Differential effect of stress on in vivo dopamine release in striatum, nucleus accumbens, and medial frontal cortex. *J Neurochem* 1989;52:1655–1658.

Abercrombie ED, Keller RW Jr, Zigmond MJ. Characterization of hippocampal norepinephrine release as measured by microdialysis perfusion: Pharmacological and behavioral studies. *Neuroscience* 1988;27:897–904.

Abercrombie ED, Nisenbaum LK, Zigmond MJ. Impact of acute and chronic stress on the release and synthesis of norepinephrine in brain: Microdialysis studies in behaving animals. In Kvetnansky R, McCarty R, Axelrod J (Eds) *Stress: Neuroendocrine and Molecular Approaches.* New York: Gordon and Breach Science Publishers, 1992, pp 29–42.

Abercrombie ED, Zigmond MJ. Partial injury to central noradrenergic neurons: Reduction of tissue norepinephrine content is greater than reduction of extracellular norepinephrine measured by microdialysis. *J Neurosci* 1989;9:4062–4067.

Abraham WT, Hensen J, Schrier RW. Elevated plasma noradrenaline concentrations in patients with low-output cardiac failure: Dependence on increased noradrenaline secretion rates. *Clin Sci* 1990;79:429–435.

Abrahamsen J, Nedergaard OA. Adrenaline released as a cotransmitter does not enhance stimulation-evoked ^{3}H-noradrenaline release from rabbit isolated aorta. *J Auton Pharmacol* 1989;9:337–346.

Abrahamsson T, Almgren O, Carlsson L. Washout of noradrenaline and its metabolites by calcium-free reperfusion after ischemia: Support for the concept of ischemia-induced noradrenaline release. *Br J Pharmacol* 1984;81:22–24.

Adams DB, Baccelli G, Mancia G, Zanchett A. Cardiovascular changes during naturally elicited fighting behavior in the cat. *Am J Physiol* 1969;216:1226–1235.

Adams MA, Bobik A, Korner PI. Differential development of vascular and cardiac hypertrophy in genetic hypertension. Relation to sympathetic function. *Hypertension* 1989;14:191–202.

Adgey AAJ, Devlin JE, Webb SW, Mulholland HC. Initiation of ventricular fibrillation outside hospital in patients with acute ischaemic heart disease. *Br Heart J* 1982;47:55–61.

Adler-Graschinsky E, Langer SZ. Possible role of a beta-adrenoceptor in the regulation of noradrenaline release by nervous stimulation through a positive feed-back mechanism. *Br J Pharmacol* 1975;53:43–50.

Agabiti-Rosei E, Alicandri C, Beschi M, Castellano M, Corea L, Beggi P, Motolese M, Muiesan G. Relationships between plasma catecholamines, renin, age and blood pressure in essential hypertension. *Cardiology* 1983;70:308–316.

Agabiti-Rosei E, Alicandri C, Fariello R, Beschi M, Boni E, Castellano M, Muiesan ML, Romanelli G, Muiesan G. Adrenergic activity in systolic hypertension. *Clin Exp Hypertens* 1982;A4:1085–1096.

Agabiti-Rosei E, Beschi M, Castellano M, Pizzocolo G, Romanelli G, Alicandri C, Muiesan G. Supine and standing plasma catecholamine in essential hypertensive patients with different renin levels. *Clin Exp Hypertens* 1984;A6:1119–1130.

Agarwal SK, Calaresu FR. Interaction of putative neurotransmitters in rostral ventrolateral medullary cardiovascular neurons. *J Auton Nerv Sys* 1992;38:159–165.

Ahlquist RP. A study of adrenotropic receptors. *Am J Physiol* 1948;153:586–600.

Ahmad J, Kham AS, Siddiqui MA. Estimation of plasma and urinary catecholamines in Guillain-Barre syndrome. *Jpn J Med* 1985;24:24–29.

Ahn SS, Marcus DR, Moore WS. Post-carotid endarterectomy hypertension: Association with elevated cranial norepinephrine. *J Vasc Surg* 1989;9:351–360.

Aksamit TR, Floras JS, Victor RG, Aylward PE. Paroxysmal hypertension due to sinoaortic baroreceptor denervation in humans. *Hypertension* 1987;9:309–314.

Albert VR, Allen JM, Joh TH. A single gene codes for aromatic L-amino acid decarboxylase in both neuronal and non-neuronal tissues. *J Biol Chem* 1987;262:9404–9411.

Albright CL, Winkleby MA, Ragland DR, Fisher J, Syme SL. Job strain and prevalence of hypertension in a biracial population of urban bus drivers. *Am J Public Health* 1992;82: 984–989.

Al-Damluji S, Bouloux P, White A, Besser M. The role of alpha-2-adrenoceptors in the control of ACTH secretion; interaction with the opioid system. *Neuroendocrinology* 1990;51:76–81.

Al-Damluji S, Francis D. Activation of central α_1-adrenoceptors in humans stimulates secretion of prolactin and TSH, as well as ACTH. *Am J Physiol* 1993;264:E208–E214.

Al-Damluji S, Francis D. Activation of central α_1-adrenoceptors in humans stimulates secretion of prolactin and TSH, as well as ACTH. *Am J Physiol* 1993;264:E208–E214.

Al-Damluji S, Perry L, Tomlin S, Bouloux P, Grossman A, Rees LH, Besser GM. Alpha-adrenergic stimulation of corticotropin secretion by a specific central mechanism in man. *Neuroendocrinology* 1987;45:68–76.

Al-Damluji S, Thomas R, White A, Besser M. Vasopressin mediates alpha 1-adrenergic stimulation of adrenocorticotropin secretion. *Endocrinology* 1990;126:1989–1995.

Al-Damluji S, White A, Besser M. Brattleboro rats have deficient adrenocorticotropin responses to activation of central α_1-adrenoceptors. *Endocrinology* 1990;127:2849–2853.

Al-Damluji S, White A. Central noradrenergic lesion impairs the adrenocorticotrophin response to release of endogenous catecholamines. *J Neuroendocrinol* 1992;4:319–323.

Al-Damluji S. Adrenergic mechanisms in the control of corticotrophin secretion. *J Endocrinol* 1988;119:5–14.

Al-Damluji S. Measuring the activity of brain adrenergic receptors in man. *J Endocrinol Invest* 1991;14:245–254.

Alexander F. Emotional factors in essential hypertension. *Psychosom Med* 1939;1:173–179.

Alexander N, De Cuir M. Role of aortic and vagus nerves in arterial baroreflex bradycardia in rabbits. *Am J Physiol* 1963;205:775–780.

Alexander RS. Tonic and reflex functions of medullary sympathetic cardiovascular centers. *J Neuropohysiol* 1946;9:205–217.

Alexander RW, Gill JR, Yamabe H, Lovenberg W, Keiser HR. Effects of dietary sodium and of acute saline infusion on the inter-relationship between dopamine excretion and adrenergic activity in man. *J Clin Invest* 1974;54:194–200.

Alfredson L, Karasek R, Theorell T. Myocardial infarction risk and psychosocial work environment: An analysis of the male Swedish working force. *Soc Sci Med* 1982;16:463–467.

Alicandri CL, Agabiti-Rosei E, Fariello R, Beschi M, Boni E, Castellano M, Montini E, Romanelli G, Zaninelli A, Muiesan G. Aortic rigidity and plasma catecholamines in essential hypertensive patients. *Clin Exp Hypertens* 1982;A4:1073–1083.

Allen EV, Adson AW. Physiologic effects of extensive sympathectomy for essential hypertension: Further observations. *Ann Intern Med* 1938;11:2151–2171.

Allenmark S, Hedman L. Cation exchange liquid chromatography with amperometric detection as a method for the analysis of endogenous catecholamine concentrations in plasma or serum. *J Liq Chromatogr* 1979;2:277–286.

Amann FW, Bolli P, Kiowski W, Buhler FR. Enhanced alpha-adrenoceptor-mediated vasoconstriction in essential hypertension. *Hypertension* 1981;3:I-I119–I123.

Amaral DG, Foss JA. Locus coeruleus lesions and learning. *Science* 1975;188:377–378.

Amaral DG, Sinnamon HM. The locus coeruleus: neurobiology of a central noadrenergic nucleus. *Prog Neurobiol* 1977;9:147–196.

Aminoff MJ. Nervous system. In Schroeder SA, Tierney LM Jr, McPhee SJ, Papadakis MA, Krupp MA (Eds) *Current Medical Diagnosis and Treatment*. Norwalk, Conn: Appleton & Lange, 1992, pp 718–775.

Amsterdam EA. Emotions, cardiac arrhythmias, and sudden death. In Byrne DG, Rosenman RH (Eds) *Anxiety and the Heart*. New York: Hemisphere Publishing Corp., 1990, pp 251–258.

Anden N-E, Grabowska-Anden M, Schwieler J. Effects of a ganglionic blocking agent on the accumulation of DOPA in peripheral organs. *Acta Physiol Scand* 1989b;136:131–132.

Anden N-E, Grabowska-Anden M, Schwieler J. Transfer of DOPA from the sympatho-adrenal system to the pancreas, liver and kidney via the blood circulation. *Acta Physiol Scand* 1989a;136:75–79.

Anden N-E, Grabowska-Anden M. Formation of deaminated metabolites of dopamine in noradrenaline neurons. *Naunyn-Schmiedeberg's Arch Pharmacol* 1983;324:1–6.

Anden N-E, Grabowska-Anden M. Synthesis and utilization of catecholamines in the rat superior cervical ganglion following changes in the nerve impulse flow. *J Neural Transmiss* 1985; 64:81–92.

Anderson DE, Kearns WD, Better WE. Progressive hypertension in dogs by avoidance conditioning and saline infusion. *Hypertension* 1983;5:286–291.

Anderson EA, Hoffman RP, Balon TW, Sinkey CA, Mark AL. Hyperinsulinemia produces both sympathetic neural activation and vasodilation in normal humans. *J Clin Ivest* 1991;87:2246–2252.

Anderson EA, Sinkey CA, Lawton WJ, Mark AL. Elevated sympathetic nerve activity in borderline hypertensive humans. Evidence from direct intraneural recordings. *Hypertension* 1989;14:177–183.

Anderson EA, Sinkey CA, Mark AL. Mental stress increases sympathetic nerve activity during sustained baroreceptor stimulation in humans. *Hypertension* 1991;17 (Suppl III):III43–III49.

Anderson EA, Wallin BG, Mark AL. Dissociation of sympathetic nerve activity in arm and leg muscle during mental stress. *Hypertension* 1987;9 (Suppl III):III114–III119.

Anderson RJ, Garcia MJ, Liebentritt DK, Kay HD. Localization of human blood phenol sulfotransferase activities: novel detection of the thermostable enzyme in granulocytes. *J Lab Clin Med* 1991;118:500–509.

Angelakos ET, King MP, Millard RW. Regional distribution of catecholamines in the hearts of various species. *Ann NY Acad Sci* 1970;156:219–240.

Antaloczy Z. Role of catecholamines in stress-induced heart disease. In Beamish RE, Panagia, V, Dhalla NS (Eds) *Pathogenesis of Stress-Induced Heart Disease*. Boston: Martinus Nijhoff Publishing, 1984, pp 213–227.

Anton AH, Sayre DF. A study of the factors affecting the alumina oxide-trihydroxyindole procedure for the analysis of catecholamines. *J Pharmacol Exp Ther* 1962;138: 360–374.

Antonaccio MJ, Halley J. Inhibition of centrally-evoked pressor responses by diazepam: Evidence for an exclusively supramedullary action. *Neuropharmacology* 1975;14:649–657.

Aoki K, Kikuchi K, Yamaji I, Nishimura M, Honma C, Kobayakawa H, Yamamoto M, Kudoh C, Shimasaki M, Sakamoto T, Wada A, Iimura O. Attenuated renal production of dopamine in patients with low renin essential hypertension. *Clin Exp Hypertens* 1989;11 (Suppl. 1): 403–409.

Aperia A, Fryckstedt J, Svensson L, Hemmings HC Jr, Nairn AC, Greengard P. Phosphorylated M_r 32,000 dopamine- and cAMP-regulated phosphoprotein inhibits N^+,K^+-ATPase activity in renal tubule cells. *Proc Natl Acad Sci USA* 1991;88:2798–2801.

Arbilla S, Langer SZ. The regulation of neurotransmitter release by α_2-adrenoceptors in the central nervous system. In Heal DJ, Marsden CA (Eds) *The Pharmacology of Noradrenaline in the Central Nervous System*. New York: Oxford University Press, 1990, pp 141–154.

Armando I, Grossman E, Hoffman A, Goldstein DS. A method for measuring concentrations of O-methyldopa (methoxytyrosine) in urine and plasma. *J Chromatogr Biomed Applic* 1991;568:45–54.

Armour JA, Hopkins DA. Anatomy of the extrinsic efferent autonomic nerves and ganglia innervating the mammalian heart. In Randall WC (Ed) *Nervous Control of Cardiovascular Function*. New York: Oxford University Press, 1984, pp 20–45.

Arnold JMO, Teasell RW, MacLeod AP, Brown JE, Carruthers SG. Increased venous alpha-adrenoceptor responsiveness in patients with reflex sympathetic dystrophy. *Ann Int Med* 1993;118:619–621.

Arnold MB. Stress and emotion. In Appley MH and Trumbull R (Eds) *Psychological Stress*. New York: Appleton-Century-Crofts, 1967, pp 123–140.

Asterita MF. *The Physiology of Stress*. New York: Human Sciences Press, Inc., 1985.

Astier B, Van Bockstaele EJ, Aston-Jones G, Pieribone VA. Anatomical evidence for multiple pathways leading from the rostral ventrolateral medulla (nucleus paragigantocellularis) to the locus coeruleus in the rat. *Neurosci Lett* 1990;118:141–146.

Astley CA, Smith OA, Ray RD, Golanov EV, Chesney MA, Chalyan VG, Taylor DJ, Bowden DM. Integrating behavior and cardiovascular responses: The code. *Am J Physiol* 1991; 261:R172–R181.

Aston-Jones G, Bloom FE. Activity of norepinephrine-containing locus coeruleus neurons in behaving rats anticipates fluctuations in the sleep-waking cycle. *J Neurosci* 1981a;1:876–886.

Aston-Jones G, Bloom FE. Norepinephrine-containing locus coeruleus neurons in behaving rats exhibit pronounced responses to non-noxious environmental stimuli. *J Neurosci* 1981b; 1:887–890.

Aston-Jones G, Ennis M, Pieribone VA, Nickell W, Shipley MT. The brain nucleus locus coeruleus: restricted afferent control of a broad efferent network. *Science* 1986;234:734–737.

Aston-Jones G, Shipley MT, Ennis M, Williams JT, Pierbone VA. Restricted afferent control of locus coeruleus neurones revealed by anatomical, physiological, and pharmacological studies. In Heal DJ, Marsden CA (Eds) *The Pharmacology of Noradrenaline in the Central Nervous System*. New York: Oxford University Press, 1990, pp 187–247.

Aston-Jones G. Behavioral functions of locus coeruleus derived from cellular attributes. *Physiol Psychol* 1985;13:118–126.

Atkinson JM, Dusting GJ, Rand MJ. Acidosis induced by catecholamines and reduction of cardiovascular responses to catecholamines in acidosis. *AJEBAK* 1972;50:847–859.

Attenborough D. *Life on Earth*. Boston: Little, Brown, 1979, pp 152–153.

Ax AF. The physiological differentiation between fear and anger in humans. *Psychosom Med* 1953;15:433–442.

Axelrod J, Reisine TD. Stress hormones: Their interaction and regulation. *Science* 1984;224: 452–459.

Axelrod J, Tomchick R. Enzymatic O-methylation of epinephrine and other catecholamines. *J Biol Chem* 1958;233:702–705.

Axelrod J, Weil-Malherbe H, Tomchick R. The physiological disposition of H^3-epinephrine and its metabolite metanephrine. *J Pharmacol Exp Therap* 1959;127:251–256.

Axelrod J. Methylation reactions in the formation and metabolism of catecholamines and other biogenic amines. *Pharmacol Rev* 1966;18:95–113.

Aylward PE, Floras JS, Leimbach WN Jr, Abboud FM. Effects of vasopressin on the circulation and its baroreflex control in healthy men. *Circulation* 1986;73:1145–1154.

Baccelli G, Albertini R, Del; Bo A, Mancia G, Zanchetti A. Role of sino-aortic reflexes in hemodynamic patterns of natural behaviour in the cat. *Am J Physiol* 1981;240:H421–H429.

Bacq ZM. La pharmacologie du système nerveux autonome, et particulièrement du sympathique, d'après la théorie neurhumorale. *Annales de physiologie et de physicochimie biologique* 1934;10:467–528.

Badoer E, Head GA, Korner PI. Effects of intracisternal and intravenous α-methyldopa and clonidine on haemodynamics and baroreceptor-heart rate reflex properties in conscious rabbits. *J Cardiovasc Pharmacol* 1983;5:760–767.

Baily RG, Leuenberger U, Leaman G, Silber D, Sinoway LI. Norepinephrine kinetics and cardiac output during nonhypotensive lower body negative pressure. *Am J Physiol* 1991;260: H1708–H1712.

Baily RG, Prophet SA, Shenberger JS, Zelis R, Sinoway LI. Direct neurohumoral evidence for isolated sympathetic nervous system activation to skeletal muscle in response to cardiopulmonary baroreceptor unloading. *Circ Res* 1990;66:1720–1728.

Bainbridge FA. The influence of venous filling upon the rate of the heart. *J Physiol* 1915;50:65–84.

Baines AD, Chan W. Production of urine free dopamine from DOPA: A micropuncture study. *Life Sci* 1980;26: 253–259.

Baines AD, Drangova R, Hatcher C. Dopamine production by isolated glomeruli and tubules from rat kidneys. *Can J Physiol Pharmacol* 1985;63:155–158.

Baines AD, Drangova R. Dopamine production by the isolated perfused rat kidney. *Can J Physiol Pharmacol* 1984;62:272–276.

Baines AD, Ho P, Drangova R. Proximal tubular dopamine production regulates basolateral Na-K-ATPase. *Am J Physiol* 1992;262:F566–F571.

Baines AD. Effects of salt intake and renal denervation on catecholamine catabolism and excretion. *Kidney Int* 1982;21:316–322.

Baines AD. Functional effects of proximal tubular dopamine production. *Am J Hypertens* 1990; 3:68S–71S.

Baker DG, Coleridge HM, Coleridge JCG, Nerdrum T. Search for a cardiac nociceptor: Stimulation by bradykinin of sympathetic afferent nerve endings in the heart of the cat. *J Physiol (Lond)* 1980;306:519–536.

Ball SG, Gunn IG, Douglas IHS. Renal handling of dopa, dopamine, norepinephrine, and epinephrine in the dog. *Am J Physiol* 1982a;242:F56–F62.

Ball SG, Gunn IG, Macarthur KJD, Douglas IHS, Inglis GC. The renal nerves in dogs: Noradrenergic and dopaminergic? *Clin Sci* 1982b;63:297s–299s.

Ball SG, Lee MR. The effect of carbidopa administration on urinary sodium excretion in man. Is dopamine an intrarenal natriuretic hormone? *Br J Clin Pharmacol* 1977;4:115–119.

Bandler R. Identification of hypothalamic and midbrain periaquaductal gray neurones mediating aggressive and defense behavior by intracerebral microinjection of excitatory amino acids. In Bandler R (Ed) *Modulation of Sensorimotor Activity during Alterations in Behavioral States*. New York: Alan R. Liss, 1985, pp 369–391.

Banister EW, Griffiths J. Blood levels of adrenergic amines during exercise. *J Appl Physiol* 1972; 33:674–676.

Banner NR, Williams M, Patel N, Chalmers J, Lightman SL, Yacoub MH. Altered cardiovascular and neurohumoral responses to head-up tilt after heart-lung transplantation. *Circulation* 1990;82:863–871.

Banwart B, Miller TD, Jones JD, Tyce GM. Plasma dopa and feeding. *Proc Soc Exp Biol Med* 1989;191:357–361.

Barber MJ, Mueller TM, Henry DP, Felten SY, Zipes DP. Transmural myocardial infarction in the dog produces sympathectomy in noninfarcted myocardium. *Circulation* 1983;67:787–796.

Barcroft H, Basnayake V, Celander O, Cobbold AF, Cunningham DJC, Jukes MGM, Young IM. The effect of carbon dioxide on the respiratory response to noradrenaline in man. *J Physiol (Lond)* 1957;137:365.

Barcroft H, Edholm OG. On the vasodilatation in human skeletal muscle during post-haemorrhagic fainting. *J Physiol (Lond)* 1945;104:161–175.

Bard P. A diencephalic mechanism for the expression of rage with special reference to the sympathetic nervous system. *Am J Physiol* 1928;84:490–516.

Bard P. Anatomical organization of the central nervous system in relation to control of the heart and blood vessels. *Physiol Rev* 1960 (Suppl. 4):3–26.

Barefoot JC, Dahlstrom WG, Williams RB. Hostility, CHD incidence, and total mortality: A 25-year follow-up study of 255 physicians. *Psychosom Med* 1983;45:59–63.

Barefoot JC, Dodge KA, Peterson BL, Dahlstrom WG. The Cook-Medley hostility scale: item conent and ability to predict survival. *Psychosom Med* 1989;51:46–57.

Barker JL, Crayton JW, Nicoll RA. Noadrenaline and acetylcholine responses of supraoptic neurosecretory cells. *J Physiol (Lond)* 1971;218:19–32.

Barman SM, Gebber GL. Sympathetic nerve rhythm of brain stem origin. *Am J Physiol* 1980; 239:R42–R47.

Barnes KL, Ferrario CM. Differential effects of angiotensin II mediated by the area postrema and the anteroventral third ventricle. In Buckley JP, Ferrario CM (Eds) *Brain Peptides and Catecholamines in Cardiovascular Regulation*. New York: Raven, 1987, pp 289–300.

Barnes RF, Raskind M, Gumprecht G, Halter JB. The effects of age on the plasma catecholamine responses to mental stress in man. *J Clin Endocrinol Metab* 1982;54:64–69.

Baroldi G, Falzi G, Mariani F. Sudden coronary death. A postmortem study in 208 selected cases compared to 97 "control" subjects. *Am Heart J* 1979;98:20–31.

Barron KW, Heesch CM. Cardiovascular effects of posterior hypothalamic stimulation in baroreflex-denervated rats. *Am J Physiol* 1990;259:H720–H727.

Bartone PT. Predictors of stress-related illness in city bus drivers. *J Occup Med* 1989;31:657–663.

Bartorelli C, Bizzi E, Libretti A, Zanchetti A. Inhibitory control of sinocarotid pressoceptive afferents on hypothalamic autonomic activity and sham rage behavior. *Arch Ital Biol* 1960;98:308–326.

Basbaum AI. Anatomical studies of the noradrenergic projection to the spinal cord dorsal horn. In Besson JM, Guillbaud (Eds) *Towards the Use of Noradrenergic Agonists for the Treatment of Pain*. New York: Elsevier Science Publishers, 1992, pp 77–89.

Basbaum CB, Heuser JE. Morphological studies of stimulated adrenergic axon varicosities in the mouse vas deferens. *J Cell Biol* 1979;80:310–344.

Bass CM. Functional cardiorespiratory syndromes. In Bass C (Ed) *Somatization: Physical Symptoms and Psychological Illness*. Oxford: Blackwell, 1990, pp 171–206.

Battelli MG. Dosage colorimetrique de la substance active des capsules surrenales. *Compt Rend Soc Biol* 1902;54:571–573.

Baylis PH, Heath DA. Plasma-arginine-vasopressin response to insulin-induced hypoglycemia. *Lancet* 1977;2:428–430.

Bayorh MA, Zukowska-Grojec Z, Kopin IJ. Effect of desipramine and cocaine on plasma norepinephrine and pressor responses to adrenergic stimulation in pithed rats. *J Clin Pharmacol* 1983;23:24–31.

Beamish RE, Dhalla NS. Involvement of catecholamines in coronary spasm under stressful conditions. In Beamish RE, Singal PK, Dhalla NS (Eds) *Stress and Heart Disease*. Boston: Martinus Nijhoof Publishing, 1985, pp 129–141.

Beamish RE, Singal PK, Ganguly PK. Stress, catecholamines, and heart disease. In Ganguly PK (Ed) *Catecholamines and Heart Disease*. Boca Raton: CRC Press, 1991, pp 231–244.

Beecher HK. Pain in men wounded in battle. *Ann Surg* 1946;123:96–105.

Beitman BD, Basha IM, Trombka LH, Jayaratna MA, Russell BD, Tarr SK. Alprazolam in the treatment of cardiology patients with atypical chest pain and panic disorder. *J Clin Psychopharmacol* 1988;8:127–130.

Belcher G, Ryall RW, Schaffner R. The differential effects of 5-hydroxytryptamine, noradrenaline and raphe stimulation on nociceptive and non-nociceptive dorsal horn interneurones in the cat. *Brain Res* 1978;151:307–321.

Bell C, Land WJ. Neurodopaminergic vasodilator control in the kidney. *Nature* 1973;246:27–29.

Bell C, Sunn N. A functional role for renal dopaminergic nerves in the dog. *J Auton Pharmacol* 1990;10 (Suppl. 1):s41–s45.

Bellin SI, Bhatnagar RK, Johnson AK. Periventricular noradrenergic systems are critical for angiotensin-induced drinking and blood pressure responses. *Brain Res* 1987;403:105–112.

Benetos A, Gavras I, Gavras H. Norepinephrine applied in the paraventricular hypothalamuc nucleus stimulates vasopressin release. *Brain Res* 1986;381:322–326.

Bennett ED, Tighe D, Wegg W. Abolition, by dopamine blockade, of the natriuretic response produced by lower-body positive pressure. *Clin Sci* 1982;63:361–366.

Bennett GW. Functional interactions between neuropeptides and noradrenaline in the brain and spinal cord. In Heal DJ, Marsden CA (Eds) *The Pharmacology of Noradrenaline in the Central Nervous System*. New York: Oxford University Press, 1990, pp 454–494.

Bennett KL, Linden RJ, Mary DASG. The atrial receptors responsible for the decrease in plasma vasopressin caused by distension of the left atrium in the dog. *Q J Exp Physiol* 1984;69: 73–81.

Bennett KL, Linden RJ, Mary DASG. The effect of stimulation of atrial receptors on the plasma concentration of vasopressin. *Q J Exp Physiol* 1983;68:579–583.

Benovic JL, Strasser RH, Caron MG, Lefkowitz RJ. Beta-adrenergic receptor kinase: identification of a novel protein kinase that phosphorylates the agonist-occupied form of the receptor. *Proc Nat Acad Sci USA* 1986;83:2797–2801.

Benschop RJ, Brosschot JF, Godaert GLR, De Smet MBM, Geenen R, Olff M, Heignen CJ, Ballieux RE. Chronic stress affects immunologic but not cardiovascular responsiveness to acute psychological stress in humans. *Am J Physiol* 1994;266:R75–R80.

Benschop RJ, Nieuwenhuis EES, Tromp EAM, Godaert GLR, Ballieux RE, van Doornen LJP. Effects of β-adrenergic blockade on immunologic and cardiovascular changes induced by mental stress. *Circulation* 1994;89:762–769.

Benson WM. Inhibition of cholinesterase by adrenaline. *Proc Soc Exp Biol Med* 1948;68:598–601.

Benvensite H, Huttmeier PC. Microdialysis—theory and application. *Prog Neurobiol* 1990;35: 195–215.

Berent H, Kuczynska K, Wocial B, Januszewicz W, Feltynowski T, Uchman B. Lipids and beta-thromboglobulin in patients with pheochromocytoma. *J Clin Hypertens* 1987;3:389–396.

Berkman LF, Syme SL. Social networks, host resistance, and mortality: a nine year follow-up study of Alameda County residents. *Am J Epidemiol* 1979;109:186–204.

Berl T, Cadnapaphornchai P, Harbottle J, Schrier R. Mechanism of suppression of vasopressin during alpha-adrenergic stimulation with norepinephrine. *J Clin Invest* 1974;53:219–227.

Bernard C. Influence du grand sympathique sur la sensibilite et sur la calorification. *C R Soc Biol (Paris)* 1852;3:162–164.

Bernard C. Lecons sur les phenomenones de la vie communs aux animaux et aux vegetaux. Paris: Ballierè, 1878.

Berne C, Fagius J, Pollare T, Hjemdahl P. The sympathetic response to euglycemic hyperinsulinemia. Evidence from microelectrode nerve recordings in healthy subjects. *Diabetologia* 1992;35:873–879.

Berridge MJ, Irvine RF. Inositol triphosphate, a novel second messenger in cellular signal transduction. *Nature* 1984;312:315–321.

Bertel O, Buhler FR, Baitsch G, Ritz R, Burkart F. Plasma adrenaline and noradrenaline in patients with acute myocardial infarction. Relationship to ventricular arrhythmias of varying severity. *Chest* 1982a;82:64–68.

Bertel O, Buhler FR, Kiowski W, Lutold BE. Decreased beta-adrenoceptor responsiveness as related to age, blood pressure, and plasma catecholamines in patients with essential hypertension. *Hypertension* 1982b;2:130–138.

Berthelot A, Hamilton CA, Petty MA, Reid JL. Central and peripheral a-adrenoceptor number and responsiveness after sinoaortic denervation in the rabbit. *J Cardiovasc Pharmacol* 1982;4:567–574.

Berthelson S, Pettinger WA. A functional basis for classification of alpha-adrenergic receptors. *Life Sci* 1977;21:595–606.

Bertorello A, Aperia A. Inhibition of proximal tubule Na^+-K^+-ATPase activity requires simultaneous activation of DA_1 and DA_2 receptors. *Am J Physiol* 1990;259:F924–F928.

Besson JM, Guillbaud (Eds) *Towards the Use of Noradrenergic Agonists for the Treatment of Pain.* New York: Elsevier Science Publishers, 1992.

Best JD, Taborsky GJ Jr, Flatness DE, Halter JB. Effect of pentobarbital anesthesia on plasma norepinephrine kinetics in dogs. *Endocrinology* 1984;115:853–857.

Bevan JA, Bevan RD, Duckles SP. Adrenergic regulation of vascular smooth muscle. In Bohr DF, Somlyo AP, Sparks HV Jr. (Eds): *Handbook of Physiology,* Sect 2: *The Cardiovascular System,* Vol II: *Vascular Smooth Muscle.* Bethesda, Md: American Physiological Society, 1980, pp 515–556.

Bevan JA, Su C. Variations of intra and perisynaptic adrenergic transmitter concentration with width of synaptic cleft in vascular tissue. *J Pharmacol Exp Ther* 1974;190:30–38.

Bevegard BS, Shepherd JT. Circulatory effects of stimulating the carotid arterial stretch receptors in man at rest and during exercise. *J Clin Ivest* 1966;45:132–142.

Biaggioni I, Goldstein DS, Atkinson T, Robertson D. Dopamine-β-hydroxylase deficiency in man. *Neurology* 1990;40:370–373.

Bian X, Seidler FJ, Slotkin TA. Fetal dexamethasone exposure interferes with establishment of cardiac noradrenergic innervation and sympathetic activity. *Teratology* 1993;47:109–117.

Bianchetti MG, Minder I, Beretta-Piccoli C, Meier A, Weidmann P. Effects of tyramine on blood pressure and plasma catecholamines in normal and hypertensive subjects. *Klin Wochenschr* 1982;60:465–470.

Bianchetti MG, Weidmann P, Beretta-Piccoli C, Rupp U, Boehringer K, Link L, Ferrier C. Disturbed noradrenergic blood pressure control in normotensive members of hypertensive families. *Br Heart J* 1984;51:306–311.

Bickerton RK, Buckley JP. Evidence for a central mechanism in angiotensin induced hypertension. *Proc Soc Exp Biol Med* 1961;106:834–836.

Bilgutay AM, Bilgutay I, Lillehei CW. Baropacing. A new concept in the treatment of hypertension. In Kezdi P (Ed) *Baroreceptors and Hypertension.* Oxford: Pergamon, 1967, pp 425–435.

Billman GE, Randall DC, Brown DR, Hall SK, Zolman JF. Hemodynamic and arrhythmogenic effects of aversive stress during myocardial ischemia. *J Auton Nerv Sys* 1990;29:193–202.

Billman GE, Randall DC. Mechanisms mediating the coronary vascular response to behavioral stress in the dog. *Circ Res* 1981;48:214–223.

Billman GE, Schwartz PJ, Stone HL. Baroreceptor control of heart rate: a predictor of sudden cardiac death. *Circulation* 1982;66:874–880.

Birch PJ, Anderson SMP, Fillenz M. Mild chronic stress leads to desensitization of presynaptic autoceptors and a long-lasting increase in noradrenaline synthesis in rat cortical synaptosomes. *Neurochem Internat* 1986;9:329–336.

Bird SJ, Kuhar MJ. Iontophoretic application of opiates to the locus coeruleus. *Brain Res* 1977;122:523–533.

Bishop VS, Hasser EM, Undesser KP. Vasopressin and sympathetic nerve activity: Involvement of the area postrema. In Buckley JP, Ferrario CM (Eds) *Brain Peptides and Catecholamines in Cardiovascular Regulation.* New York: Raven, 1987, pp 373–382.

Bjorklund A, Lindvall O. Catecholaminergic brain stem regulatory systems. In Mountcastle VB (Ed) *The Nervous System.* Sect 1. *Handbook of Physiology.* Bethesda, Md: American Physiological Society, 1986, pp 155–235.

Bjorklund A, Stenevi U. Regeneration of monoaminergic and cholinergic neurons in the mammalian central nervous system. *Physiol Rev* 1979;59:62–100.

Bjurstedt H, Rosenhamer G, Tyden G. Cardiovascular responses to changes in carotid sinus transmural pressure in man. *Acta Physiol Scand* 1975;94:497–505.

Black IB, Petito CK. Catecholamine enzymes in the degenerative neurological disease idiopathic orthostatic hypotension. *Science* 1976;192:910–912.

Blaes N, Bloissel JP. Growth-stimulating effect of catecholamines on rat aortic smooth muscle cells in culture. *J Cell Physiol* 1983;116:167–171.

Blagden C. Experiments and observations in an heated room. *Philos Trans Royal Soc* 1775;65: 111–124.

Blaschko H, Born GVR, d'Iorio A, Eade NR. Observations on the distribution of catecholamines and adenosine triphosphate in the bovine adrenal medulla. *Am J Physiol* 1956;133:548–557.

Blaschko H. The specific action of L-dopa-decarboxylase. *J Physiol (Lond)* 1939;96:50P–51P.

Blaustein MP, Hamlyn JM. Pathogenesis of essential hypertension. A link between dietary salt and high blood pressure. *Hypertension* 1991; 18:III184–III195.

Blessing WW, Goodchild AK, Dampney RAL, Chalmers JP. Cell groups in the lower brainstem of the rabbit projecting to the spinal cord, with special reference to catecholamine-containing neurons. *Brain Res* 1981;221:35–55.

Blessing WW, Hedger SC, Joh TH, Willoughby JO. Neurons in the area postrema are the only catecholamine-synthesizing cells in the medulla or pons with projections to the rostal ventrolateral medulla (C1-area) in the rabbit. *Brain Res* 1987;419:336–340.

Blessing WW, Li YW. Inhibitory vasomotor neurons in the caudal ventrolateral region of the medulla oblongata. *Prog Brain Res* 1989;81:83–97.

Blessing WW, Oliver JR, Hodgson AH, Joh TH, Willoughby JO. Neuropeptide Y-like immunoreactive C1 neurons in the rostral ventrolateral medulla of the rabbit project to sympathetic preganglionic neurons in the spinal cord. *J Auton Nerv Sys* 1987;18:121–129.

Blessing WW, Reis DJ. Inhibitory cardiovascular function of neurons in the caudal ventrolateral medulla of the rabbit: relationships to the area containing A1 noradrenergic cells. *Brain Res* 1982;253:161–171.

Blessing WW, Sved AF, Reis DJ. Destruction of noradrenergic neurons in rabbit brainstem elevates plasma vasopressin, causing hypertension. *Science* 1982;217:661–663.

Blessing WW. Depressor neurons in rabbit caudal medulla act via GABA receptors in rostral medulla. *Am J Physiol* 1988;254:H686–H692.

Bliss TVP, Goddard GV, Rives M. Reduction of long-term potentiation in the dentate gyrus of the rat following selective depletion of monoamines. *J Physiol (Lond)* 1983;334:475–491.

Blizard DA, Liang B, Emmel DK. Blood pressure, heart rate, and plasma catecholamines under resting conditions in rat strains selectively bred for differences in response to stress. *Behav Neural Biol* 1980;29:487–492.

Bloom FE, Schulman JA, Koob GF. Catecholamines and behavior. In Trendelenburg U, Weiner N (Eds) *Catecholamines II.* New York: Springer-Verlag, 1989, pp 27–88.

Bobik A, Jennings G, Jackman G, Oddie C, Korner P. Evidence for a predominantly central hypotensive effect of alpha-methyldopa in humans. *Hypertension* 1986;8:16–23.

Bodo RC, Benaglia AE. Effect of sympathin on blood sugar. *Am J Physiol* 1938;121:728–737.

Bogen DK. Simulation software for the Macintosh. *Science* 1989;246:138–142.

Bolli P, Erne P, Kiowski W, Amman FW, Buhler FR. The adrenaline-alpha 2-adrenoceptor-mediated vasoconstrictor axis. *Clin Sci* 1985;68(Suppl 10):141s–146s.

Bolli P, Erne P, Kiowski W, Ji BH, Amman FW, Buhler FR. Important contribution of postjunctional alpha-2 adrenoceptor-mediated vasoconstriction to arteriolar tone in man. *J Hypertension* 1983;1 (Suppl. 2):257–259.

Bolm-Audorff U, Schwammle J, Ehlenz K, Koop H, Kaffarnik H. Hormonal and cardiovascular variations during a public lecture. *Eur J Appl Physiol* 1986;54:669–674.

Bolm-Audorff U, Siegrist J. Occupational morbidity data in myocardial infarction. *J Occup Med* 1983;25:367–371.

Boman B. Psychosocial stress and ischemic heart disease. *Aust N Z J Psychiatry* 1982;16:265–278.

Bonisch H, Graefe K-H. Distribution kinetics of ^{3}H-(-)-noradrenaline (NA) and ^{3}H-($\pm$)-metaraminol (MA) in the perfused rabbit heart. *Naunyn-Schmeideberg's Arch Pharmacol* 1976; 293:R4.

Bonvallet M, Allen MB. Prolonged spontaneous and evoked reticular activation following bulbar lesions. *Electroencephalogr Clin Neurophysiol* 1963;15:969–988.

Boomsma F, Ausema L, Hakvoort-Cammel FG, Oosterom R, Man in't Veld AJ, Krenning EP, Hahlen K, Schalekamp MA. Combined measurements of plasma aromatic L-amino acid decarboxylase and DOPA as tumour markers in diagnosis and followup of neuroblastoma. *Eur J Cancer Clin Oncol* 1989;25:1045–1052.

Borkowski KR, Quinn P. Adrenaline and the development of spontaneous hypertension in rats. *J Auton Pharmac* 1985;5:89–100.

Borton M, Docherty JR. The effects of ageing on neuronal uptake of noradrenaline in the rat. *Naunyn-Schmiedeberg's Arch Pharmacol* 1989;340:139–143.

Boudier HS, Smeets G, Brouwer G, Van Rossum JM. Central nervous system alpha-adrenergic mechanisms and cardiovascular regulation in rats. *Arch Int Pharmacodyn Ther* 1975;213:285–293.

Boudoulas H, Reynolds JC. Mitral valve prolapse syndrome: The effect of adrenergic stimulation. *J Am Coll Cardiol* 1983;2:638–644.

Bousquet P, Feldman J, Schwartz J. Central cardiovascular effects of alpha-adrenergic drugs: Differences between catecholamines and imidazolines. *J Pharmacol Exp Ther* 1984;230:232–236.

Bousquet P, Feldman J, Tibirica E, Bricca G, Molines A, Dontenwill M, Belcourt A. New concepts on the central regulation of blood pressure. Alpha 2-adrenoceptors and "imidazoline receptors." *Am J Med* 1989;87:10S–13S.

Bousquet P, Feldman J. The blood pressure effects of alpha-adrenoceptor antagonists injected in the medullary site of action of clonidine: The nucleus reticularis lateralis. *Life Sci* 1987; 40:1045–1052.

Bouvier M, De Champlain J. Increased apparent norepinephrine release rate in anesthetized DOCA-salt hypertensive rats. *Clin Exp Hyper* 1985;A7:1629–1645.

Bouvier M, De Champlain J. Increased basal and reactive plasma norepinephrine and epinephrine levels in awake DOCA-salt hypertensive rats. *J Auton Nerv Sys* 1986;15:191–195.

Bradley T, Gewertz BL, Scott WJ, Goldberg LI. Dopamine receptor blockade does not affect the natriuresis accompanying sodium chloride infusion in dogs. *J Lab Clin Med* 1986;107:525–528.

Brady JV. Toward a behavioral biology of emotion. In Levi L (Ed) *Emotions—Their Parameters and Measurement.* New York: Raven Press, 1975, pp 17–45.

Brady LS, Whitfield HJ Jr, Fox RJ, Gold PW, Herkenham M. Long-term antidepressant administration alters corticotropin-releasing hormone, tyrosine hydroxylase, and mineralocorticoid receptor gene expression in rat brain. Therapeutic implications. *J Clin Invest* 1991; 87:831–837.

Brattstrom BH. Body temperature in reptiles. *Amer Midland Naturalist* 1965;73:376–422.

Braunwald E, Ross J, Sonnenblick EH. *Mechanisms of Contraction of the Normal and Failing Heart.* Boston: Little, Brown, 1968.

Bravo EL. Metabolic factors and the sympathetic nervous system. *Am J Hypertens* 1989;2:339S–344S.

Bravo EL, Gifford RW Jr. Pheochromocytoma: Diagnosis, localization and management. *N Engl J Med* 1984;311:1298–1303.

Bravo EL, Tarazi RC, Dustan HP, Fouad FM. The sympathetic nervous system and hypertension in primary aldosteronism. *Hypertension* 1985;7:90–96.

Bravo EL, Tarazi RC, Fouad FM, Vidt DG, Gifford RW Jr. Clonidine-suppression test: A useful aid in the diagnosis of pheochromocytoma. *N Engl J Med* 1981;305:623–626.

Brenneman AR, Kaufman S. The role of tetrahydropterines in the enzymatic conversion of tyrosine to 3,4-dihydroxyphenylalanine. *Biochem Biophys Res Commun* 1964;17:177–183.

Brezenoff HE, Giuliano R. Cardiovascular control by cholinergic mechanisms in the central nervous system. *Ann Rev Pharmacol Toxicol* 1982;22:341–381.

Briand R, Yamaguchi N, Gagne J. Plasma catecholamine and glucose concentrations during hemorrhagic hypotension in anesthetized dogs. *Am J Physiol* 1989;257:R317–R325.

Bristow JD, Honour J, Pickering GW, Sleight P, Smyth HS. Diminished baroreflex sensitivity in high blood pressure. *Circulation* 1969;39:48–54.

Bristow MR, Ginsburg R, Minobe W, Cubicciotti RS, Sageman WS, Lurie K, Billingham ME, Harrison DC, Stinson EB. Decreased catecholamine sensitivity and beta-adrenergic-receptor density in failing human hearts. *N Engl J Med* 1982;307:205–211.

Bristow MR, Ginsburg R, Umans V, Fowler M, Minobe W, Rasmussen R, Zera P, Menlove R, Shah P, Jamieson S, Stinson EB. β_1 and β_2 adrenergic-receptor subpopulations in non-failing and failing human ventricular myocardium: Coupling of both receptor subtypes to muscle contraction and selective β_1 receptor down-regulation in heart failure. *Circ Res* 1986;59:297–309.

Bristow MR, Hershberger RE, Port JD, Gilbert EM, Sandoval A, Rasmussen R, Cates AE, Feldman AM. Beta-adrenergic pathways in nonfailing and failing human ventricular myocardium. *Circulation* 1990;82:I12–I25.

Brod J, Fencl V, Hejl Z, Jirka J. Circulatory changes underlying blood pressure elevation during acute emotional stress (mental arithmetic) in normotensive and hypertensive subjects. *Clin Sci* 1959;18:269–278.

Brod J. Hemodynamic basis of acute pressor reaction and hypertension. *Br Heart J* 1963;25:227–245.

Brodde O-E. Subclassification of peripheral dopamine receptors. *J Auton Pharmacol* 1990;10 (Suppl. 1):s5–s10.

Brodie BB, Costa E. Some current views on brain monoamines. *Psychopharmacol Serv Cent Bull* 1962;2:1–25.

Brody MJ, Alper RH, O'Neill TP, Porter JP. Central neural control of the cardiovascular system. In Zanchetti A, Tarazi RC (Eds) *Handbook of Hypertension,* Vol 8: *Pathophysiology of Hypertension—Regulatory Mechanisms.* New York: Elsevier Science, 1986, pp 1–25.

Brody MJ, Johnson AK. Role of the anteroventral thrid ventricle region in fluid and electrolyte balance, arterial pressure regulation and hypertension. In Martini L, Ganon WF (Eds) *Frontiers of Neuroendocrinology.* New York: Raven Press, 1980, pp 249–292.

Brody MJ, Natelson BH. Task Force 3: Behavioral mechanisms in hypertension. *Circulation* 1987;76: Suppl 1:I95–I100.

Brody MJ, Varner KJ, Vasquez EC, Lewis SJ. Central nervous system and the pathogenesis of hypertension. Sites and mechanisms. *Hypertension* 1991;18 (Suppl III):III7–III12.

Brooks D, Fox P, Lopez R, Sleight P. The effect of mental arithmetic on blood pressure variability and baroreflex sensitivity in man. *J Physiol* 1978;280:75P–76P.

Brosnihan KB, Szilagyi JE, Ferrario CM. Effect of chronic sodium depletion on cerebrospinal fluid and plasma catecholamines. *Hypertension* 1981;3:233–239.

Brown AM. Excitation of afferent cardiac sympathetic nerve fibres during myocardial ischemia. *J Physiol (Lond)* 1967;190:35–53.

Brown AM. Regulation of heartbeat by G protein-coupled ion channels. *Am J Physiol* 1990;259: H1621–H1628.

Brown GL, Gillespie JS. The output of sympathetic transmitter from the spleen of the cat. *J Physiol (Lond)* 1957;138:81–102.

Brown JH. Atropine, scopalamine, and related antimuscarinic drugs. In Gilman AG, Rall TW, Nies AS, Taylor P (Eds) *Goodman and Gilman's The Pharmacological Basis of Therapeutics.* New York: Pergamon Press, 1990, pp 150–165.

Brown M. Simultaneous assay of noradrenaline and its deaminated metabolite, dihydroxyphenylglycol, in plasma: A simplified approach to the exclusion of pheochromocytoma in patients with borderline elevation of plasma noradrenaline concentration. *Eur J Clin Invest* 1984;14:67–72.

Brown MJ, Allison DJ, Jenner DA, Lewis PJ, Dollery CT. Increased sensitivity and accuracy of phaeochromocytoma diagnosis achieved by use of plasma-adrenaline estimations and a pentolinium-suppression test. *Lancet* 1981;1:174–177.

Brown MJ, Brown DC, Murphy MB. Hypokalemia from beta$_2$-receptor stimulation by circulating epinephrine. *N Engl J Med* 1983;309:1414–1419.

Brown MJ, Dollery CT. A specific radioenzymatic assay for dihydroxyphenylalanine (DOPA). Plasma dopa may be the precursor of urine free dopamine. *Br J Clin Pharmacol* 1981; 11:79–83.

Brown MJ, Jenner DA, Allison DJ, Dollery CT. Variations in individual organ release of noradrenaline measured by an improved radioenzymatic technique; limitations of peripheral venous measurements in the assessment of sympathetic nervous activity. *Clin Sci* 1981; 61:585–590.

Brown MR, Fisher LA. Brain peptide regulation of adrenal epinephrine secretion. *Am J Physiol* 1984;10:E41–E46.

Brown MR, Fisher LA. Corticotropin-releasing factor: Effects on the autonomic nervous system and visceral systems. *Fed Proc* 1985;44:234–248.

Brown MR, Fisher LA. Glucocorticoid suppression of the sympathetic nervous system and adrenal medulla. *Life Sci* 1986;39:1003–1012.

Brown MR, Gray TS, Fisher LA. Corticotropin-releasing factor receptor antagonist: effects on the autonomic nervous system and cardiovascular function. *Regul Peptides* 1986;16:321–329.

Brown MR, Gray TS. Peptide injections in the amygdala of conscious rats: effects on blood pressure, heart rate and plasma catecholamines. *Regul Peptides* 1988;21:95–106.

Brown MR, Hauger R, Fisher LA. Autonomic and cardiovascular effects of corticotropin-releasing factor in the spontaneously hypertensive rat. *Brain Res* 1988;441:33–40.

Brown MR. Corticotropin releasing factor: Central nervous system sites of action. *Brain Res* 1986;399:10–14.

Brown MR. Neuropeptide-mediated regulation of the neuroendocrine and autonomic responses to stress. In McCubbin JW, Kaufman PG, Nemeroff CB (Eds) *Stress, Neuropeptides, and Systemic Disease.* New York: Academic Press, 1991, pp 73–93.

Brown-Sequard CE. Experimental researches applied to physiology and pathology. *Med Exam (Phila)* 1852;8:481–504.

Brunner HG, Nelen M, Breakefield XO, Ropers HH, van Oost BA. Abnormal behavior associated with a point mutation in the structural gene for monoamine oxidase A. *Science* 1993;262: 578–580.

Brush JE Jr, Eisenhofer G, Stull R, Garty M, Maron BJ, Cannon RO III, Panza J, Epstein SE, Goldstein DS. Cardiac norepinephrine kinetics in hypertrophic cardiomyopathy. *Circulation* 1989;79:836–844.

Bucher B, Corriu C, Stoclet JC. Prejunctional opioid mu-receptors and adenosine A1-receptors on the sympathetic nerve endings of the rat tail artery interact with the alpha 2-adrenoceptors. *Naunyn-Schmiedeberg's Arch Pharmacol* 1992; 345:37–43.

Buck R. Human Motivation and Emotion. New York: John Wiley, 1988.

Budai D, Duckles SP. Opioid-induced prejunctional inhibition of vasoconstriction in the rabbit ear artery: alpha-2 adrenoceptor activation and external calcium. *J Pharmacol Exp Ther* 1989;251:497–501.

Bunag RD, Eferakeya AE. Immediate hypotensive effects of posterior hypothalamic lesions in awake rats with spontaneous, renal, or DOCA hypertension. *Cardiovasc Res* 1976;10: 663–671.

Bunag RD, Riley E. Chronic hypothalamic stimulation in awake rats fails to induce hypertension. *Hypertension* 1979;1:498–507.

Burch GE, Myers R, Abildskov JA. A new electrocardiographic pattern observed in cerebrovascular accidents. *Circulation* 1954;9:719–723.

Burch GE, Sohal RS, Sun SC, Colcolough HL. Effects of experimental intracranial hemorrhage on the ultrastructure of the myocardium of mice. *Am Heart J* 1969;77:427–429.

Burchfield SR, Woods SC, Elich MS. Pituitary adrenocortical response to chronic intermittent stress. *Physiol Behav* 1980;24:297–302.

Burke D, Sundlof G, Eriksson B-M, Dominiak P, Grobecker H, Lindblad LE. Postural effects on muscle nerve sympathetic activity in man. *J Physiol (Lond)* 1977;272:399–414.

Burnstock G, Costa M. *Adrenergic Neurons*. London: Chapman and Hall, 1975.

Burnstock G. Changes in expression of autonomic nerves in aging and disease. *J Auton Nerv Sys* 1990;30:S25–S34.

Burnstock, G. Do some nerve cells release more than one transmitter? *Neuroscience* 1976;1:239–248.

Buu NT, Duhamine J, Kuchel O. Handling of dopamine and dopamine sulfate by isolated perfused rat kidney. *Am J Physiol* 1986;250:F975–F979.

Buu NT, Kuchel O. The direct conversion of dopamine 3-O-sulfate to norepinephrine by dopamine beta-hydroxylase. *Life Sci* 1979;24:783–790.

Buu NT, Lussier C. Origin of dopamine in the rat adrenal cortex. *Am J Physiol* 1990;258:F287–F291.

Byer E, Ashman R, Toth LA. Electrocardiogram with large upright T-wave and long Q-T intervals. *Am Heart J* 1947;33:796–806.

Bylund DB, Ray-Prenger C, Murphy TJ. *Alpha*-2A- and *alpha*-2B-adrenergic receptor subtypes: Antagonist binding in tissues and cell lines containing only one subtype. *J Pharmacol Exp Ther* 1988;245:600–607.

Byrne DG, Byrne AE. Anxiety and coronary heart disease. In Byrne DG, Rosenman RH (Eds) *Anxiety and the Heart*. New York: Hemisphere Publishing, 1990, pp 213–232.

Byrum CE, Guyenet PG. Afferent and efferent connections of the A5 noradrenergic cell group in the rat. *J Comp Neurol* 1987;261:529–542.

Calaresu FR, Ciriello J, Caverson MM, Cechetto DF, Krukoff TL. Functional neuroanatomy of central pathways controlling the circulation. In Guthrie GP Jr, Kotchen TA (Eds) *Hypertension and the Brain*. New York: Futura, 1984, pp 3–21.

Callingham BA, Burgen ASV. The uptake of isoprenaline and noradrenaline by the perfused rat heart. *Mol Pharmacol* 1966;2:37–42.

Camacho A, Phillips MI. Separation of drinking and pressor responses to central angiotensin by monoamines. *Am J Physiol* 1981;240:R106–R113.

Cameron OG, Gunsher S, Hariharan M. Venous plasma epinephrine levels and the symptoms of stress. *Psychosom Med* 1990;52:411–424.

Cameron OG, Lee MA, Curtis GC, McCann DS. Endocrine and physiological changes during "spontaneous" panic attacks. *Psychoneuroendocrinology* 1987;12:321–331.

Cameron R. Inflammation and Repair. In Robbins SL (Ed) *Pathology*. Philadelphia: WB Saunders, 1967, pp 31–73.

Cameron V, Espiner EA, Nicholls MG, Donald RA, MacFarlane MR. Stress hormones in blood and cerebrospinal fluid of conscious sheep: Effect of hemorrhage. *Endocrinology* 1985; 115:1460–1465.

Cameron VA, Espiner EA, Nicholls MG, MacFarlane MR, Sadler W. Intra-cerebroventricular captopril reduces plasma ACTH and vasopressin responses to hemorrhagic stress. *Life Sci* 1986;38:553–559.

Campese VM, Romoff MS, Levitan D, Saglikes Y, Friedler RM, Massry SG. Abnormal relationship between sodium intake and sympathetic nervous system activity in salt-sensitive patients with essential hypertension. *Kidney Internat* 1982;21:371–378.

Cannon B. The effects of progressive sympathectomy on blood pressure. *Am J Physiol* 1931a; 97:592–595.

Cannon RO III, Camici PG, Epstein SE. Pathophysiological dilemma of syndrome X. *Circulation* 1992;85:883–92.

Cannon WB, Britton SW. Studies on the conditions of activity in endocrine glands. XV. Pseudoaffective medulliadrenal secretion. *Am J Physiol* 1925;72:283–294.

Cannon WB, Britton SW. The influence of motion and emotion on medulliadrenal secretion. *Am J Physiol* 1927;79:433–465.

Cannon WB, de la Paz D. Emotional stimulation of adrenal gland secretion. *Am J Physiol* 1911; 28:64–70.

Cannon WB, Lissak K. Evidence for adrenaline in adrenergic neurones. *Am J Physiol* 1939;125: 765–777.

Cannon WB, McIver MA, Bliss SW. A sympathetic and adrenal mechanism for mobilizing sugar in hypoglycemia. *Am J Physiol* 1924;69:46–66.

Cannon WB, Newton HF, Bright EM, Menkin V, Moore RM. Some aspects of the physiology of animals surviving complete exclusion of sympathetic nerve impulses. *Am J Physiol* 1929;89:84–107.

Cannon WB, Querido A, Britton SW, Bright EM. The role of adrenal secretion in the chemical control of body temperature. *Am J Physiol* 1927;79:466–507.

Cannon WB, Rapport D. Further observations on the denervated heart in relation to adrenal secretion. *Am J Physiol* 1921;58:308–337.

Cannon WB, Rosenblueth A. Studies on conditions of activity in endocrine organs. XXIX. Sympathin E and Sympathin I. *Am J Physiol* 1933;104:557–574.

Cannon WB. A law of denervation. *Am J Med Sci* 1939b;198:737–750.

Cannon WB. Again the James-Lange and thalamic theories of emotion. *Psychol Rev* 1931;38: 281–295.

Cannon WB. *Bodily Changes in Pain, Hunger, Fear and Rage.* New York: D Appleton and Co., 1929a.

Cannon WB. Organization for physiological homeostasis. *Physiol Rev* 1929b;9:399–431.

Cannon WB. The autonomic nervous system, an interpretation. The Linacre Lecture. *Lancet* 1930;i:1109–1115.

Cannon WB. The emergency function of the adrenal medulla in pain and in the major emotions. *Am J Physiol* 1914a;33:356–372.

Cannon WB. The interrelation of emotions as suggested by recent physiological researches. *Am J Psychol* 1914b;25:256–282.

Cannon WB. *The Way of an Investigator.* New York: WW Norton, 1945.

Cannon WB. *The Wisdom of the Body.* New York: WW Norton, 1939a.

Cannon WB. "Voodoo" death. *Am Anthropol* 1942;44:169–181 (reproduced in *Psychosom Med* 1957;19:182–190).

Caranasos GJ. Neurocirculatory asthenia. In Eliot RS (Ed) *Stress and the Heart.* Mount Kisco, NY: Futura, 1974, pp 219–244.

Carey RM, Siragy HM, Felder RA. Physiological modulation of renal function by the renal dopaminergic system. *J Auton Pharmacol* 1990;10 (Suppl. 1):s47–s51.

Carey RM, Thorner MO, Ortt EM. Dopaminergic inhibition of metoclopramide-induced aldosterone secretion in man. Dissociation of responses to dopamine and bromocriptine. *J Clin Ivest* 1980;66:10–18.

Carey RM, Van Loon GR, Baines AD, Ortt EM. Decreased plasma and urinary dopamine during dietary sodium depletion in man. *J Clin Endocrinol Metab* 1981;52:903–909.

Carlberg M. Evidence of dopa in the nerves of sea anemones. *J Neural Transmiss* 1983;57:75–84.

Carlsson L, Abrahamsson T, Almgren O. Local release of myocardial norepinephrine during acute ischemia: an experimental study in the isolated perfused rat heart. *J Cardiovasc Pharmacol* 1985;7:791–798.

Carlsson L, Abrahamsson T, Almgren O. Release of noradrenaline in myocardial ischemia—importance of local inactivation by neuronal and extraneuronal mechanisms. *J Cardiovasc Pharmacol* 1986;8:545–553.

Carlsson L, Graefe K-H, Trendelenburg U. Early intraneuronal mobilization and deamination of noradrenaline during global ischemia in the isolated perfused rat heart. *Naunyn-Schmiedeberg's Arch Pharmacol* 1987;336:508–518.

Carlsten A, Folkow B, Grimby G, Hamberger C-A, Thulesius O. Cardiovascular effects of direct stimulation of the carotid sinus nerve in man. *Acta Physiol Scand* 1958;44:138–145.

Carmelli D, Chesney MA, Ward MM, Rosenman RH. Twin similarity in cardiovascular stress response. *Health Psychol* 1985;4:413–423.

Carpeggiani C, Skinner JE. Coronary flow and mental stress. Experimental findings. *Circulation* 1991;83 (Suppl. II):II90–II93.

Carr DB, Sheehan DV, Surman OS, Coleman JH, Greenblatt DJ, Heninger GR, Jones KJ, Levine PH, Watkins WD. Neuroendocrine correlates of lactate-induced anxiety and their response to chronic alprazolam therapy. *Am J Psychiatry* 1986;143:483–494.

Carswell F, Hainsworth R, Ledsome JR. The effects of left atrial distension upon urine flow from the isolated perfused kidney. *Q J Exp Physiol* 1970;55:173–182.

Carty SE, Johnson RG, Vaughan T, Pallant A, Scarpa A. Amine transport into chromaffin ghosts. Kinetic measurements of net uptake of biologically and pharmacologically relevant amines using an on-line amperometric technique. *Eur J Pharmacol* 1985;147:447–452.

Carvalho ACA, Colman RW, Lees RS. Platelet function in hyperlipoproteinemia. *N Engl J Med* 1974;290:434–438.

Casiglia E, Vincenti E, Giacomello M, Plebani M, Ruffato G, Rossi GP, Zanin L, Pessina AC. Beta-endorphin levels after experimental blood loss in human subjects. Correlations with cortisol, ACTH, plasma renin activity, plasma catecholamines and blood pressure variations. *Resuscitation* 1989;18:141–143.

Cassell MD, Gray TS. The amygdala directly innervates adrenergic (C1) neurons in the ventrolateral medulla in the rat. *Neurosci Lett* 1989;97:163–168.

Cassis LA, Stitzel RE, Head RJ. Hypernoradrenergic innervation of the caudal artery of the spontaneously hypertensive rat: An influence upon neuroeffector mechanisms. *J Pharmacol Exp Therap* 1985;234:792–803.

Castagne V, Rivet JM, Mormede P. The integrity of the ventral noradrenergic bundle (VNAB) is not necessary for a normal neuroendocrine stress response. *Brain Res* 1990;511:349–352.

Casto R, Phillips MI. Neuropeptide action in nucleus tractus solitarius: Angiotensin specificity in hypertensive rats. *Am J Physiol* 1985;249:R341–R347.

Cathey C, Jones HB, Naughton J, Hammarsten JF, Wolf SG. The relationship between life stress to concentration of serum lipids in patients with coronary artery disease. *Am J Med* 1962; 244:421–441.

Cebelin MS, Hirsch CS. Human stress cardiomyopathy. Myocardial lesions in victims of homicidal assaults without internal injuries. *Hum Pathol* 1980;11:123–132.

Cedarbaum JM, Aghajanian GK. Activation of locus coeruleus neurons by peripheral stimuli: modulation by a collateral inhibitory mechanism. *Life Sci* 1978a;23:1383–1392.

Cedarbaum JM, Aghajanian GK. Afferent projections to the rat locus coeruleus as determined by a retrograde tracing technique. *J Comp Neurol* 1978b;178:1–16.

Cedarbaum JM, Aghajanian GK. Catecholamine receptors on locus coeruleus neurons: pharmacological characterization. *Eur J Pharmacol* 1977;44:375–385.

Chabal C, Jacobson L, Russell LC, Burchiel KJ. Pain response to perineuromal injection of normal saline, epinephrine, and lidocaine in humans. *Pain* 1992;49:9–12.

Chadwick RS, Goldstein DS, Keiser HR. Application of a pulse wave theory to modulation of the human brachial arterial dicrotic wave in aging and essential hypertension. *Am J Physiol* 1986;151:H1–H11.

Chai CY, Lin AMY, Hu SR, Wang JR, Kao LS, Kuo JS, Goldstein DS. Sympathoadrenal excitation and inhibition by lower brainstem stimulation in cats. *J Auton Nerv Sys* 1991;33: 35–46.

Chai CY, Share NN, Wang SX. Central control of cardiac augmentation in lower brain stem of the cat. *Am J Physiol* 1963;205:749–753.

Chai CY, Wang SC. Cardiovascular actions of diazepam in the cat. *J Pharmacol Exp Ther* 1966; 154:271–280.

Chalmers J, Pilowsky P. Brainstem and bulbospinal neurotransmitter systems in the control of blood pressure. *J Hypertens* 1991;9:675–694.

Chalmers J. Brain amines and models of experimental hypertension. *Circ Res* 1975;36:469–480.

Chan JY, Jang SF, Chan SH. Inhibition by locus coeruleus on the baroreceptor reflex response in the rat. *Neurosci Lett* 1992;144:225–228.

Chang PC, Szemeredi K, Grossman E, Kopin IJ, Goldstein DS. The fate of tritiated 6-flurodopamine in rats: A false neurotransmitter for positron emission tomographic imaging of sympathetic innervation and function. *J Pharmacol Exp Ther* 1990;255:809–817.

Chang PC, van der Krogt JA, Vermeij P, van Brummelen P. Norepinephrine removal and release in the forearm of healthy subjects. *Hypertension* 1986;8:801–809.

Chapman WP, Schroeder HR, Geyer G, Brazier MAB, Fages C, Poppen JL, Solomon HC, Yakovlev PI. Physiological evidence concerning importance of the amygdaloid nuclear region in the integration of circulatory function in man. *Science* 1954;120:949–950.

Charney DS, Heninger GR, Breier A. Noradrenergic function in panic anxiety. Effects of yohimbine in healthy subjects and patients with agoraphobia and panic disorder. *Arch Gen Psychiatry* 1984;41:751–763.

Charney DS, Heninger GR, Redmond DE Jr. Yohimbine induced anxiety and increased noradrenergic function in humans: Effects of diazepam and clonidine. *Life Sci* 1983;33:19–29.

Charney DS, Redmond DR Jr. Neurobiological mechanisms in human anxiety. Evidence supporting central noradrenergic hyperactivity. *Neuropharmacology* 1983;22:1531–1536.

Chen Y-F, Nagahama S, Winternitz SR, Oparil S. Hyperresponsiveness of monoaminergic mechanisms in DOCA/NaCl hypertensive rats. *Am J Physiol* 1985;H71–H79.

Chernow B, Lake CR, Barton M, Chobanian S, Zaloga GP, Casey LC, Fletcher JR. Sympathetic nervous system sensitivity to hemorrhagic hypotension in the subhuman primate. *J Trauma* 1984;24:229–232.

Chernow B, Lake CR, Teich S, Mougey EH, Meyergoff J, Casey LC, Fletcher JR. Hemorrhagic hypotension increases plasma beta-endorphin concentrations in the nonhuman primate. *Crit Care Med* 1986;14:505–507.

Chernow B, O'Brien JT. Overview of catecholamines in selected endocrine systems. In Ziegler MG, Lake CR (Eds) *Norepinephrine*. Baltimore: Williams and Wilkins, 1984, pp 439–470.

Chesler E, Weir EK, Braatz GA, Francis GS. Normal catecholamine and hemodynamic responses to orthostatic tilt in subjects with mitral valve prolapse. Correlation with psychologic testing. *Am J Med* 1985;78:754–760.

Chidsey CA, Braunwald E, Morrow AG, Mason DT. Myocardial norepinephrine concentration in man. Effects of reserpine and congestive heart failure. *N Engl J Med* 1963;269:653–658.

Chiueh CC, McCarty R. Sympatho-adrenal hyperreactivity to footshock stress but not to cold exposure in spontaneously hypertensive rats. *Physiol Behav* 1981;26:85–89.

Chiueh CC, Zukowska-Grojec Z, Kirk KL, Kopin IJ: 6-fluorocatecholamines as false adrenergic neurotransmitters. *J Pharmacol Exp Therap* 1983;225:529–533.

Chobanian AV, Gavras H, Gavras I, Bresnahan M, Sullivan P, Melby JC. Studies on the activity of the sympathetic nervous system in essential hypertension. *J Hum Stress* 1978;4:22–28.

Christensen NJ, Galbo H, Hansen JF, Hesse B, Richter EA, Trap-Jensen J. Catecholamines and exercise. *Diabetes* 1979;28 (Suppl 1):58–62.

Christensen NJ, Hilsted J, Hegedus L, Madsbad S. Effects of surgical stress and insulin on cardiovascular function and norepinephrine kinetics. *Am J Physiol* 1984;247:E29–E34.

Chrousos GP, Gold PW. The concepts of stress and stress system disorders. *J Am Med Assoc* 1992;267:1244–1252.

Ciriello J, Calaresu FR. Projections from buffer nerves to the nucleus of the solitary tract: an anatomical and electrophysiological study in the cat. *J Auton Nerv Sys* 1981;3:299–310.

Ciriello J, Kline RL, Zhang T-X, Caverson MM. Lesions of the paraventricular nucleus alter the development of spontaneous hypertension in the rat. *Brain Res* 1984;310:355–359.

Ciriello J, Rohlicek CV, Polosa C. Aortic baroreceptor reflex pathway: A functional mapping using [^{3}H]2-deoxyglucose autoradiography in the rat. *J Auton Nerv Sys* 1983;8:111–128.

Clarkson TB, Manuck SB, Kaplan JR. Potential role of cardiovascular reactivity in atherogenesis. In Matthews KA, Weiss SM, Detre T, Dembroski TM, Falkner B, Manuck SB, and Williams RB Jr (Eds) *Handbook of Stress, Reactivity, and Cardiovascular Disease*. New York: Wiley, 1986, pp 35–47.

Clayton PJ, Darvish HS. Course of depressive symptoms following the stress of bereavement. In Barrett J, Rose RM, Klerman GL (Eds) *Stress and Mental Disorder*. New York: Raven Press, 1979.

Clayton PJ. Mortality and morbidity in the first year of widowhood. *Arch Gen Psychiatry* 1974; 30:747–750.

Clementi WA, Durst NL, McNay JL, Keeton TK. Captopril modifies the hemodynamic and neuroendocrine responses to sodium nitroprusside in hypertensive patients. *Hypertension* 1986;8:229–237.

Clemson B, Gaul L, Gubin SS, Campsey DM, McConville J, Nussberger J, Zelis R. Prejunctional angiotensin II receptors. Facilitation of norepinephrine release in the human forearm. *J Clin Invest* 1994;93:684–691.

Cobb S, Rose RM. Hypertension, peptic ulcer, and diabetes in air traffic controllers. *J Am Med Assoc* 1973;224:489–492.

Cody RJ, Franklin KW, Kluger J, Laragh JH. Sympathetic repsonsiveness and plasma norepinephrine during therapy of chronic congestive heart failure with captopril. *Am J Med* 1982;72:791–797.

Cohen MD, Finberg J, Dibner-Dunlap M, Yuih SN, Thames MD. Effects of desipramine hydrochloride on peripheral sympathetic nerve activity. *Am J Physiol* 1990;258:R876–R882.

Cohen RA, Weisbrod RM. The endothelium inhibits norepinephrine release from adrenergic nerves of the rabbit carotid artery. *Am J Physiol* 1988;254:H871–H878.

Cohen S, Levi-Montalcini R, Hamburger V. A nerve growth-stimulating factor isolated from sarcomas 37 and 180. *Proc Nat Acad Sci USA* 1954;40:1014–1018.

Cohn JN, Archibald DG, Ziesche S, Franciosa JA, Harston WE, Tristani FE, Dunkman WB, Jacobs W, Francis GS, Flohr KH, Goldman S, Cobb FR, Shah PM, Saunders R, Fletcher RD, Loeb HS, Hughes VC, Baker B. Effect of vasodilator therapy in mortality in chronic congestive heart failure: Results of a Veterans Administration Cooperative Study (V-HeFT). *N Engl J Med* 1986;314:1547–1552.

Cohn JN, Levine BT, Olivari MT. Plasma norepinephrine as a guide to prognosis in patients with congestive heart failure. *N Engl J Med* 1984;311:819–823.

Cohn JN. Abnormalities of peripheral sympathetic nervous system control in congestive heart failure. *Circulation* 1990;82 (Suppl. I):I59–I67.

Collins S, Caron MG, Lefkowitz RJ. β_2-adrenergic receptors in hamster smooth muscle cells are transcriptionally regulated by glucocorticoids. *J Biol Chem* 1988;263:9067–9070.

Collis MG, de Mey C, Vanhoutte PM. Enhanced release of noradrenaline in the kidney of the young spontaneously hypertensive rat. *Clin Sci* 1979;57:233s–234s.

Conlay LA, Maher TJ, Wurtman RJ. Tyrosine's pressor effect is not due to tyramine formation in hypotensive rats. *Life Sci* 1984;35:1207–1212.

Conlay LA. The effects of tyrosine on blood pressure. In Kulbertus HE, Franck G (Eds) *Neurocardiology*. Mount Kisco, NY: Futura, 1988, pp 247–256.

Connor HE, Drew GM. Do adrenaline-containing neurones from the rostral ventrolateral medulla excite preganglionic sympathetic cell bodies? *J Auton Pharmac* 1987;7:87–96.

Contrada RJ, Glass DC, Krakoff LR, Krantz DS, Kehoe K, Isecke W, Collins C, Elting E. Effects of control over aversive stimulation and type A behavior on cardiovascular and plasma catecholamines responses. *Psychophysiology* 1982;19:408–419.

Conway J, Boon N, Floras J, Vann Jones J, Sleight P. Impaired control of heart rate leads to increased blood pressure variability. *J Hypertension* 1984;2:S395–S396.

Cooper A. Some experiments and observations on tying the carotid and vertebral arteries, and the pneumograstric phrenic and sympathetic nerves. *Guys Hosp Rep* 1836;1:457–472.

Cooper JR, Bloom FE, Roth RH. *The Biochemical Basis of Neuropharmacology.* New York: Oxford University Press, 1991.

Coote JH, Hilton SM, Zbrozyna AW. The pontomedullary area integrating the defense reaction in the cat and its influence on muscle blood flow. *J Physiol (Lond)* 1973;229:257–274.

Corbalan K, Verrier R, Lown B. Psychological stress and ventricular arrhythmias during myocardial infarction in the conscious dog. *Am J Cardiol* 1974;34:692–696.

Corea L, Bentivoglio M, Verdecchia P, Motolese M. Plasma norepinephrine and left ventricular hypertrophy in systemic hypertension. *Am J Cardiol* 1984;53:1299–1303.

Corea L, Bentivoglio M, Verdecchia P, Motolese M. Role of adrenergic overactivity and pressure overload in the pathogenesis of left ventricular hypertrophy in borderline and sustained essential hypertension in man. *Clin Sci* 1982;63:379s–381s.

Corea L, Bentivoglio M, Verdecchia P. Echocardiographic left ventricular hypertrophy as related to arterial pressure and plasma norepinephrine concentration in arterial hypertension. Reversal by atenolol treatment. *Hypertension* 1983;5:837–843.

Coresh J, Klag MJ, Mead LA, Liang KY, Whelton PK. Vascular reactivity in young adults and cardiovascular disease. A prospective study. *Hypertension* 1992;19:II218–II223.

Corley KC, Mauck FP, Shiel FO. Cardiac responses associated with "yoked chair" shock avoidance in squirrel monkeys. *Psychobiology* 1975;12:439–444.

Corley KC, Shiel FO, Mauck FP, Clark LS, Barber JH. Myocardial degeneration and cardiac arrest in squirrel monkey: Physiological and psychological correlates. *Psychophysiology* 1977;14:322–328.

Cornish KG, Gilmore JP, McCulloch T. Central blood volume and blood pressure in conscious primates. *Am J Physiol* 1988;254:H693–H701.

Corr PB, Gillis RA. Autonomic neural influences on the dysrhythmias resulting from myocardial infarction. *Circ Res* 1978;43:1–9.

Corr PB, Shayman JA, Kramer JB, Kipnis RJ. Increased a-adrenergic receptors in ischemic cat myocardium: A potential mediator of electrophysiological derangements. *J Clin Invest* 1981;67:1232–1236.

Corrall RJ, Frier BM. Acute hypoglycemia in man: neural control of pancreatic islet cell function. *Metabolism* 1981;30:160–164.

Cottier C, Perini C, Rauchfleisch U. Personality traits and hypertension: an overview. In Julius S, Bassett DR (Eds). *Handbook of Hypertension, Vol 9. Behavioral Factors in Hypertension.* New York: Elsevier Science, 1987, pp 123–140.

Cottingham EM, Matthews KA. Environmental events preceding sudden death in women. *Psychosom Med* 1980;42:567–574.

Cowley AW, Liard JF, Guyton AC. Role of the baroreceptor reflex in daily control of arterial blood pressure and other variables in dogs. *Circ Res* 1973;32:564–576.

Cox BF, Bishop VS. Neural and humoral mechanisms of angiotensin-dependent hypertension. *Am J Physiol* 1991;261:H1284–H1291.

Cox BF, Brody MJ. Subregions of rostral ventral medulla control arterial pressure and regional hemodynamics. *Am J Physiol* 1989;257:R635–R640.

Crary B, Hauser SL, Borysenko M, Kutz I, Hoban C, Ault KA, Weiner HL, Benson H. Epinephrine-induced changes in the distribution of lymphocyte subsets in peripheral blood of humans. *J Immunol* 1983;131:1178–1181.

Crawley JN, Ninan PT, Pickar D, Chrousos GP, Linnoila M, Skolnick P, Paul SM. Neuropharmacological antagonism of the beta-carboline-induced "anxiety" response in rhesus monkeys. *J Neurosci* 1985;5:477–485.

Creager MA, Faxon DP, Halperin JL, Melidossian CD, McCabe CH, Schick EC, Ryan TJ. Determinants of clinical response and survival in patients with congestive heart failure treated with captopril. *Am Heart J* 1982;104:1147–1154.

Cruickshank JM, Dwyer GN. Electrocardiographic changes in subarachnoid hemorrhage: role of catecholamines and effects of beta-blockade. *Br Heart J* 1974;36:395.

Cryer PE, Haymone MW, Santiago JV, Shah SD. Norepinephrine and epinephrine release and adrenergic mediation of smoking-associated hemodynamic and metabolic events. *N Engl J Med* 1976;295:573–577.

Cryer PE, Rizza RA, Haymond MW, Gerich JE. Epinephrine and norepinephrine are cleared through beta-adrenergic, but not alpha-adrenergic, mechanisms in man. *Metabolism* 1980; 29 (Suppl 1):1114–1118.

Cryer PE, Wortsman J, Shah SD, Nowak RM, Deftos LJ. Plasma chromogranin A as a marker of sympathochromaffin activity in humans. *Am J Physiol* 1991;260:E243–E246.

Cryer PE. Glucose counterregulation: prevention and correction of hypoglycemia in humans. *Am J Physiol* 1993;264:E149–E155.

Cryer PE. Physiology and pathophysiology of the human sympathoadrenal neuroendocrine system. *N Engl J Med* 1980;303:436–444.

Cubeddu LX, Hoffman IS, Davila J, Barbella YR, Ordaz P. Clonidine reduces elevated cerebrospinal fluid catecholamine levels in patients with essential hypertension. *Life Sci* 1984; 35:1365–1371.

Cuche J-L, Brochier P, Klioua N, Poirier M-F, Cuche H, Benmiloud M, Loo H, Safar M. Conjugated catecholamines in human plasma: Where are they coming from? *J Lab Clin Med* 1990;116:681–686.

Cuche J-L, Prinseau J, Selz F, Ruget G, Baglin A. Plasma free, sulfo- and glucuroconjugated catecholamines in uremic patients. *Kidney Int* 1986;30:566–572.

Cuche J-L, Prinseau J, Selz F, Ruget G, Tual J-L, Reingeissen L, Devoisin M, Baglin A, Guedon J, Fritel D. Oral load of tyrosine or L-dopa and plasma levels of free and sulfoconjugated catecholamines in healthy men. *Hypertension* 1985;7:81–89.

Cuche JL, Kuchel O, Barbeau A, Boucher R, Genest J. Relationship between the adrenergic nervous system and renin during adaptation to upright posture: A possible role for 3,4-dihydroxypheynethylamine (dopamine). *Clin Sci* 1972;43:481–491.

Cunningham ET Jr, Sawchenko PE. A circumscribed projection from the nucleus of the solitary tract to the nucleus ambiguus in the rat: Evidence for somatostatin-28-immunoreactive interneurons subserving reflex control of esophageal motility. *J Neurosci* 1989;9:1668–1682.

Cunningham ET, Sawchenko PE. Anatomical specificity of noradrenergic inputs to the paraventricular and supraoptic nuclei of the rat hypothalamus. *J Comp Neurol* 1988;274:60–76.

Curatolo PW, Robertson D. The health consequences of caffeine. *Ann Int Med* 1983;98:641–653.

Curtis AL, Drolet G, Valentino RJ. Hemodynamic stress activates locus coeruleus neurons of unanesthetized rats. *Brain Res Bull* 1993;31:737–744.

Curtis AL, Drolet G, Valentino RJ. Hemodynamic stress activates locus coeruleus neurons of unanesthetized rats. *Brain Res Bull* 1993;31:737–744.

Cutilletta AF, Erinhoff I, Heller A, Low J, Oparil S. Development of left ventricular hypertrophy in young spontaneously hypertensive rats after peripheral sympathectomy. *Circ Res* 1977; 40:428–434.

Cyon E. Die Nerven des Herzens. *Ihre Anatomie und Physiologie.* Berlin: Springer Verlag, 1907.

Dae MW, Botvinick EH. Imaging of the heart using metaiodobenzylguanidine. *J Thorac Imaging* 1990;5:31–36.

Dae MW, Herre JM, O'Connell JW, Botvinick EH, Newman D, Munoz L. Scintigraphic assessment of sympathetic innervation after transmural versus nontransmural myocardial infarction. *J Am Coll Cardiol* 1991;17:1416–1423.

Dae MW, O'Connell JW, Botvinick EH, Ahearn T, Yee E, Huberty JP, Mori H, Chin MC, Hattner RS, Herre JM, Munoz L. Scintigraphic assessment of regional cardiac adrenergic innervation. *Circulation* 1989;79:634–644.

Dahlstrom A, Fuxe K, Mya-Tu M, Zetterstrom BEM. Observations on adrenergic innervation of dog heart. *Am J Physiol* 1965;209:689–692.

Dahlstrom A, Fuxe K. Evidence for the existence of monoamine-containing neurons in the central nervous system. I. Demonstration of monoamines in the cell bodies of brain stem neurons. *Acta Physiol Scand* 1964"ppl 232:1–55.

Dahlstrom A, Fuxe K. Evidence for the existence of monoamine-containing neurons in the central nervous system. II. Experimentally induced changes in the intraneuronal amine levels of bulbospinal neuron systems. *Acta Physiol Scand* 1965"ppl 247:1–36.

Dale H. Opening Address. Ciba Foundation Symposium on Adrenergic Mechanisms, Boston: Little, Brown, 1960, pp 1–5.

Dale HH. The action of certain esters and ethers of choline, and their relation to muscarine. *J Pharmacol Exp Ther* 1914;6:147–190.

Daly I de B, Verney EB. The localisation of receptors involved in the reflex regulation of the heart rate. *J Physiol (Lond)* 1927;62:330–340.

Daly PA, Sole MJ. Myocardial catecholamines and the pathophysiology of heart failure. *Circulation* 1990;82 (Suppl. I):I35–I43.

Darlington DN, Keil LC, Dallman MF. Potentiation of hormonal responses to hemorrhage and fasting, but not hypoglycemia in conscious adrenalectomized rats. *Endocrinology* 1989; 125:1398–1406.

Darwin C. *The Expression of the Emotions in Man and Animals.* Chicago: University of Chicago Press, 1965.

Das PK. Interaction of sympathetic and parasympathetic systems under stress. In Beamish RE, Panagia, V, Dhalla NS (Eds) *Pathogenesis of Stress-Induced Heart Disease.* Boston: Martinus Nijhoff, 1984, pp 20–33.

Davies B, Sudera D, Sagnella G, Marchesi-Saviotti E, Mathias C, Bannister R, Sever P. Increased numbers of alpha receptors in sympathetic denervation supersensitivity in man. *J Clin Invest* 1982;69:779–784.

Davis BJ, Blair ML, Sladek JR Jr, Sladek CD. Effects of lesions of hypothalamic catecholamines on blood pressure, fluid balance, vasopressin and renin in the rat. *Brain Res* 1987;405:1–15.

Davydova NA, Kvetnansky R, Usakov AC. Activity of sympatho-adrenal system of cosmonauts during prolonged space flights on station ''Saljut-7.'' In Van Loon GR, Kvetnansky R, McCarty R, Axelrod J (Eds) *Stress: Neurochemical and Humoral Mechanisms.* New York: Gordon and Breach, 1989, pp 999–1013.

Davydova NA, Kvetnianski R, Ushakov AS. Characteristics of the responses of the sympatho-adrenal system in cosmonauts undergoing prolonged cosmic flight on the Saliut-7 orbital station. *Kosm Biol Aviakosm Med* 1989;23:14–20.

Dawirs RR, Teuchert-Noodt G, Kampen WU. Demonstration of dopamine-immunoreactive cells in the gastrointestinal tract of gerbils (Meriones unguiculatus). *J Histochem Cytochem* 1992;40:1197–1992.

Dawkins R. *The Blind Watchmaker.* New York: WW Norton, 1987.

Dawkins R. *The Selfish Gene.* New York: Oxford University Press, 1989.

Day TA, Renaud LP. Electrophysiological evidence that noradrenergic afferents selectively facilitate the activity of supraoptic vasopressin neurons. *Brain Res* 1984;303:233–240.

Day TA. Control of neurosecretory vasopressin cells by noradrenergic projections of the caudal ventrolateral medulla. *Prog Brain Res* 1989;81:303–317.

De Champlain J, Van Ameringen MR. Regulation of blood pressure by sympathetic nerve fibers and adrenal medulla in normotensive and hypertensive rats. *Circ Res* 1972;31:617–628.

De Champlain J. Pre- and postsynaptic adrenergic dysfunctions in hypertension. *J Hypertension* 1990; 8 (Suppl. 7):S77–S85.

De Potter WP, Dillen L, Annaert W, Tombeur K, Berghmans R, Coen EP. Evidence for the co-storage and co-release of neuropeptide Y and noradrenaline from large dense cored vesicles in sympathetic nerves of the bovine vas deferens. *Synapse* 1988;2:157–162.

De Sarro GB, Ascioti C, Froio F, Libri V, Nistrico G. Evidence that local coeruleus is the site where clonidine and drugs acting at alpha 1- and alpha 2-adrenoceptors affect sleep and arousal mechanisms. *Br J Pharmacol* 1987;90:675–685.

de Boer SF, Slangen JL, Van der Gugten J. Plasma catecholamine and corticosterone levels during active and passive shock-prod avoidance behavior in rats: effects of chlordiazepoxide. *Physiol Behav* 1990;47:1089–1098.

de Boer SF, Van der Gugten J, Slangen JL. Plasma catecholamine and corticosterone responses to predictable and unpredictable noise stress in rats. *Physiol Behav* 1989;45:789–795.

Dearry A, Gingrich JA, Falardeau P, Fremeau RT Jr, Bates MD, Caron MG. Molecular cloning and expression of the gene for a human D_1 receptor. *Nature* 1990;347:72–76.

DeCarlo DT, Gruenfeld DH. *Stress in the American Workplace.* Fort Washington, PA: LRP Publications, 1989.

DeGeest H, Levy MN, Zieske H, Lipman RI. Depression of ventricular contractility by stimulation of the vagus nerves. *Circ Res* 1965;17:222–236.

DeJong JH, Strubbe JH, Steffens AB. Hypothalamic influence on insulin and glucagon release in the rat. *Am J Physiol* 1977;233:E380–E388.

Deka-Starosta A, Garty M, Zukowska-Grojec Z, Keiser HR, Kopin IJ, Goldstein DS. Renal sympathetic nerve activity and norepinephrine release in rats. *Am J Physiol* 1989;257: R229–R236.

Delgado JMR. Circulatory effects of cortical stimulaiton. *Physiol Rev* 1960;40 (Suppl. 4):146–171.

Delitala G, Tomasi P, Virdis R. Prolactin, growth hormone and thryotropin-thyroid hormone secretion during stress states in man. In Groosman A (Ed) *Neuroendocrinology of Stress. Bailliere's Clinical Endocrinology and Metabolism.* Philadelphia: Bailliere Tindall, 1987, pp 391–414.

Delius W, Hagbarth K-E, Hongell A, Wallin BG. Manoeuvres affecting sympathetic outflow in human muscle nerves. *Acta Physiol Scand* 1972b;84:82–94.

Delius W, Hagbarth K-E, Hongell A, Wallin BG. Manoeuvres affecting sympathetic outflow in human skin nerves. *Acta Physiol Scand* 1972a;84:177–186.

Dembroski TM, Costa PT. Assessment of cornary-prone behavior. A current overview. *Ann Behav Med* 1988;10:60–63.

DeQuattro V, Campese V, Miura Y, Meijer D. Increased plasma catecholamines in high renin hypertension. *Am J Cardiol* 1976;38:801–804.

DeQuattro V, Loo R, Foti A. Sympathoadrenal responses to stress: The linking of type A behavior pattern to ischemic heart disease. *Clin Exp Hyper* 1985;7:469–481.

DeQuattro V, Nagatsu T, Mendez A, Verska J. Determinants of cardiac noradrenaline depletion in human congestive failure. *Cardiovasc Res* 1973;7:344–350.

DeQuattro V, Sullivan P, Minagawa R, Kopin IJ, Bornheimer J, Foti A, Barndt R. Central and peripheral noradrenergic tone in primary hypertension. *Fed Proc* 1984;43:47–51.

DeSilva RA, Verrier RL, Lown B. The effects of psychological stress and vagal stimulation with morphine on vulnerability to ventricular fibrillation (VF) in the conscious dog. *Am Heart J* 1978;95:197–203.

Devinsky O, Emoto S, Goldstein DS, Stull R, Porter RJ, Theodore WH, Nadi NS. Cerebrospinal fluid levels of dopa, catechols, and monoamine metabolites in patients with epilepsy. *Epilepsia* 1992;33:263–270.

Dhariwal KR, Black CDV, Levine M. Semidehydroascorbic acid as an intermediate in norepinephrine biosynthesis in chromaffin granules. *J Biol Chem* 1991;266:12908–12914.

DiBona GF, Wilcox CS. The kidney and the sympathetic nervous system. In Bannister R, Mathias CJ (Eds) *Autonomic Failure*. New York: Oxford University Press, 1992, pp 178–196.

Dietl H, Sinha JN, Philippu A. Presynaptic regulation of the release of catecholamines in the cat hypothalamus. *Brain Res* 1981;208:213–218.

Dietl H. Temporal relationship between noradrenaline release in the central amygdala and plasma noradrenaline secretion in rats and tree shrews. *Neurosci Lett* 1985;55:41–46.

Dilraj A, Botha JH, Rambiritch V, Miller R, van Dellen JR. Levels of catecholamine in plasma and cerebrospinal fluid in aneurysmal subarachnoid hemorrhage. *Neurosurgery* 1992;31:42–50.

Dimsdale JE, Herd JA, Hartley LH. Epinephrine mediated increases in plasma cholesterol. *Psychosom Med* 1983;45:227–232.

Dimsdale JE, Herd JA. Variability of plasma lipids in response to emotional arousal. *Psychosom Med* 1982;44:413–430.

Dimsdale JE, Moss J. Plasma catecholamines in stress and exercise. *J Am Med Assoc* 1980;243:340–342.

Dimsdale JE, Ziegler M, Mills P, Berry C. Prediction of salt sensitivity. *Am J Hypertens* 1990a;3:429–435.

Dimsdale JE, Ziegler M, Mills P, Delehanty SG, Berry C. Effects of salt, race, and hypertension on reactivity to stressors. *Hypertension* 1990b;16:573–580.

Dimsdale JE, Ziegler MG. What do plasma and urinary measures of catecholamines tell us about human response to stressors? *Circulation* 1991;83 (Suppl II): II36–II42.

Dinerstein RJ, Vannice J, Henderson RC, Roth LJ, Goldberg LI, Hoffmann PC. Histofluorescence techniques provide evidence for dopamine-containing neuronal elements in canine kidney. *Science* 1979;205:497–499.

Ding Y-S, Fowler JS, Dewey SL, Logan J, Schlyer DJ, Gatley SJ, Volkow ND, King PT, Wolf AP. Comparison of high specific acitivity (−) and (+)-6-[^{18}F]fluoronorepinephrine and 6-[^{18}F]fluorodopamine in baboons: Heart uptake, metabolism and the effect of desipramine. *J Nucl Med* 1993;34:619–629.

Dionne R, Goldstein DS, Wirdzek PR, Keiser HR, Dubner R. Effects of diazepam premedication and epinephrine-containing local anesthetic on circulatory and plasma catecholamine responses to minor surgery. *Anesthes Analg* 1984;63:640–646.

Dittmar C. Ein neuer Beweis fur die Reizbarkeit der centripatelen Fasern des Ruckenmarks. *Sachs Akad Wiss Sitz* 1870;22:18–45.

Djojosugito AM, Folkow B, Kylstra P, Lisander B, Tuttle RS. Differentiated interaction between the hypothalamic defense reaction and baroreceptor reflexes. I. Effects on heart rate and regional flow resistance. *Acta Physiol Scand* 1970;78:376–385.

Doba N, Reis DJ. Acute fulminating neurogenic hypertension produced by brainstem lesions in rat. *Circ Res* 1973;32:584–593.

Docherty JR, McGrath JC. Inhibition of sympathetic transmission in rat heart by clonidine: The roles of stimulation frequency, endogenous feedback and noradrenaline re-uptake. *Naunyn-Schmiedeberg's Arch Pharmacol* 1979;309:225–233.

Dominiak P, Grobecker H. Elevated plasma catecholamines in young hypertensive and hyperkinetic patients: Effect of pindolol. *Br J Clin Pharmacol* 1982;13:381S–390S.

Dominiak P, Kees F, Grobecker H. Circulating and tissue catecholamines in rats with chronic neurogenic hypertension. *Bas Res Cardiol* 1986;81:20–28.

Donald DE, Shepherd JT. Reflexes from the heart and lungs: Physiological curiosities or important regulatory mechanisms. *Cardiovasc Res* 1978;12:446–469.

Donohue SJ, Head RJ, Stitzel RE. Elevated nerve growth factor levels in young spontaneously hypertensive rats. *Hypertension* 1989;14:421–426.

Dorward PK, Rudd CD. Influence of brain renin-angiotensin system on renal sympathetic and cardiac baroreflexes in conscious rabbits. *Am J Physiol* 1991;260:H770–H778.

Downing SE, Lee JC. Contribution of α-adrenoceptor activation to the pathogenesis of norepinephrine cardiomyopathy. *Circ Res* 1983;52:471–478.

Doxey JC, Everitt J. Inhibitory effects of clonidine on responses to sympathetic nerve stimulaiton in the pithed rat. *Br J Pharmacol* 1977;61:559–566.

Doyle AE, Smirk FH. The neurogenic component in hypertension. *Circulation* 1955;12:543–552.

Draper AJ, Kendall HE, Redfern PH. The chronic effect of β-adrenoceptor antagonists on the efflux of tritiated noradrenaline from sympathetic nerves of the pithed rat. *J Auton Pharmacol* 1986;5:259–268.

Drew GM, Whiting SB. Evidence for two distinct types of postsynaptic α-adrenoceptor in vascular smooth muscle in vivo. *Br J Pharmacol* 1979;67:207–215.

Drolet G, Bouvier M, De Champlain J. Enhanced sympathoadrenal reactivity to haemorrhagic stress in DOCA-salt hypertensive rats. *J Hypertension* 1989;7:237–242.

Drummond PD, Finch PM, Smythe GA. Reflex sympathetic dystrophy: the significance of differing plasma catecholamine concentrations in affected and unaffected limbs. *Brain* 1991; 114:2025–2036.

Drummond PD, Lance JW. Facial flushing and sweating mediated by the sympathetic nervous system. *Brain* 1987;110:793–803.

Due BR, Schwaber JS. Bulbar origin of catecholaminergic projections to the central amygdaloid nucleus in the rat. *Neurosci Abst* 1990;No. 234.22.

Duncan MW, Compton P, Lazarus L, Smythe GA. Measurement of norepinephrine and 3,4-dihydroxyphenylglycol in urine and plasma for the diagnosis of pheochromocytoma. *N Engl J Med* 1988;319:136–142.

Dunnette J, Weinshilboum R. Inheritance of low immunoreactive human plasma dopamine-β-hydroxylase: Radioimmunoassay studies. *J Clin Invest* 1977;60:1080–1087.

DuPen S, Eisenach JC, Allin D, Zaccaro D. Epidural clonidine for intractable cancer pain. *Regional Anesthesia* 1993; 18 (Suppl.):23.

Duprez D, De Pue N, Clement DL. Peripheral vascular responses during carotid baroreceptor stimulation in normotensive and hypertensive subjects. *Clin Sci* 1987;73:635–640.

Dworkin BR, Filewich RJ, Miller NE, Craigmyle N, Pickering TG. Baroreceptor activation reduces reactivity to noxious stimulation: Implications for hypertension. *Science* 1979; 205:1299–1301.

Eaton WW, Sigal JJ, Weinfeld M. Impairment in Holocaust survivors after 33 years: Data from an unbiased community sample. *Am J Psychiatry* 1982;139:773–777.

Ebert PA, Allgood RJ, Sabiston DC. Effect of cardiac denervation on arrhythmia following coronary artery occlusion. *Surg Forum* 1967;18:114–115.

Ebert PA, Vanderveek RB, Allgood RJ, Sabiston DC Jr. Effect of chronic cardiac denervation on arrhythmias after coronary artery ligation. *Cardiovasc Rev* 1970;4:141–147.

Eckert E, Henseling M, Gescher A, Trendelenburg U. Stereoselectivity of the distribution of labelled noradrenaline in rabbit aortic strips after inhibition of the noradrenaline-metabolizing enzymes. *Naunyn-Schmiedeberg's Arch Pharmacol* 1976;292:219–229.

Edlund MJ, Swann AC, Davis CM. Plasma MHPG in untreated panic disorder. *Biol Psychiatry* 1987;22:1488–1491.

Edwards BS, Zimmerman RS, Schwab TR, Heublein DM, Burnett JC Jr. Atrial stretch, not pressure, is the prime determinant controlling the acute release of atrial natriuretic factor. *Circ Res* 1988;62:191–195.

Egan B, Fitzpatrick A, Julius S. The heart and the regulation of renin. *Circulation* 1987;75 (Suppl. I):I130–I133.

Egan B, Julius S. Vascular hypertrophy in borderline hypertension: Relationship to blood pressure and sympathetic drive. *Clin Exp Hyper* 1985;A7:243–255.

Egan BM, Panis R, Hinderliter A, Schork N, Julius S. Mechanism of increased alpha adrenergic vasoconstriction in human essential hypertension. *J Clin Invest* 1987;80:812–817.

Eibl-Eibesfeldt I. *Ethology: The Biology of Behavior*. New York: Holt, Rinehart and Winston, 1970.

Eide I, Kolloch R, DeQuattro V, Miano L, Dugger R, Van der Meulen J. Raised cerebrospinal fluid norepinephrine in some patients with primary hypertension. *Hypertension* 1979;1: 255–260.

Eilam R, Malach R, Bergmann F, Segal M. *Hypertension* induced by hypothalamic transplantation from genetically hypertensive to normotensive rats. *J Neurosci* 1991;11:401–411.

Eisenach J, Detweiler D, Hood D. Hemodynamic and analgesic actions of epidurally administered clonidine. *Anesthesiology* 1993;78:277–287.

Eisenhofer G, Brush JE, Cannon RO III, Stull R, Kopin IJ, Goldstein DS. Plasma dihydroxyphenylalanine and total body and regional noradrenergic activity in humans. *J Clin Endocrinol Metab* 1989;68:247–255.

Eisenhofer G, Cox HS, Esler MD. Noradrenaline reuptake and plasma dihydroxyphenylglycol during sustained changes in sympathetic activity in rabbits. *J Auton Nerv Sys* 1991;32: 217–232.

Eisenhofer G, Cox HS, Esler MD. Parallel increases in noradrenaline reuptake and release into plasma during activation of the sympathetic nervous system in rabbits. *Naunyn-Schmiedeberg's Arch Pharmacol* 1990;342:328–335.

Eisenhofer G, Esler MD, Cox HS, Meredith IT, Jennings GL, Angus JA, Brush JE Jr, Goldstein DS. Differences in the neuronal removal of circulating epinephrine and norepinephrine. *J Clin Endocrinol Metab* 1990;70:1710–1720.

Eisenhofer G, Esler MD, Goldstein DS, Kopin IJ. Neuronal uptake, metabolism, and release of tritium-labeled norepinephrine during assessment of its plasma kinetics. *Am J Physiol* 1991;261:E505–E515.

Eisenhofer G, Esler MD, Meredith IT, Dart A, Cannon RO III, Quyyumi AA, Lambert G, Chin J, Jennings GL, Goldstein DS. Sympathetic nervous function in the human heart as assessed by cardiac spillovers of dihydroxyphenylglycol and norepinephrine. *Circulation* 1992;85:1775–1785.

Eisenhofer G, Goldstein DS, Kopin IJ. Plasma dihydroxyphenylglycol for estimation of noradrenaline neuronal reuptake in the sympathetic nervous system in vivo. *Clin Sci* 1989; 76:171–182.

Eisenhofer G, Goldstein DS, Ropchak TG, Nguyen HQ, Keiser HR, Kopin IJ. Source and physiological significance of plasma 3,4-dihydroxyphenylglycol and 3-methoxy-4-hydroxyphenylglycol. *J Auton Nerv Sys* 1988;24:1–14.

Eisenhofer G, Goldstein DS, Stull R, Keiser HR, Sunderland T, Murphy DL, Kopin IJ. Simultaneous liquid chromatographic determination of 3,4-dihydroxyphenylglycol, catecholamines, and 3,4-dihydroxyphenylalanine in plasma and their responses to inhibition of monoamine oxidase. *Clin Chem* 1986;32:2030–2033.

Eisenhofer G, Goldstein DS, Stull RW, Gold PW, Keiser HR, Kopin IJ. Dissociation between corticotropin and catecholamine responses to isoprenaline in humans. *Clin Exp Pharmacol Physiology* 1987;14:337–341.

Eisenhofer G, Hovevey-Sion D, Kopin IJ, Miletich R, Kirk KL, Finn R, Goldstein DS. Neuronal uptake and metabolism of 2- and 6-Fluorodopamine: False neurotransmitters for positron emission tomographic imaging of sympathetically innervated tissues. *J Pharmacol Exp Therap* 1989;248:419–427.

Eisenhofer G, Ropchak T, Nguyen H, Keiser HR, Kopin IJ, Goldstein DS. Source and physiological significance of plasma 3,4-dihydroxyphenylalanine in the rat. *J Neurochem* 1988; 51:1210–1213.

Eisenhofer G, Saigusa T, Esler MD, Cox HS, Angus JA, Dorward PK. Central sympathoinhibition and peripheral neuronal uptake blockade after desipramine in rabbits. *Am J Physiol* 1991; 260:R824–R832.

Eisenhofer G, Smolich JJ, Esler MD. Disposition of endogenous adrenaline compared to noradrenaline released by cardiac sympathetic nerves in the anaesthetized dog. *Naunyn-Schmiedeberg's Arch Pharmacol* 1992;345:160–171.

Ekas RD, Steenberg ML, Lokhandwala MF. Increased presynaptic α-adrenoceptor-mediated regulation of noradrenaline release in the isolated perfused kidney of spontaneously hypertensive rats. *Clin Sci* 1982;63:309s–311s.

Ekas RD, Steenberg ML, Woods MS, Lokhandwala MF. Presynaptic alpha- and beta-adrenoceptor stimulation and norepinephrine release in the spontaneously hypertensive rat. *Hypertension* 1983;5:198–204.

Ekeberg O, Kjeldsen E, Greenwood DT, Enger E. Correlations between psychological and physiological responses to acute flight phobia stress. *Scand J Clin Lab Invest* 1990;50:671–677.

Ekman P, Levenson RW, Friesen WV. Autonomic nervous system activity distinguishes among emotions. *Science* 1983;221:1208–1210.

Elam M, Svensson TH, Thoren P. Differentiated cardiovascular afferent regulation of locus coeruleus neurons and sympathetic nerves. *Brain Res* 1985;358:77–84.

Elam M, Svensson TH, Thoren P. Locus coeruleus neurons and sympathetic nerves: activation by cutaneous sensory afferents. *Brain Res* 1986;375:117–125.

Elam M, Thoren P, Svensson TH. Locus coeruleus neurons and sympathetic nerves: Activation by visceral afferents. *Brain Res* 1986;375:117–125.

Elam M, Yao T, Svensson TH, Thoren P. Regulation of locus coeruleus neurons and splanchnic, sympathetic nerves by cardiovascular afferents. *Brain Res* 1984;290:281–287.

Elayan H, Kennedy B, Ziegler MG. Cardiac atria and ventricles contain different inducible adrenaline synthesizing enzymes. *Cardiovasc Res* 1990;24:53–56.

Eldrup E, Christensen NJ, Andreasen J, Hilsted J. Plasma dihydroxyphenylalanine (DOPA) is independent of sympathetic activity in humans. *Eur J Clin Invest* 1989;19:514–517.

Eldrup E, Richter AE, Christensen NJ. Dopa, norepinephrine, and dopamine in rat tissues: no effect of sympathectomy on muscle dopa. *Am J Physiol* 1989;256:E284–E287.

Eliasson K, Hjemdahl P, Kahan T. Circulatory and sympathoadrenal responses to stress in borderline and established hypertension. *J Hypertension* 1983;1:131-139.

Eliasson S, Folkow B, Lindren O, Uvnas B. Activation of sympathetic vasodilator nerves to the skeletal muscles in the cat by hypothalamic stimulation. *Acta Physiol Scand* 1951;23:333–351.

Eliot RS (Ed) *Stress and the Heart. Mechanisms, Measurements, and Management.* Mount Kisco, NY: Futura, 1988.

Eliot RS, Buell, JC. Utilization of a new objective, non-physical stress test. In Beamish RE, Singal PK, Dhalla NS (Eds) *Stress and Heart Disease.* Boston: Martinus Nijhoof, 1985, pp 116–126.

Eliot RS, Clayton FC, Pieper GM, Todd GL. Influence of environmental stress on the pathogenesis of sudden cardiac death. *Fed Proc* 1977;36:1719–1724.

Eliot RS, Todd GL, Clayton FC, Pieper GM. Experimental catecholamine-induced acute myocardial necrosis. *Adv Cardiol* 1978;25:107–118.

Eliot RS. *Behavior and Cardiovascular Disease.* Kalamazoo, MI: Upjohn Co., 1989.

Eliot RS. Detection and management of brain-heart interrelations. *J Am Coll Cardiol* 1988;12:1101–1105.

Eliot RS. Twentieth century stress and the heart. In Eliot RS (Ed) *Stress and the Heart.* Mount Kisco, NY: Futura, 1974, pp 7–12.

Ellenbogen KA, Mohanty PK, Rea R, Szentpetery S, Thames MD. Reversal of arterial baroreflex abnormalities after orthotopic cardiac transplantation. *Circulation* 1987;76:IV–60.

Elliott TR. On the action of adrenalin. *J Physiol* 1904;31:xx–xxi.

Ellison GD, Zanchetti A. Specific appearance of sympathetic cholinergic vasodilatation in muscles during conditioned movements. *Nature* 1971;232:124–125.

Elmadjian F, Hope JM, Lamson ET. Excretion of epinephrine and norepinephrine in various emotional states. *J Clin Endocrinol Metab* 1965;17:608–620.

Ely DL, Mostardi RA. The effect of recent life events stress, life assets, and temperament pattern on cardiovascular risk factors for Akron City police officers. *J Human Stress* 1986;12:77–91.

Emorine LJ, Marullo S, Briend-Sutren M-M, Patey G, Tate K, Delavier-Klutchko C, Strosberg AD. Molecular characterization of the human β3-adrenergic receptor. *Science* 1989;245:1118–1121.

Emoto H, Yokoo H, Yoshida M, Tanaka M. Corticotropin-releasing factor enhances noradrenaline release in the rat hypothalamus assessed by intracerebral microdialysis. *Brain Res* 1993;601:286–288.

Engel GL. Psychologic distress, vasodepressor (vasovagal) syncope, and sudden death. *Ann Int Med* 1978;89:403–412.

Engel GL. Sudden and rapid death during psychological stress: Folklore or folk wisdom? *Ann Int Med* 1971;74:771–782.

Engelman K, Portnoy B, Lovenberg W. A sensitive and specific double-isotope derivative method for the determination of catecholamines in biological specimens. *Am J Med* Sci 1968; 255:259–268.

Engelman K, Portnoy B. A sensitive double-isotope derivative assay for norepinephrine and epinephrine. *Circ Res* 1970;26:53–57.

Ennis M, Aston-Jones G. A potent excitatory input to the nucleus locus coeruleus from the ventrolateral medulla. *Neurosci Lett* 1986;71:299–305.

Ennis M, Aston-Jones G. Potent inhibitory input to locus coeruleus from the nulceus prepositus hypoglossi. *Brain Res Bull* 1989;22:793–803.

Epstein M, Johnson G, DeNunzio AG. Effects of water immersion on plasma catecholamines in normal humans. *J Appl Physiol* 1983;54:244–248.

Epstein M, Norsk P, Loutzenhiser R. Effects of water immersion on atrial natriuretic peptide release in humans. *Am J Nephrol* 1989;9:1–24.

Epstein SE, Beiser GD, Goldstein RE, Stampfer M, Wechsler AS, Glick G, Braunwald E. Circulatory effects of electrical stimulation of the carotid sinus nerves in man. *Circulation* 1969;40:269–276.

Erickson JS, Eiden LE, Hoffman BJ. Expression cloning of a reserpine-sensitive vesicular monoamine transporter. *Proc Natl Acad Sci USA* 1992;89:10993–10997.

Eriksson E, Dellborg M, Soderpalm B, Carlsson M, Nilsson C. Growth hormone responses to clonidine and GRF in spontaneously hypertensive rats: neuroendocrine evidence for enhanced responsiveness of brain alpha 2-adrenoceptors in genetical hypertension. *Life Sci* 1986;39:2103–2109.

Eriksson T, Granerus AK, Linde A, Carlsson A. "On-off" phenomenon in Parkinson's disease: Relationship between dopa and other large neutral amino acids in plasma. *Neurology* 1988;38:1245–1248.

Erne P, Bolli P, Burgisser E, Buhler FR. Correlation of platelet calcium with blood pressure. Effect of antihypertensive therapy. *N Engl J Med* 1984;310:1084–1088.

Ernsberger P, Meeley MP, Reis DJ. An endogenous clonidine-like substance binds preferentially to imidazole binding sites in the ventrolateral medulla labeled by ^{3}H-*para*-aminoclonidine. *J Hypertension* 1986;4 (Suppl. 5):S109–S111.

Esler M, Eisenhofer G, Dart A, Chin J, Cox H, Lambert G, Jennings G. Adrenaline release by the human heart. *Clin Exp Pharmacol Physiol* 1991;18:67–70.

Esler M, Ferrier C, Lambert G, Eisenhofer G, Cox H, Jennings G. Biochemical evidence of sympathetic hyperactivity in human hypertension. *Hypertension* 1991;17 (Suppl III): III29–III35.

Esler M, Hasking GJ, Willett IR, Leonard PW, Jennings GL. Noradrenaline release and sympathetic nervous system activity. *J Hypertension* 1985;3:117–129.

Esler M, Jackman G, Bobik A, Kelleher D, Jennings G, Leonard P, Skews H, Korner P. Determination of norepinephrine apparent release rate and clearance in humans. *Life Sci* 1979; 25:1461–1470.

Esler M, Jackman G, Bobik A, Leonard P, Kelleher D, Skews H, Jennings G, Korner P. Norepinephrine kinetics in essential hypertension. Defective neuronal uptake of norepinephrine in some patients. *Hypertension* 1981;3:149–156.

Esler M, Jennings G, Biviano B, Lambert G, Hasking G. Mechanism of elevated plasma noradrenaline in the course of essential hypertension. *J Cardiovasc Pharmacol* 1986;8 (Suppl 5):S39–S43.

Esler M, Jennings G, Korner P, Blombery P, Burke F, Willett I, Leonard P. Total, and organ-specific, noradrenaline plasma kinetics in essential hypertension. *Clin Exper Hyper* 1984a; 6:507–521.

Esler M, Jennings G, Korner P, Blombery P, Sacharias N, Leonard P. Measurement of total and organ-specific norepinephrine kinetics in humans. *Am J Physiol* 1984b;247:E21–E28.

Esler M, Jennings G, Korner P, Willett I, Dudley F, Hasking G, Anderson W, Lambert G. Assessment of human sympathetic nervous system activity from measurements of nor-epinephrine turnover. *Hypertension* 1988;11:3–20.

Esler M, Jennings G, Lambert G, Meredith I, Horne M, Eisenhofer G. Overflow of catecholamine neurotransmitters to the circulation: Source, fate, and functions. *Physiol Rev* 1990;70: 963–985.

Esler M, Jennings G, Lambert G. Measurements of overall and cardiac norepinephrine release into plasma during cognitive challenge. *Psychoneuroendocrinology* 1989b;14:477–481.

Esler M, Jennings G, Lambert G. Noradrenaline release and the pathophysiology of primary human hypertension. *Am J Hypertens* 1989a;2(3 Pt. 2):140S–146S.

Esler M, Jennings G, Leonard P, Sacharias N, Burke F, Johns J, Blombery P. Contribution of individual organs to total noradrenaline release in humans. *Acta Physiol Scand* 1984; Suppl. 527:11–16.

Esler M, Jennings GL, Lambert GW. Release of noradrenaline into the cerebrovascular circulation in patients with primary hypertension. *J Hypertens* 1988;6:S494–S496.

Esler M, Julius S, Zweifler A, Randall O, Harburg E, Gardiner H, DeQuattro V. Mild high-renin essential hypertension: neurogenic human hypertension. *N Engl J Med* 1977;296:405–411.

Esler M, Lambert G, Jennings G. Increased regional sympathetic nervous activity in human hypertension: Causes and consequences. *J Hypertens* 1990;8 (Suppl. 7):S53–S57.

Esler M. Assessment of sympathetic nervous function in humans from noradrenaline plasma kinetics. *Clin Sci* 1982;62:247–254.

Esler MD, Wallin G, Dorward PK, Eisenhofer G, Westerman R, Meredith I, Lambert G, Cox HS, Jennings G. Effects of desipramine on sympathetic nerve firing and norepinephrine spillover to plasma in humans. *Am J Physiol* 1991;260:R817–R823.

Evans DE, Alter WA, Shotsky SA, Gunby EN. Cardiac arrhythmias resulting from experimental head injury. *J Neurosurg* 1976;45:609–616.

Evans PJ, Dieguez C, Rees LH, Hall R, Scanlon MF. The effect of cholinergic blockade on the ACTH, beta-endorphin and cortisol responses to insulin-induced hypoglycemia. *Clin Endocrinol* 1986;24:687–691.

Everitt BJ, Robbins TW, Selden NRW. Functions of the locus coeruleus noradrenergic system: a neurobiological and behavioural synthesis. In Heal DJ, Marsden CA (Eds) *The Pharmacology of Noradrenaline in the Central Nervous System*. New York: Oxford University Press, 1990, pp 349–378.

Evinger MJ, Joh TH. Strain-specific differences in transcription of the gene for the epinephrine-synthesizing enzyme phenylethanolamine N-methyltransferase. *Brain Res Mol Brain Res* 1989;5:141–147.

Eyster JAE, Meek WJ. Cardiac irregularities in morphine poisoning in the dog. *Heart* 1912;4: 59–66.

Fabris B, Caretta R, Fischetti F, Bellini G, Giraldi T, Campanacci L. Baroreflex sensitivity in spontaneously hypertensive rats acutely treated with clonidine or guanfacine. In Lown B, Malliani A, Prosdocimi M (Eds) *Neural Mechanisms and Cardiovascular Disease*. New York: Springer Verlag, 1986, pp 557–558.

Factor SM, Minase T, Cho S, Dominitz R, Sonnenblick EH. Microvascular spasm in cardiomyopathic Syrian hamster: A preventable cause of focal myocardial necrosis. *Circulation* 1982;66:342–354.

Faden AI, Holaday JW. Opiate antagonists: A role in the treatment of hypovolemic shock. *Science* 1979;205:317–318.

Fagius J, Berne C. Changes of sympathetic nerve activity induced by 2-deoxy-D-glucose infusion in humans. *Am J Physiol* 1989;256:E714–E720.

Fagius J, Kay R. Low ambient temperature increases baroreflex-governed sympathetic outflow to muscle vessels in humans. *Acta Physiol Scand* 1991;142:201–209.

Fagius J, Wallin BG, Sundlof G, Nerhed C, Englesson S. Sympathetic outflow in man after anaesthesia of the glossopharyngeal and vagus nerves. *Brain* 1985;108:423–438.

Fagius J, Wallin BG. Long-term variability and reproducibility of resting human muscle nerve sympathetic activity at rest, as reassessed after a decade. *Clin Auton Res* 1993;3:201–205.

Fain JN, Garcia-Sainz JA. Role of phosphotidylinositol turnover in alpha-1 and of adenylate cyclase inhibition in alpha-2 effects of catecholamines. *Life Sci* 1980;26:1183–1194.

Falck B, Hillarp N-A, Thieme G, Torp A. Fluorescence of catecholamines and related compounds condensed with formaldehyde. *J Histochem Cytochem* 1962;10:348–354.

Falck B. Observations on the possibilities of the cellular localization of monoamines by a fluorescence method. *Acta Physiol Scand* 1962; Suppl. 197:1–25.

Falckh PH, Harkin LA, Head RJ. Resistance vessel gene expression of nerve growth factor is elevated in young spontaneously hypertensive rats. *J Hypertens* 1992;10:913–918.

Falkner B, Kushner H, Gaddo O, Angelakos ET. Cardiovascular characteristics in adolescents who develop essential hypertension. *Hypertension* 1981;3:521–527.

Falkner B, Onesti G, Angelakos E. Effect of salt loading on the cardiovascular response to stress in adolescents. *Hypertension* 1981;3 (Suppl. 2):II195–II199.

Falkner B, Onesti G, Angelakos ET, Fernandes M, Langman C. Cardiovascular response to mental stress in normal adolescents with hypertensive parents. *Hypertension* 1979;1:23–30.

Falkner B, Onesti G, Hamstra B. Stress response characteristics of adolescents with high genetic risk for essential hypertension: a five year follow-up. *Clin Exp Hyper* 1981;3:583–591.

Fani K, Jimenez FA, De Soto F. Heart morphological changes in rats placed in a crowded environment. *J Toxicol Environ Health* 1977;421–429.

Farabollini F. Behavioral and endocrine aspects of dominance and submissiveness in male rabbits. *Agress Behav* 1987;13:247–258.

Farrell PA, Ebert TJ, Kampine JP. Naloxone augments muscle sympathetic nerve activity during isometric exercise in humans. *Am J Physiol* 1991;260:E379–E388.

Farsang C, Kunos G. Naloxone reverses the antihypertensive effect of clonidine. *Br J Pharmacol* 1979;67:161–164.

Faucheux B, Buu NT, Kuchel O. Effects of saline and albumin on plasma and urinary catecholamines in dogs. *Am J Physiol* 1977;232:F123–F127.

Favier RJ, Desplanches D, Pequignot JM, Peyrin L, Flandrois R. Effects of hypoxia on catecholamine and cardiorespiratory responses in exercising dogs. *Respir Physiol* 1985;61:167–177.

Fedida D, Shimoni Y, Giles WR. A novel effect of norepinephrine on cardiac cells is mediated by alpha$_1$-adrenoceptors. *Am J Physiol* 1989;256:H1500–H1504.

Feigl EO. Carotid sinus reflex control of coronary blood flow. *Circ Res* 1968;23:223–237.

Feigl EO. Parasympathetic control of coronary blood flow in dogs. *Circ Res* 1969;25:509–519.

Felder RB, Thames MD. Responses to activation of cardiac sympathetic afferents with epicardial bradykinin. *Am J Physiol* 1982;242:H148–H153.

Felder RB, Thames MD. The cardiocardiac sympathetic reflex during coronary occlusion in anesthetized dogs. *Circ Res* 1981;48:685–692.

Feldman PD, Moises HC. Electrophysiological evidence for alpha 1- and alpha 2-adrenoceptors in solitary tract nucleus. *Am J Physiol* 1988;254:H756–H762.

Feldman S, Conforti N, Melamed E. Involvement of ventral noradrenergic bundle in corticosterone secretion following neural stimuli. *Neuropharmacology* 1988;27:129–133.

Fell D, Derbyshire DR, Maile CJ, Larsson I-M, Ellis R, Achola KJ, Smith G. Measurement of plasma catecholamine concentrations. An assessment of anxiety. *Br J Anaesth* 1985;57: 770–774.

Ferguson AV, Renaud LP. Hypothalamic paraventricular nucleus lesions decrease pressor responses to subfornical organ stimulation. *Brain Res* 1984;305:361–364.

Fernandez de Molina A, Hunsperger RW. Organization of the subcortical system governing defense and flight reactions in the cat. *J Physiol (Lond)* 1962;160:200–213.

Ferrans VJ, Hibbs RG, Walsh JJ, Burch GE. Histochemical and electron microscopic studies on the cardiac necroses produced by sympathomimetic agents. *Ann NY Acad Sci* 1969;156: 309–332.

Ferrans VJ, Van Vleet JF. Morphological aspects of myocardial lesions associated with stress. In Beamish RE, Singal PK, Dhalla NS (Eds) *Stress and Heart Disease.* Boston: Martinus Nijhoof, 1985, pp 211–227.

Ferrari P, Weidmann P, Ferrier C, Dietler R, Hollmann R, Piso RJ, Wey J, Shaw S. Dysregulation of atrial natriuretic factor in hypertension-prone man. *J Clin Endocrinol Metab* 1990;71: 944–951.

Ferrier C, Cox H, Esler M. Elevated total body noradrenaline spillover in normotensive members of hypertensive families. *Clin Sci* 1993;84:225–230.

Feuerstein G, Gutman Y. Preferential secretion of adrenaline or noradrenaline by the cat adrenal *in vivo* in response to different stimuli. *Br J Pharmacol* 1971;43:764–775.

Feuerstein G, Hassan AH, Faden AI. TRF: Cardiovascular and sympathetic modulation in brain nuclei of the rat. *Peptides* 1983;4:617–620.

Feuerstein G, Jimerson DC, Kopin IJ. Prostaglandins, catecholamines, and cardiovascular responses to hemorrhage. *Am J Physiol* 1981;240:R166–R174.

Fillenz M. Fine structure of noradrenaline storage vesicles in nerve terminals of the rat vas deferens. *Phil Trans Roy Soc Lond* 1971;B261;319–323.

Fillenz M. *Noradrenergic Neurons.* New York: Cambridge University Press, 1990.

Fischer JE, Horst WD, Kopin IJ. Norepinephrine metabolism in hypertrophied rat hearts. *Nature* 1965;207:951–953.

Fisher LA. Corticotropin-releasing factor: Central nervous system effects on baroreflex control of heart rate. *Life Sci* 1988;42:2645–2649.

Fleckenstein A, Doring HJ, Leder O. The significance of high-energy phosphate exhaustion in the etiology of isoproterenol-induced cardiac necrosis and its prevention by iproveratril, compound D 600 or prenylamine. In Lamarche M, Royer R (Eds) *International Symposium on Drug and Metabolism of Myocardium and Striated Muscle.* University of Nancy, France, 1969, pp 11–22.

Flemstrom G, Safsten B, Jedstedt G. Stimulation of mucosal alkaline secretion in rat duodenum by dopamine and dopaminergic compounds. *Gastroenterology* 1993;104:825–833.

Floras JS, Aylward PE, Abboud FM, Mark AL. Inhibition of muscle sympathetic nerve activity in humans by arginine vasopressin. *Hypertension* 1987;10:409–416.

Floras JS, Aylward PE, Victor RG, Mark AL, Abboud FM. Epinephrine facilitates neurogenic vasoconstriction in humans. *J Clin Invest* 1988a;81:1265–1274.

Floras JS, Hassan MO, Jones JV, Osikowska BA, Sever PS, Sleight P. Consequences of impaired arterial baroreflexes in essential hypertension: Effects on pressor responses, plasma noradrenaline and blood pressure variability. *J Hypertens* 1988b;6:525–535.

Floras JS, Legault L, Morali GA, Hara K, Blendis LM. Increased sympathetic outflow in çirrhosis and ascites: Direct evidence from intraneural recordings. *Ann Int Med* 1991;114:373–380.

Floras JS, Sole MJ, Morris BL. Desipramine blocks augmented neurogenic vasoconstrictor responses to epinephrine. *Hypertension* 1990;15:132–139.

Floras JS. Epinephrine and the genesis of hypertension. *Hypertension* 1992;19:1–18.

Flordellis CS, Handy DE, Bresnahan MR, Zannis VI, Gavras H. Cloning and expression of a rat brain α_{2B}-adrenergic receptor. *Proc Natl Acad Sci USA* 1991;88:1019–1023.

Fluharty SJ, Rabow LE, Stricker EM, Zigmond MJ. Tyrosine hydroxylase activity in the sympathoadrenal system under basal and stressful conditions: Effect of 6-hydroxydopamine. *J Pharmacol Exp Ther* 1985a;235:354–360.

Fluharty SJ, Snyder GL, Zigmond MJ, Stricker EM. Tyrosine hydroxylase activity and catecholamine biosynthesis in the adrenal medulla of rats during stress. *J Pharmacol Exp Ther* 1985b;233:32–38.

Foley PJ, Tacker WA, Wortsman J, Frank S, Cryer PE. Plasma catecholamine and serum cortisol responses to experimental cardiac arrest in dogs. *Am J Physiol* 1987;253:E283–E289.

Folkow B, Di Bona GF, Hjemdahl P, Thoren PH, Wallin BG. Measurement of plasma norepinephrine concentrations in human primary hypertension: A word of caution on their applicability for assessing neurogenic contributions. *Hypertension* 1983;5:399–403.

Folkow B, Hallback-Norlander M, Martner J, Nordborg C. Influence of amygdala lesions on cardiovascular responses to alerting stimuli, on behaviour and on blood pressure development in spontaneously hypertensive rats. *Acta Physiol Scand* 1982;116:133–139.

Folkow B, Karlstrom G. Age- and pressure dependent changes of systemic resistance vessels concerning the relationships between geometric design, wall distensibility, vascular reactivity and smooth muscle sensitivity. *Acta Physiol Scand* 1984;122:17–33.

Folkow B, Rubinstein EH. Cardiovascular effects of acute and chronic stimulation of the hypothalamic defense area in the rat. *Acta Physiol Scand* 1966;68:48–57.

Folkow B, Uvnas B. The distribution and functional significance of sympathetic vasodilators to the hind limbs of the cat. *Acta Physiol Scand* 1948;15:389–400.

Folkow B, von Euler US. Selective activation of noradrenaline and adrenaline producing cells in the cat's adrenal gland by hypothalamic stimulation. *Circ Res* 1954;2:191–195.

Folkow B. Physiological aspects of primary hypertension. *Physiol Rev* 1982;62:347–504.

Folkow B. Physiology of behavior and blood pressure regulation in animals. In Julius S, Bassett DR (Eds). *Handbook of Hypertension*, Vol 9. *Behavioral Factors in Hypertension*. New York: Elsevier Science, 1987, pp 1–18.

Folkow B. Stress, hypothalamic function and neuroendocrine consequences. *Acta Med Scand* 1988; Suppl. 723:61–69.

Foote SL, Aston-Jones G, Bloom FE. Impulse activity of locus coeruleus neurons in awake rats and squirrel monkeys is a function of sensory stimulation and arousal. *Proc Natl Acad Sci USA* 1980;77:3033–3037.

Foote SL, Bloom FE, Aston-Jones G. Nucleus locus coeruleus: New evidence of anatomical and physiological specificity. *Physiol Rev* 1983;63:844–914.

Fornai F, Blandizzi C, del Tacca M. Central alpha-2 adrenoceptors regulate central and peripheral functions. *Pharmacol Res* 1990;22:541–554.

Forsman L, Lindblad LE. Effect of mental stress on baroreceptor-mediated changes in blood pressure and heart rate and on plasma catecholamines and subjective responses in healthy men and women. *Psychosom Med* 1983;45:435–445.

Fort P, el Mansari M, Salvert D, Jouvet M. Lower brainstem afferents to the cat posterior hypothalamus: A double-labeling study. *Brain Res Bull* 1990;24:437–455.

Fowlis RAF, Sang CT, Lundy PM, Ahuja SP, Colhoun H. Experimental coronary artery ligation in conscious dogs six months after bilateral cardiac sympathectomy. *Am Heart J* 1974; 88:748–757.

Fozard JR, Mohring J, Palfreyman MG, Koch-Weser J. Mechanisms of the antihypertensive action of DL-alpha-monofluoromethyldopa: implications for the role of the sympathetic nervous system in maintenance of elevated blood pressure in spontaneously hypertensive rats. *J Cardiovasc Pharmacol* 1981;3:1038–1049.

Fozard JR, Spedding M, Palfreyman MG, Wagner J, Mohring J, Koch-Weser J. Depression of sympathetic nervous function by DL-alpha-monofluoromethyldopa, an enzyme-activated, irreversible inhibitor of L-aromatic amino acid decarboxylase. *J Cardiovasc Pharmacol* 1980;2:229–245.

Franciosa JA, Schwartz DE. Acute hemodynamic effects of norepinephrine inhibition in patients with severe chronic congestive heart failure. *J Am Coll Cardiol* 1989;14:624–630.

Francis GS, Benedict C, Johnstone DE, Kirlin PC, Nicklas J, Liang C-S, Kubo SH, Rudin-Toretsky E, Yusuf S. Comparison of neuroendocrine activation in patients with left ventricular dysfunction with and without congestive heart failure. *Circulation* 1990;82:1724–1729.

Francis GS, Cohn JN. The autonomic nervous system in congestive heart failure. *Ann Rev Med* 1986;37:235–247.

Francis GS, Olivari MT, Goldsmith SR, Levine TB, Pierpont G, Cohn JN. The acute response of plasma norepinephrine, renin activity, and arginine vasopressin to short-term nitroprusside and nitroprusside withdrawal in patients with congestive heart failure. *Am Heart J* 1983;106:1315–1320.

Frandsen H, Berne C, Fagius J, Niklasson F, Christensen NJ, Hilsted J. Plasma volume substitution does not inhibit plasma noradrenaline and muscle nerve sympathetic responses to insulin-induced hypoglycaemia in healthy humans. *Scand J Clin Lab Invest* 1989;49:573–581.

Frankenhaeuser M, Jarpe G, Matell G. Effects of intravenous infusions of adrenaline and noradrenaline on certain psychological and physiological functions. *Acta Physiol Scand* 1961;51:175–186.

Frankenhaeuser M. Experimental approaches to the study of catecholamines and emotion. In Levi L (Ed) *Emotions—Their Parameters and Measurement*. New York: Raven Press. 1975, pp 209–234.

Frankenhaeuser M. The sympathetic-adrenal and pituitary-adrenal response to challenge: Comparison between the sexes. In Dembroski TM, Schmidt TH, Blumchen G (Eds) *Biobehavioral Bases of Coronary Heart Disease*. Basel: Karger, 1983, pp 91–105.

Fraser J, Nadeau J, Robertson D, Wood AJ. Regulation of human leukocyte beta receptors by endogenous catecholamines: relationship of leukocyte beta receptor density to the cardiac sensitivity to isoproterenol. *J Clin Invest* 1981;67:1777–1784.

Fraser R, Connell JM, Inglis G, Kenyon CJ, Tree M. The role of dopamine in the control of corticosteroid secretion and metabolism. *J Steroid Biochem* 1989;32:217–222.

Freeman ZS. Stress and hypertension—a critical review. *Med J Aust* 1990;153:621–625.

Friberg P, Meredith I, Jennings G, Lambert G, Fazio V, Esler M. Evidence for increased renal norepinephrine overflow during sodium restriction in humans. *Hypertension* 1990;16: 121–130.

Friedman M, Rosenman RH, Carroll V. Changes in the serum cholesterol and blood clotting time in man subjected to cyclic variation of occupational stress. *Circulation* 1958;17:852–861.

Friedman M. Studies concerning the etiology and pathogenesis of neurocirculatory asthenia. III. The cardiovascular manifestations of neurocirculatory asthenia. *Am Heart J* 1945;30:478–491.

Friedman R, Iwai J. Genetic predisposition and stress-induced hypertension. *Science* 1976;193: 161–162.

Friedman S, Kaufman S. 3,4-Dihydroxyphenylethylamine β-hydroxylase. Physical properties, copper content, and role of copper in the catalytic activity. *J Biol Chem* 1965;240:4763–4773.

Friedman WF, Pool PE, Jacobowitz D, Seagren SC, Braunwald E. Sympathetic innervation of the developing rat heart. Biochemical and histochemical comparisons of fetal, neonatal, and adult myocardium. *Circ Res* 1968;23:25–32.

Frielle T, Collins S, Daniel KW, Caron MG, Lefkowitz RJ, Kobilka BK. Cloning of the cDNA for the β_1-adrenergic receptor. *Proc Nat Acad Sci USA* 1987;84:7920–7924.

Frishman WH, Furberg CD, Friedewald WT. β-adrenergic blockade for survivors of acute myocardial infarction. *N Engl J Med* 1984;310:830–837.

Fritschy J-M, Grzanna R. Distribution of locus coeruleus axons within the rat brainstem demonstrated by Phaseolus vulgaris leucoagglutinin anterograde tracing in combination with dopamine-β-hydroxylase immunofluorescence. *J Comp Neurol* 1990;293:616–631.

Fritschy J-M, Lyons WE, Mullen CA, Kosofsky BE, Mooliver ME, Grzanna R. Distribution of locus coeruleus axons in the rat spinal cord: A combined anterograde transport and immunohistochemical study. *Brain Res* 1987;437:176–180.

Frohlich ED, Tarazi RC, Dustan HP. Hyperdynamic beta-adrenergic circulatory state. *Arch Int Med* 1969;123:1–7.

Frohlich ED. Beta-adrenergic blockade in circulatory regulation of hyperkinetic states. *Am J Cardiol* 1977;27:195–199.

Frye RL, Braunwald E. Studies on Starling's law of the heart. I. The circulatory response to acute hypervolemia and its modification by ganglion blockade. *J Clin Invest* 1960;39:1043–1050.

Fujino K. *Brain* catecholamines in spontaneously hypertensive and DOCA-salt hypertensive rats. *Acta Med Okayama* 1984;38:325–340.

Fujita T, Henry WL, Bartter FC, Lake CR, Delea CS. Factors influencing blood pressure in salt-sensitive patients with hypertension. *Am J Med* 1980;69:334–344.

Fujita T, Noda H, Ando K. Sodium susceptibility and potassium effects in young patients with borderline hypertension. *Circulation* 1984;69:468–476.

Fulton JF. *Frontal Lobotomy and Affective Behavior.* New York: Norton, 1951.

Fulton JF. *Selected Readings in the History of Physiology.* Baltimore, MD: CC Thomas, 1930.

Funkenstein DH. Nor-epinephrine-like and epinephrine-like substances in relation to human behavior. *J Mental Dis* 1956;124:58–68.

Furchgott RF. Role of endothelium in responses of vascular smooth muscle. *Circ Res* 1983;53: 557–573.

Gaffney TE, Braunwald E. Importance of the adrenergic nervous system in the support of circulatory function in patients with congestive heart failure. *Am J Med* 1963;34:320–324.

Gale A, Edwards JA. Individual differences. In Coles MGH, Donhin E, Porges SW (Eds) *Psy-*

chophysiology: Systems, Processes, and Applications. New York: Guilford Press, 1986, pp 431–507.

Galloway MP, Westfall TC. The release of endogenous norepinephrine from the coccygeal artery of spontaneously hypertensive and Wistar-Kyoto rats. *Circ Res* 1982;51:225–232.

Galosy RA, Clarke LE, Vasko MR, Crawford IL. Neurophysiology and neuropharmacology of cardiovascular regulation and stress. *Neurosci Biobehav Rev* 1981;5:137–175.

Gammage MD, Wilkins MR, Lewis HM, Murray RG, Littler WA. Effects of lower body positive pressure on plasma atrial natriuretic peptide and sodium excretion in cardiac transplant patients. *Circulation* 1987;76:IV–136 (Abstract).

Ganau A, Devereux RB, Atlas SA, Pecker M, Roman MJ, Vargiu P, Cody RJ, Laragh JH. Plasma atrial natriuretic factor in essential hypertension: relation to cardiac size, function and systemic hemodynamics. *J Am Coll Cardiol* 1989;14:715–724.

Ganguly PK, Anderson WA. Involvement of the sympathetic nervous system in the development of cardiac hypertrophy: A fresh look at an old problem. *J Auton Pharmacol* 1989;9:367–378.

Ganten D, Hermann K, Bayer C, Unger T, Lang RE. Angiotensin synthesis in the brain and increased turnover in hypertensive rats. *Science* 1983;221:869–871.

Garber AJ, Cryer PE, Santiago JV, Haymond MW. Pagliara AS, Kipnis DM. The role of adrenergic mechanisms in the substrate and hormonal response to insulin-induced hypoglycemia in man. *J Clin Invest* 1976;58:7–15.

Garty M, Deka-Starosta A, Chang P, Kopin IJ, Goldstein DS. Effects of clonidine on renal sympathetic nerve activity and norepinephrine spillover. *J Pharmacol Exp Ther* 1990; 254:1068–1074.

Garty M, Deka-Starosta A, Chang PC, Eisenhofer G, Zukowska-Grojec Z, Stull R, Kopin IJ, Goldstein DS. Plasma levels of catechols during reflexive changes in sympathetic nerve activity. *Neurochem Res* 1989;14:523–531.

Garty M, Deka-Starosta A, Stull R, Kopin IJ, Goldstein DS. Plasma levels of catechols after fasting in intact or adrenal-demedullated rats. *J Auton Nerv Sys* 1989;26:181–184.

Garty M, Stull R, Kopin IJ, Goldstein DS. Skin color, aging, and plasma dopa levels. *J Auton Nerv Sys* 1989;26:261–263.

Garvey JL, Melville KI. Cardiovascular effects of lateral hypothalamic stimulation in normal and coronary-ligated dogs. *J Cardiovasc Surg* 1969;10:377–385.

Gaskell WH. On the innervation of the heart. *J Physiol (Lond)* 1883-1884;4:43–127.

Gaumann DM, Yaksh TL, Tyce GM, Lucas DL. Opioids preserve the adrenal medullary response evoked by severe hemorrhage: Studies on adrenal catecholamine and met-enkephalin secretion in halothane anesthetized cats. *Anesthesiology* 1988;68:743–753.

Gauthier P, Nadeau R, De Champlain J. Acute and chronic cardiovascular effects of 6-hydroxydopamine in dogs. *Circ Res* 1972;31:207–217.

Gebber GL, Barman SM. Rhythmogenesis in the sympathetic nervous system. *Fed Proc* 1980; 39:2526–2530.

Gebber GL, Snyder DW. Hypothalamic control of baroreceptor reflexes. *Am J Physiol* 1969;218: 124–131.

Gebber GL. Brainstem systems involved in cardiovascular regulation. In Randall WC (Ed) *Nervous Conrol of Cardiovascular Function.* New York: Oxford University Press, 1984, pp 346–368.

Genovese A, Chiariello M, Bozzaotre M, Latte S, De Alfieri W, Condorelli M. Adrenergic activity as a modulating factor in the genesis of myocardial hypertrophy in the rat. *Exp Molec Pathol* 1984;41:390–396.

Genovesi S, Pieruzzi F, Wijnmaalen P, Centonza L, Golin R, Zanchetti A, Stella A. Renal afferents signaling diuretic activity in the cat. *Circ Res* 1993;73:906–913.

George DT, Kaye WH, Goldstein DS, Brewerton TD, Jimerson DC. Altered norepinephrine regulation in bulimia: Effects of pharmacological challenge with isoproterenol. *Psychiatry Res* 1990;33:1–10.

Gero J, Gerova M. Significance of the individual parameters of pulsating pressure in stimulation of baroreceptors. In Kezdi P (Ed) *Baroreceptors and Hypertension.* Oxford, UK: Pergamon, 1967, pp 17–30.

Gerrard JN, Peterson DA. The contribution of platelets to stress-related cardiovascular disease. In Beamish RE, Singal PK, Dhalla NS (Eds) *Stress and Heart Disease.* Boston: Martinus Nijhoof, 1985, pp 331–346.

Giannattasio C, Del Bo A, Cattaneo BM, Cuspidi C, Gronda E, Frigerio M, Mangiavacchi M, Marabini M, De Vita C, Grassi G, Zanchetti A, Mancia G. Reflex vasopressin and renin modulation by cardiac receptors in humans. *Hypertension* 1993;21:461–469.

Gidding SS, Rocchini AP, Beekman R, Szpunar CA, Moorehead C, Behrendt D, Rosenthal A. Therapeutic effect of propranolol on paradoxical hypertension after repair of coarctation of the aorta. *N Engl J Med* 1985;312:1224–1228.

Gilbey MP, Coote JH, Fleetwood-Walker S, Petersen DF. The influence of the paraventricular-spinal pathway, and oxytocin and vasopressin on sympathetic preganglionic neurones. *Brain Res* 1982;251:283–290.

Gill G. Study of mortality and autopsy findings amongst former prisoners of the Japanese. *J Roy Army Med Corps* 1983;129:11–13.

Gill JR Jr, Grossman E, Goldstein DS. High urinary dopa excretion and low urinary dopamine: dopa ratio in salt-sensitive hypertension. *Hypertension* 1991;18:614–621.

Gill JR Jr, Gullner G, Lake CR, Lakatua DJ, Lan G. Plasma and urinary catecholamines in salt-sensitive idiopathic hypertension. *Hypertension* 1988;11:312–319.

Gillis RA. Role of the nervous system in the arrhythmias produced by coronary occlusion in the cat. *Am Heart J* 1971;81:677–684.

Gimpl MP, Brickman AL, Kaufman MP, Schneiderman N. Temporal relationships of barosensory attenuation in conscious rabbits. *Am J Physiol* 1976;230:1480–1486.

Giros B, el Mestikaway S, Bertrand L, Caron MG. Cloning and functional characterization of a cocaine-sensitive dopamine transporter. *FEBS Lett* 1991;295:149–154.

Giubbini R, Galli M, Campini R, Bosimino A, Bencivelli W, Tavazzi L. Effects of mental stress on myocardial perfusion in patients with ischemic heart disease. *Circulation* 1991;83 (Suppl. II):II100–II107.

Glaser B, Vinik AI, Valtysson G, Zoghlin G. Truncal vagotomy abolishes the somatostatin response to insulin-induced hypoglycemia in man. *J Clin Endocrinol Metab* 1981;52: 823–825.

Glass DC, Krakoff LR, Contrada R, Hilton WF, Kehoe K Mannucci EG, Collins C, Snow B, Elting E. Effect of harassment and competition upon cardiovascular and plasma catecholamine responses in type A and type B individuals. *Psychophysiology* 1980;17:453–463.

Glatzer NN. *Jerusalem and Rome. The Writings of Josephus.* New York: Meridian Books, 1960.

Glaubinger G, Lefkowitz RJ. Elevated β-adrenergic receptor number after chronic propranolol treatment. *Biochem Biophys Res Commun* 1977;78:720–725.

Glavin GB. Dopamine and gastroprotection. The brain-gut axis. *Dig Dis Sci* 1991;36:1670–1672.

Glavin GB. Dopamine: A stress modulator in the brain and gut. *Gen Pharmac* 1992;23:1023–1026.

Glowiniak JV, Turner FE, Gray LL, Palac RT, Lagunas-Solar MC, Woodward WR. Iodine-123 metaiodobenzylguanidine imaging of the heart in idiopathic congestive cardiomyopathy and cardiac transplants. *J Nucl Med* 1989;30:1182–1191.

Glowinski J, Kopin IJ, Axelrod J. *Metabolism* of ³H-norepinephrine in the rat brain. *J Neurochem* 1965;12:25–30.

Godfraind T. Calcium exchange in vascular smooth muscle, action of noradrenaline and lanthanum. *J Physiol (Lond)* 1976;260:21–35.

Goetz KL, Wang BC, Geer PG, Leadley RJ Jr, Reinhardt HW. Atrial stretch increases sodium excretion independently of release of atrial peptides. *Am J Physiol* 1986;250:R946–R950.

Gold MS, Redmond DR Jr, Kleber HD. Clonidine blocks acute opiate-withdrawal symptoms. *Lancet* 1978;ii:599–602.

Gold PW, Goodwin FK, Chrousos GP. Clinical and biochemical manifestations of depression. Relation to the neurobiology of stress. *N Engl J Med* 1988;319:348–353, 413–420.

Goldberg LI, Rajfer EI. Dopamine receptors: Applications in clinical cardiology. *Circulation* 1985;72:245–248.

Goldberg LI. Dopamine receptors and hypertension. Physiologic and pharmacologic implications. *Am J Med* 1984;77, 37–44.

Goldberg MR, Hollister AS, Robertson D. Influence of yohimbine on blood pressure, autonomic reflexes, and plasma catecholamines in humans. *Hypertension* 1983;5:772–778.

Goldberg MR, Jackson RV, Krakau J, Island DP, Robertson D. Influence of yohimbine on release of anterior pituitary hormones. *Life Sci* 1986;39:395–398.

Goldfien A. Effects of glucose deprivation on the sympathetic outflow to the adrenal medulla and adipose tissue. *Pharmacol Rev* 1966;18:303–311.

Goldsmith SR, Hasking GJ. Effect of a pressor infusion of angiotensin II on sympathetic activity and heart rate in normal humans. *Circ Res* 1991;68:263–268.

Goldsmith SR, Iber C, McArthur CD, Davies SF. Influence of acid-based status on plasma catecholamines during exercise in normal humans. *Am J Physiol* 1990;258:R1411–R1416.

Goldstein DS. Arterial baroreflex sensitivity, plasma catecholamines, and pressor responsiveness in essential hypertension. *Circulation* 1983a;68:234–240.

Goldstein DS. Catecholamines in plasma and cerebrospinal fluid: Sources and meanings. In Buckley JP, Ferrario CM (Eds) *Brain Peptides and Catecholamines in Cardiovascular Regulation in Normal and Disease States.* New York: Raven Press, 1987a, pp 15–25.

Goldstein DS. Plasma catecholamines in essential hypertension: An analytical review. *Hypertension* 1983b;5:86–99.

Goldstein DS. Plasma norepinephrine as an indicator of sympathetic neural activity in clinical cardiology. *Am J Cardiol* 1981b;48:1147–1154.

Goldstein DS. Plasma norepinephrine in essential hypertension: A study of the studies. *Hypertension* 1981a;3:48–52.

Goldstein DS. Plasma norepinephrine in essential hypertension: The elusive measurement. *Trends Autonom Pharmacol* 1985;3:331–349.

Goldstein DS. Stress-induced activation of the sympathetic nervous system. In Grossman A (Ed) *Neuroendocrinology of Stress.* East Sussex, UK: Bailliere Tindall, 1987b, pp 253–278.

Goldstein DS. The electrocardiogram in stroke: Relationship to pathophysiologic type and comparison with prior tracings. *Stroke* 1979;3:253–259.

Goldstein DS, Bonner RF, Zimlichman R, Zahn TP, Cannon RO III, Rosing DR, Stull R, Keiser HR. Indices of sympathetic vascular innervation in sympathectomized patients. *J Autonom Nerv Sys* 1986;15:309–318.

Goldstein DS, Breier A, Wolkowitz OM, Pickar D, Lenders JWM. Plasma levels of catechols and ACTH during acute glucopenia in humans. *Clin Autonom Res* 1992; 2:359–366.

Goldstein DS, Brush JE Jr, Eisenhofer G, Stull R, Esler M. In vivo measurement of neuronal uptake of norepinephrine in the human heart. *Circulation* 1988;78:41–48.

Goldstein DS, Cannon RO III, Quyyumi A, Chang P, Duncan M, Brush JE Jr, Eisenhofer G. Regional extraction of circulating norepinephrine, dopa, and dihydroxyphenylglycol in humans. *J Auton Nerv Sys* 1991;34:17–36.

Goldstein DS, Chang PC, Eisenhofer G, Miletich R, Finn R, Bacher J, Kirk KL, Bacharach S, Kopin IJ. Positron emission tomographic imaging of cardiac sympathetic innervation and function. *Circulation* 1990;81:1606–1621.

Goldstein DS, Dionne R, Sweet J, Gracely R, Brewer HB Jr, Gregg R, Keiser HR. Circulatory, plasma catecholamine, cortisol, lipid, and psychological responses to a real-life stress (wisdom tooth extractions): Effects of diazepam sedation and of inclusion of epinephrine with the local anesthetic. *Psychosom Med* 1982;44:259–271.

Goldstein DS, Eisenhofer G, Dunn BB, Armando I, Lenders J, Grossman E, Holmes C, Kirk KL, Bacharach S, Adams R, Herscovitch P, Kopin IJ. Positron emission tomographic imaging of cardiac sympathetic innervation using 6-[^{18}F]fluorodopamine: Initial findings in humans. *J Am Coll Cardiol* 1993;22:1961–1971.

Goldstein DS, Eisenhofer G, Garty M, Sax FL, Keiser HR, Kopin IJ. Pharmacologic and tracer methods to study sympathetic function in primary hypertension. *Clin Exp Hypertens* 1989; A11 (Suppl. 1):173–189.

Goldstein DS, Eisenhofer G, Sax FL, Keiser HR, Kopin IJ. Plasma norepinephrine pharmaco-kinetics during mental challenge. *Psychosom Med* 1987;48:591–605.

Goldstein DS, Eisenhofer G, Stull R, Folio CJ, Keiser HR, Kopin IJ. Plasma dihydroxyphenyl-glycol and the intraneuronal disposition of norepinephrine in humans. *J Clin Invest* 1988; 81:213–220.

Goldstein DS, Feuerstein GZ, Izzo JL Jr, Kopin IJ, Keiser HR. Validity and reliability of liquid chromatography with electrochemical detection for measuring plasma levels of norepi-nephrine and epinephrine in man. *Life Sci* 1981;28:467–475.

Goldstein DS, Garty M, Bagdy G, Szemeredi K, Sternberg EM, Listwak S, Deka-Starosta A, Hoffman A, Chang PC, Stull R, Gold PW, Kopin IJ. Role of CRH in glucopenia-induced adrenomedullary activation in rats. *J Neuroendocrinol* 1993;5:475–486.

Goldstein DS, Grossman E, Armando I, Wolfovitz E, Folio CJ, Holmes C, Keiser HR. Correlates of urinary excretion of catechols in humans. *Biogenic Amines* 1993;10:3–17.

Goldstein DS, Grossman E, Listwak S, Folio CJ. Sympathetic reactivity during a yohimbine challenge test in essential hypertension. *Hypertension* 1991;18 (Suppl. III):III40–III48.

Goldstein DS, Grossman E, Tamrat M, Chang PC, Eisenhofer G, Bacher J, Kirk KL, Bacharach S, Kopin IJ. Positron emission imaging of cardiac sympathetic innervation and function using [^{18}F]-fluorodopamine: Effects of chemical sympathectomy by 6-hydroxydopamine. *J Hypertens* 1991;9:417–423.

Goldstein DS, Harris AH, Brady JV. Baroreflex sensitivity during operant blood pressure con-ditioning. *Biofeedback Self-Regul* 1977;2:127–138.

Goldstein DS, Horwitz D, Keiser HR, Polinsky RJ, Kopin IJ. Plasma ^{3}H-l-norepinephrine, ^{14}C-d-norepinephrine, and ^{3}H-d,l-isoproterenol kinetics in essential hypertension. *J Clin Invest* 1983;72:1748–1758.

Goldstein DS, Horwitz D, Keiser HR. Comparison of techniques for measuring baroreflex sen-sitivity in man. *Circulation* 1982;66:432–439.

Goldstein DS, Keiser HR. Neural circulatory control in the hyperdynamic circulation syndrome. *Am Heart J* 1985;109:387–390.

Goldstein DS, Keiser HR. Pressor and depressor responses after cholinergic blockade in man. *Am Heart J* 1984;107:974–979.

Goldstein DS, Kopin IJ. The autonomic nervous system and catecholamines in normal blood pressure control and in hypertension. In Laragh JH, Brenner BM (Eds) *Hypertension: Pathophysiology, Diagnosis and Management*. New York: Raven Press, 1990, pp 711–747.

Goldstein DS, Lake CR, Chernow B, Ziegler MG, Coleman MD, Taylor AA, Mitchell JR, Kopin IJ, Keiser HR. Age-dependence of hypertensive-normotensive differences in plasma norepinephrine. *Hypertension* 1983;5:100–104.

Goldstein DS, Lake CR. Plasma norepinephrine and epinephrine levels in essential hypertension. *Fed Proc* 1984;43:57–61.

Goldstein DS, Levinson PD, Zimlichman R, Pitterman A, Stull R. Keiser HR. Clonidine suppression testing in essential hypertension. *Ann Int Med* 1985;102:42–48.

Goldstein DS, McCarty R, Polinsky RJ, Kopin IJ. Relationship between plasma norepinephrine and sympathetic neural activity. *Hypertension* 1983;5:552–559.

Goldstein DS, Nadi NS, Stull R, Wyler AR, Porter RJ. Catecholamines and DOPA in epileptogenic and non-epileptogenic regions of the human brain. *J Neurochem* 1988;50:225–229.

Goldstein DS, Nurnberger J Jr, Gershon ES, Simmons S, Polinsky R, Keiser HR. Effects of injected sympathomimetic amines on plasma catecholamines and circulatory variables in man. *Life Sci* 1983;32:1057–1063.

Goldstein DS, Polinsky RJ, Garty M, Robertson D, Biaggioni I, Brown RT, Stull R, Kopin IJ. Patterns of plasma levels of catechols in neurogenic orthostatic hypotension. *Ann Neurol* 1989;26:558–563.

Goldstein DS, Spanarkel M, Pitterman A, Toltzis R, Gratz E, Epstein S, Keiser HR. Circulatory control mechanisms in vasodepressor syncope. *Am Heart J* 1982;104:1071–1075.

Goldstein DS, Stull R, Eisenhofer G, Gill JR Jr. Urinary excretion of DOPA and dopamine during alterations in dietary salt intake in humans. *Clin Sci* 1989;76:517–522.

Goldstein DS, Stull R, Eisenhofer G, Sisson, JC, Weder A, Averbuch SD, Keiser HR. Plasma levels of dihydroxyphenylalanine and catecholamines in patients with neuroblastoma or pheochromocytoma. *Ann Int Med* 1986;105:887–888.

Goldstein DS, Stull R, Markey SP, Marks ES, Keiser HR. Dihydrocaffeic acid: a common contaminant in the liquid chromatographic-electrochemical measurement of plasma catecholamines in man. *J Chromatog* 1984;311:148–153.

Goldstein DS, Stull RW, Zimlichman R, Levison PD, Smith H, Keiser HR. Simultaneous measurement of DOPA, DOPAC, and catecholamines in plasma by liquid chromatography with electrochemical detection. *Clin Chem* 1984;30:815–816.

Goldstein DS, Udelsman R, Eisenhofer G, Keiser HR, Kopin IJ. Neuronal source of plasma dihydroxyphenylalanine. *J Clin Endocrinol Metab* 1987;64:856–861.

Goldstein DS, Zimlichman R, Kelly G, Stull R, Bacher JD, Keiser HR. Effect of ganglion blockade on cerebrospinal fluid norepinephrine. *J Neurochem* 1987;49:1484–1490.

Goldstein DS, Zimlichman R, Stull R, Folio J, Levinson PD, Keiser HR, Kopin IJ. Measurement of regional neuronal removal of norepinephrine in man. *J Clin Invest* 1985;76:15–21.

Goldstein DS, Zimlichman R, Stull R, Keiser HR, Kopin IJ. Estimation of intrasynaptic norepinephrine concentrations in man. *Hypertension* 1986b;8:471–475.

Goldstein DS, Zimlichman R, Stull R, Keiser HR. Plasma catecholamine and hemodynamic responses during isoproterenol infusions in man. *Clin Pharmacol Ther* 1986a;40:233–238.

Goltz F. Der Hund ohne Grosshirn. *Pflugers Arch* 1892;51:570–614.

Gonon F, Bao JX, Msghina M, Suaud-Chagny MF, Stjarne L. Fast and local electrochemical monitoring of noradrenaline release from sympathetic terminals in isolated rat tail artery. *J Neurochem* 1993;60:1251–1257.

Goodwin JF. The frontiers of cardiomyopathy. *Br Heart J* 1980;48:1–18.

Govier WC. Prolongation of myocardial functional refractory period by phenylephrine. *Life Sci* 1967;6:1367–1371.

Graafsma SJ, Hectors MP, van Tits LJ, Rodrigues de Miranda JF, Thien T. The relationship between adrenaline and beta 2-adrenoceptors on human lymphocytes. *Br J Clin Pharmacol* 1990;30 (Suppl. 1):145S–147S.

Graafsma SJ, van Tits LJ, van Heijst P, Reyenga J, Lenders JW, Thien T. Adrenoceptors on blood cells in patients with essential hypertension before and after mental stress. *J Hypertens* 1989;7:519–524.

Graefe K-H, Bonisch H. The transport of amines across the axonal membranes of noradrenergic and dopaminergic neurones. In Trendelenburg U, Weiner N (Eds) *Catecholamines I*. New York: Springer-Verlag, 1988, pp 193–245.

Graefe K-H, Henseling M. Neuronal and extraneuronal uptake and metabolism of catecholamines. *Gen Pharmac* 1983;14:27–33.

Graefe K-H, Stefano FJE, Langer SZ. Stereoselectivity in the metabolism of 3H-noradrenaline during uptake into and efflux from the isolated rat vas deferens. *Naunyn-Schmiedeberg's Arch Pharmacol* 1977;299:225–238.

Graefe K-H. The disposition of ^{3}H-(-)-noradrenaline in the perfused cat and rabbit heart. *Naunyn-Schmiedeberg's Arch Pharmacol* 1981;318:71–82.

Graessler J, Kvetnansky R, Jezova D, Dobrakovova M, van Loon GR. Prior immobilization stress alters adrenal hormone responses to hemorrhage in rats. *Am J Physiol* 1989;257:R661–R667.

Graham JDP. High blood pressure after battle. *Lancet* 1945;1:239–240.

Graham TE, Sathasivam P, MacNaughton KW. Influence of cold, exercise, and caffeine on catecholamines and metabolism in men. *J Appl Physiol* 1991;70:2052–2058.

Granata AR, Kumada M, Reis DJ. Sympathoinhibition by A1-noradrenergic neurons is mediated by neurons in the C1 area of the rostral medulla. *J Auton Nerv Sys* 1985;14:387–395.

Granata AR, Numao Y, Kumada M, Reis DJ. A1 noradrenergic neurons tonically inhibit sympathoexcitatory neurons of C1 area in rat brain stem. *Brain Res* 1986;377:127–146.

Granata AR, Ruggiero DA, Park DH, Joh TH, Reis DJ. *Brain* stem area with C1 epinephrine neurons mediates baroreflex vasopressor responses. *Am J Physiol* 1985;248:H547–H567.

Grant JA, Scrutton MC. Positive interaction between agonists in the aggregation response of human blood platelets: Interaction between ADP, adrenaline and vasopressin. *Br J Haem* 1980;44:109–125.

Grant SJ, Redmond DE. Neuronal activity of the locus coeruleus in awake *Macaca arctoides*. *Exp Neurol* 1984;84:701–708.

Grassler J, Jezova D, Kvetnansky R, Scheuch DW. Hormonal responses to hemorrhage and their relationship to individual hemorrhagic shock susceptibility. *Endocrinol Exp* 1990;24:105–116.

Gray JA. *The Neuropsychology of Anxiety*. Oxford, UK: Clarendon Press, 1982.

Gray TS. Amygdala: Role in autonomic and neuroendocrine responses to stress. In McCubbin

JW, Kaufman PG, Nemeroff CB (Eds) *Stress, Neuropeptides, and Systemic Disease.* New York: Academic Press, 1991b, pp 37–53.

Gray TS. Limbic pathways and neurotransmitters as mediators of autonomic and neuroendocrine responses to stress. In Brown MR, Koob GF, Rivier C (Eds) *Stress. Neurobiology and Neuroendocrinology.* New York: Marcel Dekker, 1991a, pp 73–89.

Green AR. The effects of antidepressant drugs on noradrenergic receptor mechanisms in the central nervous system. In Heal DJ, Marsden CA (Eds) *The Pharmacology of Noradrenaline in the Central Nervous System.* New York: Oxford University Press, 1990, pp 316–348.

Green JR, Duisberg REH, McGrath WB. Focal epilepsy of psychomotor type. A preliminary report of observation on effects of surgical therapy. *J Neurosurg* 1951;8:151–172.

Greenberg S, Wilborn W. Effect of chronic administration of clonidine and propranolol on the myocardium of spontaneously hypertensive rats. *Arch Int Pharmacodyn Ther* 1982c;255: 141–161.

Greenberg S, Wilborn W. Effect of clonidine and propranolol on venous smooth muscle from spontaneously hypertensive rats. *Arch Int Pharmacodyn Ther* 1982b;258:234–259.

Greenberg S, Wilborn W. Functional and structural changes in veins in spontaneous hypertension. *Arch Int Pharmacodyn Ther* 1982a;258:203–233.

Greenberg S. Effect of chronic administration of clonidine, propranolol and alpha-methyldopa on extensibility and biochemical properties of the veins in renal and spontaneous hypertension. *J Pharmacol Exp Ther* 1981;218:779–790.

Greene WA, Goldstein S, Moss AJ. Psychosocial aspects of sudden death. *Arch Int Med* 1972; 129:725–731.

Greenhoot JH, Reichenbach DD. Cardiac injury and subarachnoid hemorrhage. *J Neurosurg* 1969;30:521–531.

Greenough A, Lagercrantz H, Pool J, Dahlin I. Plasma catecholamine levels in preterm infants. Effect of birth asphyxia and Apgar score. *Acta Paediatr Scand* 1987;76:54–59.

Greenwald JE, Apkon M, Hruska KA, Needleman P. Stretch-induced atriopeptin secretion in the isolated rat myocyte and its negative mdoulation by calcium. *J Clin Invest* 1989;83:1061–1065.

Grignani G, Soffiantino F, Zucchella M, Pacchiarini L, Tacconi F, Bonomi E, Pastoris A, Sbaffi A, Fratino P, Tavazzi L. Platelet activation by emotional stress in patients with coronary artery disease. *Circulation* 1991;83 (Suppl. II):II128–II136.

Grobecker H, Roizen MF, Weise V, Saavedra JM, Kopin IJ. Sympathoadrenal medullary activity in young, spontaneously hypertensive rats. *Nature* 1975;258–267.

Grobecker H, Saavedra J, Weise V. Biosynthetic enzyme activities and catecholamines in adrenal glands of genetic and experimental hypertensive rats. *Clin Sci* 1982;63:113s–116s.

Gross PM, Wainman DS, Shaver SW, Wall KM, Ferguson AV. Metabolic activation of efferent pathways from the rat area postrema. *Am J Physiol* 1990;258:R788–797.

Gross-Isseroff R, Dillon KA, Fieldust SJ, Biegon A. Autoradiographic analysis of α_1-noradrenergic receptors in the human brain postmortem. Effect of suicide. *Arch Gen Psychiatry* 1990;47:1049–1053.

Grossman E, Chang PC, Hoffman A, Tamrat M, Goldstein DS. Evidence for functional α_2-adrenoceptors on vascular sympathetic nerve endings in the human forearm. *Circ Res* 1991a;69:887–897.

Grossman E, Chang PC, Hoffman A, Tamrat M, Kopin IJ, Goldstein DS. Forearm kinetics of plasma norepinephrine: Dependence on regional blood flow and the site of infusion of the tracer. *Am J Physiol* 1991b;260:R946–R952.

Grossman E, Goldstein DS, Hoffman A, Keiser HR. Glucagon and clonidine testing in the diagnosis of pheochromocytoma. *Hypertension* 1991;17:733–741.

Grossman E, Goldstein DS, Hoffman A, Wacks IR, Epstein M. Neurohormonal effects of water immersion in humans. *Am J Physiol* 1992;262:R993–R999.

Grossman E, Hoffman A, Armando I, Kopin IJ. Goldstein DS. Sympathoadrenal contribution to plasma dopa. *Clin Sci* 1992;83:65–74.

Grossman E, Hoffman A, Chang PC, Keiser HR, Goldstein DS. Increased spillover of dopa into arterial blood during dietary salt loading. *Clin Sci* 1990;78:423–429.

Grossman E, Oren S, Garavaglia GE, Schmieder R, Messerli FH. Disparate hemodynamic and sympathoadrenergic responses to isometric and mental stress in essential hypertension. *Am J Cardiol* 1989;64:42–44.

Grossman E, Rea RF, Hoffman A, Goldstein DS. Yohimbine increases sympathetic nerve activity and norepinephrine spillover in normal volunteers. *Am J Physiol* 1991;260:R142–R147.

Grossman E, Rosenthal T, Peleg E, Holmes C, Goldstein DS. Oral yohimbine increases blood pressure and sympathetic outflow in hypertensives. *J Cardiovasc Pharmacol* 1993;22: 22–26.

Grossman SH, David D, Gunnells JC, Shand DG. Plasma norepinephrine in the evaluation of baroreceptor function in humans. *Hypertension* 1982;4:566–571.

Grundy SM, Griffin AC. Effects of periodic mental stress on serum cholesterol levels. *Circulation* 1959;19:496–498.

Gulati A. Down-regulation of α_2-adrenoceptors in ventrolateral medulla of spontaneously hypertensive rats. *Life Sci* 1991;48:1199–1206.

Gullichsen E, Nelimarkka O, Scheinin M, Antila K, Leppaluoto J, Niinikoski J. Plasma levels of atrial natriuretic factor and catecholamines in endotoxin shock in dogs. *Acta Chir Scand* 1989;155:567–571.

Guo GB, Schmid PG, Abboud FM. Sites at which vasopressin facilitates the arterial baroreflexes in rabbits. *Am J Physiol* 1986;251:H644–H655.

Guo GB, Sharabi FM, Abboud FM, Schmid PG. Vasopressin augments baroreflex inhibition of lumbar sympathetic nerve activity in rabbits. *Circulation* 1982;66 (Suppl. 2):34.

Guo GB, Thames MD, Abboud FM. Arterial baroreflexes in renal hypertensive rabbits: Selectivity and redundancy of baroreceptor influence on heart rate, vascular resistance, and lumbar sympathetic activity. *Circ Res* 1983;53:223–234.

Guo GB, Thames MD, Abboud FM. Differential baroreflex control of heart rate and vascular resistance in rabbits. Relative role of carotid, aortic, and cardiopulmonary baroreceptors. *Circ Res* 1982;50:554–565.

Gupta BN, Abboud AL, Floras JS, Aylward PE, Abboud FM. Vasopressin facilitates inhibition of renal nerve activity mediated through vagal afferents. *Am J Physiol* 1987;253:H1–H7.

Gurguis GNM, Uhde TW. Plasma 3-methoxy-4-hydroxyphenylethylene glycol (MHPG) and growth hormone responses to yohimbine in panic disorder patients and normal controls. *Psychoneuroendocrinology* 1990;15:217–224.

Gurtu S, Sinha JN, and Bhargava KP. Involvement of alpha-2-adrenoceptors of nucleus tractus solitarius in baroreflex mediated bradycardia. *Naunyn-Schmiedeberg's Arch Pharmacol* 1982;321:38–43.

Guyenet PG, Cabot JB. Inhibition of sympathetic preganglionic neurons by catecholamines and clonidine: mediation by an adrenergic receptor. *J Neurosci* 1981;1:908–917.

Guyenet PG, Filtz TM, Donaldson SR. Role of excitatory amino acids in rat vagal and sympathetic baroreflexes. *Brain Res* 1987;407:272–284.

Guyenet PG, Stronetta RL. Inhibition of sympathetic preganglionic discharges by epinephrine and α-methylepinephrine. *Brain Res* 1982;235:271–283.

Guyenet PG, Young BS. Projections of nucleus paragigantocellularis to locus coeruleus and other structures in rat. *Brain Res* 1987;406:171–184.

Guyenet PG. The coeruleospinal noradrenergic neurons: anatomical and electrophysiological studies in the rat. *Brain Res* 1980;189:121–133.

Guyton AC. Abnormal renal function and autoregulation in essential hypertension. *Hypertension* 1991;18 (Suppl. III):III40–III48.

Guz A, Noble MIM, Widdicombe JG, Trenchard D, Mushin WW, Makey AR. The role of vagal and glossopharyngeal afferent nerves in respiratory sensation, control of breathing and arterial pressure regulation in conscious man. *Clin Sci* 1966;30:161–170.

Guzzetti S, Piccaluga E, Casati R, Masu AM, Longoni P, Tinelli M, Cerutti S, Pagani M, Malliani A. Sympathetic predominance in essential hypertension: a study employing spectral analysis of heart rate variability. *J Hypertens* 1988;6:711–717.

Gwinup G, Steinberg T, King CG, Vernikos-Danellis J. Vasopressin-induced ACTH secretion in man. *J Clin Endocrinol Metab* 1967;27:927–930.

Haass M, Cheng B, Richardt G, Lang RE, Schomig A. Characterization and presynaptic modulation of stimulation-evoked exocytotic co-release of noradrenaline and neuropeptide Y in guinea pig heart. *Naunyn-Schmiedeberg's Arch Pharmacol* 1989a;339:71–78.

Haass M, Rock M, Richardt G, Schomig A. Neuropeptide Y differentiates between exocytotic and nonexocytotic release in guinea-pig heart. *Naunyn-Schmiedeberg's Arch Pharmacol* 1989b;340:509–515.

Haeusler G. Activation of central pathway of the baroreceptor reflex, a possible mechanism of the hypotensive action of clonidine. *Naunyn-Schmiedeberg's Arch Pharmacol* 1973;278:231–246.

Haeusler G. Clonidine-induced inhibition of sympathetic nerve activity: no indication of a central presynaptic or an indirect sympathomimetic mode of action. *Naunyn-Schmiedeberg's Arch Pharmacol* 1974;286:97–111.

Haft JI, Arkel YS. Effect of emotional stress on platelet aggregation in humans. *Chest* 1976;70:501–505.

Hagbarth KE, Vallbo AB. Pulse and respiratory grouping of sympathetic impulses in human muscle nerves. *Acta Physiol Scand* 1968;74:96–108.

Hagege J, Wahbe F, Wiemeyer A, Richet G. Dopamine in rat kidney slices—its production and its histofluorescent localization. *Contrib Nephrol* 1985;49:140–144.

Haggendal J, Harley LH, Saltin B. Arterial noradrenaline concentration during exercise in relation to the relative work levels. *Scand J Clin Lab Invest* 1970;26:337–342.

Hainsworth R. Reflexes from the heart. *Physiol Rev* 1991;71:617–658.

Halbrugge T, Friedgen B, Ludwig J, Graefe K-H. Effects of catechol-O-methyltransferase inhibition on the plasma clearance of noradrenaline and the formation of 3,4-dihydroxyphenylglycol in the rabbit. *Naunyn-Schmiedeberg's Arch Pharmacol* 1993;347:162–170.

Halbrugge T, Wolfel R, Graefe KH. Plasma 3,4-dihydroxyphenylglycol as a tool to assess the role of neuronal uptake in the anaesthetized rabbit. *Naunyn-Schmiedeberg's Arch Pharmacol* 1989;340:726–732.

Hall RE, Livingston RR, Bloor MD. Orbital cortical influences on cardiovascular dynamics and myocardial structure in conscious monkeys. *J Neurosurg* 1977;46:638–647.

Hall RE, Sybers HD, Greenhoot JH, Bloor CM. Myocardial alterations after hypothalamic stimulation in the intact conscious dog. *Am Heart J* 1974;88:770–776.

Hallback-Nordlander M. Left/right ventricular weight ratio: an estimate of cardiac adaptation to hypertension. *Clin Sci* 1980;59:415s–417s.

Halliday GM, Li YW, Joh TH, Cotton RG, Howe PR, Geffen LB, Blessing WW. Distribution of monoamine-synthesizing neurons in the human medulla oblongata. *J Comp Neurol* 1988;273:301–317.

Hammermeister KE, Reichenbach DD. QRS changes, pulmonary edema, and myocardial necrosis associated with subarachnoid hemorrhage. *Am Heart J* 1969;78:94–100.

Hano T, Jeng Y, Rho J. Norepinephrine release and reuptake by hypothalamic synaptosomes of spontaneously hypertensive rats. *Hypertension* 1989;13:25–255.

Hanson PG. *The Joy of Stress*. Toronto: Hanson Stress Management Org, 1985.

Harden TK, Cotton CU, Walden GL, Lutton JK, Perkins JP. Catecholamine-induced alteration in sedimentation behavior of membrane bound β-adrenergic receptors. *Science* 1980;210: 441–443.

Harfstrand A, Fuxe K, Cintra A, Agnati LF, Zini I, Wikstrom AC, Okret S, Yu ZY, Goldstein M, Steinbusch H, Verhofstad A, Gustafsson JA. Glucocorticoid receptor immunoreactivity in monoaminergic neurons of rat brain. *Proc Natl Acad Sci USA* 1986;83:9779–9783.

Hargreaves KM, Dionne RA, Mueller GP, Goldstein DS, Dubner R. Naloxone, fentanyl and diazepam modify plasma beta-endorphin levels during surgery. *Clin Pharmacol Ther* 1986;40:165–171.

Harland D, Gardiner SM, Bennett T. Cardiovascular and dipsogenic effects of angiotensin II administered i.c.v. in Long Evans and Brattleboro rats. *Brain Res* 1988;455:58–64.

Harrap SB, Louis WJ, Doyle AE. Failure of psychosocial stress to induce chronic hypertension in the rat. *J Hypertens* 1984;2:653–662.

Harris AP, Koehler RC, Gleason CA, Jones MD Jr, Traystman RJ. Cerebral and peripheral circulatory responses to intracranial hypertension in fetal sheep. *Circ Res* 1989;64:991–1000.

Harris AS, Estandia A, Tillotson RF. Ventricular ectopic rhythms and ventricular fibrillation following cardiac sympathectomy and coronary occlusion. *Am J Physiol* 1951;65:505–512.

Harris P. Cardiac oedema and physical stress. In Beamish RE, Singal PK, Dhalla NS (Eds) *Stress and Heart Disease*. Boston: Martinus Nijhoof, 1985, pp 327–330.

Harris P. Evolution and the cardiac patient. *Cardiovasc Res* 1983;17:313–319, 373–378, 437–445.

Hart BB, Stamford GG, Ziegler MG, Lake CR, Chernow B. Catecholamines: Study of interspecies variation. *Crit Care Med* 1989;17:1203–1222.

Harvey JN, Casson IF, Clayden AD, Cope GF, Perkins CM, Lee MR. A paradoxical fall in urine dopamine output when patients with essential hypertension are given added dietary salt. *Clin Sci* 1984;67:83–88.

Haselton JR, Guyenet PG. Electrophysiological characteristics of putative C1 adrenergic neurons in the rat. *Neuroscience* 1989;30:199–214.

Hasking GJ, Esler MD, Jennings GL, Burton D, Korner PI. Norepinephrine spillover to plasma in patients with congestive heart failure: evidence of increased overall and cardiorenal sympathetic nervous activity. *Circulation* 1986;73:615–621.

Hasser EM, DiCarlo SE, Applegate RJ, Bishop VS. Osmotically released vasopressin augments cardiopulmonary reflex inhibition of the circulation. *Am J Physiol* 1988;254:R815–R820.

Hasser EM, Nelson DO, Haywood JR, Bishop VS. Inhibition of renal sympathetic nervous activity by area postrema stimulation in rabbits. *Am J Physiol* 1987;253:H91–H99.

Hatzinikolaou P, Gavras I, North WG, Brunner HR, Gavras H. Interaction of the sympathetic nervous sytem with vasopressin and renin in the maintenance of blood pressure in rats. *Clin Sci* 1982;63:313s–317s.

Havel PJ, Mundinger TO, Veith RC, Dunning BE, Taborsky GJ Jr. Corelease of galanin and NE from pnacreatic sympathetic nerves during severe hypoglycemia in dogs. *Am J Physiol* 1992;263:E8–E16.

Hawking SW. *A Brief History of Time.* New York: Bantam Books, 1988.

Hawkins WE, Clower BR. Myocardial damage after head trauma and simulated intracranial hemorrhage in mice: The role of the autonomic nervous system. *Cardiovasc Res* 1971;5: 524–529.

Hawley RJ, Major LF, Schulman EA, Lake CR. CSF levels of norepinphrine during alcohol withdrawal. *Arch Neurol* 1981;38:289–292.

Hayes JR, Adrill J, Kennedy TL, Shanks RG, Buchanan KD. Stimulation of gastrin release by catecholamines. *Lancet* 1972;1:819–821.

Haynes SG, Feinlieb M, Levine S, Scotch N, Kannel WB. The relationship of psychosocial factors to coronary heart disease in the Framingham Study. II. Prevalence of coronary heart disease. *Am J Epidemiol* 1978;107:384–402.

Head GA. Cardiovascular functions of central noradrenergic neurons in rabbits. *Clin Exp Pharmacol Physiol* 1991;18:51–54.

Heal DJ. The effects of drugs on behavioural models of central noradrenergic function. In Heal DJ, Marsden CA (Eds) *The Pharmacology of Noradrenaline in the Central Nervous System.* New York: Oxford University Press, 1990, pp 266–315.

Hearn MD, Murray EM, Luepker RU. Hostility, coronary heart disease, and total mortality: A 33-year follow-up study of university students. *J Behav Med* 1989;12:105–121.

Heathers GP, Yamada KA, Pogwizd SM, Corr PB. The contribution of a- and β-adrenergic mechanisms in the genesis of arrhythmias during myocardial ischemia and reperfusion. In Kulbertus HE, Franck G (Eds) *Neurocardiology.* Mount Kisco, NY: Futura, 1988, pp 143–178.

Hecker MH, Chesney MA, Black GW, Frautschi N. Coronary-prone behaviors in the Western Collaborative Group Study. *Psychosom Med* 1988;50:153–164.

Hedberg A, Minneman KP, Molinoff PB. Differential distribution of Beta-1 and Beta-2 adrenergic receptors in cat and guinea pig heart. *J Pharmacol Exp Ther* 1980;212:503–508.

Hedqvist P. Modulating effect of prostaglandin E-2 on noradrenaline release from the isolated cat spleen. *Acta Physiol Scand* 1969;75:511–512.

Hegde SS, Lokhandwala MF. Stimulation of renal dopamine production during acute volume expansion requires the presence of intact vagi but not renal nerves. *Clin Exp Hyper* 1992; A14:1169–1187.

Heilman KM, Schwartz HD, Watson RT. Hypoarousal in patients with the neglect syndrome and emotional indifference. *Neurology* 1978;28:229–232.

Heise A, Kroneberg G. Central nervous alpha adrenergic receptors and the mode of action of alpha methyl dopa. *Naunyn-Schmiedeberg's Arch Pharmacol* 1973;279:285–300.

Helander A, Tottmar O. Effects of ethanol, acetaldehyde and disulfiram on the metabolism of biogenic aldehydes in isolated human blood cells and platelets. *Biochem Pharmacol* 1987; 36:3981–3985.

Helin P, Lorenzen I, Garbarsch C, Matthiessen E. Arteriosclerosis in rabbit aortia induced by noradrenaline. *Atherosclerosis* 1970;12:125–132.

Helke CJ, O'Donohue TL, Jacobowitz DM. Substance P as a baro- and chemoreceptor afferent neurotransmitter: Immunocytochemical and neurochemical evidence in the rat. *Peptides* 1980;1:1–9.

Hendley ED, Cierpial MA, McCarty R. Sympathetic-adrenal medullary response to stress in hyperactive and hypertensive rats. *Physiol Behav* 1988;44:47–51.

Hennessy JW, Levine S. Stress, arousal, and the pituitary-adrenal system: A psychoendocrine hypothesis. *Prog Psychobiol Physiol Psychol* 1979;8:133–178.

Henquet JW, van Baak M, Schols M, Rahn KH. Studies on the autonomic nervous system in borderline hypertension. *Eur J Clin Pharmacol* 1982;22:285–288.

Henriksen O, Skagen K. Local and central sympathetic vasoconstrictor reflexes in human limbs during orthostatic stress. In Christensen NJ, Henriksen O, Lassen NA (Eds) *The Sympathoadrenal System. Physiology and Pathophysiology.* New York: Raven Press, 1986. pp 83–91.

Henry D, Dentino M, Gibbs P, Weinberger M. Vascular compartmentalization of plasma norepinephrine in normal man. *J Lab Clin Med* 1979;94:429–437.

Henry DP, Starman BJ, Johnson DG, Williams RH. A sensitive radioenzymatic assay for norepinephrine in tissues and plasma. *Life Sci* 1975;16:375–384.

Henry JP, Grim CE. Psychosocial mechanisms of primary hypertension. *J Hypertens* 1990;8:783–793.

Henry JP, Liu Y-Y, Nadra WE, Qian C-g, Mormede P, Lemaire V, Ely D, Hendley ED. Psychosocial stress can induce chronic hypertensiion in normotensive strains of rats. *Hypertension* 1993;21:714–723.

Henry JP, Stephens PM, Ely DL. Psychosocial hypertension and the defence and defeat reactions. *J Hypertens* 1986;4:687–697.

Henry JP. Biological basis of the stress response. *Integ Physiol Behav Sci* 1992;27:66–83.

Henseling M, Trendelenburg U. Stereselectivity of the accumulation and metabolism of noradrenaline in rabbit aortic strips. *Naunyn-Schmiedeberg's Arch Pharmacol* 1978;302:195–206.

Herbert H, Moga MM, Saper CB. Connections of the parabrachial nucleus with the nucleus of the solitary tract and the medullary reticular formation in the rat. *J Comp Neurol* 1990;293:540–580.

Herbert H, Saper CB. Cholecystokinin-, galanin-, and corticotropin-releasing factor-like immunoreactive projections from the nucleus of the solitary tract to the parabrachial nucleus in the rat. *J Comp Neurol* 1990;293:581–598.

Herd JA. Cardiovascular response to stress. *Physiol Rev* 1991;71:305–330.

Herd JA. Neuroendocrine mechanisms in coronary heart disease. In Matthews KA, Weiss SM, Detre T, Dembroski TM, Falkner B, Manuck SB, Williams RB Jr (Eds) *Handbook of Stress, Reactivity, and Cardiovascular Disease.* New York: John Wiley, 1986, pp 49–70.

Hering HE. *Die Karotissinusreflexe auf Herz und Gefasse.* Dresden: Steinkopff, 1927.

Hermiller JB, Magorien RD, Leithe NE, Unverferth DV, Leier CV. Clonidine in congestive heart failure. *Am J Cardiol* 1983;51:791–795.

Hertting G, Wurster S, Allgaier C. Regulatory proteins in presynaptic function. *Ann NY Acad Sci* 1990;604:289–304.

Hertz JH (Ed) *The Pentateuch and Haftorahs.* London: Soncino Press, 1985.

Heseltine D, Potter JF, Hartley G, Macdonald IA, James OFW. Blood pressure, heart rate and neuroendocrine responses to a high carbohydrate and a high fat meal in healthy young subjects. *Clin Sci* 1990;79:517–522.

Hess WR. *Das Zwischenhirn.* Basel: B Schwabe, 1949.

Heymans C, Neil E. *Reflexogenic Areas of the Cardiovascular System.* Boston: Little, Brown, 1958.

Hieble JP, Sulpizio AC, Nichols AJ, Willette RN, Ruffolo RR Jr. Pharmacologic characterization of SK&F 104078, a novel α_2-adrenoceptor antagonist which discriminates between pre- and postjunctional α_2-adrenoceptors. *J Pharmacol Exp Ther* 1988;247:645–652.

Higaki J, Ogihara T, Nakamaru M, Shima K, Kumahara Y. Responses of active and inactive plasma renin to insulin-induced hypoglycemia in normal subjects. *Jpn Heart J* 1984;25: 565–570.

Hillarp N-A. The release of catechol amines from the amine containing granules of the adrenal medulla. *Acta Physiol Scand* 1958;43:292–302.

Hillhouse EW, Milton NG. Effect of noradrenaline and gamma-aminobutyric acid on the secretion of corticotropin-releasing factor-41 and arginine vasopressin from the rat hypothalamus in vitro. *J Endocrinol* 1989;122:719–723.

Hilsted J, Christensen NJ, Larsen S. Norepinephrine kinetics during insulin-induced hypoglycemia. *Metabolism* 1985b;34:300–302.

Hilsted J, Christensen NJ, Larsen S. Plasma clearance of noradrenaline does not change with age in normal subjects. *Clin Physiol* 1985a;5:443–446.

Hilsted J, Christensen NJ, Madsbad S. Whole body clearance of norepinephrine. The significance of arterial sampling and of surgical stress. *J Clin Invest* 1983;71:500–505.

Hilton SM, Smith PR. Ventral medullary neurones excited from the hypothalamic and midbrain defense areas. *J Auton Nerv Sys* 1984;11:35–42.

Hilton SM, Zbrozyna AW. Amygdaloid region for defence reactions and its efferent pathway to the brain stem. *J Physiol (Lond)* 1963;165:160–173.

Hilton SM. Hypothalamic control of the cardiovascular responses in fear and rage. *Sci Basis Med Annu Rev* 1965;217–238.

Hilton SM. Inhibition of baroreceptor reflexes on hypothalamic stimulation. *J Physiol (Lond)* 1963;165:56P–57P.

Hilton SM. Ways of viewing the central nervous control of the circulation—old and new. *Brain Res* 1975;66:235–251.

Himms-Hagen J. Sympathetic regulation of metabolism. *Pharmacol Rev* 1967;19:367–461.

Hiner B. Tilt-table testing in the diagnosis of unexplained syncope. *Proceedings, Third International Symposium on Autonomic Disorders*. Nashville, Tenn: Vanderbilt University, 1992 (Abstract).

Hines EA, Brown GE. The cold pressor test for measuring reactibility of the blood pressure: Data concerning 571 normal and hypertensive subjects. *Am Heart J* 1936;11:1–9.

Hjemdahl P, Daleskog M, Kahan T. Determination of plasma catecholamines by high performance liquid chromatography with electrochemical detection: comparison with a radioenzymatic method. *Life Sci* 1979;25:131–135.

Hjemdahl P, Fagius J, Freyschuss U, Wallin BG, Daleskog M, Bohlin G, Perski A. Muscle sympathetic activity and norepinephrine release during mental challenge in humans. *Am J Physiol* 1989;257:E654–E664.

Hjemdahl P, Freychuss U, Juhlin-Dannfelt A, Linde B. Differentiated sympathetic activation during mental stress evoked by the Stroop test. *Acta Physiol Scand* 1984;(Suppl 527): 25–29.

Hockman CH, Mauck HP, Hoff EC. ECG changes resulting from cerebral stimulation. II. A spectrum of ventricular arrhythmias of sympathetic origin. *Am Heart J* 1966;71:695–701.

Hoeldtke RS, Cilmi KM. Effects of aging on catecholamine metabolism. *J Clin Endocrinol Metab* 1985;60:479–484.

Hoeldtke RS, Stetson PL. In in vivo tritium release assay of human dopamine beta-hydroxylase. *J Clin Endocrinol Metab* 1980;51:810–815.

Hoffman BB, Lefkowitz RJ. Catecholamines and sympathomimetic drugs. In Gilman AG, Rall TW, Nies AS, Taylor P (Eds) *Goodman and Gilman's The Pharmacological Basis of Therapeutics*. New York: Pergamon Press, 1990, pp 187–220.

Hokfelt T, Fuxe K, Goldstein M, Johansson O. Immunohistochemical evidence for the existence of adrenaline neurons in the rat brain. *Brain Res* 1974;66:235–251.

Hokfelt T, Lundberg JM, Tatemoto K, Mutt V, Terenius L, Polak J, Bloom S, Sasek C, Elde R, Goldstein M. Neuropeptide Y (NPY)- and FMRFamide neuropeptide-like immunoreactivities in catecholamine neurons of the rat medulla oblongata. *Acta Physiol Scand* 1983; 117:315–318.

Holets VR. The anatomy and function of noradrenaline in the mammalian brain. In Heal DJ, Marsden CA (Eds) *The Pharmacology of Noradrenaline in the Central Nervous System*. New York: Oxford University Press, 1990, pp 1–40.

Holland KN, Brill RW, Chang RKC, Sibert JR, Fournier DA. Physiological and behavioural thermoregulation in bigeye tuna *(Thunnus obesus)*. *Nature* 1992;358:410–411.

Hollander W, Michaelson AL, Wilkins RW. Serotonin and antiserotonins. I. Their circulatory, respiratory and renal effects in man. *Circulation* 1957;16:246–255.

Hollenberg M, Carriere S, Barger AC. Biphasic action of acetylcholine on ventricular myocardium. *Circ Res* 1965;16:527–536.

Hollenberg NK, Borucki LJ, Adams DF. The renal vasculature in early essential hypertension. Evidence for a pathogenetic role. *Medicine* 1978;57:167–176.

Hollenberg NK, Sandor T. Vasomotion of renal blood flow in essential hypertension. Oscillations in xenon transit. *Hypertension* 1984;6:579–585.

Hollenberg NK, Williams GH, Adams DF. Essential hypertension: Abnormal renal, vascular and endocrine responses to a mild psychological stimulus. *Hypertension* 1981;3:11–17.

Hollister AS, Onrot J, Lonce S, Naudeau JH, Robertson D. Plasma catecholamine modulation of alpha$_2$ adrenoceptor agonist affinity and sensitivty in normotensive and hypertensive human platelets. *J Clin Invest* 1986;77:1416–1421.

Holmes TH, Rahe RH. The social readjustment rating scale. *J Psychosom Res* 1967;11:213–218.

Holzbauer M, Sharman DF. The distribution of catecholamines in vertebrates. In Eichler O, Farah A, Herken H, Welch AD (Eds) *Handbook of Experimental Pharmacology*. XXXIII. New York: Springer-Verlag, 1972, pp 110–185.

Honda T, Ninomiya I, Azumi T. Cardiac sympathetic nerve activity and catecholamine kinetics in cat hearts. *Am J Physiol* 1987;252:H879–H885.

Horikoshi Y, Tajima I, Igarashi H, Inui M, Kasahara K, Noguchi T. The adreno-sympathetic system, the genetic predisposition to hypertension, and stress. *Am J Med* Sci 1985;289: 186–191.

Horn EM, Bilezikian JP. Mechanisms of abnormal transmembrane signaling of the β-adrenergic receptor in congestive heart failure. *Circulation* 1990;82 (Suppl. I):I26–I34.

Horwitz D, Clineschmidt BV, van Buren JM, Ommaya AK. Temporal arteries from hypertensive and normotensive man. *Circ Res* 1974;34, 35:I109–I115.

Horwitz D, Fox SM, Goldberg LI. Effects of dopamine in man. *Circ Res* 1962;10:237–243.

Hosotani R, Chowdhury P, Huang YS, Rayford PL. Neural mechanisms of pancreatic polypeptide release in conscious dogs. *Am J Physiol* 1989;257:G134–G137.

Hossmann V, Maling TJ, Hamilton CA, Reid JL, Dollery CT. Sedative and cardiovascular effects of clonidine and nitrazepam. *Clin Pharmacol Ther* 1980;28:167–176.

Hovevey-Sion D, Eisenhofer G, Kopin IJ, Kirk KL, Chang PC, Szemeredi K, Goldstein DS. Metabolic fate of injected [^{3}H]-dopamine and [^{3}H]-2-fluorodopamine in rats. *Neuropharmacology* 1989;28:791–797.

Hovevey-Sion D, Harvey-White J, Kopin IJ, Goldstein DS. Measurement of homovanillic acid in small volumes of plasma using liquid chromatography with electrochemical detection. *J Chromatog* 1988;426:141–147.

Hovevey-Sion D, Kopin IJ, Stull RW, Goldstein DS. Effects of monoamine oxidase inhibitors on levels of catechols and homovanillic acid in striatum and plasma. *Neuropharmacology* 1989;28:791–797.

Howe PRC, Rogers PF, Morris MJ, Chalmers JP, Smith RM. Plasma catecholamines and neuropeptide-Y as indicators of sympathetic nerve activity in normotensive and stroke-prone spontaneously hypertensive rats. *J Cardiovasc Pharmacol* 1986;8:1113–1121.

Howe PRC. Blood pressure control by neurotransmitters in the medulla oblongata and spinal cord. *J Auton Nerv Sys* 1985;12:95–115.

Huangfu D, Hwang L-J, Riley TA, Guyenet PG. Splanchnic nerve response to A5 area stimulation in rats. *Am J Physiol* 1992;263:R437–R446.

Hubbard JW, Cox RH, Sanders BJ Lawler JE. Changes in cardiac output and vascular resistance during behavioral stress in the rat. *Am J Physiol* 1986b;251:R82–R90.

Hubbard JW, Cox RH, Sanders BJ Lawler JE. The effects of intracerebroventricular injection of clonidine on conditioned pressor and adrenergic responses in rats. *Neuropharmacology* 1986a;25:963–972.

Huchet A-M, Chelly J, Schmitt H. Role of alpha 1- and alpha 2-adrenoceptors in the modulation of the baroreflex vagal bradycardia. *Eur J Pharmacol* 1981;71:455–461.

Huchet A-M, Huguet F, Ostermann G, Bakri-Logeais F, Schmitt H, Narcisse G. Central α_1-adrenoceptors and cardiovascular control in normotensive and spontaneously hypertensive rats. *Eur J Pharmacol* 1983;95:207–213.

Hughes J, Roth RH. Evidence that angiotensin enhances transmitter release during sympathetic nerve stimulation. *Br J Pharmacol* 1971;41:239–255.

Hull CL. *Principles of Behavior.* New York: Appleton, 1943.

Hume WR, Bevan JA. The structure of the peripheral adrenergic synapse and its functional implications. In Ziegler MG, Lake CR. (Eds) *Norepinephrine.* Baltimore: Williams and Wilkins, 1984, pp 47–54.

Humphrey DR Neuronal activity in the medulla oblongata of the cat evoked by stimulation of the carotid sinus nerve. In Kezdi P (Ed) *Baroreceptors and Hypertension.* Oxford, UK: Pergamon, 1967, pp 131–167.

Humphrey SJ, McCall RB. Evidence that L-glutamic acid mediates baroreceptor function in the cat. *Clin Exp Hyper* 1984;6:1311–1329.

Hunt D, Gore I. Myocardial lesions following experimental intracranial hemorrhage. Prevention with propranolol. *Am Heart J* 1972;83:232–236.

Hunter LW, Rorie DK, Tyce GM. Dihydroxyphenylalanine and dopamine are released from portal vein together with noradrenaline and dihydroxyphenylglycol during nerve stimulation. *J Neurochem* 1992;59:972–982.

Husebye E, Kjeldsen SE, Lande K, Gjesdal K, Os I, Eide I. Increased arterial adrenaline is related to pain in uncomplicated myocardial infarction. *J Intern Med* 1990;228:617–622.

Hyland K, Clayton PT. Aromatic L-amino acid decarboxylase deficiency: Diagnostic methodology. *Clin Chem* 1992;38:2405–2410.

Hyland K, Surtees RA, Rodeck C, Clayton PT. Aromatic L-amino acid decarboxylase deficiency: Clinical features, diagnosis, and treatment of a new inborn error of neurotransmitter amine synthesis. *Neurology* 1992;42:1980–1989.

Iimura O, Kikuchi K, Sato S. Plasma noradrenaline concentration and pressor response to infused noradrenaline in patients with borderline hypertension, and mild or moderate essential hypertension. *Jpn Circ J* 1984;48:159–167.

Iimura O, Shimamoto K, Ura N. Dopaminergic activity and water-sodium handling in the kidneys of essential hypertensive subjects: Is renal dopaminergic acitivity suppressed at the pre-hypertensive stage? *J Cardiovasc Pharmacol* 1990;16 (Suppl. 7):S56–S58.

Ikeda J, Haneda T, Kanda H, Hiramoto T, Furuyama M, Sakuma T, Shirato K, Takishima T. Influence of reduced presynaptic myocardial norepinephrine stores on left ventricular contractility. *J Auton Nerv Sys* 1991;34:231–238.

Imaizumi T, Granata AR, Benarroch EE, Sved AF, Reis DJ. Contributions of arginine vasopressin and the sympathetic nervous system to the fulminating hypertension after destruction of neurons of caudal ventrolateral medulla of the rat. *J Hypertens* 1985;3:491–501.

Imaizumi T, Takeshita A, Higashi H, Nakamura M. Alpha-ANP alters reflex control of lumbar and renal sympathetic nerve activity and heart rate. *Am J Physiol* 1987;253:H1136–H1140.

Imaizumi T, Thames MD Influence of intravenous and intracerebroventricular vasopressin on baroreflex control of renal nerve traffic. *Circ Res* 1986;58:17–25.

Imperato-McGinley J, Gautier T, Ehlers K, Zullo MA, Goldstein DS, Vaughan ED Jr. Reversibility of catecholamine-induced cardiomyopathy in a child with a pheochromocytoma. *N Engl J Med* 1987;316:793–797.

Indolfi C, Piscione F, Villari B, Russolillo E, Rendina V, Golino P, Condorelli M, Chiariello M. Role of α_2-adrenoceptors in normal and atherosclerotic human coronary circulation. *Circulation* 1992;86:1116–1124.

Inoue H, Zipes DP. Results of sympathetic denervation in the canine heart: Supersensitivity that may be arrhythmogenic. *Circulation* 1987;75:877–887.

Insel TR, Aloi JA, Goldstein DS, Wood JH, Jimerson DC. Plasma cortisol and catecholamine responses to intra-cerebroventricular administration of CRF to rhesus monkeys. *Life Sci* 1984;34:1873–1878.

Iosa D, DeQuattro V, De-Ping Lee D, Elkayam U, Caeiro T, Palmero H. Pathogenesis of cardiac neuro-myopathy in Chagas' disease and the role of the autonomic nervous system. *J Auton Nerv Sys* 1990;30:S83–S88.

Iosa D, DeQuattro V, Lee DD, Elkayam U, Palmero H. Plasma norepinephrine in Chagas' cardiomyopathy: A marker of progressive dysautonomia. *Am Heart J* 1989;117:882–887.

Iovino M, Vanacore A, Steardo L. Alpha$_2$-adrenergic stimulation within the nucleus tractus solitarius attenuates vasopressin release induced by depletion of cardiovascular volume. *Pharmacol Biochem Behav* 1990;37:821–824.

Iriuchijima J. Sympathetic discharge rate in spontaneously hypertensive rats. *Jpn Heart J* 1973;14:350–356.

Ito K, Sato S, Shimamura K, Swenson RS. Reflex changes in sympatho-adrenal medullary functions in response to baroreceptor stimulation in anesthetized rats. *J Auton Nerv Sys* 1984;10:295–303.

Itoh Y, Oishi R, Nishibori M, Saeki K. *In vivo* measurement of noradrenaline and 3,4-dihydroxyphenylethyleneglycol in the rat hypothalamus by microdialysis: Effects of various drugs affecting noradrenaline metabolism. *J Pharmacol Exp Ther* 1990;255:1090–1097.

Iversen LL, Rossor MN, Reynolds GP, Hills R, Roth M, Mountjoy CQ, Foote SL, Morrison JH, Bloom FE. Loss of pigmented dopamine-beta-hydroxylase positive cells from locus coeruleus in senile dementia of Alzheimer's type. *Neurosci Lett* 1983;39:95–100.

Iversen LL. Catecholamine uptake processes. *Br Med Bull* 1973;29:130–135.

Iversen LL. *The Uptake and Storage of Noradrenaline in Sympathetic Nerves.* Cambridge, UK: Cambridge University Press, 1967.

Iwata J, LeDoux JE, Meeley MP, Arneric S, Reis DJ. Intrinsic neurons in the amygdaloid field projected to by the medical geniculate body mediate emotional responses conditioned to acoustic stimuli. *Brain Res* 1986a;383:195–214.

Iwata J, LeDoux JE, Reis DJ. Destruction of intrinsic neurons in the lateral hypothalamus disrupts the classical conditioning of autonomic but not behavioral emotional responses in the rat. *Brain Res* 1986b;368:161–166.

Izard CE, Haynes OM, Chisolm G, Baak K. Emotional determinants of infant-mother attachment. *Child Devel* 1991;62:906–917.

Izard CE, Huebner RR, Risser D, McGinnes GC, Dougherty LM. The young infant's ability to produce discreet emotion expressions. *Devel Psychol* 1980;16:132–140.

Izard CE. Emotions as motivations: An evolutionary-developmental perspective. In Dienthier RA (Ed) *Nebraska Symposium on Motivation 1978.* Lincoln, Neb: University of Nebraska Press, 1979.

Izard CE. Facial expressions and the regulation of emotions. *J Pers Soc Psychol* 1990;58:487–498.

Izzo JL Jr, Smith RJ, Larrabee PS, Kallay MC. Plasma norepinephrine and age as determinants of systemic hemodynamics in men with established hypertension. *Hypertension* 1987;9:415–419.

Izzo JL Jr. Sympathoadrenal activity, catecholamines, and the pathogenesis of vasculopathic hypertensive target-organ damage. *Am J Hypertens* 1989;2:305S–312S.

Jacobowitz D, Kent KM, Fleisch JH. Histofluorescent study of catecholamine-containing elements in cholinergic ganglia from the calf and dog lung. *Proc Soc Exp Biol Med* 1973;144:464–466.

Jacobowitz D. Histochemical studies of the relationship of chromaffin cells and adrenergic nerve fibers to the cardiac ganglia of several species. *J Pharmacol Exp Ther* 1967;158:227–240.

Jacobowitz DM, Ziegler MG, Thomas JA. In vivo uptake of antibody to dopamine β-hydroxylase into sympathetic elements. *Brain Res* 1975;91:165–170.

Jacobs BL. Locus coeruleus neuronal activity in behaving animals. In Heal DJ, Marsden CA (Eds) *The Pharmacology of Noradrenaline in the Central Nervous System.* New York: Oxford University Press, 1990, pp 248–265.

Jacobs S, Ostfeld A. An epidemiological review of the mortality of bereavement. *J Psychosom Med* 1977;39:344–357.

Jacobsen J, Sfelt S, Sheikh S, Warberg J, Secher NH. Cardiovascular and endocrine responses to haemorrhage in the pig. *Acta Physiol Scand* 1990;138:167–173.

James TN. Primary and seconary cardioneuropathies and their functional significance. *J Am Coll Cardiol* 1983;2:983–1002.

Janowsky DS, Risch SC, Huey LY, Kennedy B, Ziegler M. Effects of physostigmine on pulse, blood pressure, and serum epinephrine levels. *Am J Psychiatry* 1985;142:738–740.

Jarrott B. Changes in central catecholaminergic neurons in cardiovascular diseases. In Ganguly PK (Ed) *Catecholamines and Heart Disease.* Boca Raton: CRC Press, 1991, pp 177–200.

Jasmin G, Solymoss B, Proscheck L. Therapeutic trials in hamster dystrophy. *Ann NY Acad Sci* 1979;317:338–348.

Jay GW, Leestma JE. Sudden death in epilepsy: A comprehensive review of the literature and proposed mechanisms. *Acta Neurol Scand* 1981;63 (Suppl. 2):1–66.

Jeffrey RF, Macdonald TM, Rutter M, Freestone S, Brown J, Samson RR, Lee MR. The effect of intravenous frusemide on urine dopamine in normal volunteers: studies with indomethacin and carbidopa. *Clin Sci* 1987;73:151–157.

Jenkins CD. Psychological risk factors for coronary heart disease. *Acta Med Scand* 1982;660: 123–136.

Jenkins CD. Recent evidence supporting psychosocial fisk factors for coronary disease. *N Engl J Med* 1976;294:987 and 1033.

Jensen KS, Bie P, Secher NH, Astrup A, Christensen NJ, Warberg J, Giese J, Schwartz TW. Regulatory mechanisms in hypotensive central hypovolemia in man. In Lown B, Malliani A, Prosdocimi M (Eds) *Neural Mechanisms and Cardiovascular Disease*. New York: Springer Verlag, 1986, pp 605–606.

Jeske I, Morrison SF, Cravo SL, Reis DJ. Identification of baroreceptor reflex interneurons in the caudal ventrolateral medulla. *Am J Physiol* 1993;264:R169–R178.

Jezova D, Kvetnansky R, Kovacs K, Oprsalova Z, Vigas M, Makara GB. Insulin-induced hypoglycemia activates the release of adrenocorticotropin predominantly via central and propranolol insensitive mechanisms. *Endocrinology* 1987;120:409:409–415.

Joanny P, Steinberg J, Zamora AJ, Conte-Devolx B, Millet Y, Oliver C. Corticotropin-releasing factor release from in vitro superfused and incubated rat hypothalamus. Effect of potassium, norepinephrine, and dopamine. *Peptides* 1989;10:903–911.

Joh TH, Park DH, Reis DJ. Direct phosphorylation of brain tyrosine hydroxylase by cyclic AMP-dependent protein kinase: Mechanism of enzyme activation. *Proc Nat Acad Sci USA* 1978; 75:4744–4748.

Johannessen JN, Goldstein DS, Oliver J, Markey SP. Prolonged changes in plasma catecholamine metabolites following a single infusion of an MPTP analog. *Life Sci* 1990;47:1895–1901.

Johansson GL, Jonsson L, Lannek N, Blomgren L, Lindberg P, Poupa O. Severe stress-cardiopathy in pigs. *Am Heart J* 1974;87:451–457.

Johnson DA, Pinto JMB, Kirby DA, Lown B. Catecholamines in cerebrospinal fluid are increased by behavioral arousal and myocardial ischemia. *Am J Physiol* 1992;263:H83–H87.

Johnson GA, Peuler JD, Baker CA. Plasma catecholamines in normotensive subjects. *Curr Ther Res* 1977;21:898–908.

Johnson GL, Wolfe BB, Harden TK, Molinoff PB, Perkins JP. Role of beta-adrenergic receptors in catecholamine-induced desensitization of adenylate cyclase in human astrocytoma cells. *J Biol Chem* 1978;253:1472–1480.

Johnson J, Leventhal H. The effects of accurate expectations and behavioral instructions on reactions during a noxious medical examination. *J Pers Soc Psychol* 1974;29:710–718.

Johnson RH, Lambie DG, Spalding JMK. *Neurocardiology. The Interrelationships between Dysfunction in the Nervous and Cardiovascular Systems*. Philadelphia, Pa: WB Saunders Co., 1984.

Johnson TS, Young JB, Landsberg L. Sympathoadrenal responses to acute and chronic hypoxia in the rat. *J Clin Invest* 1983;71:1263–1272.

Johnston DW. Stress management in the treatment of mild primary hypertension. *Hypertension* 1991;17 (Suppl. III):III63–III68.

Jones CJH, DeFily DV, Patterson JL, Chilian WM. Endothelium-dependent relaxation competes with α_1- and α_2-adrenergic constriction in the canine epicardial coronary microcirculation. *Circulation* 1993;87;1264–1274.

Jones CR, Hoyer D, Palacios JM. Adrenoceptor autoradiography. In Heal DJ, Marsden CA (Eds) *The Pharmacology of Noradrenaline in the Central Nervous System*. New York: Oxford University Press, 1990, pp 41–75.

Jones SL, Gebhart GF. Characterization of coeruleospinal inhibition of the nociceptive tail-flick reflex in the rat: Mediation by spinal alpha$_2$-adrenoceptors. *Brain Res* 1986;364:315–330.

Jonkers R, Boxtel CJV, Oosterhuis B. β2-adrenoceptor-mediated hypokalemia and its abolishment by oxprenolol. *Clin Pharmacol Ther* 1987;42:627–633.

Jonnesco T. Traiement chirurgical de l'angine de poitrine par la resection du sympathetic cervico-thoracique. *Press Med* 1921;20:193–194.

Jorgensen LS, Bonlokke L, Christensen NJ. Life strain, life events, and autonomic response to a psychological stressor in patients with chronic upper abdominal pain. *Scand J Gastroenterol* 1986;21:605–613.

Jorgensen LS, Bonlokke L, Christensen NJ. Plasma adrenaline and noradrenaline during mental stress and isometric exercise in man. The role of arterial sampling. *Scand J Clin Lab Invest* 1985;45:447–452.

Jouvet M. The role of monoamines and acetylcholine-containing neurons in the regulation of the sleep-waking cycle. *Ergeb Physiol* 1972;64:166–307.

Jubelin BC, Kannan MS. Neurons from neonatal hypertensive rats exhibit abnormal membrane properties in vitro. *Am J Physiol* 1990;259:C389–C396.

Judy WV, Watanabe AM, Henry DP, Besch HR Jr, Murphy WR, Hockel G. Sympathetic nerve activity. Role in regulation of blood pressure in the spontaneously hypertensive rat. *Circ Res* 1976;38:II21–II29.

Julien C, Kandza P, Barres C, Lo M, Cerutti C, Sassard J. Effects of sympathectomy on blood pressure and its variability in conscious rats. *Am J Physiol* 1990;259:H1337–H1342.

Julius S, Esler M. Autonomic nervous cardiovascular regulation in borderline hypertension. *Am J Cardiol* 1975;36:685–696.

Julius S, Jones K, Schork N, Johnson E, Krause L, Nazzaro P, Zemva A. Independence of pressure reactivity from pressure levels in Tecumseh, Michigan. *Hypertension* 1991;17 (Suppl. III):III12–III21.

Julius S, Li Y, Brant L, Krause L, Buda AJ. Neurogenic pressor episodes fail to cause hypertension, but do induce cardiac hypertrophy. *Hypertension* 1989;13:422–429.

Julius S, Pascual AV, London R. Role of parasympathetic inhibition in the hyperkinetic type of borderline hypertension. *Circulation* 1971;44:413–418.

Julius S. Changing role of the autonomic nervous system in human hypertension. *J Hypertens* 1990;9 (Suppl. 7):S59–S65.

Juorio AV, Chedrese PJ. The concentration of dopamine and related monoamines in arteries and some other tissues of the sheep. *Comp Biochem Physiol* 1990;95C:35–37.

Kagedal B, Goldstein DS. Catecholamines and their metabolites. *J Chromatog* 1988;429:177–233.

Kagia T, Hori M, Iwakura K, Iwai K, Watanabe Y, Uchida S, Yoshida H, Kitabatake A, Inoue M, Kamada T. Role of increased α$_1$-adrenergic activity in cardiomyopathic Syrian hamster. *Am J Physiol* 1991;260:H80–H88.

Kalen P, Kokaia M, Lindvall O, Bjorklund A. Basic characteristics of noradrenaline release in the hippocampus of intact and 6-hydroxydopamine lesioned rats as studied by in vivo microdialysis. *Brain Res* 1988;474:374–379.

Kaler SG, Goldstein DS, Holmes C, Salerno JA, Gahl WA. Plasma and cerebrospinal fluid neurochemical pattern in Menkes' disease. *Ann Neurol* 1993;33:171–175.

Kalia M, Fuxe K, Goldstein M. Rat medulla oblongata. II. Dopaminergic, noradrenergic (A1 and A2) and adrenergic neurons, nerve fibers, and presumptive terminal processes. *J Comp Neurol* 1985a;233:308–332.

Kalia M, Fuxe K, Goldstein M. Rat medulla oblongata. III. Adrenergic (C1 and C2) neurons, nerve fibers and presumptive terminal processes. *J Comp Neurol* 1985b;233:333–349.

Kalia M. *Brain* stem localization of vagal preganglionic neurons. *J Autonom Nerv Sys* 1981;3: 451–481.

Kalin NH. The neurobiology of fear. *Scientific American,* May, 1993:94–101.

Kampine JP, Kostreva DR. The abdominal sympathetic afferent fibers and their reflex function. In Lown B, Malliani A, Prosdocimi M (Eds) *Neural Mechanisms and Cardiovascular Disease.* New York: Springer Verlag, 1986, pp 47–61.

Kanbe T, Nara Y, Tagami M, Yamori Y. Studies of hypertension-induced vascular hypertrophy in cultured smooth muscle cells from spontaneously hypertensive rats. *Hypertension* 1983;5:887–892.

Kandel ER, Tauc L. Mechanism of heterosynaptic facilitation in the giant cell of the abdominal ganglion of Aplysia depilans. *J Physiol (Lond)* 1965;181:28–47.

Kandel ER. From metapsychology to molecular biology: Explorations into the nature of anxiety. *Am J Psychiatry* 1983;140:1277–1293.

Kaneko K, Okada K, Ishikawa S-E, Kuzuya T, Saito T. Role of atrial natriuretic peptide in natriuresis in volume-expanded rats. *Am J Physiol* 1987;253:R877–R882.

Kaneto AK, Kosaka K, Nakao K. Effects of stimulation of vagus nerve on insulin secretion. *Endocrinology* 1967;80:530–536.

Kannan H, Hayashida Y, Yamashita H. Increase in sympathetic outflow by paraventricular nucleus stimulation in awake rats. *Am J Physiol* 1989;256:R1325–R1330.

Kaplan GP, Hartman BK, Creveling CR. Immunohistochemical demonstration of catechol-O-methyltransferase in mammalian brain. *Brain Res* 1979;167:241–250.

Kaplan JR, Manuck SB, Clarkson TB. Lusso FM, Taub DM, Miller EW. Social stress and atherosclerosis in normocholesterolemic monkeys. *Science* 1983;220:733–735.

Kaplan JR, Manuck SB, Clarkson TB. Social status, environment, and atherosclerosis in cynomolgus monkeys. *Atherosclerosis* 1982;2:359–368.

Kapp BS, Markgraf CG, Schwaber JS, Bilyk-Spafford T. The organization of dorsal medullary projections to the central amygdaloid nucleus and parabrachial nuclei in the rabbit. *Neuroscience* 1989;30:717–732.

Kappagoda CT, Linden RJ, Snow HM. Effect of stimulating right atrial receptors on urine flow in the dog. *J Physiol (Lond)* 1973;235:493–502.

Karasek R, Baker D, Marxer F, Albom A, Theorell T. Job decision latitude, job demands, and cardiovascular disease: A prospective study of Swedish men. *Am J Pub Health* 1981;71: 694–705.

Karasek RA, Theorell TG, Schwarts J, Pieper C, Alfredsson L. Job psychological factors and coronary heart disease: Swedish retrospective findings and U.S. prevalence findings using a new occupational inference method. *Adv Cardiol* 1982;29:62–67.

Karim F, Kidd C, Malpus CM, Penna PE. The effects of stimulation of the left atrial receptors on sympathetic efferent nerve activity. *J Physiol (Lond)* 1972;227:254–260.

Karlsberg RP, Cryer PE, Roberts R. Serial plasma catecholamine response early in the course of clinical acute myocardial infarction: Relationship to infarct extent and mortality. *Am Heart J* 1981;102:24–29.

Karmazyn M, Beamish RE, Dhalla NS. Involvement of calcium in coronary vasoconstriction due to prolonged hypoxia. *Am Heart J* 1984;107:293–297.

Karmazyn M, Beamish RE, Fliegel L, Dhalla NS. Adrenochrome-induced coronary artery constriction in the rat heart. *J Pharmacol Exp Ther* 1981;219:225–230.

Kaszaki J, Nagy S, Tarnoky K, Laczi F, Vecsernyes M, Boros M. Humoral changes in shock induced by cardiac tamponade. *Circ Shock* 1989;29:143–153.

Kaufman LJ, Vollmer RR. Low sodium diet augments plasma and tissue catecholamine levels in pithed rats. *Clin Exp Hyper* 1984;A6:1543–1558.

Kaufman LN, Young JB, Landsberg L. Differential catecholamine responses to dietary intake: effects of macronutrients on dopamine and epinephrine excretion in the rat. *Metabolism* 1989;38:91–99.

Kaufman S, Milstien S, Bartholome K. New forms of phenylketonuria. *Lancet* 1975;2:708.

Kaufman S, Stelfox J. Atrial stretch-induced diuresis in Brattleboro rats. *Am J Physiol* 1987;252: R503–R506.

Kaufman S. Influence of right atrial stretch on plasma renin activity in the conscious rat. *Can J Physiol Pharmacol* 1987;65:257–259.

Kaufmann H, Oribe E, Miller M, Knott P, Wiltshire-Clement M, Yahr MD. Hypotension-induced vasopressin release distinguishes between pure autonomic failure and multiple system atrophy with autonomic failure. *Neurology* 1992;42:590–593.

Kawano Y, Fukiyama K, Takeya Y, Abe I, Kawasaki T, Omae T. Augmented sympathetic nervous function in young subjects with borderline hypertension. *Jpn Circ J* 1982;46: 483–485.

Kawasaki S, Takeda K, Tanaka M, Itoh H, Kirata M, Nakata T, Hayashi J, Oguro M, Sasaki S, Nakagawa M. Enhanced norepinephrine release in hypothalamus form locus coeruleus in SHR. *Jpn Heart J* 1991;32:255–262.

Keehn RJ, Goldberg ID, Beebe GW. Twenty-four year mortality follow-up of Army veterans with disability separations for psychoneurosis in 1944. *Psychosom Med* 1974;36:27–46.

Keim KL, Sigg EB. Activation of central sympathetic neurons by angiotensin II. *Life Sci* 1971; 10:565–574.

Keller W. *The Bible as History.* New York: Bantam Books, 1980.

Keller-Wood ME, Wade CE, Shinsako J, Keil LC, van Loon GR, Dallman MF. Insulin-induced hypoglycemia in conscious dogs: effect of maintaining carotid arterial glucose levels on the adrenocorticotropin, epinephrine, and vasopressin responses. *Endocrinology* 1983; 112:624–632.

Kendrick KM, Leng G. Haemorrhage-induced release of noradrenaline, 5-hydroxytryptamine and uric acid in the supraoptic nucleus of the rat measured by microdialysis. *Brain Res* 1987; 440:402–406.

Keng LB. On the nervous supply of the dog's heart. *J Physiol (Lond)* 1893;14:407–482.

Kennedy B, Elayan H, Ziegler MG. Epinephrine synthesis by rat arteries. *Am J Hypertens* 1991; 4:45–50.

Kennedy B, Elayan H, Ziegler MG. Lung epinephrine synthesis. *Am J Physiol* 1990;258:L227–L231.

Kennedy B, Janowsky DS, Risch SC, Ziegler MG. Central cholinergic stimulation causes adrenal epinephrine release. *J Clin Invest* 1984;74:972–975.

Kent KM, Smith ER, Redwood DR, Epstein SE. Electrical stability of acutely ischemic myocardium: influence of heart rate and vagal stimulation. *Circulation* 1973;47:291–298.

Keogh AM, Baron DW, Hickie JB. Prognostic guides in patients with idiopathic or ischemic dilated cardiomyopathy assessed for cardiac transplantation. *Am J Cardiol* 1990;65:903–908.

Kern KB, Elchisak MA, Sanders AB, Badylak SF, Tacker WA, Ewy GA. Plasma catecholamines and resuscitation from prolonged cardiac arrest. *Crit Care Med* 1989;17:786–791.

Kerr D, Macdonald IA, Tattersall RB. Influence of duration of hypoglycemia on the hormonal counterregulatory response in normal subjects. *J Clin Endocrinol Metab* 1989;68:1118–1122.

Kety SS. The biogenic amines in the central nervous system: Their possible roles in arousal, emotion and learning. In Schmitt FO (Ed) *The Neurosciences*. New York: Rockefeller University Press, 1970, pp 324–336.

Keys A, Taylor ML, Blackburn HW, Brozek J, Anderson J, Simonsor E. Mortality and coronary heart disease among men studied for 23 years. *Arch Int Med* 1971;128:201–214.

Keys A. The individual risk of coronary heart disease. *Ann NY Acad Sci* 1966;134:1046–1063.

Kezdi P. Resetting of the carotid sinus in experimental renal hypertension. In Kezdi P (Ed) *Baroreceptors and Hypertension*. Oxford, UK: Pergamon, 1967, pp 301–306.

Khan MI, Hamilton JT, Manning GW. Protective effect of beta-adrenoceptor blockade in experimental coronary occlusion in conscious dogs. *Am J Cardiol* 1972;30:832–837.

Kilty JE, Lorang D, Amara SG. Cloning and expression of a cocaine-sensitive rat dopamine transporter. *Science* 1991;254:578–579.

Kim YD, Lake CR, Lees DE, Schuette WH, Bull JM, Weise V, Kopin IJ. Hemodynamic and plasma catecholamine responses to hyperthermic cancer therapy in humans. *Am J Physiol* 1979;237:H570–H574.

King BD, Sack D, Kichuk MR, Hintze TH. Absence of hypertension despite chronic marked elevations in plasma norepinephrine in conscious dogs. *Hypertension* 1987;9:582–590.

King KA, Mackie G, Pang CCY, Wall RA. Central vasopressin in the modulation of catecholamine release in conscious rats. *Can J Physiol Pharmacol* 1985;63:1501–1505.

Kirby DA, Pinto JMB, Hottinger S, Johnson DA, Lown B. Behavioral arousal enhances inducibility and rate of ventricular tachycardia. *Am J Physiol* 1991;261:H1734–H1739.

Kirshner N. Biosynthesis of adrenaline from noradrenaline. *Pharmacol Rev* 1959;11:350–357.

Kirshner N. Uptake of catecholamines by a particulate fraction of the adrenal medulla. *J Biol Chem* 1962;327:2311–2317.

Klein RL. Chemical composition of the large noradrenergic vesicles. In Klein RL, Lagercrantz H, Zimmerman H (Eds) *Neurotransmitter Vesicles*. New York: Academic Press, 1982, pp 133–174.

Kligfield P. John Hunter, angina pectoris and medical education. *Am J Cardiol* 1980;45:367–369.

Kluger J, Cody RJ, Laragh JH. The contributions of sympathetic tone and the renin-angiotensin system to severe chronic congestive heart failure: response to specific inhibitors (prazosin and captopril). *Am J Cardiol* 1982;49:1667–1674.

Kluver H, Bucy P. Preliminary analysis of functions of the temporal lobes in monkeys. *Arch Neurol Psychiat* 1939;42:979–100.

Knuepfer MM, Printz MM, Stock G. Increased sensitivity to arousal in spontaneously hypertensive rats is partially dependent upon the amygdala. *Clin Exp Hypertens* 1991;13:505–523.

Knutson L, Knutson TW, Flemstrom G. Endogenous dopamine and duodenal bicarbonate secretion in humans. *Gastroenterology* 1993;104:1409–1413.

Kobilka BK, Kobilka TS, Yang-Feng TL, Francke U, Caron MG, Lefkowitz RJ, Regan JW. Cloning, sequencing and expression of the gene encoding for the human platelet α_2-adrenergic receptor. *Science* 1987;238:650–656.

Kobler J. *The Reluctant Surgeon. A Biography of John Hunter*. New York: Doubleday and Co., 1960.

Koch E, Mies A. Chronisches arterilles Hochdruck durch experimentelle Dauerausschaltung der Blutdruckzugler. *Krankheitsforschung* 1929;7:241–256.

Koepke JP, Di Bona GF. Central adrenergic receptor control of renal function in conscious hypertensive rats. *Hypertension* 1986;8:133–141.

Koepke JP, Di Bona GF. Central beta-adrenergic receptors mediate renal nerve activity during stress in conscious spontaneously hypertensive rats. *Hypertension* 1985b;7:350–356.

Koepke JP, Di Bona GF. High sodium intake enhances renal nerve and antinatriuretic responses to stress in spontaneously hypertensive rats. *Hypertension* 1985a;7:357–363.

Koepke JP, Jones S, Di Bona GF. Alpha 2-adrenoceptors in amygdala control renal sympathetic nerve activity and renal function in conscious spontaneously hypertensive rats. *Brain Res* 1987;404:80–88.

Koepke JP, Jones S, Di Bona GF. Hypothalamic beta 2-adrenoceptor control of renal sympathetic nerve activity and urinary sodium excretion in conscious, spontaneously hypertensive rats. *Circ Res* 1986;58:241–248.

Koizumi F, Ohneda M, Ohneda A. Role of autonomic nervous system in the response of plasm pancreatic polypeptide to glycopenia in dogs. *Tohoku J Exp Med* 1990;162:355–362.

Koizumi K, Kollai M. Control of reciprocal and non-reciprocal action of vagal and sympathetic efferents: Study of centrally induced reactions. *J Auton Nerv Sys* 1981;3:483–501.

Kolin A, Norris JW. Myocardial damage from acute cerebral lesions. *Stroke* 1984;15:990–993.

Kolman BS, Verrier RL, Lown B. Effect of vagus nerve stimulaiton upon excitability of the canine ventricle. *Am J Cardiol* 1976;37:1041–1045.

Komersaroff PA, Funder JW, Differential glucocorticoid effects on catecholamine responses to stress. *Am J Physiol* 1994;266:E118–E128.

Kondo M. Autoradiographic study of ^{3}H-DOPA uptake by superior cervical and stellate ganglia of spontaneously hypertensive rats during the prehypertensive stage. *Virchows Arch B* 1987;54:190–193.

Koob GF. Drugs of abuse: Anatomy, pharmacology and function of reward pathways. *Trends Pharmacol Sci* 1992;13:177–184.

Koolen MI, den Boer EB-V, van Brummelen P. Clinical biochemical and haemodynamic correlates of sodium sensitivity in essential hypertension. *J Hypertens* 1983;1 (Suppl 2):21–23.

Koolen MI, van Brummelen P.Adrenergic activity and peripheral hemodynamics in relation to sodium sensitivity in patients with essential hypertension. *Hypertension* 1984;6:820–825.

Kopia GA, Kopaciewics LJ, Ruffolo RR. Alpha-adrenoceptor regulation of coronary artery blood flow in normal and stenotic canine coronary arteries. *J Pharmacol Exp Ther* 1986;239:641–647.

Kopin IJ, Breese GR, Krauss KR, Weise VK. Selective release of newly synthesized norepinephrine from the cat spleen during sympathetic nerve stimulation. *J Pharmacol Exp Ther* 1968;161:271–278.

Kopin IJ, Fischer JE, Musacchio J, Horst WD. Evidence for a false neurochemical transmitter as a mechanism for the hypotensive effect of monoamine oxidase inhibitors. *Biochemistry* 1964;52:716–721.

Kopin IJ, Gordon EK. Origin of norepinephrine in the heart. *Nature* 1963;199:1289.

Kopin IJ, Weise VK. Effect of reserpine and metaraminol on excretion of homovanillic acid and 3-methoxy-4-hydroxyphenylglycol in the rat. *Biochem Pharmacol* 1968;17:1461–1464.

Kopin IJ, Zukowska-Grojec Z, Bayorh MA, Goldstein DS. Estimation of intrasynaptic norepinephrine concentrations at vascular neuroeffector junctions in vivo. *Naunyn-Schmiedeberg's Arch Pharmacol* 1984;325:298–305.

Kopin IJ. Catecholamine metabolism: Basic aspects and and clinical significance. *Pharmacol Rev* 1985;37:333-364.

Kopin IJ. Plasma levels of catecholamines and dopamine-β-hydroxylase. In Trendelenburg U, Weiner N (Eds) *Catecholamines* II. New York: Springer-Verlag, 1989, pp 211–275.

Kopin IJ. Technique for the study of alternate metabolic pathways: Epinephrine metabolism in man. *Science* 1960;131:1372–1374.

Koren MJ, Devereux RB, Casale PN, Savage DD, Laragh JH. Relation of left ventricular mass and geometry to morbidity and mortality in uncomplicated essential hypertension. *Ann Int Med* 1991;114:345–352.

Korn SJ, McCarthy KD. Modulation of cyclic AMP accumulation by α_2-adrenergic receptors in astroglial cell cultures. *Fed Proc* 1981;40:1–45.

Korner PI, Angus JA. Central nervous control of blood pressure in relation to antihypertensive drug treatment. In Austin DE (Ed) *Antihypertensive Drugs*. New York: Pergamon Press, 1982, pp 61–96.

Korner PI, Bobik A, Angus JA, Adams MA, Friberg P. Resistance control in hypertension. *J Hypertens* 1989;7 (Suppl.):S125–S134.

Korner PI, Bobik A, Oddie C, Friberg P. Sympathoadrenal system is critical for structural changes in genetic hypertension. *Hypertension* 1993;22:243–252.

Korner PI, Oliver JR, Sleight P, Chalmers JP, Robinson JS. Effects of clonidine on the baroreceptor-heart rate reflex and on single aortic baroreceptor fibre discharge. *Eur J Pharmacol* 1974;28:189–198.

Korner PI, Shaw J, Uther JB, West MJ, McRitchie RJ, Richards JG. Autonomic and non-autonomic circulatory components in essential hypertension in man. *Circulation* 1973;48: 107–117.

Korner PI. Causal and homeostatic factors in hypertension. *Clin Sci* 1982;63 (Suppl. 8):S52–S55.

Kotchen TA, Hartley LH, Rice TW, Mougey EH, Jones LG, Mason JW. Renin, norepinephrine, and epinephrine responses to graded exercise. *J Appl Physiol* 1971;31:178–184.

Koulu M, Saavedra JM, Niwa M, Linnoila M. Increased catecholamine metabolism in the locus coeruleus of young spontaneously hypertensive rats. *Brain Res* 1986;369:361–364.

Kowasaki H, Cline WH, Su C. Enhanced angiotensin-mediated facilitation of adrenergic neurotransmission in spontaneously hypertensive rats. *J Pharmacol Exp Ther* 1982;221:112–116.

Krantz DS, Lazar JD. The stress concept: issues and measurement. In Julius S, Bassett DR (Eds) *Behavioral Factors in Hypertension*. New York: Elsevier Science, 1987, pp 43–58.

Krantz DS, Manuck SB. Acute psychophysiologic reactivity and risk of cardiovascular disease: a review and methodologic critique. *Psychol Bull* 1984;96:435–464.

Krieger JE, Liard J-F, Cowley AW Jr. Hemodynamics, fluid volume, and hormonal responses to chronic high-salt intake in dogs. *Am J Physiol* 1990;259:H1629–H1636.

Krishna GG, Danovitch GM, Beck FW, Sowers JR. Dopaminergic mediation of the natriuretic response to volume expansion. *J Lab Clinical Med* 1985;105, 214–218.

Kubo T, Misu Y. Pharmacological characterization of the alpha-adrenoceptors responsible for a decrease of blood pressure in the nucleus tractus solitarii of the rat. *Naunyn-Schmiedeberg's Arch Pharmacol* 1981;317:120–125.

Kuchel O, Buu NT, Hamet P, Larochelle P, Bourque M, Genest J. Catecholamine sulfates and platelet phenolsulfotransferase activity in essential hypertension. *J Lab Clin Med* 1984; 104:238–244.

Kuchel O, Buu NT, Hamet P, Larochelle P, Bourque M, Genest J. Essential hypertension with low conjugated catecholamines imitates pheochromocytoma. *Hypertension* 1981;3:347–355.

Kuchel O, Buu NT, Neemen J. The platelet phenolsulfotransferase is not indispensable for the sulfoconjugation of plasma catecholamines. *Endocrine Res* 1985;11:225–232.

Kuchel O, Buu NT, Unger T, Genest J. Free and conjugated catecholamines in human hypertension. *Clin Sci* 1978;55:77s–80s.

Kuchel O, Buu NT, Unger T, Lis M, Genest J. Free and conjugated plasma and urinary dopamine in human hypertension. *J Clin Endocrinol Metab* 1979;48:425–429.

Kuchel O, Cusson JR, Laroachelle P, Buu NT, Genest J. Posture- and emotion-induced severe hypertensive paroxysms with baroreceptor dysfunction. *J Hypertens* 1987;5:277–283.

Kuhar MJ, Unnerstall JR. Mapping receptors for α_2-agonists in the central nervous system. *J Cardiovasc Pharmacol* 1984;6:S536–S542.

Kukreja RS, Datta BN, Cakravarti RN. Catecholamine-induced aggravation of aortic and coronary atherosclerosis in monkeys. *Atherosclerosis* 1981;40:291–298.

Kulbertus HE, Franck G (Eds) *Neurocardiology.* Mount Kisco, NY: Futura, 1988.

Kumada M, Sagawa K. Modulation of carotid sinus baroreceptor reflex by central gray stimulation. *Nippon Seirigaku Zasshi* 1974;36:147–148.

Kumada M, Schramm LP, Altmansberger RA, Sagawa K. Modulation of carotid sinus baroreceptor reflex by hypothalamic defense response. *Am J Physiol* 1975;228:34–45.

Kumagai H, Averill DB, Ferrario CM. Renal nerve activity in rats with spontaneous hypertension: effect of converting enzyme inhibitor. *Am J Physiol* 1992;263:R109–R115.

Kunihara M, Oshima T. Effects of epinephrine on plasma cholesterol levels in rats. *J Lipid Res* 1983;24:639–644.

Kurosawa M, Sato A, Swenson RS, Takahashi Y. Sympatho-adrenal medullary functions in response to intracerebroventricularly injected corticotropin-releasing factor in anesthetized rats. *Brain Res* 1986;367:250–257.

Kvetnansky R, Armando I, Weise VK, Holmes C, Fukuhara K, Deka-Starosta A, Kopin IJ, Goldstein DS. Plasma DOPA responses during stress: Dependence on sympathoadrenal activity and tyrosine hydroxylation. *J Pharmacol Exp Ther* 1992;261:899–909.

Kvetnansky R, Davydova NA, Noskov VB, Vigas M, Popova IA, Usakov AC, Macho L, Grigoriev AI. Plasma and urine catecholamine levels in cosmonauts during long-term stay on space station Salyut-7. *Acta Astronautica* 1988;17:181–186.

Kvetnansky R, Fukuhara K, Pacak K, Cizza G, Goldstein DS, Kopin IJ. Endogenous glucocorticoids restrain catecholamine synthesis and release at rest and during immobilization stress in rats. *Endocrinology* 1993;133:1411–1419.

Kvetnansky R, Gewirtz GP, Weise VK, Kopin IJ. Enhanced synthesis of adrenal dopamine beta-hydroxylase induced by repeated immobilization in rats. *Molec Pharmacol* 1971;7:81–86.

Kvetnansky R, Goldstein DS, Weise VK, Holmes C, Szemeredi K, Bagdy G, Kopin IJ. Effects of handling or immobilization on plasma levels of dopa, catecholamines, and metabolites in rats. *J Neurochem* 1992;58:2296–2302.

Kvetnansky R, Mikulaj L. Adrenal and urinary catecholamines in rat during adaptation to repeated immobilization stress. *Endocrinology* 1970;87:738–743.

Kvetnansky R, Nemeth S, Vigas M, Oprsalova Z, Jurcovicova J. Plasma catecholamines in rats during adaptation to intermittent exposure to different stressors. In Usdin E, Kvetnansky R, Axelrod J (Eds) *Stress: The Role of Catecholamines and Other Neurotransmitters.* New York: Gordon and Breach, 1984, pp 537–562.

Kvetnansky R, Torda T. Heart adrenergic system activity in rats during adaptation to repeated stress. In Beamish RE, Panagia, V, Dhalla NS (Eds) *Pathogenesis of Stress-Induced Heart Disease.* Boston: Martinus Nijhoff, 1984, pp 3–19.

Kvetnansky R, Weise VK, Gewirtz GP, Kopin IJ. Synthesis of adrenal catecholamines in rats during and after immobilization stress. *Endocrinology* 1971;89:46–49.

Kvetnansky R, Weise VK, Kopin IJ. Elevation of adrenal tyrosine hydroxylase and phenyle-thanolamine-N-methyl transferase by repeated immobilization of rats. *Endocrinology*1970;87:744–749.

L'Abbate A, Carpeggiani C, Trivella MG, Simonetti I, Biagini A. Myocardial ischemia induced by emotion in patients with angina pectoris. In Beamish RE, Singal PK, Dhalla NS (Eds) *Stress and Heart Disease*. Boston: Martinus Nijhoof, 1985, pp 81–98.

Lacey JI, Lacey BC. Some autonomic-central nervous system interrelationships. In Black P (Ed) *Physiological Correlates of Emotion*. New York: Academic Press, 1970, pp 205–227.

Lacey JI, Lacey BC. Verification and extension of the principle of autonomic response-stereotypy. *Am J Psychol* 1958;71:50–73.

Lacey JI. Somatic response patterning and stress: some revisions of activation theory. In Appley MH, Trumble R (Eds) *Psychological Stress*. New York: Appleton-Century-Crofts, 1967, pp 14–42.

Lachuer J, Gaillet S, Barbagli B, Buda M, Tappaz M. Differential early time course activation of the brainstem catecholaminergic groups in response to various stresses. *Neuroendocrinology* 1991;53:589–596.

Lake CR, Chernow B, Goldstein DS, Coleman M, Ziegler MG. Plasma catecholamine levels in normal subjects and in patients with secondary hypertension. *Fed Proc* 1984;43:52–56.

Lake CR, Gullner HG, Polinsky RJ, Ebert MH, Ziegler MG, Bartter FC. Essential hypertension: Central and peripheral norepinephrine. *Science* 1981;211:955–957.

Lake CR, Major LF, Ziegler MH, Kopin IJ. Increased sympathetic nervous system activity in alcoholic patients treated with disulfiram. *Am J Psychiatry* 1977;134:1411–1414.

Lake CR, Polinsky RJ, Gullner H-G, Ebert MH, Ziegler MG, Bartter FC, Kopin IJ. Dissociation between central and peripheral noradrenergic activity in essential hypertension. *Clin Sci* 1980;59:229s–233s.

Lake CR, Sternberg DE, van Kammen DP, Ballenger JC, Ziegler MG, Post RM, Kopin IJ, Bunney WE. Schizophrenia: Elevated cerebrospinal fluid norepinephrine. *Science* 1980;207:331–333.

Lake CR, Wood JH, Ziegler MG, Ebert MH, Kopin IJ. Probenecid-induced norepinephrine elevations in plasma and CSF. *Arch Gen Psychiatry* 1978;35:237–240.

Lake CR, Ziegler MG, Coleman MD, Kopin IJ. Hydrochlorothiazide-induced sympathetic hyperactivity in hypertensive patients. *Clin Pharmacol Ther* 1979;26:428–432.

Lake CR, Ziegler MG, Coleman MD, Kopin IJ. Lack of correlation of plasma norepinephrine and dopamine-beta-hydroxylase in hypertensive and normotensive subjects. *Circ Res* 1977;41:865–869.

Lake CR, Ziegler MG, Kopin IJ. Use of plasma norepinephrine for evaluation of sympathetic neuronal function in man. *Life Sci* 1976;18:1315–1325.

Lake CR, Ziegler MG. Effect of acute volume alterations on norepinephrine and dopamine-beta-hydroxylase in normotensive and hypertensive subjects. *Circulation* 1978;57:774–778.

Laks MM, Morady F, Swan HJC. Myocardial hypertrophy produced by chronic infusion of subhypertensive doses of norepinephrine in the dog. *Chest* 1973;64:75–78.

Laks MM. Functional status of the sympathetic nervous system in cardiovascular disease—The role of norepinephrine in the production of physiologic and pathologic hypertrophy. In Ganguly PK (Ed) *Catecholamines and Heart Disease*. Boca Raton: CRC Press, 1991, pp 103–122.

Lands AM, Luduena FP, Buzzo HH. Differentiation of receptors responsive to isoproterenol. *Life Sci* 1967;6:2241–2249.

Langer SZ, Adler E, Enero MA, Stefano FJE. The role of the a-receptor in regulating noradrenaline overflow by nerve stimulation. *Proc Int Un Physiol Sci* 1971;9:335.

Langer SZ, Lehmann, J. Presynaptic receptors on catecholamine neurones. In Trendelenburg U, Weiner N (Eds) *Catecholamines* II. New York: Springer-Verlag, 1989, pp 419–507.

Langer SZ, Massingham R, Shepperson NB. Presence of post-synaptic alpha 2-adrenoceptors of predominantly extrasynaptic location in the vascular smooth muscle of the dog hind-limb. *Clin Sci* 1980;59:225s–228s.

Langer SZ. Presynaptic regulation of catecholamine release. *Biochem Pharmacol* 1974;23:1793–1800.

Langer SZ. Presynaptic regulation of the release of catecholamines. *Pharmacol Rev* 1981;32:337–362.

Langer SZ. The metabolism of [^{3}H]noradrenaline released by electrical stimulation from the isolated nictitating membrane of the cat and from the vas deferens of the rat. *J Physiol (Lond)* 1970;208:515–546.

Langman J. *Medical Embryology.* Baltimore: Williams & Wilkins, 1969.

Langosch W, Brodner G, Borcherding H. Psychological and vocational longterm outcomes of cardiac rehabilitation with post-infarction patients under the age of forty. *Psychother Psychosom* 1983;40:115–128.

Lanzmann C. Shoah. *An Oral History of the Holocaust.* New York: Pantheon Books, 1985.

Lappe R, Henry D, Willis L. Contribution of renal sympathetic nerves to the urinary excretion of norepinephrine. *Can J Physiol Pharmacol* 1982;60:1067–1072.

Larsson PT, Hjemdahl P, Olsson G, Angelin B, Hornstra G. Platelet aggregability in humans: contrasting in vivo and in vitro findings during sympatho-adrenal activation and relationship to serum lipids. *Eur J Clin Invest* 1990;20:398–405.

Lathers CM, Tumer N, Schoffstall JM. Plasma catecholamines, pH, and blood pressure during cardiac arrest in pigs. *Resuscitation* 1989;18:59–74.

Lauria P, Sharma VN, Vanjani S. Effect of prolonged stress of repeated electric shock on rat myocardium. *Ind J Physiol Pharmacol* 1972;16:315–318.

Lavian G, Di Bona G, Finberg JPM. Inhibition of sympathetic nerve activity by acute administration of the tricyclic antidepressant desipramine. *Eur J Pharmacol* 1991;194:153–159.

Lavicky J, Dunn AJ. Corticotropin-releasing factor stimulates catecholamine release in hypothalamus and prefrontal contrex in freely moving rats as assessed by microdialysis. *J Neurochem* 1993;60:602–612.

Lawler JE, Barker GF, Hubbard JW, Schaub RG. Effects of stress on blood pressure and cardiac pathology in rats with borderline hypertension. *Hypertension* 1981;3:496–505.

Lawrence AM. Glucagon provocation test for pheochromocytoma. *Ann Int Med* 1967;66:1091–1096.

Lay DC Jr, Friend TH, Randel RD, Bowers CL, Grissom KK, Jenkins OC. Behavioral and physiological effects of freeze or hot-iron branding on crossbred cattle. *J Anim Sci* 1992;70:330–336.

Lazarus RS. *Emotion and Adaptation.* New York: Oxford University Press, 1991.

Lazarus RS. *Psychological Stress and the Coping Process.* New York: McGraw-Hill, 1966.

Leatham A. Carotid sinus syncope. *Br Heart J* 1982;47:409–410.

LeBlanc JJ, Cote M, Jobin M, Labrie A. Plasma catecholamines and cardiovascular responses to cold and mental activity. *J Appl Physiol* 1979;47:1207–1211.

Ledsome JR, Linden RJ. A reflex increase in heart rate from distension of the pulmonary vein-atrial junctions. *J Physiol (Lond)* 1964;170:456–473.

Ledsome JR, Ngsee J, Wilson N. Plasma vasopressin concentration in the anesthetized dog before, during and after atrial distension. *J Physiol (Lond)* 1983;338:413–421.

Lee DD, Kimura S, DeQuattro V, Davison G. Relaxation therapy lowers blood pressure more effectively in hypertensives with raised plasma norepinephrine and blunts pressor response to anger. *Clin Exp Hyper* 1989;11 (Suppl. 1):191–198.

Lee JC, Sponenberg DP. The contribution of the alpha adrenoceptor system to the pathogenesis of norepinephrine cardiomyopathy. In Beamish RE, Panagia, V, Dhalla NS (Eds) *Pathogenesis of Stress-Induced Heart Disease.* Boston: Martinus Nijhoff, 1984, pp 251–260.

Lee RMKW, Triggle CR, Cheung DWT, Coughlin MD. Structural and functional consequence of neonatal sympathectomy on the blood vessels of spontaneously hypertensive rats. *Hypertension* 1987;10:328–338.

Leeb-Lundberg LM, Cotecchia S, De Blasi A, Caron MG, Lefkowitz RJ. Regulation of adrenergic receptor function by phosphorylation. I. Agonist-promoted desensitization and phosphorylation of α_1-adrenergic receptors coupled to inositol phospholipid metabolism in DDT, MF-2 smooth muscle cells. *J Biol Chem* 1987;262:3098–3105.

Lefkowitz RJ, Hoffman BB, Taylor P. Drugs acting at synaptic and neuroeffector junctional sites. In Gilman AG, Rall TW, Nies AS, Taylor P (Eds) *Goodman and Gilman's The Pharmacological Basis of Therapeutics.* New York: Pergamon, 1990, pp 84–121.

Leier CV, Binkley PF, Cody RF. α-adrenergic component of the sympathetic nervous system in congestive heart failure. *Circulation* 1990;82 (Suppl. I):I68–I76.

Leimbach WN, Wallin BG, Victor RG, Aylward PE, Sundlof G, Mark AL. Direct evidence from intraneuronal recordings for increased central sympathetic outflow in patients with heart failure. *Circulation* 1986;73:913–919.

Leitz FH, Stefano FJE. Effect of ouabain and desipramine on the uptake and storage of norepinephrine and metaraminol. *Eur J Pharmacol* 1970;11:278–285.

Lekan H, Gary HE Jr, Eisenberg HM. Cerebral metabolic and hormonal activations during hemorrhage in sinoaortic-denervated rats. *Am J Physiol* 1990;259:R305–R312.

Lenders JWM, de Boo T, Lemmens WA, Willemsen JJ, Thien T. Cardiovascular responsiveness to norepinephrine in mild essential hypertension. *Am J Cardiol* 1989b;63:1231–1234.

Lenders JWM, Eisenhofer G, Armando I, Keiser HR, Goldstein DS, Kopin IJ. Determination of plasma metanephrines by liquid chromatography with electrochemical detection. *Clin Chem* 1993;39:97–103.

Lenders JWM, Fast JH, Blankers J, De Boo T, Lemmens WAJ, Thien T. Normal sympathetic neural activity in patients with mitral valve prolapse. *Clin Cardiol* 1986;9:177–182.

Lenders JWM, Kvetnansky R, Pacak K, Goldstein DS, Kopin IJ, Eisenhofer G. Extraneuronal metabolism of endogenous and exogenous norepinephrine and epinephrine in rats. *J Pharmacol Exp Ther* 1993;266:288–293.

Lenders JWM, Willemsen JJ, Beissel T, Kloppenborg PWC, Thien T, Benrad TJ. Value of the plasma norepinephrine/3,4-dihydroxyphenylglycol ratio for the diagnosis of pheochromocytoma. *Am J Med* 1992;92;147–152.

Lenders JWM, Willemsen JJ, de Boo T, Lemmens WAJ, Thien T. Disparate effects of mental stress on plasma noradrenaline in young normotensive and hypertensive subjects. *J Hypertens* 1989a;7:317–323.

LeNoble LM, Lappe RW, Brody MJ, Struyker-Boudier HA, Smits JF. Selective efferent chemical sympathectomy of rat kidneys. Selective destruction of renal afferent versus efferent nerves in rats. *Am J Physiol* 1985;249:R496–R501.

Lenz HJ, Raedler A, Greten H, Brown MR. CRF initiates actions within the brain that are observed in response to stress. *Am J Physiol* 1987;252:R34–R39.

Leone C, Gordon FJ. Is L-glutamate a neurotransmitter of baroreceptor information in the nucleus of the tractus solitarius? *J Pharmacol Exp Ther* 1989;250:953–962.

Leriche RL, Hermann L, Fontaine R. Ligature de la coronaire gauche et fonction de colur apres enervation sympathique. *Compt Rend Soc de Biol* 1931;107:547–548.

Lerner P, Major LF, Dendel PS, Ziegler MG. Differential effects of DL-propranolol on norepinephrine in cerebrospinal fluid and plasma. *Brain Res* 1981;223:444–447.

Leszczyszyn DJ, Jankowski JA, Viveros OH, Diliberto EJ Jr, Near JA, Wightman RM. Nicotinic receptor-mediated catecholamine secretion from individual chromaffin cells. Chemical evidence for exocytosis. *J Biol Chem* 1990;265:14736–14737.

Leszczyszyn DJ, Jankowski JA, Viveros OH, Diliberto EJ Jr, Near JA, Wightman RM. Secretion of catecholamines from individual adrenal medullary chromaffin cells. *J Neurochem* 1991; 56:1855–1863.

Letizia C, Scavo D. Meta-iodobenzylguanidine seen inthe diagnosis of pathologic conditions of the adrenal medulla (pheochromocytoma). *Arch Int Med* 1990;150:1541–1542.

Leuenberger U, Gleeson K, Wroblewski K, Prophet S, Zelis R, Zwilliach C, Sinoway L. Norepinephrine clearance is increased during acute hypoxemia in humans. *Am J Physiol* 1991; 261:H1659–H1664.

Levav I, Abrahamson JH. Emotional distress among concentration camp survivors: A community study in Jersusalem. *Psychol Med* 1984;14:215–218.

Levi L. The urinary output of adrenaline and noradrenaline during pleasant and unpleasant emotional states. A preliminary study. *Psychosom Med* 1965;27:80–85.

Levi-Montalcini R. The nerve growth factor 35 years later. *Science* 1987;237:1154–1162.

Levin BE, Hubschmann OR. Dorsal column stimulation: Effect on human cerebrospinal fluid and plasma catecholamines. *Neurology* 1980;30:65–71.

Levin BE, Sullivan AC. Glucose, insulin and sympathoadrenal activation. *J Auton Nerv Sys* 1987; 20:233–242.

Levin BE. Glucose increases rat plasma norepinephrine levels by direct action in the brain. *Am J Physiol* 1991;261:R1351–R1357.

Levine ES, Litto WJ, Jacobs BL. Activity of cat locus coeruleus noradrenergic neurons during the defense reaction. *Brain Res* 1990;531:189–195.

Levine S, Coe C, Wiener S. The psychoneuroendocrinology of stress: A psychobiological perspective. In Levine S, Brush R (Eds) *Psychoendocrinology*. New York: Academic Press, 1989, pp 181–207.

Levine S, Ursin H. What is stress? In Brown MR, Koob GF, Rivier C (Eds) *Stress. Neurobiology and Neuroendocrinology*. New York: Marcel Dekker, 1991, pp 3–21.

Levine TB, Cohn JN. Determinants of acute and long-term response to converting enzyme inhibitors in congestive heart failure. *Am Heart J* 1982;104 (5 Pt. 2):1159–1164.

Levine TB, Olivari MT, Cohn JN. Dissociation of the responses of the renin-angiotensin system and sympathetic nervous system to a vasodilator stimulus in congestive heart failure. *Int J Cardiol* 1986a;12:165–173.

Levine TB, Olivari MT, Cohn JN. Effects of orthotopic heart transplantation on sympathetic control mechanisms in congestive heart failure. *Am J Cardiol* 1986b;58:1035–1040.

Levinson PD, Goldstein DS, Munson PJ, Gill JR Jr, Keiser HR. Endocrine, renal, and hemodynamic responses to graded dopamine infusions in normal subjects. *J Clin Endocrinol Metab* 1985;60:621–826.

Levitan IB. Phosphorylation of ion channels. *J Memb Biol* 1985;87:177–190.

Levitt P, Moore RY. Origin and organization of brainstem catecholamine innervation in the rat. *J Comp Neurol* 1979;186:505–528.

Levy MN, Blattberg B. Effect of vagal stimulation on the overflow of norepinephrine into the coronary sinus during cardiac sympathetic nerve stimulation in the dog. *Circ Res* 1976; 38:81–84.

Levy MN, Martin P. Parasympathetic control of the heart. In Randall WC (Ed) *Nervous Control of Cardiovascular Function.* New York: Oxford University Press, 1984, pp 68–94.

Levy MN, Zieske H. Autonomic control of cardiac pacemaker activity and atrioventricular transmission. *J Appl Physiol* 1969;27:465–470.

Levy MN. Sympathetic-parasympathetic interactions in the heart. *Circ Res* 1971;29:437–445.

Levy MN. Sympathetic-parasympathetic interactions in the heart. In Kulbertus HE, Franck G (Eds) *Neurocardiology.* Mount Kisco, NY: Futura, 1988, pp 85–98.

Lewis SJ, Verberne AJ, Robinson TG, Jarrott B, Louis WJ, Beart PM. Excitotoxin-induced lesions of the central but not basolateral nucleus of the amygdala modulate the baroreceptor heart rate reflex in conscious rats. *Brain Res* 1989;494:232–240.

Li P, Lovick TA. Excitatory projections from hypothalamic and midbrain defense regions to nucleus paragigantocellularis lateralis in the rat. *Exp Neurol* 1985;89:543–553.

Li YW, Halliday GM, Joh TH, Geffen LB, Blessing WW. Tyrosine hydroxylase-containing neurons in the supraoptic and paraventricular nuclei of the adult human. *Brain Res* 1988; 461:75–86.

Liang C-S, Fan T-H M, Sullebarger JT, Sakamoto S. Decreased adrenergic neuronal uptake activity in experimental right heart failure. A chamber-specific contributor to beta-adrenoceptor downregulation. *J Clin Invest* 1989;84:1267–1275.

Liard J-F. Renal denervation delays blood pressure increase in the spontaneously hypertensive rat. *Experientia* 1977;33:339–340.

Light KC, Koepke JP, Obrist PA, Willis PW. Psychological stress induces sodium and fluid retention in men at high risk for hypertension. *Science* 1983;220:429–431.

Liljefors I, Rahe RH. An identical twin study of psychosocial factors in coronary heart disease in Sweden. *Psychosom Med* 1970;32:523–542.

Lillywhite HB. Snakes, blood circulation and gravity. *Sci Am,* December, 1988, pp 92–98.

Limas CJ, Limas C. Cardiac adrenergic receptors in cardiovascular diseases. In Ganguly PK (Ed) *Catecholamines and Heart Disease.* Boca Raton: CRC Press, 1991, pp 201–216.

Limbird LE. Receptors linked to inhibition of adenylate cyclase: additional signaling mechanisms. *FASEB J* 1988;2:2686–2695.

Linares OA, Zech LA, Jacquez JA, Rosen SG, Sanfield JA, Morrow LA, Supiano MA, Halter JB. Effect of sodium-restricted diet and posture on norepinephrine kinetics in humans. *Am J Physiol* 1988;254:E222–E230.

Linden CH, Vellman WP, Rumack B. Yohimbine: A new street drug. *Ann Emerg Med* 1985;14: 1002–1004.

Linden RJ, Kappagoda CT. *Atrial Receptors.* Cambridge, UK: Cambridge University Press, 1982.

Linden RJ, Sreeharan N. Humoral nature of urine response to stimulation of atrial receptors. *Q J Exp Physiol* 1981;66:431–438.

Linden RJ. Sensory endings in the heart with comment on excitatory reflexes. In Lown B, Malliani A, Prosdocimi M (Eds) *Neural Mechanisms and Cardiovascular Disease.* New York: Springer Verlag, 1986, pp 11–33.

Lindmar R, Loffelholz K, Muscholl E. Muscarinic mechanism inhibiting the release of noradrenaline from peripheral adrenergic nerve fibers by nicotinic agents. *Br J Pharmacol* 1968; 32:280–294.

Lindvall M, Edvinsson L, Owman C. Sympathetic nervous control of cerebrospinal fluid production from the choroid plexus. *Science* 1978;201:176–178.

Lindvall O, Bjorklund A. The organization of the ascending catecholamine neuron sysems in the rat brain as revealed by the glyoxylic acid fluorescence method. *Acta Physiol Scand* 1974; Suppl 412:1–48.

Little RA, Frayn KN, Randall PE, Yates DW. Plasma catecholamines and cardiac arrest. *Lancet* 1985;ii:509–510.

Liu Y, Peter D, Roghani A, Shuldiner S, Prive GG, Eisenberg D, Brecha N, Edwards RH. A cDNA that suppresses MPP$^+$ toxicity encodes a vesicular amine transporter. *Cell* 1992; 70:539–551.

Llinas R, McGuiness TL, Leonard CS, Sugimori M, Greengard P. Intraterminal injection of synapsin I or calcium/calmodulin-dependent protein kinase II alters neurotransmitter release at the squid giant synapse. *Proc Nat Acad Sci USA* 1985;82:3035–3039.

Lo M, Julien C, Barres C, Boomsma F, Cerutti C, Vincent M, Sassard J. Blood pressure maintenance in hypertensive sympathectomized rats. I. Adrenal medullary catecholamines. *Am J Physiol* 1991a;261:R1045–R1051.

Lo M, Julien C, Barres C, Boomsma F, Cerutti C, Vincent M, Sassard J. Blood pressure maintenance in hypertensive sympathectomized rats. II. Renin-angiotensin system and vasopressin. *Am J Physiol* 1991b;261:R1052–R1056.

Loewi O, Navratil E. Uber humorale Ubertragbarkeit der Herzenvenwirkung. X. Mitteilung. Uber das Schicksal des Vagusstoffs. *Pflugers Arch* 1926;214:678–688.

Loewi O. Uber humorale Ubertragbarkeit der Herzenvenwirkung. *Pflugers Arch* 1921;189:239–242.

Loewy AD, Marson L, Parkiknson D, Perry MA, Sawyer WB. Descending noradrenergic pathways involved in the A5 depressor response. *Brain Res* 1986;386:313–324.

Loewy AD, McKellar S, Saper CB. Direct projections from the A5 catecholamine cell group to the intermediolateral cell column. *Brain Res* 1979;174:309–314.

Loffesholz K, Muscholl E. Muscarinic inhibition of the noradrenaline release evoked by postganglionic sympathetic nerve stimulation. *Naunyn-Schmiedeberg's Arch Pharmakol Exp Pathol* 1969;263:1–15.

Lokhandwala MF, Hegde SS. Cardiovascular pharmacology of dopamine receptor agonists. In Amenta F (Ed) *Peripheral Dopamine Pathophysiology*. Boca Raton, FL: CRC Press, 1990, pp 63–77.

Lombardi C, Missale C, De Cotiis R, Spedini C, Pizzoccolo G, Memo M, Albertini A, Spano PF. Inhibition of the aldosterone response to sodium depletion in man by stimulation of dopamine DA2 receptors. *Eur J Clin Pharmacol* 1988;35:323–326.

Lombardi F, Verrier RL, Lown B. Relationship between sympathetic neural activity, coronary dynamics and vulnerability to ventricular fibrillation during myocardial ischemia and reperfusion. *Am Heart J* 1983;105:958–965.

Lorenz K. *King Solomon's Ring*. New York: Thomas Y Crowell, 1952.

Lorenz K. *On Aggression.* New York: Bantam, 1963.

Lovenberg W, Bruckwick EA, Hanbauer I. ATP, cyclic-AMP, and magnesium increase the affinity of rat striatal tyrosine hydroxylase for its cofactor. *Proc Natl Acad Sci USA* 1982;72: 2955–2958.

Low JM, Harvey JT, Prys-Roberts C, Dagnino J. Studies of aneasthesia in relation to hypertension. VII: Adrenergic responses to laryngoscopy. *Br J Anaesth* 1986;58:471–477.

Lown B, Verrier RL. Neural activity and ventricular fibrillation. *N Engl J Med* 1976;294:1165–1170.

Ludbrook J, Faris IB, Iannos J, Jamieson GG, Russell WJ. Lack of effect of isometric handgrip exercise on the responses of the carotic baroreceptor reflex in man. *Clin Sci Mol Med* 1978;55:189–194.

Ludwig J Gerlich M, Halbrugge T, Graefe KH. Plasma norepinephrine and dihydroxyphenylglycol in essential hypertension. *Hypertension* 1991;17:546–552.

Ludwig J Gerlich M, Halbrugge T, Graefe KH. The synaptic noradrenaline concentraiton in humans as estimated from simultaneous measurements of plasma noradrenaline and dihydroxyphenylglycol (DOPEG). *J Neural Transm Suppl.* 1990;32:441–445.

Ludwig J, Gerhardt T, Halbrugge T, Walter J, Graefe K-H. Plasma concentrations of noradrenaline and 3,4-dihydroxyphenylethyleneglycol under conditions of enhanced sympathetic activity. *Eur J Clin Pharmacol* 1988;35:261–267.

Ludwig J, Halbrugge T, Gerlich M, Grafe K-H. Estimation of noradrenaline concentrations in the axoplasm of noradrenergic neurones in man. *Clin Auton Res* 1992;2:159–164.

Ludwig J, Halbrugge T, Vey G, Walter J, Graefe K-H. Haemodynamics as a determinant of the pharmacokinetics of and the plasma catecholamine responses to isoprenaline. *Eur J Clin Pharmacol* 1989;37:493–500.

Luft FC, Demmert G, Rohmeiss P, Unger T. Baroreceptor reflex effect on sympathetic nerve activity in stroke-prone spontaneously hypertensive rats. *J Auton Nerv Sys* 1986;17:199–209.

Luft FC, Miller JZ, Weinberger MH, Grim CE, Daugherty SA, Christian JC. Influence of genetic variance on sodium sensitivity of blood pressure. *Klin Wochenschr* 1987;65:101–109.

Luft FC, Rankin LI, Henry DP, Bloch R, Grim CE, Weyman AE, Murray RH, Weinberger MH. Plasma and urinary norepinephrine values at extremes of sodium intake in normal man. *Hypertension* 1979;1:261–266.

Luft FC, Unger T, Lang RE, Ganten D. Chemical messengers and transmitters in the brain and cardiovascular regulation. In Zanchetti A, Tarazi RC (Eds) *Handbook of Hypertension, Vol 8: Pathophysiology of Hypertension—Regulatory Mechanisms.* New York: Elsevier Science, 1986, pp 26–46.

Luger A, Deuster PA, Kyle SB, Gallucci WT, Montgomery LC, Gold PW, Loriaux L, Chrousos GP. Acute hypothalamic-pituitary-adrenal responses to the stress of treadmill exercise. Physiological adaptations to physical training. *N Engl J Med* 1987;316:1309–1315.

Lund-Johansen P. Central hemodynamics in essential hypertension at rest and during exercise: a 20-year follow-up study. *J Hypertens* 1989;7 (Suppl. 6):S52–S55.

Lund-Johansen P. Hemodynamic patterns in the natural history of borderline hypertension. *J Cardiovasc Pharmacol* 1986;8 (Suppl. 5):S8–S14.

Lundberg U, Fredrikson M, Wallin L, Melin B, Frankenhaeuser M. Blood lipids as related to cardiovascular and neuroendocrine functions under different conditions in healthy males and females. *Pharmacol Biochem Behav* 1989;33:381–386.

Lundin S, Hallback-Nordlander M. Background of hyperkinetic circulatory state in young spontaneously hypertensive rats. *Cardiovasc Res* 1982;14:561.

Lundin S, Rickstein S-E, Thoren P. Interaction between mental stress and baroreceptor control of heart rate and sympathetic activity in conscious spontaneously hypertensive (SHR) and normotensive (WKY) rats. *J Hypertens* 1983;1 (Suppl. 2):68–70.

Lundin S, Rickstein S-E, Thoren P. Interaction between "mental" stress and baroreceptor reflexes concerning effects on heart rate, mean arterial pressure and renal sympathetic activity in conscious spontaneously hypertensive rats. *Acta Physiol Scand* 1984;120:273–281.

Lundin S, Thoren P. Renal function and sympathetic activity during mental stress in normotensive and spontaneously hypertensive rats. *Acta Physiol Scand* 1982;115:115–124.

Lundin S, Thoren P. Renal function and sympathetic activity during mental stress in spontaneously hypertensive rats. *Clin Sci* 1982;63:327s–330s.

Luque JM, Guillamon A, Hwang BH. Quantitative autoradiographic study on tyrosine hydroxylase mRNA with in situ hybridization and α_2 adrenergic receptor binding in the locus coeruleus of the spontaneously hypertensive rat. *Neurosci Lett* 1991;131:163–166.

Lvgren NA, Poulsen J, Schwartz TW. Impaired pancreatic innervation after selective gastric vagotomy. Reduction of the pancreatic polypeptide response to food and insulin hypoglycemia. *Scand J Gastroenterol* 1981;16:811–816.

Macallum AB. The paleochemistry of the body fluids and tissues. *Physiol Rev* 1926;6:316–357.

Mace PJE, Watson RDS, Skan W, Littler WA. Inhibition of the baroreceptor heart rate reflex by angiotensin II in normal man. *Cardiovasc Res* 1985;19:525–527.

MacGilchrist AJ, Hawksby C, Howes LG, Reid JL. Rise in plasma noradrenaline with age results from an increase in spillover rate. *Gerontology* 1989;35:7–13.

Machado BH, Brody MJ. Mechanisms of pressor response produced by stimulation of nucleus ambiguus. *Am J Physiol* 1990;259:R955–R962.

Maclean PD. The limbic system (''visceral brain'') and emotional behavior. *Arch Neurol Psychiatry* 1955;73:130–134.

Maclean PD. The triune brain, emotion and scientific bias. In Schmitt FO (Ed) *The Neurosciences, Second Study Program.* New York: Rockefeller University Press, 1970, pp 336–348.

Magnus K, Matroos AW, Strackee J. The self-employed and the self-driven: Two coronary-prone subpopulations from the Zeist study. *Am J Epidemiol* 1983;118:799–805.

Majewski H, Tung LH, Rand MJ. Adrenaline activation of prejunctional beta-adrenoceptors and hypertension. *J Cardiovasc Pharmacol* 1982;4:99–106.

Majewski H, Tung LH, Rand MJ. *Hypertension* through adrenaline activation of prejunctional beta-adrenoceptors. *Clin Exp Pharmacol Physiol* 1981;8:463–468.

Makara GB, Kvetnansky R, Jezova D, Jindra A, Kakucska I, Oprasalova Z. Plasma catecholamines do not participate in pituitary-adrenal activation by immobilization stress in rats with transection of nerve fibers to the median eminence. *Endocrinology* 1986;119:1757–1762.

Malliani A, Lombardi F, Pagani M, Cerutti S. The neural regulation of circulation explored in the frequency domain. *J Auton Nerv Sys* 1990;30:S103–S108.

Malliani A, Pagani M, Lombardi F, Furlan R, Guzzetti S, Cerutti S. Spectral analysis to assess increased sympathetic tone in arterial hypertension. *Hypertension* 1991;17 (Suppl. III): III36–III42.

Malliani A, Pagani M, Lombardi F. Positive feedback reflexes. In Zanchetti A, Tarazi RC (Eds) *Handbook of Hypertension,* Vol 8: *Pathophysiology of Hypertension—Regulatory Mechanisms.* New York: Elsevier Science, 1986, pp 69–81.

Malliani A, Schwartz PJ, Zanchetti A. A sympathetic reflex elicited by experimental coronary occlusion. *Am J Physiol* 1969;217:703–709.

Malliani A. Homeostasis and instability: The hypothesis of tonic interaction in the cardiovascular regulation of negative and positive feedback mechanisms. In Lown B, Malliani A, Prosdocimi M (Eds) *Neural Mechanisms and Cardiovascular Disease.* New York: Springer Verlag, 1986, pp 1–9.

Malmfors T. Studies on adrenergic nerves. *Acta Physiol Scand* 1965;64 (Suppl. 248):1–93.

Man in't Veld AJ, Boomsma H, Moleman P, Schalekamp MADH. Congenital dopamine-beta-hydroxylase deficiency. *Lancet* 1987;1:183–188.

Mancia G, Baccelli G, Zanchetti A. Hemodynamic responses to different emotional stimuli in the cat: patterns and mechanisms. *Am J Physiol* 1972;223:925–933.

Mangiapane ML, Brody MJ. Mechanisms of hemodynamic responses to electrical stimulation of subfornical organ. *Am J Physiol* 1986;250:R1117–R1122.

Mangiapane ML, Brody MJ. Vasoconstrictor and vasodilator sites within anteroventral third ventricle region. *Am J Physiol* 1987;253:R827–R831.

Manning GW, McEachern CG, Hall GE. Reflex coronary artery spasm following sudden occlusion of coronary branches. *Arch Int Med* 1939;64:661–674.

Manning JW, Cotten MD. Mechanisms of cardiac arrhythmias induced by diencephalic stimulation. *Am J Physiol* 1962;203:1120–1124.

Manuck SB, Kaplan JR, Clarkson TB. Behaviorally-induced heart rate reactivity and atherosclerosis in cynomolgus monkeys. *Psychosom Med* 1983;45:95–108.

Mark AL, Kerber RE. Augmentation of cardiopulmonary baroreflex control of forearm vascular resistance in borderline hypertension. *Hypertension* 1982;4:39–46.

Mark AL. Regulation of sympathetic nerve activity in mild human hypertension. *J Hypertens* 1990;8 (Suppl. 7):S67–S75.

Markovitz JH, Matthews KA, Wing RR, Kuller LH, Meilahn EN. Psychological, biological and health behavior predictors of blood pressure changes in middle-aged women. *J Hypertens* 1991;9:399–406.

Marmot MG, Syme SL. Acculturation and coronary heart disease in Japanese-Americans. *Am J Epidemiol* 1976;104:225–247.

Marsden CA. A critical assessment of methods for monitoring noradrenaline release *in vivo.* In Heal DJ, Marsden CA (Eds) *The Pharmacology of Noradrenaline in the Central Nervous System.* New York: Oxford University Press, 1990, pp 155–186.

Marson L, Kiritsy-Roy JA, Bobbitt FA, Van Loon GR. Cardiovascular and sympathoadrenal responses to intacerebral opioid peptides: Receptor specific effects at rest and during stress. In Van Loon GR, Kvetnansky R, McCarty R, Axelrod J (Eds) *Stress. Neurochemical and Humoral Mechanisms.* New York: Gordon and Breach, 1989, pp 583–597.

Martin PR, Ebert MH, Gordon EK, Linnoila M, Kopin IJ. Effects of clonidine on central and peripheral catecholamine metabolism. *Clin Pharmacol Ther* 1984;35:322–327.

Martin SM, Malkinson TJ, Bauce LG, Veale WL, Pittman QJ. Plasma catecholamines in conscious rabbits after central administration of vasopressin. *Brain Res* 1988;457:192–195.

Martin WR. Opioid antagonists. *Pharmacol Rev* 1967;19:463–521.

Marty J, Gauzit R, Lefevre P, Couderc E, Farinotti R, Henzel C, Desmonts JM. Effects of diazepam and midazolam on baroreflex control of heart rate and on sympathetic activity in humans. *Anesth Anal* 1986;65:113–119.

Maseri A, L'Abbate A, Baroldi G, Chierchia S, Marzilli M, Ballestra MM, Severi S, Parodi O, Biagini A, Distante A, Pesola A. Coronary vasospasm as a possible cause of myocardial infarction: A conclusion derived from the study of "preinfarction" angina. *N Engl J Med* 1978;1271–1277.

Maseri A, Severi S, Marzullo P. Role of coronary arterial spasms in sudden coronary ischemic death. *Ann NY Acad Sci* 1982;382:204–216.

Mason JW, Maher JT, Hartley LH, Mougey E, Perlow MJ, Jones LG. Selectivity of corticosteroid and catecholamine response to various natural stimuli. In Serban G (Ed) *Psychopathology of Human Adaptation.* New York: Plenum Press, 1976.

Mason JW. A historical view of the stress field. II. *J Hum Stress* 1975a;1:6–12, 22–36.

Mason JW. A re-evaluation of the concept of 'non-specificity' in stress theory. *J Psychiatr Res* 1971;8:323–333.

Mason JW. Emotion as reflected in patterns of endocrine integration. In Levi L (Ed) *Emotions: Their Parameters and Measurement.* New York: Raven Press, 1975b, pp 143–181.

Mason ST, Angel A. Anaesthesia: The role of adrenergic mechanisms. *Eur J Pharmacol* 1983; 91:29–39.

Mason ST, Corcoran ME. Catecholamines and convulsions. *Brain Res* 1979;170:497–507.

Mason ST, Iversen SD. Theories of the dorsal bundle extinction effect. *Brain Res Rev* 1979;1: 107–137.

Mason ST. *Catecholamines and Behaviour.* Cambridge, UK: Cambridge University Press, 1984.

Masserano JM, Vaulliet PR, Tank AW, Weiner N. The role of tyrosine hydroxylase in the regulation of catecholamine synthesis. In Trendelenburg U, Weiner N (Eds) *Catecholamines II.* New York: Springer-Verlag, 1989, pp 427–469.

Massumi RA, Mason DT, Amsterdam EA, Demaria AN, Miller AR, Scheinman MN, Zelis R. Ventricular fibrillation and tachycardia after intravenous atropine for the treatment of bradycardia. *N Engl J Med* 1972;287:336–338.

Masuo K, Ogihara T, Kumahara Y, Tamatodani A, Wada H. Increased plasma norepinephrine in young patients with essential hypertension under three sodium intakes. *Hypertension* 1984;6:315–321.

Masuyama Y, Tsuda K, Kuchii M, Nishio I. Peripheral neural mechanism of hypertension in rat models—peripheral sympathetic neurotransmission in hypertension. *J Hypertens* 1986a; 4:S189–S192.

Masuyama Y, Ueno Y, Arita M, Suruda H, Mohara O. Changes of plasma and cerebrospinal fluid noradrenaline during frusemide administration and acute renal artery constriction in dogs. *Clin Sci* 1982b;63:343s–345s.

Masuyama Y. Responses to antihypertensive agents in relation to the pathogenic factors in essential hypertension. *Jpn J Med* 1982;21:158–160.

Mathias CJ, Bannister R. Investigation of autonomic disorders. In Bannister R, Mathias CJ (Eds) *Autonomic Failure.* New York: Oxford University Press, 1992, pp 255–290.

Mathias CJ, Christensen NJ, Corbett JL, Frankel HL, Spaulding JMK. Plasma catecholamines during paroxysmal neurogenic hypertension in quadriplegic man. *Circ Res* 1976;39:204–208.

Mathias CJ, Frankel HL. Autonomic failure in tetraplegia. In: Bannister R (Ed) *Autonomic Failure.* New York: Oxford University Press, 1983, pp 453–488.

Mathias CJ. Role of the sympathetic efferent nerves in blood pressure regulation and in hypertension. *Hypertension* 1991;18 (Suppl III):III22–III30.

Matoba T, Adachi K, Ito T, Yamashita Y, Chiba M, Odawara K, Inuzuka S, Toshima H. Cardiac hypertrophy in surgically denervated dogs with aortic stenosis. *Experientia* 1984;40:73–75.

Matsukawa K, Gotoh E, Hasegawa O, Shionoiri H, Tochikubo O, Ishii M. Reduced baroreflex changes in muscle sympathetic nerve activity during blood pressure elevation in essential hypertension. *J Hypertens* 1991a;9:537–542.

Matsukawa K, Honda T, Ninomiya I. Renal sympathetic nerve activity and plasma catecholamines during eating in cats. *Am J Physiol* 1989;257:R1034–R1039.

Matsukawa T, Gotoh E, Uneda S, Miyajima E, Shionoiri H, Tochikubo O, Ishii M. Augmented sympathetic nerve activity in response to stressors in young borderline hypertensive men. *Acta Physiol Scand* 1991b;141:157–165.

Matsukawa T, Miyajima E, Yameda Y, Uneda S, Tochikubo O, Kaneko Y. Increased response of muscle sympathetic nerve activity to cold pressor test in borderline hypertension. *Clin Exp Hyper* 1987;A9:829.

Matsumoto M, Togashi H, Yoshioka M, Morii K, Hirokami M, Tochihara M, Ikeda T, Saito Y,

Saito H. Significant correlation between cerebrospinal fluid and brain levels of norepinephrine, serotonin and acetylcholine in anesthetized rats. *Life Sci* 1991;48:823–829.

Matta RJ, Lawler JE, Lown B. Ventricular electrical instability in the conscious dog. Effects of psychologic stress and beta adrenergic blockade. *Am J Cardiol* 1976;38:594–598.

Matthews KA, Haynes SG. Type A behavior pattern and coronary disease risk. Update and critical evaluation. *Am J Epidemiol* 1986;123:923–960.

Mauck HO, Hockman CH, Hoff EC. ECG changes after cerebral stimulation of the mesencephalic reticular formation. *Am Heart J* 1964;68:98–101.

May GS, Eberlein KA, Furberg CD, Passamani ER, DeMets DL. Secondary prevention after myocardial infarction: A review of long-term trials. *Prog Cardiovasc Dis* 1982;24:331–335.

Mayer N, Zimpfer M, Kotai E, Placheta P. Enflurane alters compensatory hemodynamic and humoral responses to hemorrhage. *Circ Shock* 1990;30:165–178.

McAllen RM, Neil JJ, Loewy AD. Effects of kainic acid applied to the ventral surface of the medulla oblongata on vasomotor tone, the baroreceptor reflex and hypothalamic autonomic responses. *Brain Res* 1982;238:65–76.

McAllen RM. Identification and properties of sub-retrofacial bulbospinal neurones: A descending cardiovascular pathway. *J Auton Nerv Sys* 1986;17:151–164.

McCall RB, Schuette MR, Humphrey SJ, Lahti RA, Barsuhn C. Evidence for a central sympathoexcitatory action of alpha-2 adrenergic antagonists. *J Pharmacol Exp Ther* 1983;224:501–507.

McCall RB. Central neurotransmitters involved in cardiovascular regulation. In Antonaccio MJ (Ed) *Cardiovascular Pharmacology*. New York: Raven Press, 1990, pp 161–200.

McCall RB. GABA-mediated inhibition of sympathoexcitatory neurons by midline medullary stimulation. *Am J Physiol* 1988;255:R605–R615.

McCance AJ, Forfar JC. Cardiac and whole body [^{3}H]noradrenaline kinetics in ischaemic heart disease: contrast between unstable anginal syndromes and pacing induced ischaemia. *Br Heart J* 1989b;61:238–247.

McCance AJ, Forfar JC. Plasma noradrenaline as an index of sympathetic tone in coronary arterial disease: The confounding infuence of clearance of noradrenaline. *Int J Cardiol* 1990;26:335–342.

McCance AJ, Forfar JC. Selective enhancement of the cardiac sympathetic response to exercise by anginal chest pain in humans. *Circulation* 1989a;80:1642–1651.

McCance AJ. Assessment of sympathoneural activity in clinical research. *Life Sci* 1991;48:713–721.

McCarty R, Konarska M, Stewart RE. Adaptation to stress: A learned response? In Kvetnansky R, McCarty R, Axelrod J (Eds) *Stress: Neuroendocrine and Molecular Approaches*. New York: Gordon and Breach, 1992, pp 521–535.

McCarty R, Kopin IJ. Alterations in plasma catecholamines and behavior during acute stress in spontaneously hypertensive and Wistar-Kyoto normotensive rats. *Life Sci* 1978;22:997–1005.

McCarty R. Physiological and behavioral responses of New Zealand hypertensive and normotensive rats to stress. *Physiol Behav* 1981;28:103–108.

McCubbin JW, Green JH, Page IH. Baroreceptor function in chronic renal hypertension. *Circ Res* 1956;4:205–210.

McCubbin JW, Kaneko Y, Page IH. Ability of serotonin and norepinephrine to mimic the central effects of reserpine on vasomotor activity. *Circ Res* 1960;8:849–858.

McDonald RH Jr, Goldberg LI, McNay JL, Tuttle EP Jr. Effects of dopamine in man: Augmentation of sodium excretion, glomerular filtration rate, and renal plasma flow. *J Clin Invest* 1964;43:1116–1124.

McEwen BS, Lambdin LT, Rainbow TC, De Nicola AF. Aldosterone effects on salt appetite in adrenalectomized rats. *Neuroendocrinology* 1986;43:38-43.

McFarlan D (Ed) *The Guiness Book of World Records*. New York: Bantam Books, 1992.

McGrady A, Higgins JT Jr. Prediction of response to biofeedback-assisted relaxation in hypertensives: Development of a hypertensive predictor profile (HYPP). *Psychosom Med* 1989; 51:277-284.

McGrath BP, Lim SP, Leversha L, Shanahan A. Myocardial and peripheral catecholamine responses to acute coronary artery constriction before and after propranolol treatment in the anesthetized dog. *Cardiovasc Res* 1981;15:28–34.

McKellar S, Loewy AD. Efferent projections of the A1 catecholamine group in the rat: An autoradiographic study. *Brain Res* 1982;241:11–29.

McNair JL, Clower BR, Sandford RA. The effects of reserpine pretreatment on myocardial damage associated with simulated intracranial hemorrhage in mice. *Eur J Pharmacol* 1970;9:1–6.

McWhirter N. *Guiness Book of World Records*. New York: Bantam, 1980, p. 665.

Medvedev OS, Delle M, Thoren P. 2-deoxy-D-glucose-induced central glycopenia differentially influences renal and adrenal nerve activity in awake SHR rats. *Clin Exp Hyper* 1988;A10 (Suppl. 1):375–381.

Meeley MP, Ernsberger PR, Granata AR, Reis DJ. An endogenous clonidine-displacing substance from bovine brain: receptor binding and hypotensive actions in the ventrolateral medulla. *Life Sci* 1986;38:1119–1126.

Meerson FZ, Khalfen ES, Liamina NP. Effects of stress and exercise on rhythm activity of the heart and state of adrenergic regulation in patients with neurocirculatory dystonia. *Kardiologiia* 1990;30:56–59.

Meert TF, Noorduin H, Vercauteren M, De Kock M. Pharmacological interactions between α_2-adrenergic agonists and opioids. *Reg Anesthe* 1993; 18 (Suppl.):27.

Meisel SR, Kutz I, Dayan KI, Pauzner H, Chetboun I, Arbel Y, David D. Effect of Iraqi missile war on incidence of acute myocardial infarction and sudden death in Israeli citizens. *Lancet* 1991;338:660–661, 1991.

Melcher A, Donald DE. Maintained ability of carotid baroreflex to regulate arterial pressure during exercise. *Am J Physiol* 1981;241:H838–H849.

Meller ST, Gebhart GF. A critical review of the afferent pathways and the potential chemical mediators involved in cardiac pain. *Neuroscience* 1992;48:501–524.

Melville KI, Blum B, Shister HE, Silver MD. Cardiac ischemic changes in arrhythmias induced by hypothalamic stimulation. *Am J Cardiol* 1963;12:781–791.

Melville KI, Garvey HL, Shister H, Knaack J. Central nervous system stimulation and cardiac ischemic changes in monkeys. *Ann NY Acad Sci* 1969;156:241–260.

Meredith IT, Broughton A, Jennings GL, Esler MD. Evidence of a selective increase in cardiac sympathetic activity in patients with sustained ventricular arrhythmias. *N Engl J Med* 1991;325:618–624.

Meredith IT, Eisenhofer G, Lambert GW, Jennings GL, Thompson J, Esler MD. Plasma norepinephrine responses to head-up tilt are misleading in autonomic failure. *Hypertension* 1992;19:628–633.

Meredith IT, Esler MD, Lambert GW, Jennings GL, Eisenhofer G. Biochemical evidence of sympathetic denervation of the heart in pure autonomic failure. *Clin Auton Res* 1991;1: 187–194.

Mermet C, Suaud-Chagny MF, Gonon F. Electrically evoked noradrenaline release in the rat hypothalamic paraventricular nucleus studied by in vivo electrochemistry: Autoregulation by alpha-2 receptors. *Neuroscience* 1990;34:423–432.

Metz SA, Halter JB, Porte D, Jr, Robertson RP. Autonomic epilepsy: Clonidine blockade of paroxysmal catecholamine release and flushing. *Ann Int Med* 1978;88:189–193.

Micalizzi ER, Pals DT. Evaluation of plasma norepinephrine as an index of sympathetic neuron function in the conscious, unrestrained rat. *Life Sci* 1979;24:2071–2076.

Michel MC, Brodde O-E, Schnepel B, Behrendt J, Tschada R, Motulsky HJ, Insel PA. [^{3}H]Idazoxan and some other α_2-adrenergic drugs also bind with high affinity to a nonadrenergic site. *Molec Pharmacol* 1989;35:324–330.

Michel MC, Regan JW, Gerhardt MA, Neubig RR, Insel PA, Motulsky HJ. Nonadrenergic [^{3}H]idazoxan binding sites are physically distinct from α_2-adrenergic receptors. *Molec Pharmacol* 1990;37:65–68.

Mifflin SW, Felder RB. Synaptic mechanisms regulating cardiovascular afferent inputs to solitary tract nucleus. *Am J Physiol* 1990;259:H653–H661.

Mikami H, Bumpus FM, Ferrario CM. Hierarchy of blood pressure control mechanisms after spinal sympathectomy. *J Hypertens* Suppl 1983;1:62–65.

Mikami H, Bumpus FM, Ferrario CM. Hierarchy of blood pressure control mechanisms after spinal sympathectomy. *J Hypertens* 1983;1 (Suppl 2):62–65.

Miki K, Hayashida Y, Sagawa S, Shiraki K. Renal sympathetic nerve activity and natriuresis during water immersion in conscious dogs. *Am J Physiol* 1989;256:R299–R305.

Milei J, Nunez RB, Bolomo NJ. Isoproterenol-induced ^{45}Ca uptake into myocardium of rats. *Res Exp Med* 1979;176:117–121.

Miller J. *The Body in Question.* New York: Vintage Books, 1978.

Miller JA, Floras JS, Skorecki KL, Blendis LM, Logan AG. Renal and humoral responses to sustained cardiopulmonary deactivation in humans. *Am J Physiol* 1991;260:R642–R648.

Miller JZ, Luft FC, Grim CE, Henry DP, Christian JC, Weinberger MH. Genetic influences on plasma and urinary norepinephrine after volume expansion and contraction in normal men. *J Clin Endocrinol Metab* 1980;50:219–222.

Miller NE. Learning of visceral and glandular responses. *Science* 1969;163:434–445.

Millhorn DE, Guyenet P, Kiley JP. Neurobiology of brain stem cardiopulmonary control mechanisms. *J Appl Physiol* 1990;69:1916–1920.

Mills DCB, Roberts GCK. Effects of adrenaline on human blood platelets. *J Physiol (Lond)* 1967;193:443–453.

Mills E, Wang SC. Liberation of antidiuretic hormone: location of ascending pathways. *Am J Physiol* 1964;207:1399–1404.

Minami M, Sano M, Togashi H, Endo T, Saito I, Nomura A, Saito H, Nakamura N, Kurimoto F, Sakurai H. The factors affecting plasma catecholamines concentration in rats and man. *Nippon Yakurigaku Zasshi* 1984;83:17–31.

Minardo JD, Tuli MM, Mock BH, Weiner RE, Pride HP, Wellman HN, Zipes DP. Scintigraphic and electrophysiological evidence of canine sympathetic denervation and reinnervation produced by myocardial infarction or phenol application. *Circulation* 1988;78:1008–1019.

Miner LL, Kaplan BB. Trans-synaptic regulation of rat adrenal tyrosine hydroxylase gene expression during cold stress. In Kvetnansky R, McCarty R, Axelrod J (Eds) *Stress: Neuroendocrine and Molecular Approaches.* New York: Gordon and Breach, 1992, pp 313–324.

Minisi AJ, Thames MD. Activation of cardiac sympathetic afferents during coronary occlusion. Evidence for reflex activation of sympathetic nervous system during transmural myocardial ischemia in the dog. *Circulation* 1991;84:357–367.

Minneman KP, Hegstrand LR, Molinoff PB. Simultaneous determination of beta$_1$ and beta$_2$ adrenergic receptors in tissues containing both receptor subtypes. *Mol Pharmacol* 1979;16:34–46.

Minneman KP, Pittman RN, Molinoff PB. Beta-adrenergic receptor subtypes: properties, distribution and regulation. *Ann Rev Neurosci* 1981;4:419–461.

Minson J, Chalmers J, Kapoor V, Cain M, Caon A. Relative importance of sympathetic nerves and of circulating adrenaline and vasopressin in mediating hypertension after lesions of the caudal ventrolateral medulla in the rat. *J Hypertens* 1986;4:273–281.

Mirowski M, Mower MM, Reid PR. The automatic impantable defibillator. *Am Heart J* 1980; 100:1089–1092.

Missale C, Lombardi C, De Cotiis R, Memo M, Carruba MO, Spano PF. Dopaminergic receptor mechanisms modulating the renin-angiotensin system and aldosterone secretion: An overview. *J Cardiovasc Pharmacol* 1989;14:S29–S39.

Missale C, Memo M, Liberini P, Spano P. Dopamine selectively inhibits angiotensin II-induced aldosterone secretion by interacting with D-2 receptors. *J Pharmacol Exp Ther* 1988;246: 1137–1143.

Mitrakou A, Mokan M, Bolli G, Veneman T, Jenssen T, Cryer P, Gerich J. Evidence against the hypothesis that hyperinsulinemia increases sympathetic nervous system activity in man. *Metabolism* 1992;41:198–200.

Miura M, Reis DJ. A blood pressure response from fastigial nucleus and its relay pathway in brainstem. *Am J Physiol* 1970;219:1330–1336.

Miura M, Reis DJ. Termination and secondary projections of carotid sinus nerve in the cat brainstem. *Am J Physiol* 1969;217:142–153.

Miura Y, DeQuattro V. Biochemical evaluation of sympathetic nerve tone in essential hypertension. *Jpn Circ J* 1975;39:583–589.

Miyawaki T, Kawamura H, Komatsu K, Yasugi T. Chemical stimulation of the locus coeruleus: inhibitory effects on hemodynamics and renal symapthetic nerve activity. *Brain Res* 1991; 568:101–108.

Mohanty PK, Thames MD, Arrowood JA, Sowers JR, McNamara C, Szentpetery S. Impairment of cardiopulmonary baroreflex after cardiac transplantation in humans. *Circulation* 1987; 75:914–921.

Mohring J, Kintz J, Schoun J, McNeill JR. Pressor responsiveness and cardiovascular reflex activity in spontaneously hypertensive and normotensive rats during vasopressin infusion. *J Cardiovasc Pharmacol* 1981;3:948–957.

Mohrman DE, Feigl EO. Competition between sympathetic vasoconstriction and metabolic vasodilation in the canine coronary circulation. *Circ Res* 1978;42:79–86.

Molderings G, Likungu J, Zerkowski HR, Gothert M. Presynaptic beta 2-adrenoceptors on the sympathetic nerve fibres of the human saphenous vein: no evidence for involvement in adrenaline-mediated positive feedback loop regulating noradrenergic transmission. *Naunyn Schmiedeberg's Arch Pharmacol* 1988a;337:408–14.

Molderings GJ, Likungu J, Hentrich F, Gothert M. Facilitatory presynaptic angiotensin receptors on the sympathetic nerves of the human saphenous vein and pulmonary artery. Potential involvement in beta-adrenoceptor-mediated facilitation of noradrenaline release. *Naunyn Schmiedeberg's Arch Pharmacol* 1988b;338:228–33.

Morgan DA, Balon TW, Ginsberg BH, Mark AL. Nonuniform regional sympathetic nerve responses to hyperinsulinemia in rats. *Am J Physiol* 1993;264:R423–R427.

Morgan DA, Thoren P, Wilczynski EA, Victor RG, Mark AL. Serotonergic mechanisms mediate renal sympathoinhibition during severe hemorrhage in rats. *Am J Physiol* 1988;255:H496–H502.

Mori H, Pisarri TE, Aldea GS, Husseini WK, Dae MW, Stevens MB, Hill AC, Coleridge HM, Hoffman JI. Usefulness and limitations of regional cardiac sympathectomy by phenol. *Am J Physiol* 1989;257:H1523–H1533.

Morilak DA, Fornal C, Jacobs BL. Effects of physiological manipulations on locus coeruleus neuronal activity in freely moving cats. II. Cardiovascular challenge. *Brain Res* 1987; 422:24–31.

Morita H, Nishida Y, Motochigawa H, Uemura N, Hosomi H, Vatner SF. Opiate receptor-mediated decrease in renal nerve activity during hypotensive hemorrhage in conscious rabbits. *Circ Res* 1988;63:165–172.

Morita H, Vatner SF. Effects of hemorrhage on renal nerve activity in conscious dogs. *Circ Res* 1985a;57:788–793.

Morita H, Vatner SF. Effects of volume expansion on renal nerve activity, renal blood flow and sodium and water excretion in conscious dogs. *Am J Physiol* 1985b;249:F680–F687.

Morita K, Nakanishi A, Oka M. In vitro activation of bovine adrenal tyrosine hydroxylase by rabbit skeletal muscle actin: Evidence for a possible role of cytoskeletal elements as an activator for cytoplasmic enzymes. *Biochim Biophys Acta* 1989;993:21–26.

Morlin C, Wallin BG, Eriksson BM. Muscle sympathetic activity and plasma noradrenaline in normotensive and hypertensive man. *Acta Physiol Scand* 1983;119:117–121.

Mormede P, Rivet JM, Gaillard R, Corder R. Involvement of neuropeptide Y in neuroendocrine stress responses. Central and peripheral studies. *J Neural Transm* 1990 (Suppl. 29):65–75.

Morpurgo C. Pharmacological modifications of sympathetic responses by hypothalamic stimulation in the rat. *Br J Pharmacol* 1968;34:532–542.

Morris M, Salom P, Steinberg H, Sykes EA, Bouloux P, Newbould E, McLoughlin L, Besser GM, Grossman A. Endogenous opioids modulate the cardiovascular response to mental stress. *Psychoneuroendocrinology* 1990;15:185–192.

Morris MJ, Woodcock EA. Central a-adrenoceptors and blood pressure regulation in the rat. *Clin Exp Pharmacol Physiol* 1982;9:303–307.

Morrison SF, Gebber GL. Raphe neurons with sympathetic-related activity: baroreceptor responses and spinal connections. *Am J Physiol* 1984;246:R338–R348.

Morrison SF, Whitehorn D. Baroreceptor reflex gain is not diminished in spontaneous hypertension. *Am J Physiol* 1982;243:R500–R505.

Morrow LA, Linares OA, Hill TJ, Sanfield JA, Supiano MA, Rosen SG, Halter JB. Age differences in the plasma clearance mechanisms for epinephrine and norpeinephrine in humans. *J Clin Endocrinol Metab* 1987;65:508–511.

Morse DR, Schacterle GR, Esposito JV, Chod SD, Furst ML, DiPonziano J, Zaydenberg M. Stress, meditation and saliva: A study of separate salivary gland secretions in endodontic patients. *J Oral Med* 1983;38:150–160.

Motulsky HJ, Shattil SJ, Ferry N, Rozansky D, Insel PA. Desensitization of epinephrine-initiated platelet aggregation does not alter binding to α_2-adrenergic receptor or receptor coupling to adenylate cyclase. *Molec Pharmacol* 1986;29:1–6.

Moura D, Azevedo I, Guimaraes S. Differential distribution in, and release from, sympathetic nerve endings of endogenous noradrenaline and recently incorporated catecholamines. *Naunyn-Schmiedeberg's Arch Pharmacol* 1990;342:153–159.

Mueller RA, Millward DK, Woods JW. Circulating catecholamines, plasma renin and dopamine-beta-hydroxylase activity with postural stress. *Pharmacol Biochem Behav* 1974;2:757–761.

Muller JE, Stone PH, Turi ZG, Rutherford JD, Czeisler CA, Parker C, Poole WK, Passamani E, Roberts R, Robertson T, Sobel BE, Willerson JT, Braunwald E, and the MILIS Study Group. Circadian variation in the frequency of onset of acute myocardial infarction. *N Engl J Med* 1985;313:1315–1322.

Munch PA, Andresen MC, Brown AM. Rapid resetting of aortic baroreceptor in vitro. *Am J Physiol* 1983;244:H672–H680.

Munch PA, Brown AM. Role of the vessel wall in acute resetting of aortic baroreceptors. *Am J Physiol* 1985;248:H843–H852.

Mundal R, Erikssen J, Rodahl K. Latent ischemic heart disease in sea captains. *Scand J Work Environ Health* 1982;8:178–184.

Munjack DJ, Baltazar PL, DeQuattro V, Sobin P, Palmer R, Zulueta A, Crocker B, Usigli R, Buckwalter G, Leonard M. Generalized anxiety disorder: Some biochemical aspects. *Psychiatry Res* 1990;32:35–43.

Murad F, Chi YM, Rall TW, Sutherland EW. Adenylcyclase III. The effect of catecholamines and choline esters on the formation of adenosine-3'-5'-phosphate by preparations from cardiac muscle and liver. *J Biol Chem* 1962;237:1233–1238.

Murphy DL, Sims KB, Karoum F, Garrick NA, de la Chapelle A, Sankila EM, Norio R, Breakefield XO. Plasma amine oxidase activities in Norrie disease patients with an X-chromosomal deletion affecting monoamine oxidase. *J Neural Transm Gen Sect* 1991;83:1–12.

Murphy W, Mann R, McGrath BP, Bell C. Neuronal antibodies and autonomic failure. *Lancet* 1993;342:563.

Murray MJ, Offord KP, Yaksh TL. Physiologic and plasma hormone correlates of survival in endotoxic dogs: Effects of opiate antagonists. *Crit Care Med* 1989;17:39–47.

Muscholl E. Peripheral muscarinic control of norepinephrine release in the cardiovascular system. *Am J Physiol* 1980;239:H713–720.

Myers MG, De Champlain J. Effects of atenolol and hydroxhlorothiazide on blood pressure and plasma catecholamines in essential hypertension. *Hypertension* 1983;5:591–596.

Myers MG, Norris JW, Hachinski VC, Sole MJ. Plasma norepinephrine in stroke. *Stroke* 1981;12:200–204.

Myers MG, Norris JW, Hachinski VC, Weingert ME, Sole MJ. Cardiac sequelae of acute stroke. *Stroke* 1982;13:838–842.

Myers MG. Clonidine-induced facilitation of baroreceptor reflex. *Br Med J* 1977;2:802-803.

Nadeau RA, De Champlain J. Plasma catecholamines in acute myocardial infarction. *Am Heart J* 1979;98:548–554.

Nagatsu M, Zile MR, Tsutsui H, Schmid PG, DeFreyte G, Cooper G IV, Carabello BA. Native β-adrenergic support for left ventricular dysfunction in experimental mitral regurgitation normalizes indexes of pump and contractile function. *Circulation* 1994;89:818–826.

Nagatsu T, Levitt M, Udenfriend S. Tyrosine hydroxylase: The initial step in norepinephrine biosynthesis. *J Biol Chem* 1964;239:2910–2917.

Nagatsu T. Genes of human catecholamine synthesizing enzymes and their regulation in stress. In Kvetnansky R, McCarty R, Axelrod J (Eds) *Stress: Neuroendocrine and Molecular Approaches*. New York: Gordon and Breach, 1992, pp 287–295.

Nakada T, Kimura M, Watanabe H, Yamori Y, Lovenberg W. Increased non-collagen protein synthesis in the posterior cerebral artery in spontaneously hypertensive rats. *J Hypertens* 1986;4 (Suppl 3):S93–S95.

Nakamura K, Gerold M, Thoenen H. Genetically hypertensive rats: relationship between the development of hypertension and the changes in norepinephrine turnover of peripheral and central adrenergic neurons. *Naunyn-Schmiedeberg's Arch Pharmacol* 1971;271:157–169.

Nakamura K, Nakamura K. Role of brainstem and spinal noradrenergic and adrenergic neurons in the development and maintenance of hypertension in spontaneously hypertensive rats. *Naunyn-Schmiedeberg's Arch Pharmacol* 1978;305:127–133.

Nakata T, Berard W, Kogosov E, Alexander N. Hypothalamic NE release and cardiovascular response to NaCl in sinoaortic-denervated rats. *Am J Physiol* 1991;260:R733–R738.

Nanda EN, Boyle FC, Gillespie JS, Johnson RH, Keogh HJ. Idiopathic orthostatic hypotension from failure of noradrenaline release in a patient with vasomotor innervation. *J Neurol Neurosurg Psychiatry* 1977;40:11–19.

Narabayashi H, Nagao T, Saito Y, Yoshida M, Nagahata M. Stereotaxic amygdalotomy for behavior disorders. *Arch Neurol* 1963;9:1–16.

Natelson BH, Creighton D, McCarty R, Tapp WN, Pitman D, Ottenweller JE. Adrenal hormonal indices of stress in laboratory rats. *Physiol Behav* 1987;39:117–125.

Natelson BH. Neurocardiology. An interdisciplinary area for the 80s. *Arch Neurol* 1985;42:178–184.

Nathan MA, Reis DJ. Chronic labile hypertension produced by lesions of the nucleus tractus solitarii in the cat. *Circ Res* 1977;40:72–81.

Nathan MA, Reis DJ. Fulminating arterial hypertension elicited either by lesions or by electrical stimulation of the rostral hypothalamus in the rat. *Brain Res* 1981;211:91.

Nathan MA, Tucker LW, Severini WH, Reis DJ. Enhancement of conditioned arterial pressure responses in cats after brainstem lesions. *Science* 1978;201:71–73.

Nauta WJH, Kuypers HGJM. Some ascending pathways in the brain stem reticular formation. In Jasper JJ, Proctor LD, Knighton RS, Noshay WC, Costello RT (Eds) *Reticular Formation of the Brain*. Boston: Little Brown, 1958, pp 3–30.

Navone F, Jahn R, Di Gioia G, Stukenbrok H, Greengard P, De Camilli P. Protein p38: An integral membrane protein specific for small vesicles of neurons and neuroendocrine cells. *J Cell Biol* 1986;103:2511–2527.

Neil-Dwyer G, Water P, Cruickshank JM, Doshi B, O'Gorman P. Effect of propranolol and phentolamine on myocardial necrosis after subarachnoid hemorrhage. *Br Med J* 1978; 990–992.

Nestler EJ, Greengard P. Protein phosphorylation and the regulation of neuronal function. In Sigel GJ, Agranoff BW, Albers RW, Molinoff PB (Eds) *Basic Neurochemistry*. New York: Raven Press, 1989, pp 373–398.

Nestler EJ, McMahon A, Sabban EL, Tallman JF, Duman RS. Chronic antidepressant administration decreases the expression of tyrosine hydroxylase in the rat locus coeruleus. *Proc Natl Acad Sci USA* 1990;87:7522–7526.

Newling RP, Fletcher PJ, Contis M, Shaw J. Noradrenaline and cardiac hypertrophy in the rat: changes in morphology, blood pressure and ventricular performance. *J Hypertens* 1989; 7:561–567.

Nichols AJ, Ruffolo RR Jr. a-Adrenoceptor subclassification. In Ruffolo RR Jr (Ed) *α-Adrenoceptors: Molecular Biology, Biochemistry and Pharmacology*. Basel: Karger, 1991, pp 1–23.

Niehoff DL, Kuhar MJ. Benzodiazepine receptors: Localization in rat amygdala. *J Neurosci* 1983; 3:2091–2097.

Nijima A. The effect of 2-deoxy-D-glucose and D-glucose on the efferent discharge rate of sympathetic nerves. *J Physiol (Lond)* 1975;251:231–243.

Ninan PT, Insel TM, Cohen RM, Cook JM, Skolnick P, Paul SM. Benzodiazepine receptor-mediated experimental "anxiety" in primates. *Science* 1982;218:1332–1334.

Ninomiya I, Nisimaru N, Irisawa H. Sympathetic nerve activity to the spleen, kidney, and heart in response to baroceptor input. *Am J Physiol* 1971;221:1346–1351.

Nisenbaum LK, Abercrombie ED. Enhanced tyrosine hydroxylation in hippocampus of chronically stressed rats upon exposure to a novel stressor. *J Neurochem* 1992;58:276–281.

Nisenbaum LK, Zigmond MJ, Sved AF, Abercrombie ED. Prior exposure to chronic stress results in enhanced synthesis and release of hippocampal norepinephrine in response to a novel stressor. *J Neurosci* 1991;11:1478–1484.

Nissinen E, Linden I-B, Schultz E, Pohto P. Biochemical and pharmacological properties of a peripherally acting catechol-O-methyltransferase inhibitor Entcapone. *Naunyn-Schmiedeberg's Arch Pharmacol* 1992;346:262–266.

Nomura M, Ohtsuji Nm Nagata Y. Changes in the alpha-adrenoceptors in the medulla oblongata including nucleus tractus solitarii of spontaneously hypertensive rats. *Neurochem Res* 1985;10:1143–1154.

Nordborg C, Johansson BB. Morphometric study on cerebral vessels in spontaneously hypertensive rats. *Stroke* 1982;11:266–270.

Norris JW, Hachinski VS, Myers MG, Callow J, Wong T, Moore RW. Serum cardiac enzymes in stroke. *Stroke* 1979;10:548–553.

Norsk P, Epstein M. Effects of water immersion on arginine vasopressin release in humans. *J Appl Physiol* 1988;64:1–10.

Northrup JK, Sternweis PC, Smigel MD, Schleifer LS, Ross EM, Gilman AG. Purification of the regulatory component of adenylate cyclase. *Proc Nat Scad Sci USA* 1980;77:6516–6520.

Noshiro T, Saigusa T, Way D, Dorward PK, McGrath BP. Norepinephrine spillover faithfully reflects renal sympathetic nerve activity in conscious rabbits. *Am J Physiol* 1991;261:F44–F50.

Nowicki S, Levin G, Enero MA. Involvement of renal dopamine synthesis in the diuretic effect of furosemide in normohydrated rats. *J Pharmacol Exp Ther* 1993;264:1377–1380.

O'Benar JD, Hannon JP, Peterson JL, Bossone CA. Beta-endorphin, ACTH, and cortisol response to hemorrhage in conscious pigs. *Am J Physiol* 1987;252:R953–R958.

O'Connor DT, Bernstein KN. Human chromogranin A, the major catecholamine storage vesicle soluble protein: purification from catecholamine storage vesicles of pheochromocytoma, quantitation by RIA, and evaluation of plasma chromogranin A as an index of exocytotic sympathoadrenal activity in normal and hypertensive man. *Hypertension* 1984;6:787 (Abstract).

O'Donnell L, O'Meara N, Owens D, Johnson A, Collins P, Tomkin G. Plasma catecholamines and lipoproteins in chronic psychological stress. *J R Soc Med* 1987;80:339–342.

Oates NS, Ball SG, Perkins CM, Lee MR. Plasma and urine dopamine in man given sodium chloride in the diet. *Clin Sci* 1979;56:261–264.

Oberg B, Thoren P. Increased activity in left ventricular receptors during hemorrhage or occlusion of caval veins in the cat. A possible cause of vasovagal reaction. *Acta Physiol Scand* 1972;85:164–173.

Ogawa H, Matsuno T, Tsuchiya S, Ban M, Minaguchi K. Plasma levels of norepinephrine, cyclic AMP and cyclic GMP in essential hypertension. *Jpn Circ J* 1981;45:654–660.

Ohashi H, Miura Y, Kimura S, Ishizuka Y, Sugawara T, Toriyabe S, Noshiro T, Takahashi M, Sano N, Watanabe H, Yoshinaga K. Effects of dietary potassium on the hemodynamics and plasma norepinephrine kinetics in patients with essential hypertension. *Jpn Circ J* 1985;49:1019–1027.

Ohlstein EH, Kruse LI, Ezekiel M, Sherman SS, Erickson R, DeWolf WE Jr, Berkowitz BA. Cardiovascular effects of a new potent dopamine β-hydroxylase inhibitor in spontaneously hypertensive rats. *J Pharmacol Exp Ther* 1987;241:554–559.

Ohyanagi M, Faber JE, Nishigaki K. Differential activation of α_1- and α_2-adrenoceptors on microvascular smooth muscle during sympathetic nerve stimulation. *Circ Res* 1991;68: 232–244.

Okamoto K, Nosaka S, Yamori Y, Matsumoto M. Participation of neural factor in the pathogenesis of hypertension in the spontaneously hypertensive rat. *Jpn Heart J* 1967;8:168–180.

Olanow CW. An introduction to the free radical hypothesis in Parkinson's disease. *Ann Neurol* 1992;32:S2–S9.

Olivari MT, Levine TB, Cohn JN. Abnormal neurohumoral response to nitroprusside infusion in congestive heart failure. *J Am Coll Cardiol* 1983;2:411–417.

Oliver G, Schafer EA. On the physiological action of extract of the suprarenal capsules. *J Physiol (Lond)* 1895;17:ix–xiv.

Oliver JA, Pinto J, Sciacca RR, Cannon PJ. Basal norepinephrine overflow into the renal vein: Effect of renal nerve stimulation. *Am J Physiol* 1980;239:F371–F377.

Olschowka JA, Molliver ME, Grzanna R, Rice FL, Coyle JT. Ultrastructural demonstration of noradrenergic synapses in the rat central nervous system by dopamine-β-hydroxylase immunocytochemistry. *J Histochem Cytochem* 1981;29:271–280.

Oparil S, Vassaux C, Sanders CA, Haber E. Role of renin in acute postural homeostasis. *Circulation* 1970;41:89–95.

Os I, Kjeldsen E, Westheim A, Jackson MB, Akesson I, Frederichsen P, Eide I, Leren P. The effect of sodium depletion and potassium supplementation on vasopressin, renin and catecholamines in hypertensive men. *Acta Med Scand* 1986;220:195–203.

Osborn JL, Holdaas H, Thames MD, Di Bona GF. Renal adrenoceptor mediation of antinatriuretic and renin responses to low frequency renal nerve stimulation in the dog. *Circ Res* 1983; 53:298–305.

Osler W. The Lumleian lectures on angina pectoris. *Lancet* 1910;1:697–699 and 839–844.

Ostman-Smith I. Adaptive changes in the sympathetic nervous system and some effector organs of the rat following long term exercise or cold acclimation and the role of cardiac sympathetic nerves in the genesis of compensatory cardiac hypertrophy. *Acta Physiol Scand* 1980;108 (Suppl 477):1–118.

Ostman-Smith I. Cardiac sympathetic nerves as the final common pathway in the induction of adaptive cardiac hypertrophy. *Clin Sci* 1981;61:265–272.

Outschoorn AS, Vogt M. The nature of cardiac sympathin in the dog. *Br J Pharmacol* 1952;7: 319–324.

Owsjannikow P. Die tonischen und reflectorischen Centren der Gefassnerven. *Sachs Akad Wiss Sitz* 1871;23:135–147.

Pacak K, Armando I, Fukuhara K, Kvetnansky R, Palkovits M, Kopin IJ, Goldstein DS. Noradrenergic activation in the paraventricular nucleus during acute and chronic immobilization stress in rats: An *in vivo* microdialysis study. *Brain Res* 1992b;589:91–96.

Pacak K, Armando I, Komoly S, Fukuhara K, Weise VK, Holmes C, Kopin IJ, Goldstein DS.

Hypercortisolemia inhibits yohimbine-induced release of norepinephrine in the postero-lateral hypothalamus of conscious rats. *Endocrinology* 1992a;131:1369–1376.

Pacak K, Palkovits M, Kvetnansky R, Fukuhara K, Armando I, Kopin IJ, Goldstein DS. Effects of single or repeated immobilization on release of norepinephrine and its metabolites in the central nucleus of the amygdala in conscious rats. *Neuroendocrinology* 1993; 57:626–633.

Pacak K, Palkovits M, Kvetnansky R, Kopin IJ, Goldstein DS. Effects of brainstem hemisections on in vivo synthesis and release of catecholamines in the paraventricular nucleus of the hypothalamus. *Neuroendocrinology* 1993; 58:196–201.

Pacak K, Yadid G, Jakab J, Lenders JWM, Kopin IJ, Goldstein DS. *In vivo* hypothalamic release and synthesis of catecholamines in spontaneously hypertensive rats. *Hypertension* 1993; 22:467–478.

Pacholczyk T, Blakely RD, Amara SG. Expression cloning of a cocaine- and antidepressant-sensitive human noradrenaline transporter. *Nature* 1991;350:350–354.

Packer M. Role of the sympathetic nervous system in chronic heart failure. A historical and philosophical perspective. *Circulation* 1990;82 (Suppl I):I1–I16.

Packer M. Sudden unexpected death in patients with congestive heart failure: A second frontier. *Circulation* 1985;72:681–685.

Paddu PE, Pasternac A, Tabau JF, Krol R, Farley L, DeChamplain J. QT interval prolongation and increased plasma catecholamine levels in patients with mitral valve prolapse. *Am Heart J* 1983;105:422–428.

Pagani M, Lombardi F, Guzzetti S, Rimoldi O, Furlan R, Pizzinelli P, Sandrone G, Malfatto G, Dell'Orto S, Piccaluga E, Turiel M, Baselli G, Cerutti S, Malliani A. Power spectral analysis of heart rate and arterial pressure variabilities as a marker of sympatho-vagal interaction in man and conscious dog. *Circ Res* 1986;59:178–193.

Page IH, McCubbin JW. Mechanisms by which ganglioplegics and atropine enhance cardiovascular responsiveness. *Am J Physiol* 1963;205:1–9.

Paintal AS. A study of right and left atrial receptors. *J Physiol (Lond)* 1953;120:596–610.

Pak CH. Plasma adrenaline and noradrenaline concentrations of the spontaneously hypertensive rat. *Jpn Heart J* 1981;22:987–995.

Palermo A, Costantini C, Mara G, Libretti A. Role of the sympathetic nervous system in spontaneous hypertension: changes in central adrenoceptors and plasma catecholamine levels. *Clin Sci* 1981;61:195s–198s.

Palkovitz M, Brownstein MJ. Catecholamines in the central nervous system. In Trendelenburg U, Weiner N (Eds) *Catecholamines* II. New York: Springer-Verlag, 1989, pp 1–26.

Pandey RC, Srivastava RD, Bathnagar UN. Effect of unilateral stellate ganglion blockade and stimulation on experimental arrhythmias. *Int J Physiol Pharmacol* 1979;23:305–314.

Panksepp J, Pollack A, Krost KP, Meeker R, Ritter M. Feeding in response to repeated protamine zinc insulin injections. *Physiol Behav* 1975;14:487–493.

Papez JW. A proposed mechanism of emotion. *Arch Neurol Psychiatry* 1937;38:725–743.

Parkes CM, Benjamin B, Fitzgerald RG. Broken heart: A statistical study of increased mortality among widowers. *Br Med J* 1969;1:740–743.

Parkes CM, Brown RJ. Health after bereavement: A controlled study of young Boston widows and widowers. *Psychosom Med* 1972;34:449–461.

Parkes DG, Coghlan JP, McDougall JG, Tyers MR, Scoggins BA. Hemodynamic interactions of atrial natiuretic factor with the sympathetic nervous system in sheep. *Clin Exp Hyper* 1990;A12:383–398.

Parmer RJ, Cervenka JH, Sone RA. Baroreflex sensitivity and heredity in essential hypertension. *Circulation* 1992;85:497–503.

Partridge WM, Oldendorf WH. Transport of metabolic substrates through the blood-brain barrier. *J Neurochem* 1977;28:5–12.

Pascual J, del Arco C, Gonzalez AM, Pazos A. Quantitative light microscopic autoradiographic localization of α_2-adrenoceptors in the human brain. *Brain Res* 1992;585:116–127.

Passon PG, Peuler JD. A simplified radiometric assay for plasma norepinephrine and epinephrine. *Anal Biochem* 1973;51:618–631.

Pasternac A, Tabau JF, Paddu PE, Krol RB, De Champlain J. Increased plasma catecholamine levels in patients with symptomatic mitral valve prolapse. *Am J Med* 1982;73:783–790.

Paul SM, Crawley JN, Skolnick P. The neurobiology of anxiety: The role of the GABA/benzo-diazepine receptor complex. In Berger PA, Brodie KH (Eds) *American Handbook of Psychiatry,* Vol 8. New York: Basic Books, 1986, pp 581–596.

Pauletto P, Scannapieco G, Pessina AC. Sympathetic drive and vascular damage in hypertension and atherosclerosis. *Hypertension* 1991;17 (Suppl III):III75–III81.

Pavlov IP. *Conditioned Reflexes: An Investigation of the Physiological Activity of the Cerebral Cortex.* London: Oxford University Press, 1927.

Pavlov IP. Uber centrifugalen Nerven des Herzens. *Arch Physiol (Leipzig)* 1887;498–569.

Pazos A, Gonzalez AM, Pascual J, Mean JJ, Barturen F, Garcia-Sevilla JA. Alpha 2-adrenoceptors in human forebrain: Autoradiographic visualization and biochemical parameters using the agonist [³H]UK-14304. *Brain Res* 1988;475:361–365.

Pearse AGE. Histochemistry and electron microscopy of obstructive cardiomyopathy. In Wolstenhome GEW, O'Connor M (Eds) *Cardiomyopathies. Ciba Foundation Symposium.* Boston: Little, Brown, 1964, pp 132–171.

Peart WS. The nature of splenic sympathin. *J Physiol (Lond)* 1949;108:491–501.

Peiss CN. Central control of sympathetic cardioacceleration in the cat. *J Physiol (Lond)* 1960; 151:225–237.

Pelleg A, Burnstock G. Physiological importance of ATP released from nerve terminals and its degradation to adenosine in humans. *Circulation* 1990;82:2269–2272.

Pentecost BL, Austen WG. Beta-adrenergic blockade in experimental myocardial infarction. *Am Heart J* 1966;72:790–796.

Perini C, Muller FB, Buhler FR. Suppressed aggression accelerates early development of essential hypertension. *J Hypertens* 1991;9:499–503.

Perini C, Muller FB, Rauschfleisch U, Battegay R, Buhler FR. Effects of psychological and physical covariates on plasma catecholamines in borderline hypertensives and offspring of hypertensive parents. *Clin Exp Hypertens* 1990a;A12:137–150.

Perini C, Muller FB, Rauschfleisch U, Battegay R, Hobi V, Buhler FR. Psychosomatic factors in borderline hypertensive subjects and offspring of hypertensive parents. *Hypertension* 1990b;16:627–634.

Perloff JK. Pathogenesis of hypertrophic cardiomyopathy; hypothesis and speculations. *Am Heart J* 1981;101:219.

Peronnet F, Nadeau R, Boudreau G, Cardinal R, Lamontagne D, Yamaguchi N, De Champlain J. Epinephrine release from the heart during left stellate ganlgion stimulation in dogs. *Am J Physiol* 1988;254:R659–R662.

Perry JC, Garson A Jr. The child with recurrent syncope: Autonomic function testing and beta-adrenergic hypersensitivity. *J Am Coll Cardiol* 1991;17:1168–1171.

Persson B, Andersson OK, Hjemdahl P, Wysocki M, Agerwall S, Wallin G. Adrenaline infusion in man increases muscle sympathetic nerve activity and noradrenaline overflow to plasma. *J Hypertens* 1989;7:747–756.

Pert CB, Snyder SH. Opiate receptor: Demonstration in nervous tissue. *Science* 1973;179:1011–1014.

Peruzzi D, Hendley ED, Forehand CJ. Hypertrophy of stellate ganglion cells in hypertensive, but not hyperactive, rats. *Am J Physiol* 1991;261:R979–R984.

Peskind ER, Raskind MA, Wilkinson CW, Flatness DE, Halter JB. Peripheral sympathectomy and adrenal medullectomy do not alter cerebrospinal fluid norepinephrine. *Brain Res* 1986;367:258–264.

Petch MC, Nayler WG. Concentration of catecholamines in human cardiac muscle. *Br Heart J* 1979a;41:340–344.

Petch MC, Nayler WG. Uptake of catecholamines by human cardiac muscle in vitro. *Br Heart J* 1979b;41:336–339.

Peters JP. The role of sodium in the production of edema. *N Engl J Med* 1948;239:353–362.

Petraglia F, Bakalakis S, Facchinetti F, Volpe A, Muller BE, Genazzani AR. Effects of sodium valproate and diazepam on beta-endorphin, beta-lipotropin and cortisol secretion induced by hypoglycemic stress in humans. *Neuroendocrinology* 1986;44:320–325.

Pettibone DJ, Mueller GP. a-adrenergic stimulation by clonidine increases plasma concentrations of immunoreactive β-endorphin in rats. *Endocrinology* 1981;109:798–1802.

Peuler JD, Johnson GA. Simultaneous single isotope radioenzymatic assay of plasma norepinephrine, epinephrine and dopamine. *Life Sci* 1977;21:625–636.

Pfeifer MA, Ward K, Malpass T, Stratton J, Halter J, Evans M, Beiter H, Harker LA, Porte D Jr. Variations in circulating catecholamines fail to alter human platelet alpha-2-adrenergic receptor number or affinity for [^{3}H]yohimbine or [^{3}H]dihydroergocryptine. *J Clin Invest* 1984;74:1063–1072.

Philippu A, Matthaei A. Transport and storage of catecholamines in vesicles. In Trendelenburg U, Weiner N (Eds) *Catecholamines* I. New York: Springer-Verlag, 1988, pp 1–42.

Philippu A, Przuntek H, Heyd G, Burger A. Central effects of sympathomimetic amines on the blood pressure. *Eur J Pharmacol* 1971;15:200–208.

Pi F, Garcia-Sevilla JA. α_2-autoreceptor-mediated modulation of tyrosine hydroxylase activity in noradrenergic regions of the rat brain in vivo. *Naunyn-Schmiedeberg's Arch Pharmacol* 1992;345:653–660.

Pickering TG, Gerin W. Reactivity and the role of behavioral factors in hypertension. A critical review. *Ann Behav Med* 1990;12:3–16.

Pickering TG, Sleight P. Baroreceptors and hypertension. *Prog Brain Res* 1977;47:43–60.

Pickering TG. Does psychological stress contribute to the development of hypertension and coronary heart disease? *Eur J Clin Pharmacol* 1990;39 (Suppl. 1):S1–S7.

Pieribone VA, Aston-Jones G, Bohn MC. Adrenergic and non-adrenergic neurons in the C1 and C3 areas project to locus coeruleus: A fluorescent double labeling study. *Neurosci Lett* 1988;85:297–303.

Pierpont GL, Francis GS, DeMaster EG, Levine TB, Bolman RM, Cohn JN. Elevated left ventricular myocardial dopamine in preterminal idiopathic dilated cardiomyopathy. *Am J Cardiol* 1983;52:1033–1035.

Pierpont GL. The contribution of animal models to understanding neuroadrenergic responses to heart failure. In Ganguly PK (Ed) *Catecholamines and Heart Disease*. Boca Raton, Fla: CRC Press, 1991, pp 73–86.

Pilowsky PM, Jiang C, Lipski J. An intracellular study of respiratory neurons in the rostral ventrolateral medulla of the rat and their relationship to catecholaine-containing neurons. *J Comp Neurol* 1990;301:604–617.

Pitts DK, Marwah J. Cocaine modulation of central monoaminergic neurotransmission. *Pharmacol Biochem Behav* 1987;26:453–461.

Planz G, Planz R. Dopamine-β-hydroxylase, adrenaline, noradrenaline, and dopamine in the venous blood of adrenal gland in man: A comparison with levels in the periphery of the circulation. *Experientia* 1979;35:207–208.

Planz G. Adrenaline and noradrenaline concentration in blood of suprarenal and renal venin in man with normal blood pressure and with essential hypertension. *Klin Wochenschr* 1978; 56:1109–1112.

Plotsky PM, Bruhn TO, Vale W. Hypophysiotropic regulation of adrenocorticotropin secretion in response to insulin-induced hypoglycemia. *Endocrinology* 1985;117:323–329.

Plotsky PM. Facilitation of immunoreactive corticotropin-releasing factor secretion into the hypophyseal-portal circulation after activation of catecholaminergic pathways or central norepinephrine injection. *Endocrinology* 1987;121:924–930.

Polinksy RJ, Goldstein DS, Brown RT, Keiser HR, Kopin IJ. Decreased sympathetic neuronal uptake in idiopathic orthostatic hypotension. *Ann Neurol* 1985;18:48–53.

Polinsky RJ, Jimerson DC, Kopin IJ. Chronic autonomic failure: CSF and plasma 3-methoxy-4-hydroxyphenylglycol. *Neurology* 1984;34:979-983.

Polinsky RJ, Kopin IJ, Ebert MH, Weise V. Pharmacologic distinction of different orthostatic hypotension syndromes. *Neurology* 1981;31:1–7.

Polinsky RJ, McRae A, Baser SM, Dahlstrom A. Antibody in the CSF of patients with multiple system atrophy reacts specifically with rat locus ceruleus. *J Neurol Sci* 1991;106:96–104.

Polinsky RJ, Samaras GM, Kopin IJ. Sympathetic neural prosthesis for managing orthostatic hypotension. *Lancet* 1983;1:901–904.

Polinsky RJ. Neuropharmacological investigation of autonomic failure. In Bannister R, Mathias CJ (Eds) *Autonomic Failure*. New York: Oxford University Press, 1992, pp 334–358.

Pool JL. Neurophysiological symposium; visceral brain of man. *J Neurosurg* 1954;11:45–63.

Pool PE, Covell JW, Levitt M, Gibb J, Braunwald E. Reduction of cardiac tyrosine hydroxylase activity in experimental congestive heart failure. *Circ Res* 1967;20:349–353.

Porte D, Robertson RP. Control of insulin secretion by catecholamines, stress and the sympathetic nervous system. *Fed Proc* 1973;32:1792–1796.

Porte D. Sympathetic regulation of insulin secretion. *Arch Int Med* 1969;123:252–260.

Porter ID, Whitehouse BJ, Price GM, Hinson JP, Vinson GP. Effects of dopamine, high potassium concentration and field stimulation on the secretion of aldosterone by the perfused rat adrenal gland. *J Endocrinol* 1992;133:275–282.

Porter JC, Kedzierski W, Aguila-Mansilla N, Kozlowski GP. Stimulation of molecular events associated with secretion by catecholaminergic cells in culture. In Kvetnansky R, McCarty R, Axelrod J (Eds) *Stress: Neuroendocrine and Molecular Approaches*. New York: Gordon and Breach, 1992, pp 351–362.

Porter JP, Brody MJ. A comparison of the hemodynamic effects produced by electrical stimulation of subnuclei of the paraventricular nucleus. *Brain Res* 1986b;375:20–29.

Porter JP, Brody MJ. Neural projections from paraventricular nucleus that subserve vasomotor functions. *Am J Physiol* 1985;248:R271–R281.

Porter JP, Brody MJ. Spinal vasopressin mechanisms of cardiovascular regulation. *Am J Physiol* 1986a;251:R510–R517.

Powers RE, Struble RG, Casanova MF, O'Connor DT, Kitt CA, Price DL. Innervation of human hippocampus by noradrenergic systems: Normal anatomy and structural abnormalities in aging and in Alzheimer's disease. *Neuroscience* 1988;25:401–417.

Premel-Cabic A, Spiesser R, Bigorgne JC, Fressinaud P, Allain P. Concentration plasmatique de noradrenaline dans l'hypertension arterielle essentielle. *La Presse Med* 1987;16:811–814.

Price HL. Circulating adrenaline and noradrenaline during diethyl ether anaesthesia in man. *Clin Sci* 1957;16:377–387.

Price K, Smith SE. Cheese reaction and tyramine. *Lancet* 1971;1 (690):130–131.

Prince CR, Anisman H. Situation specific effects of stressor controllability on plasma corticosterone changes in mice. *Physiol Biochem Behav* 1990;37:613–621.

Prinzmetal M, Kennamer R, Merliss R, Wada T, Bor N. Angina pectoris: I. A variant form of angina pectoris. *Am J Med* 1959;27:375–388.

Probst A, Cortex R, Palacios JM. Distribution of α_2-adrenergic receptors in the human brainstem: An autoradiographic study using [^{3}H]p-aminoclonidine. *Eur J Pharmacol* 1985;106:477–488.

Proud VK, Hsia YE, Wolf B. Disorders of amino acid metabolism. In Siegel GJ, Agranoff BW, Albers RW, Molinoff PB (Eds) *Basic Neurochemistry*. New York: Raven Press, 1989, pp 733–763.

Provoost AP, De Jong W. Differential development of renal, DOCA-salt, and spontaneous hypertension in the rat after neonatal sympathectomy. *Clin Exp Hyper* 1978;1:177–189.

Puritz R, Lightman SL, Wilcox CS, Forsling M, Bannister R. Blood presure and vasopressin in progressive autonomic failure: Response to postural stimulation, l-dopa and naloxone. *Brain* 1983;106:503–511.

Qualy JM, Westfall TC. Age-dependent overflow of endogenous norepinephrine from paraventricular hypothalamic nucleus of hypertensive rats. *Am J Physiol* 1993;265:H39–H46.

Qualy JM, Westfall TC. Release of norepinephrine from the paraventricular hypothalamic nucleus of hypertensive rats. *Am J Physiol* 1988;254:H993–H1003.

Quillen EW Jr, Cowley AW Jr. Influence of volume changes on osmolality-vasopressin relationships in conscious dogs. *Am J Physiol* 1983;244:H73–H79.

Raab W, Chaplin JP, Bajusz E. Myocardial necroses produced in domesticated rats and in wild rats by sensory and emotional stresses. *Proc Soc Exp Biol Med* 1964;116:881–893.

Raab W, Stark E, MacMillan WH, Gigee WR. Sympathogenic origin and anti-adrenergic prevention of stress-induced myocardial lesions. *Am J Cardiol* 1961;8:203–211.

Raab W. Emotional and sensory stress factors in myocardial pathology. Neurogenic and hormonal mechanisms in pathogenesis, therapy, and prevention. *Am Heart J* 1966;72:538–564.

Radjfer J, Aronson WJ, Bush PA, Dorey FJ, Ignarro LJ. Nitric oxide as a mediator of relaxation of the corpus cavernosum in response to nonadrenergic, noncholinergic neurotransmission. *N Engl J Med* 1992;326:90–94.

Radosevich PM, Lacy DB, Brown LL, Williams PE, Abumrad NN. Effects of insulin-induced hypoglycemia on plasma and cerebrospinal fluid levels of ir-beta-endorphins, ACTH, cortisol, norepinephrine, insulin and glucose in the conscious dog. *Brain Res* 1988;458:325–338.

Rahe RH, Mahan JL, Arthur RJ. Prediction of near-future health change from subjects preceeding life changes. *J Psychosom Res* 1970;14:401–406.

Rahe RH, Romo M, Bennett L, Siltanen P. Recent life changes, myocardial infarction and abrupt coronary death. *Arch Int Med* 1974;133:221–228.

Rahe RH. Life changes and near-future illness reports. in Levi L (Ed) *Emotions—Their Parameters and Measurement*. New York: Raven Press, 1975, pp 511–529.

Rainbow TC, Biegon A. Quantitative autoradiography of [^{3}H]prazosin binding sites in rat fore-brain. *Neurosci Lett* 1983;40:221–226.

Rainbow TC, Parsons B, Wolfe BB. Quantitative autoradiography of beta 1- and beta 2-adrenergic receptors in rat brain. *Proc Nat Acad Sci USA* 1984;81:1585–1589.

Raizner AE, Cahine RA, Ishimori T, Verani MS, Zacca N, Jamal N, Miller RR, Luchi RJ. Provocation of coronary artery spasm by the cold pressor test: Hemodynamic, arteriographic and quantitative angiographic observations. *Circulation* 1980;65:1171–1177.

Raj PP, Kelly JF, Cannella J, McConn K. Multidisciplinary management of reflex sympathetic dystrophy. *Pain Digest* 1992:2:267–273.

Raja SN. Reflex sympathetic dystrophy: Pathophysiological basis for therapy. *Pain Digest* 1992; 2:274–280.

Rajfer SI, Davis FR. Role of dopamine receptors and the utility of dopamine agonists in heart failure. *Circulation* 1990;82 (Suppl I):I97–I102.

Rand MJ, Majewski H. Adrenaline mediates a positive feedback loop in noradrenergic transmission: its possible role in development of hypertension. *Clin Exp Hyper* 1984;A6:347–370.

Randall DC, Brown DR, Raisch RM, Yingling JD, Randall WC. SA nodal parasympathectomy delineates autonomic control of heart rate power spectrum. *Am J Physiol* 1991;260:H985–H988.

Randall WC. Selective autonomic innervation of the heart. In Randall WC (Ed) *Nervous Control of Cardiovascular Function*. New York: Oxford University Press, 1984, pp 46–67.

Rankin AJ, Kelpin BG, Courneya CA, Wilson N, Ledsome JR. Plasma vasopressin response to haemorrhage in the anaesthetized rabbit. *Can J Physiol Pharmacol* 1986;64:904–908.

Ranson SW, Billingsley PR. Vasomotor reactions from stimulation of the floor of the fourth ventricle. *Am J Physiol* 1916;41:85–90.

Rao DD, McKelvy J, Kebabian J, MacKenzie RG. Two forms of the reat D2 dopamine receptor as revealed by the polymerase chain reaction. *FEBS Lett* 1990;263:18–22.

Rappaport EB, Young JB, Landsberg L. Effects of 2-deoxy-D-glucose on the cardiac sympathetic nerves and the adrenal medulla in the rat: Further evidence for a dissociation of sympathetic nervous system and adrenal medullary responses. *Endocrinology* 1982;110:650–656.

Rascher W, Dietz R, Schomig A, Voss U, Gross F. Effects of neonatal sympathectomy by 6-hydroxydopamine on blood pressure and intravascular volume in young stroke-prone spontaneously hypertensive rats. *Clin Exp Pharmacol Physiol* 1983;10:27–33.

Rasmussen K, Jacobs BL. Single unit activity of locus coeruleus neurons in the freely moving cat. II. Conditioning and pharmacologic studies. *Brain Res* 1986;23:335–344.

Rasmussen K, Morilak DA, Jacobs BL. Single unit activity of locus coeruleus neurons in the freely moving cat. I. During naturalistic behaviors and in response to simple and complex stimuli. *Brain Res* 1986;371:324–334.

Ratcliffe ML, Cronin MTI. Changing frequency of atherosclerosis in mammals and birds in the Philadelphia Zoological Gardens. *Circulation* 1958;18:41–52.

Ratge D, Bauersfeld W, Wisser H. The relationship of free and conjugated catecholamines in plasma and cerebrospinal fluid in cerebral and meningeal disease. *J Neural Transm* 1985; 62:267–284.

Ratge D, Kohse KP, Steegmuller U, Wisser H. Distribution of free and conjugated catecholamines between plasma, platelets and erythrocytes: Different effects of intravenous and oral catecholamine administrations. *J Pharmacol Exp Ther* 1991;257:232–238.

Raymond JR, Hnatowich M, Lefkowitz RJ, Caron MG. Adrenergic receptors. Models for regulation of signal transduction processes. *Hypertension* 1990;15:119–131.

Rea RF, Eckberg DL, Fritsch JM, Goldstein DS. Relation of plasma norepinephrine and sympathetic traffic during hypotension in man. *Am J Physiol* 1990;258:R982–R986.

Rea RF, Eckberg DL. Carotid baroreceptor-muscle sympathetic relation in humans. *Am J Physiol* 1987;253:R929–R934.

Rea RF, Hamdan M. Baroreflex control of muscle sympathetic nerve activity in borderline hypertension. *Circulation* 1990;82:856–862.

Rea RF, Wallin BG. Sympathetic nerve activity in arm and leg muscles during lower body negative pressure in humans. *J Appl Physiol* 1989;66:2778–2781.

Rector TS, Olivari MT, Levine TB, Francis GS, Cohn JN. Predicting survival for an individual with congestive heart failure using the plasma norepinephrine concentration. *Am Heart J* 1987;114:148–152.

Reddy SYR, Yaksh TL. Spinal noradrenergic terminal system mediates antinociception. *Brain Res* 1980;189:391–401.

Redmond DE Hr, Huang YH, Snyder DR, Maas JW. Behavioral effects of stimulation of the locus coeruelus in the stump tail monkey (Macaca arctoides). *Brain Res* 1976;116:502–510.

Redmond DE Hr, Huang YH. New evidence for a locus coeruleus-norepinephrine connection with anxiety. *Life Sci* 1979;25:2149–2162.

Rees WD, Lutkins SG. Mortality of bereavement. *Br Med J* 1976;4:13.

Regitz V, Bossaller C, Strasser R, Schuler S, Hetzer R, Fleck E. Myocardial catecholamine content after heart transplantation. *Circulation* 1992;82:620–623.

Regunathan S, Meeley MP, Reis DJ. Clonidine-displacing substance from bovine brain binds to imidazoline receptors and releases catecholamines in adrenal chromaffin cells. *Mol Pharmacol* 1991;40:884–888.

Reich P, DeSilva RA, Lown B, Murawski BJ. Acute psychological disturbances preceding life-threatening ventricular arrhythmias. *J Am Med Assoc* 1981;246:233–235.

Reichenbach DD, Benditt EP. Catecholamines and cardiomypathy: The pathogenesis and potential importance of myofibrillar degeneration. *Hum Pathol* 1970;1:125–150.

Reid JL, Wing LMH, Mathias CJ, Frankel HL, Neill E. The central hypotensive effect of clonidine. Studies in tetraplegic subjects. *Clin Pharmacol Ther* 1977;21:375–381.

Reid JL, Zivin JA, Kopin IJ. Central and peripheral adrenergic mechanisms in the development of deoxycorticosterone-saline hypertension in rats. *Circ Res* 1975;37:569–579.

Reis DJ, Granata AR, Joh TH, Ross CA, Ruggiero DA, Park DH. Brain stem catecholamine mechanisms in tonic and reflex control of blood pressure. *Hypertension* 1984;6 (5 Pt 2): II7–II15.

Reis DJ, Gunne L-M. Brain catecholamines: Relation to the defense reaction evoked by brain stimulation in the cat. *Science* 1965;156:1768–1770.

Reis DJ, Joh TH. Long term regulation of brain tyrosine hydroxylase. In Usdin E, Weiner N, Youdim MBH (Eds) *Structure and Function of Monoamine Enzymes*. New York: Marcel Dekker, 1977, pp 169–192.

Reis DJ, Ledoux JE. Some central neural mechanisms governing resting and behaviorally coupled control of blood pressure. *Circulation* 1987;76 (Suppl I):I2–I9.

Reis DJ, Morrison S, Ruggiero DA. The C1 area of the brainstem in tonic and reflex control of blood pressure. State of the art lecture. *Hypertension* 1988;11 (Suppl I): I8–I13.

Reiser MF, Brust AA, Ferris EB. Life situation, emotions, and the course of patients with arterial hypertension. *Psychosom Med* 1951;13:133–139.

Reison DS, Oliver JA, Sciacca RR, Cannon PJ. Release of norepinephrine from sympathetic nerve efferents by bilateral carotid occlusion. *Am J Physiol* 1983;245:H635–H639.

Rengo F, Perez G, Chiariello M, De Caprio L, Sacca L, Trimarco B, Condorelli M. Studies on the hemodynamic changes in the perfused hindlimb induced by electrostimulation of the sinus nerve in the dog. *Life Sci* 1976;19:1387–1398.

Rennick BR, Pryor MZ. Effects of autonomic drugs on renal tubular transport of catecholamines in the chicken. *J Pharmacol Exp Ther* 1965;148:262–269.

Review Panel on Coronary-Prone Behavior and Coronary Heart Disease: Coronary prone behavior and coronary heart disease: A critical review. *Circulation* 1981;63:1199–1215.

Reynolds RC. Community and occupational influences in stress at Cape Kennedy: Relationships to heart disease. In Eliot RS (Ed) *Stress and the Heart*. Mount Kisco, NY: Futura, 1974, pp 33–49.

Ricci DR, Orlick AE, Cipriano PR, Guthaner DF, Harrison DC. Altered adrenergic activity in coronary arterial spasm: Insight into mechanism based on study of coronary hemodynamics and electrocardiogram. *Am J Cardiol* 1979;43:1073–1079.

Richardson KC. The fine structure of autonomic nerve endings in smooth muscle of the rat vas deferens. *J Anat* 1962;96:427–442.

Riche D, De Pommery J, Menetrey D. Neuropeptides and catecholamines in efferent projections of the nuclei of the solitary tract in the rat. *J Comp Neurol* 1990;293:399–424.

Richet G, Wahbe F, Hagege J, Wiemeyer W. Extraneuronal production of dopamine by kidney slices in normo and hypertensive rats. *Clin Exp Hyper* 1987;9 (Suppl 1):127–134.

Ring-Larsen H, Hesse B, Henriksen JH, Christensen NJ. Sympathetic nervous activity and renal and systemic hemodynamics in cirrhosis: Plasma norepinephrine concentration, hepatic extraction, and renal release. *Hepatology* 1982;2:304–310.

Rissanen V, Romo M, Seltanen P. Premonitory symptoms and stress factors preceding sudden death from ischemic heart disease. *Acta Med Scand* 1978;204:389.

Ritchie CM, Sheridan B, Fraser R, Hadden DR, Kennedy AL, Riddell J, Atkinson AB. Studies on the pathogenesis of hypertension in Cushing's disease and acromegaly. *Q J Med* 1990; 76:855–867.

Rivet J-M, Stinu L, Le Moal M, Mormede P. 6-hydroxydopamine lesion of ventral tegmental area dopaminergic cell bodies does not impair neuroendocrine responses to environmental stimuli. *J Neuroendocrinol* 1990;2:733–736.

Robert F, Lambas-Senas L, Ortemann C, Pujol J-F, Renaud B. Microdialysis monitoring of 3,4-dihydroxyphenylalanine accumulation after decarboxylation inhibition: A means to estimate in vivo changes in tyrosine hydroxylase activity of the rat locus ceruleus. *J Neurochem* 1993;60:721–729.

Robertson D, Frolich JC, Carr RK, Watson JT, Hollifield JW, Shand DG, Oates JA. Effects of caffeine on plasma renin activity, catecholamines, and blood pressure. *N Engl J Med* 1978;298:181–186.

Robertson D, Goldberg MR, Hollister AS, Wade D, Robertson RM. Clonidine raises blood pressure in severe idiopathic orthostatic hypotension. *Am J Med* 1983;74:193–200.

Robertson D, Goldberg MR, Onrot J, Hollister AS, Wiley R, Thompson JG Jr, Robertson RM. Isolated failure of autonomic noradrenergic neurotransmission. Evidence for impaired beta-hydroxylation of dopamine. *N Engl J Med* 1986;314:1494–1497.

Robertson D, Hollister AS, Biaggioni I, Netterville JL, Mosqueda-Garcia R, Robertson RM. Arterial baroreflex failure in man. *Clin Auton Res* 1993;3:212.

Robertson D, Shand DG, Hollifield JW, Nies AS, Frolich JC, Oates JA. Alterations in the responses of the sympathetic nervous system and renin in borderline hypertension. *Hypertension* 1979;1:118–124.

Robertson D, Wade D, Workman R, Woolsey RL, Oates JA. Tolerance to the humoral and hemodynamic effects of caffeine in man. *J Clin Invest* 1981;67:1111–1117.

Robertson DA, Johnson GA, Robertson RM, Nies AS, Shand DG, Oates JA. Comparative assessment of stimuli that release neuronal and adrenomedullary catecholamines in man. *Circulation* 1979;59:637–643.

Robertson GL, Berl T. Pathophysiology of water metabolism. In Brenner BM, Rector FC Jr (Eds) *The Kidney.* Philadelphia: WB Saunders, 1991, pp 677–736.

Robertson RM, Bernard Y, Robertson D. Arterial and coronary sinus catecholamines in the course of spontaneous coronary artery spasm. *Am Heart J* 1983;105:901–906.

Robertson RM, Killian TJ, Biaggioni I, Haile V, Mosqueda-Garcia R. Sympathetic nervous system activity is increased by acetylcholinesterase inhibition in humans. *Clin Auton Res* 1993;3:217.

Rockhold RW, Acuff CG, Clower BR. Excitotoxic lesions of the paraventricular hypothalamus: Metabolic and cardiac effects. *Neuropharmacology* 1990;29:663–673.

Roder S, Ciriello J. Innervation of the amygdaloid complex by catecholaminergic cell groups of the ventrolateral medulla. *J Comp Neurol* 1993;332:105–122.

Rogers PF, Head GA, Lungershausen YK, Howe PRC. Effects of depleting central and peripheral adrenaline stores on blood pressure in stroke-prone spontaneously hypertensive rats. *J Auton Nerv Sys* 1991;34:9–16.

Roizen MF, Weise V, Grobecker H, Kopin IJ. Plasma catecholamines and dopamine-beta-hydroxylase activity in spontaneously hypertensive rats. *Life Sci* 1975;17:283–288.

Romoff MS, Keusch G, Campese VM, Wang M-S, Friedler RM, Weidmann P, Massry SG. Effect of sodium intake on plasma catecholamines in normal subjects. *J Clin Endocrinol Metab* 1979;48:26–31.

Rooney DP, Edgar JD, Sheridan B, Atkinson AB, Bell PM. The effects of low dose insulin infusions on the renin angiotensin and sympathetic nervous systems in normal man. *Eur J Clin Invest* 1991;21:430–435.

Rose CE Jr, Althaus JA, Kaiser DL, Miller ED, Carey RM. Acute hypoxemia and hypercapnia: Increase in plasma catecholamines in conscious dogs. *Am J Physiol* 1983;245:H924–H929.

Rose CP, Burgess JH, Cousineau D. Tracer norepinephrine kinetics in coronary circulation of patients with heart failure secondary to chronic pressure and volume overload. *J Clin Invest* 1985;76:1740–1747.

Rosell S, Axelrod J, Kopin IJ. Release of tritiated epinephrine following sympathetic nerve stimulation. *Nature* 1964;201:301.

Rosen SG, Supiano MA, Perry TJ, Linares OA, Hogikyan RV, Smith MA, Halter JB. β-Adrenergic blockade decreases norepinephrine release in humans. *Am J Physiol* 1990;258: E999–E1005.

Rosenblueth A, Simeone FA. The interrelations of vagal and accelerator effects on the cardiac rate. *Am J Physiol* 1934;110:42–55.

Rosengren A, Orth-Gomer K, Wedel H, Wilhelmsen L. Stressful life events, social support, and mortality in men. *Br Med J* 1993;307:1102–1105.

Rosenman RH, Brand RJ, Jenkins CD, Friedman M, Straus R, Wurm M. Coronary heart disease in the Western Collaborative Group Study: Final follow-up experience of 8 1/2 years. *J Am Med Assoc* 1975;233:872–877.

Rosenman RH, Friedman M, Straus R, Wurm M, Hahn R, Kositchek R, Werthessen N. A pre-
    dictive study of coronary heart disease. *J Am Med Assoc* 1964;189:15–22.

Rosenman RH. Pathogenesis of mitral valve prolapse and its relationship to anxiety. In Byrne
    DG, Rosenman RH (Eds) *Anxiety and the Heart.* New York: Hemisphere Publishing,
    1990, pp 295–346.

Ross CA, Ruggiero DA, Joh TH, Park DH, Reis DJ. Rostral ventrolateral medulla: Selective
    projections to the thoracic autonomic cell columns from the region containing C1 adren-
    aline neurons. *J Comp Neurol* 1984a;228:168–185.

Ross CA, Ruggiero DA, Park DH, Joh TH, Sved AF, Fernandez-Pardal J, Saavedra JM , Reis
    DJ. Tonic vasomotor control by the rostral ventrolateral medulla: Effect of electrical or
    chemical stimulation of the area containing C1 adrenaline neurons on arterial pressure,
    heart rate, and plasma catecholamines and vasopressin. *J Neurosci* 1984b;4:474–494.

Ross CA, Ruggiero DA, Reis DJ. Projections from the nucleus tractus solitarii to the rostral
    ventrolateral medulla. *J Comp Neurol* 1985;242:511–534.

Rossi L. Neuroanatomopathology of the cardiovascular system. In Kulbertus HE, Franck G (Eds)
    Neurocardiology. Mount Kisco, NY: Futura, 1988, pp 25–55.

Rostrup M, Mundal HH, Westheim A, Eide I. Awareness of high blood pressure increases arterial
    plasma catecholamines, platelet noradrenaline and adrenergic responses to mental stress.
    J Hypertens 1991;9:159–166.

Routledge C, Marsden CA. Electrical stimulation of the C1 region of the rostral ventrolateral
    medulla of the rat increases mean arterial pressure and adrenaline release in the posterior
    hypothalamus. *Neuroscience* 1987;20:457–466.

Rowe BP, Nasjlettia A. The effect of angiotensin II infusion on plasma catecholamines in the
    conscious rabbit. *Proc Soc Exp Biol Med* 1981;168:1101–1113.

Rowell LB, Seals DR. Sympathetic activity during graded central hypovolemia in hypoxemic
    humans. *Am J Physiol* 1990;259:H1197–H1206.

Rowell LB. *Human Circulation Regulation during Physical Stress.* New York: Oxford University
    Press, 1986.

Roy A, Pickar D, Linnoila M, Chrousos GP, Gold PW. Cerebrospinal fluid corticotropin-releasing
    hormone in depression: Relationship to noradrenergic function. *Psychiatry Res* 1987;20:
    229–37.

Rozanski A, Bairey CN, Krantz DS, Friedman J, Resser KJ, Morell M, Hilton-Chalfen S, Hestrin
    L, Bietendorg J, Berman DS. Mental stress and the induction of silent myocardial ischemia
    in patients with coronary artery disease. *N Engl J Med* 1988;318:1005–1112.

Rozanski A, Krantz DS, Bairey CN. Ventricular responses to mental stress testing in patients
    with coronary artery disease. Pathophysiological implications. *Circulation* 1991;83
    (Suppl II):II137–II144.

Rubin Z, McNeil EB. *Psychology: Being Human.* New York: Harper & Row, 1987.

Ruddel H, Schmieder R, von Eiff AW, Peters TK, Zerbst E. The impact of electrical carotid sinus
    nerve stimulation on BP reactions during mental stress and ambulatory BP monitoring in
    patients with CHD and malignant hypertension. In Lown B, Malliani A, Prosdocimi M
    (Eds) *Neural Mechanisms and Cardiovascular Disease.* New York: Springer Verlag,
    1986, pp 599–601.

Rudman D, Moffitt SD, Fernhoff PM, Blackston RD, Faraj BA. Epinephrine deficiency in hypo-
    corticotropic hypopituitary children. *J Clin Endocrinol Metab* 1981;53:722–728.

Ruffolo RR Jr, Sulpizio AC, Nichols AJ, DeMarinis RM, Hieble JP. Pharmacological differen-
    tiation between pre- and postjunctional alpha 2-adrenoceptors by SK & F 104078. *Nau-
    nyn-Schmiedeberg's Arch Pharmacol* 1987;336:415–418.

Russek HI. Emotional stress and coronary heart disease in American physicians. *Am J Med Sci* 1960;39:711–721.

Ryan KO, Thornton RM, Proppe DW. Vasopressin contributes to maintenance of arterial blood pressure in dehydrated baboons. *Am J Physiol* 1989;256:H486–H492.

Ryan TJ, Fallon JT. Case records of the Massachusetts General Hospital. A 44-year-old women with substernal pain and pulmonary edema after severe emotional stress. *N Engl J Med* 1986;314:1240–1247.

Sabban E, Kvetnansky R, McMahon A, Fukuhara K, Kilbourne E, Kopin IJ. Stressors regulate mRNA levels of tyrosine hydroxylase and dopamine β-hydroxylase in adrenals both *in vivo* and in PC12 cells. In Kvetnansky R, McCarty R, Axelrod J (Eds) *Stress: Neuroendocrine and Molecular Approaches.* New York: Gordon and Breach, 1992, pp 325–335.

Sacks FM, Dzau VJ. Adrenergic effect on plasma lipoprotein metabolism. *Am J Med* 1986;80 (Suppl 2A):71–81.

Sadeghi HM, Eikenburg DC. Chronic epinephrine treatment fails to alter prejunctional adrenoceptor modulation of sympathetic neurotransmission in the rat mesentery. *J Pharmacol Exp Ther* 1992;261:924–930.

Sadoshima S, Yoshida F, Ibayashi S, Fujii K, Yao H, Fujishima M. Effect of chronic sympathetic denervation on cerebral circulation during development of hypertension in spontaneously hypertensive rats. *J Hypertens* 1986;4 (Suppl 3):S85–S87.

Saelens JK, Schoen MS, Kovacsics GB. An enzyme assay for norepinephrine in brain tissue. *Biochem Pharmacol* 1967;16:1043–1049.

Sagnella GA, Markandu ND, Shore AC, MacGregor GA. Changes in plasma immunoreactive atrial natriuretic peptide in response to saline infusion or to alterations in dietary sodium intake in normal subjects. *J Hypertens* 1986;4 (Suppl 2):S115–S118.

Saini V, Carr DB, Hagestad EL, Lown B, Verrier RL. Antifibrillatory mechanism of the narcotic agonist fentanyl. *Am Heart J* 1988;115:598–605.

Saito I, Takeshita E, Saruta T, Nagano S, Sekihara T. Plasma prolactin, renin and catecholamines in young normotensive and borderline hypertensive subjects. *J Hypertens* 1984;2:61–64.

Sakai K, Yoshimoto Y, Luppi PH, Fort P, el Mansari M, Jouvet M. Lower brainstem afferents to the cat posterior hypothalamus: A double labeling study. *Brain Res Bull* 1990;24:437–455.

Sales SM, House J. Job dissatisfaction as a possible risk factor in coronary heart disease. *J Chron Dis* 1971;23:861–873.

Salgado HC, Krieger EM. Reversibility of baroreceptor adaptation in chronic hypertension. *Clin Sci Mol Med* 1973;45:123s–126s.

Salt PJ. Inhibition of noradrenaline uptake 2 in the isolated rat heart by steroids, clonidine and methoxylated phenylethylamines. *Eur J Pharmacol* 1972;20:329–340.

Samuels MA. Electrocardiographic manifestations of neurological disease: A unifying hypothesis. In Beamish RE, Singal PK, Dhalla NS (Eds) *Stress and Heart Disease.* Boston: Martinus Nijhoff, 1985, pp 154–166.

Sanders JS, Mark AL, Ferguson DW. Evidence for cholinergically mediated vasodilation at the beginning of isometric exercise in humans. *Circulation* 1989a;79:815–824.

Sanders JS, Mark AL, Ferguson DW. Importance of aortic baroreflex in regulation of sympathetic responses during hypotension. Evidence from direct sympathetic nerve recordings in humans. *Circulation* 1989b;79:83–92.

Sandler M. Catecholamine synthesis and metabolism in man: Clinical implications. In Eichler O, Farah A, Herken H, Welch AD (Eds) *Handbook of Experimental Pharmacology.* XXXIII. New York: Springer-Verlag, 1972, pp 843–899.

Sanford SC. Central adrenoceptors in response to adaptation to stress. In Heal DJ, Marsden CA (Eds) *The Pharmacology of Noradrenaline in the Central Nervous System.* New York: Oxford University Press, 1990, pp 379–422.

Sano N, Way D, McGrath BP. Renal sympathetic nerve activity measured by norepinephrine spillover rate in response to changes in blood pressure in conscious rabbits. *Clin Exp Pharmacol Physiol* 1989;16:319–322.

Saper CB, Swanson LW, Cowan WM. The efferent connections of the ventromedial nucleus of the hypothalamus of the rat. *J Comp Neurol* 1976;169:409–442.

Sapolsky RM. Adrenocortical function, social rank, and personality among wild baboons. *Biol Psychiatry* 1990b;28:862–878.

Sapolsky RM. Stress in the wild. *Sci Am* (January) 1990a, pp 116–123.

Saslow G, Gressel GC, Shobe FO, DuBois PH, Schroeder HA. Possible etiologic relevance of personality factors in arterial hypertension. *Psychosom Med* 1950;12:292–302.

Sassa H. Mechanism of myocardial catecholamine depletion in cardiac hypertrophy and failure in rabbits. *Jpn Circ J* 1971;35:391–403.

Satinoff E, Rutstein J. Behavioral thermoregulation in rats with anterior hypothalamic lesions. *J Comp Physiol Psychol* 1970;71:77–82.

Saul LJ. Hostility in cases of essential hypertension. *Psychosom Med* 1939;1:153–161.

Savard P, Cardinal R, Nadeau RA, Armour JA. Epicardial distribution of ST segment and T wave changes produced by stimulation of intrathoracic ganglia or cardiopulmonary nerves in dogs. *J Auton Nerv Sys* 1991;34:47–58.

Sawchenko PE, Swanson LW. Central noradrenergic pathways for the integration of hypothalamic neuroendocrine and autonomic responses. *Science* 1981a;214:685–687.

Sawchenko PE, Swanson LW. Immunohistochemical identification of neurons in the paraventricular nucleus of the hypothalamus that project to the medulla or to the spinal cord in the rat. *J Comp Neurol* 1981b;196:271–285.

Sawchenko PE, Swanson LW. The organization of noradrenergic pathways from the brainstem to the paraventricular and supraoptic nuclei in the rat. *Brain Res* 1982;4:275–325.

Sawchenko PE. A tale of three peptides: Corticotropin-releasing factor-, oxytocin-, and vasopressin-containing pathways mediating integrated hypothalamic responses to stress. In McCubbin JW, Kaufman PG, Nemeroff CB (Eds) *Stress, Neuropeptides, and Systemic Disease.* New York: Academic Press, 1991, pp 3–17.

Saynavalammi P, Vaalasti A, Pyykonen M-L, Ylitalo P, Vapaatalo H. The effect of renal sympathectomy on blood pressure and plasma renin activity in spontaneously hypertensive and normotensive rats. *Acta Physiol Scand* 1982;115:289–293.

Schaal SF, Wallace AG, Sealy WC. Protective influence of cardiac denervation against arrhythmias of myocardial infarction. *Cardiovasc Res* 1969;3:241–244.

Schachter S, Singer J. Cognitive, social, and physiological determinants of emotional state. *Psychol Rev* 1962;69:379–399.

Schadt JC, Ludbrook J. Hemodynamic and neurohumoral responses to acute hypovolemia in conscious mammals. *Am J Physiol* 1991;260:H305–H318.

Schauer UJ, Schauer I. Inhibition of human lecithin:cholesterol acyltransferase activity by catecholamines in vitro. *Biomed Biochim Acta* 1989;48:849–852.

Scherrer U, Vissing S, Morgan BJ, Hanson P, Victor RG. Vasovagal syncope after infusion of a vasodilator in a heart-transplant recipient. *N Engl J Med* 1990a;322:602–604.

Scherrer U, Vissing S, Morgan BJ, Rollins JA, Tindall RS, Ring S, Hanson P, Mohanty PK, Victor RG. Cyclosporine-induced sympathetic activation and hypertension after heart transplantation. *N Engl J Med* 1990b;323:693–699.

Scheurink AJW, Steffens AB, Gaykema RPA. Hypothalamic adrenoceptors mediate sympatho-adrenal activity in exercising rats. *Am J Physiol* 1990;259:R470–R477.

Schlor K-H, Stumpf H, Stock G. Baroreceptor reflex during arousal induced by electrical stimulation of the amygdala or by natural stimuli. *J Auton Nerv Sys* 1984;10:157–165.

Schmid PG, Lund DD, Davis JA, Whiteis CA, Bhatnagar RK, Roskoski R Jr. Selective sympathetic neural changes in hypertrophied right ventricle. *Am J Physiol* 1982;234:H175–H180.

Schmidt RM, Kumada M, Sagawa K. Cardiovascular responses to various pulsatile pressures in the carotid sinus. *Am J Physiol* 1972;223:1–7.

Schnall PL, Pieper C, Schwartz JE, Karasek RA, Schlussel Y, Devereux RB, Ganau A, Alderman M, Warren K, Pickering TG. The relationship between 'job strain,' workplace diastolic blood pressure, and left ventricular mass index. Results of a case-control study. *J Am Med Assoc* 1990;263:1929–1935.

Schomig A, Fischer S, Kunz T, Richardt G, Schomig E. Nonexocytotic release of endogenous noradrenaline in the ischemic and anoxic rat heart: Mechanism and metabolic requirements. *Circ Res* 1987;60:194–205.

Schomig A, Richardt G. Cardiac sympathetic activity in myocardial ischemia: Release and effects of noradrenaline. In Heusch G, Ross J Jr (Eds) *Adrenergic Mechanisms in Myocardial Ischemia*. New York: Springer Verlag Darmstadt, 1990, pp 9–30.

Schomig A. Adrenergic mechanisms in myocardial infarction: cardiac and systemic catecholamine release. *J Cardiovasc Pharmacol* 1988; (Suppl 1): S1–S7.

Schramm LP, Chornoboy ES. Sympathetic activity in spontaneously hypertensive rats after spinal transection. *Am J Physiol* 1982;243:R506–R511.

Schrier RW. Body fluid volume regulation in health and disease: A unifying hypothesis. *Ann Int Med* 1990;113:155–159.

Schulkin J. *Sodium Hunger.* New York: Cambridge University Press, 1992.

Schultz HD, Fater DC, Sundet WD, Geer PG, Goetz KL. Reflexes elicited by acute stretch of atrial vs. pulmonary receptors in conscious dogs. *Am J Physiol* 1982;242:H1065–H1076.

Schwaber JS, Kapp BS, Higgins G. The origin and extent of direct amygdala projections to the region of the dorsal motor nucleus of the vagus and the nucleus of the solitary tract. *Neurosci Lett* 1980;20:15–20.

Schwaiger M, Guibourg H, Rosenspire K, McClanahan T, Gallagher K, Hutchins G, Wieland DM. Effect of regional myocardial ischemia on sympathetic nervous system as assessed by fluorine-18-metaraminol. *J Nucl Med* 1990a;31:1352–1357.

Schwaiger M, Hutchins GD, Kalff V, Rosenspire K, Haka MS, Mallette S, Deeb M, Abrams GD, Wieland D. Evidence for regional catecholamine uptake and storage sites in the transplanted human heart by positron emission tomography. *J Clin Invest* 1991;87:1681–1690.

Schwaiger M, Kalff V, Rosenspire K, Haka MS, Molina E, Hutchins GD, Deeb M, Wolfe E Jr, Wieland DM. Noninvasive evaluation of sympathetic nervous system in human heart by positron emission tomography. *Circulation* 1990b;82:457–464.

Schwartz NS, Clutter WE, Shah SD, Cryer PE. Glycemic thresholds for activation of glucose counterregulatory systems are higher than the threshold for symptoms. *J Clin Invest* 1987; 79:777–781.

Schwartz PJ, Stone HL, Brown AM. Effects of unilateral stellate ganglion blockade on the arrhythmias associated with coronary occlusion. *Am Heart J* 1976;92:589–599.

Schwartz PJ, Stromba-Badiale M. Parasympathetic nervous system and malignant arrhythmias.

In Kulbertus HE, Franck G (Eds) *Neurocardiology*. Mount Kisco, NY: Futura, 1988, pp 179–200.

Schwartz PJ, Zaza A, Locati E, Moss AJ. Stress and sudden death. The case of the long QT syndrome. *Circulation* 1991;83 (Suppl II):II71–II80.

Schwartz PJ. Idiopathic long QT syndrome: Progress and questions. *Am Heart J* 1985;109:399–411.

Schwartzmann RJ. Reflex sympathetic dystrophy and causalgia. *Neurol Clin* 1992;10:953–973.

Schwarzenbrunner U, Schmidle T, Obendorf D, Scherman D, Hook V, Fischer-Colbrie R, Winkler H. Sympathetic axons and nerve terminals: The protein composition of small and large dense-core and of a third type of vesicles. *Neuroscience* 1990;37:819–827.

Scott TM, Pang SC. The correlation between the development of sympathetic innervation and the development of medial hypertrophy in jejunal arteries in normotensive and spontaneously hypertensive rats. *J Auton Nerv Sys* 1983;8:25–32.

Scriven AJI, Dollery CT, Murphy MB, Macquin I, Brown MJ. Blood pressure and plasma norepinephrine concentrations after endogenous norepinephrine release by tyramine. *Clin Pharmacol Therap* 1983;33:710–716.

Seals D, Victor R, Mark A. Plasma norepinephrine and muscle sympathetic discharge during rhythmic exercise in humans. *J Appl Physiol* 1988;65:940–944.

Seals DR. Sympathetic neural adjustments to stress in physically trained and untrained humans. *Hypertension* 1991;17:36–43.

Seckl JR, Haddock JA, Dunne MJ, Lightman SL. Opioid-mediated inhibition of oxytocin during insulin-induced hypoglycemic stimulation of vasopressin in man. *Acta Endocrinol* 1988; 118:77–81.

Seckl JR, Williams TDM, Lightman SL. Oral hypertonic saline causes transient fall of vasopressin in humans. *Am J Physiol* 1986;251:R214–R217.

Segal M, Bloom FE. The action of norepinephrine in the rat hippocampus. *Brain Res* 1976;107:499–525.

Segar WE, Moore WW. The regulation of antidiuretic hormone release in man. Effects of change in position and ambient temperature on blood ADH levels. *J Clin Invest* 1968;47:2143–2151.

Seino Y, Shimai S, Tanaka K, Takano T, Hayakawa H. Cardiovacular circulatory adjustments and renal function in acute heart failure. *Jpn Circ J* 1989;53:180–190.

Seligman MEP, Maier SF. Failure to escape traumatic shock. *J Exper Psychol* 1967;74:1–9.

Seller H, Illert M. The localization of the first synapse in the carotid sinus baroreceptor reflex pathway and its alteration of the afferent input. *Pflugers Arch* 1969;306:1–19.

Selye H. A syndrome produced by diverse nocuous agents. *Nature* 1936;138:32.

Selye H. *Stress without Distress*. New York: New American Library, 1974.

Selye H. Stress: Eustress, distress, and human perspectives. In Day SB (Ed) *Life Stress*. Vol III. *Companion to the Life Sciences*. New York: Van Nostrand Reinhold, 1982, pp 3–13.

Selye H. *The Chemical Prevention of Cardiac Necrosis*. New York: Ronald Press, 1958.

Selye H. *The Physiology and Pathology of Exposure to Stress. A Treatise Based on the Concepts of the General-Adaptation Syndrome and the Diseases of Adaptation*. Montreal, Canada: Acta, 1950.

Selye H. *The Stress of Life*. New York: McGraw-Hill, 1956.

Senba EK, Matsunaga K, Tohyama M, Noguchi K. Stress-induced c-fos expression in the rat brain: Activation mechanism of sympathetic pathway. *Brain Res Bull* 1993;31:329–344.

Seri I, Kone BC, Gullans SR, Aperia A, Brenner BM, Ballermann BJ. Locally formed dopamine inhibits Na-K-ATPase activity in rat renal cortical tubule cells. *Am J Physiol* 1988;255: F666–F673.

Sewell WH, Koth DR, Huggins CE. Ventricular fibrillation in dogs after sudden return of flow to the coronary artery. *Surgery* 1955;38:1050–1053.

Shade RE, Bishop VS, Haywood JR, Hamm CK. Cardiovascular and neuroendocrine responses to baroreceptor denervation in baboons. *Am J Physiol* 1990;258:R930–R938.

Shah SD, Tse TF, Clutter WE, Cryer PE. The human sympathochromaffin system. *Am J Physiol* 1984;247:E380–E384.

Share NN, Melville KI. Centrally mediated sympathetic cardiovascular responses induced by intraventricular norepinephrine. *J Pharmacol Exp Ther* 1963;141:15–21.

Sharma AD, Saffitz JE, Lee BI, Sobel BE, Corr PB. Alpha adrenergic-mediated accumulation of calcium in reperfused myocardium. *J Clin Invest* 1983;72:802–818.

Sharma VS, Barar FS. Restraint stress as it influences the myocardium of rat. *Indian J Med Res* 1966;54:1102–1107.

Sharpey-Schaefer EP. Syncope. *Br Med J* 1956;1:506–509.

Shattil SJ, Anaya-Galindo R, Bennett J, Colman RW, Cooper RA. Platelet hypersensitivity induced by cholesterol incorporation. *J Clin Invest* 1975;55:636–643.

Shekelle R, Gale M, Ostfeld A. Hostility, risk of coronary heart disease and mortality. *Psychosom Med* 1983;45:109–114.

Shekelle RB, Hulley SB, Neaton JD, Billings JH, Borhani NO, Gerace TA, Jacobs DR, Lasser NL, Mittlemark MB, Stamler J. The MRFIT behavior pattern study. II. Type A behavior and incidence of coronary heart disease. *Am J Epidemiol* 1985;122:559–570.

Shepherd AM, Pinkley W, Lin MS, McNay JL, Keeton TK. Activation of the renin-angiotensin system by sodium nitroprusside in essential hypertension. *J Cardiovasc Pharmacol* 1984; 6:201–205.

Shepherd AMM, Irvine NA. Differential hemodynamic and sympathoadrenal effects of sodium nitroprusside and hydralazine in hypertensive subjects. *J Cardiovasc Pharmacol* 1986;8: 527–533.

Shepherd JT, Vanhoutte PM. *The Human Cardiovascular System.* New York: Raven Press, 1979.

Shepherd JT. Increased systemic vascular resistance and primary hypertension: The expanding complexity. *J Hypertens* 1990;8 (Suppl 7):S15–S27.

Sheridan DJ, Penkoske PA, Sobel BE, Corr PB. Alpha-adrenergic contributions to dysrhythmia during myocardial ischemia and reperfusion in cats. *J Clin Invest* 1980;65:161–171.

Shigeno T. Norepinephrine in cerebrospinal fluid of patients with cerebral vasospasm. *J Neurosurg* 1982;56:344–349.

Shikuma R, Yoshimura M, Kambara S, Yamazaki H, Takashina R, Takahashi H, Takeda K, Ijichi H. Dopaminergic modulation of salt sensitivity in patients with essential hypertension. *Life Sci* 1986;38:915–921.

Shimada S, Kitayama S, Lin CL, Patel A, Nanthakumar E, Gregor P, Kuhar M, Uhl G. Cloning and expression of a cocaine-sensitive dopamine transporter complementary DNA. *Science* 1991;254:576–578.

Shore AC, Markandu ND, Sagnella GA, Singer DRJ, Forsling ML, Buckley MG, Sugden AL, MacGregor GA. Endocrine and renal response to water loading and water restriction in normal man. *Clin Sci* 1988;75:171–177.

Shy GM, Drager GA. A neurological syndrome associated with orthostatic hypotension. *Arch Neurol* 1960;3:511–527.

Sibley DR, Lefkowitz RJ. Molecular mechanisms of receptor desensitization using the β-adrenergic receptor-coupled adenylate cyclase system as a model. *Nature* 1985;317:124–129.

Sibley DR, Monsma FJ Jr. Molecular biology of dopamine receptors. *Trends Pharmacol Sci* 1992;13:61–69.

Siciliano H. Les effets de la compression des carotides sur la pression, sur le coeur et sur la respiration. *Arch Ital Biol* 1900;33:338–344.

Siegel A, Edinger H, Dotto M. Effects of electrical stimulatino of the lateral aspect of the prefrontal cortex upon attack behavior in rats. *Brain Res* 1975;93:473–484.

Siegel A, Edinger H, Lowenthal H. Effects of electrical stimulation of the medial aspect of the prefrontal cortex upon attack behavior in cats. *Brain Res* 1974;66:467–479.

Siegel S. Conditioning of insulin effects. *J Comp Physiol Psychol* 1972;78:233–241.

Sigg EB, Keim KL, Kepner. Selective effect of diazepam on certain central sympathetic components. *Neuropharmacology* 1971;10:621–629.

Sigg EB, Sigg TD. Hypothalamic stimulation of preganglionic autonomic activity and its modification by chlorpromazine, diazepam and pentobarbital. *Int J Neuropharmacol* 1969;8: 567–572.

Sigg EB. The organization and functions of the central sympathetic nervous system. In Levi L (Ed) *Emotions—Their Parameters and Measurement.* New York: Raven Press, 1975, pp 93–122.

Silverberg AB, Shah SD, Haymond MW, Cryer PE. Norepinephrine: hormone and neurotransmitter in man. *Am J Physiol* 1978;234:E252–E256.

Silverman AJ, Oldfield B, Hou-Yu A, Zimmerman EA. The noradrenergic innervation of vasopressin neurons in the paraventricular nucleus of the hypothalamus: An ultrastructural study using radioautography and immunocytochemistry. *Brain Res* 1985;325:215–219.

Sim MK, Hsu TP. Levels of dopamine and 3,4-dihydroxyphenylacetic acid in the adenohypophysis of normo- and hypertensive rats. *Clin Exp Hypertens* 1990;A12:343–353.

Simon OR, Schramm LP. The spinal course and medullary termination of myelinated renal afferents in the rat. *Brain Res* 1984;290:239–247.

Simon RP. Physiologic consequences of status epilepticus. *Epilepsia* 1985;26 (Suppl 1):S58–S66.

Simpson P, McGrath A, Savion S. Myocyte hypertrophy in neonatal heart cultures and its regulation by serum and by catecholamines. *Circ Res* 1982;51:787–801.

Singal PK, Beamish RE, Dhalla NS. Potential oxidative pathways of catecholamines in the formation of lipid peroxides and genesis of heart disease. *Adv Exp Med Biol* 1983;161:391–401.

Singal PK, Dhillon KS, Beamish RE, Kapur N, Dhalla NS. Myocardial cell damage and cardiovascular changes due to i.v. infusion of adrenochrome in rats. *Br J Pathol* 1982;63:167–176.

Singal PK, Kapur N, Dhillon KS, Beamish RE, Dhalla NS. Role of free radicals in catecholamine-induced cardiomyopathy. *Can J Physiol Pharmacol* 1982;60:1390–1397.

Singewald N, Schneider C, Philippu A. Effects of blood pressure changes on the catecholamine release in the locus coeruleus of cats anesthetized with pentobarbital or chloralose. *Naunyn-Schmiedeberg's Arch Pharmacol* 1993;348:242–248.

Siragy HM, Felder RA, Howell NL, Chevalier RL, Peach MJ, Carey RM. Evidence that intrarenal dopamine acts as a paracrine substance at the renal tubule. *Am J Physiol* 1989;257:F469–F477.

Siren A-L, Paakkari P, Goldstein DS, Feuerstein G. Mechanisms of central hemodynamic and sympathetic regulation by mu opioid receptors: Effects of dermorphin in the conscious rat. *J Pharmacol Exp Ther* 1989;248:596–604.

Sisson JC, Wieland DM. Radiolabeled meta-iodobenzylguanidine: Pharmacology and clinical studies. *Am J Physiol Imaging* 1986;1:96–103.

Skinner JE, Lie JT, Entman ML. Modification of ventricular fibrillation latency following coronary artery occlusion in the conscious pig: The effects of psychological stress and beta-adrenergic blockade. *Circulation* 1975;51:656–667.

Skinner JE, Reed JC. Blockade of a frontocortical-brainstem pathway prevents ventricular fibrillation of the ischemic heart in pigs. *Am J Physiol* 1981;240:H156–H163.

Skinner JE. Psychosocial stress and sudden cardiac death: brain mechanisms. In Beamish RE, Singal PK, Dhalla NS (Eds) *Stress and Heart Disease*. Boston: Martinus Nijhoff, 1985, pp 44–59.

Skoog P, Mansson J, Thoren P. Changes in renal sympathetic outflow during hypotensive haemorrhage in rats. *Acta Physiol Scand* 1985;125:655–660.

Skrabal F, Herholz, Neumayer M, Ledochowski M, Schwarz S, Hamberger L. Enhanced sympathetic responsiveness as a cause of salt sensitivity in normal man. *J Hypertens* 1983;1 (Suppl 2):162–164.

Sleight P, Fox P, Lopez R, Brooks DE. The effect of mental arithmetic on blood pressure variability and baroreflex sensitivity in man. *Clin Sci Mol Med* 1978;55 (Suppl 4):381s–382s.

Sleight P, Robinson JL, Brooks D, Rees PM. Characteristics of single carotid sinus baroreceptor fibres and whole nerve activity in the normotensive and the renal hypertensive dog. *Circ Res* 1977;41:750–758.

Sleight P. Disorders of neural control of the cardiovascular system: clinical implications of cardiovascular reflexes. In Zanchetti A, Tarazi RC (Eds) *Handbook of Hypertension*, Vol 8: *Pathophysiology of Hypertension—Regulatory Mechanisms*. New York: Elsevier Science, 1986, pp 82–95.

Slotkin TA, Kirshner N. Uptake, storage, and distribution of amines in bovine adrenal medullary vesicles. *Mol Pharmacol* 1971;7:581–592.

Smith AD. Mechanisms involved in the release of noradrenaline from sympathetic nerves. *Br Med Bull* 1973;29:123–129.

Smith JK, Barron KW. Cardiovascular effects of L-glutamate and tetrodotoxin microinjected into the rostral and caudal ventrolateral medulla in normotensive and spontaneously hypertensive rats. *Brain Res* 1990c;506:1–8.

Smith JK, Barron KW. GABAergic responses in ventrolateral medulla in spontaneously hypertensive rats. *Am J Physiol* 1990a;258:R450–R456.

Smith JK, Barron KW. The rostral and caudal ventrolateral medulla in young spontaneously hypertensive rats. *Brain Res* 1990b;506:153–158.

Smith M, Ray CT. Cardiac arrhythmias, increased intracranial pressure, and the autonomic nervous system. *Chest* 1972;61:125–133.

Smith MA, Brady LS, Glowa J, Gold PW, Herkenham M. Effects of stress and adrenalectomy on tyrosine hydroxylase mRNA levels in the locus ceruleus by in situ hybridization. *Brain Res* 1991;544:26–32.

Smith ML, Ellenbogen KA, Eckberg DL. Sympathoinhibition and hypotension in carotid sinus hypersensitivity. *Clin Auton Res* 1992;2:389–392.

Smith OA, Astley CA, Chesney MA, Taylor DJ, Spelman FA. Personality, stress and cardiovascular disease: Human and nonhuman primates. In Lown B, Malliani A, Prosdocimi M (Eds) *Neural Mechanisms and Cardiovascular Disease*. New York: Springer Verlag, 1986, pp 471–484.

Smith OA, DeVito JL, Astley CA. Neurons controlling cardiovascular responses to emotion are located in lateral hypothalamus-perifornical region. *Am J Physiol* 1990;259:R943–R954.

Smith OA, DeVito JL. Central neural integration for the control of autonomic responses associated with emotion. *Ann Rev Neurosci* 1984;4:43–65.

Smith OA, Golanov E, Astley CA, Chalyan V, Spelman FA, Urmancheeva T, Bowden DM, Chesney MA. Behavior and the cardiovascular system. In Kulbertus HE, Franck G (Eds) *Neurocardiology*. Mount Kisco, NY: Futura, 1988, pp 279–289.

Smith R, Owens PC, Lovelock M, Chan EC, Falconer J. Acute hemorrhagic stress in conscious sheep elevates immunoreactive beta-endorphin in plasma but not in cerebrospinal fluid. *Endocrinology* 1986;118:2572–2576.

Smits P, Lender JWM, Willemsen JJ, Thien T. Adenosine attenuates the response to sympathetic stimuli in humans. *Hypertension* 1991;18:216–223.

Smyth HS, Sleight P, Pickering GW. Reflex regulation of arterial pressure during sleep in man: quantitative method of assessing baroreflex sensitivity. *Circ Res* 1969;24:109–121.

Snyder DW, Nathan MA, Reis DJ. Chronic lability of arterial pressure produced by selective destruction of the catecholamine innervation of the nucleus tractus solitarii in the rat. *Circ Res* 1978;43:662–671.

Snyder SH. Adenosine as a neuromodulator. *Ann Rev Neurosci* 1985;8:103–124.

Soares-da-Silva P, Fernandes MH. Sodium-dependence and ouabain-sensitivity of the synthesis of dopamine in renal tissues of the rat. *Br J Pharmacol* 1992;105:811–816.

Sokoloff P, Giros B, MArtres MP, Bouthenet ML, Schwartz JC. Molecular cloning and characteristics of a novel dopamine receptor (D3) as a target for neuroleptics. *Nature* 1990;347: 146–151.

Sole MJ, Drobac M, Schwartz L, Hussain MN, Vaughan-Neil EF. The extraction of circulating catecholamines by the lungs in normal man and in patients with pulmonary hypertension. *Circulation* 1979;60:160–163.

Sole MJ, Factor SM. Hamster cardiomyopathy: A genetically-transmitted sympathetic dystrophy? In Beamish RE, Panagia, V, Dhalla NS (Eds) *Pathogenesis of Stress-Induced Heart Disease*. Boston: Martinus Nijhoff, 1984, pp 34–43.

Sole MJ, Helke CJ, Jacobowitz DM. Increased dopamine in the failing hamster heart: Transvesicular transport of dopamine limits the rate of norepinephrine synthesis. *Am J Cardiol* 1982;49:1682–1690.

Sole MJ, Lo C-M, Laird CW, Sonnenblick EH, Wurtman RJ. Norepinephrine turnover in the heart and spleen of the cardiomyopathic Syrian hamster. *Circ Res* 1975;37:855–862.

Sole MJ. Sympathetic innervation of the failing heart: Pathophysiological implications. In Kulbertus HE, Franck G (Eds) *Neurocardiology*. Mount Kisco, NY: Futura, 1988, pp 201–209.

Somers VK, Dyken ME, Mark AL, Abboud FM. Sympathetic-nerve activity during sleep in normal subjects. *N Engl J Med* 1993;328:303–307.

Somers VK, Mark AL, Zavala DC, Abboud FM. Contrasting effects of hypoxia and hypercapnia on ventilation and sympathetic activity in humans. *J Appl Physiol* 1989a;67:2101–2106.

Somers VK, Mark AL, Zavala DC, Abboud FM. Influence of ventilation and hypocapnia on sympathetic nerve responses to hypoxia in normal humans. *J Appl Physiol* 1989b;67: 2095–2100.

Somiya H, Tonoue T. Neuropeptides as central integrators of autonomic nerve activity: Effects of TRH, SRIF, VIP and bombesin on gastric and adrenal nerves. *Regul Pept* 1984;9:47–52.

Sommers-Flanagan J, Greenberg RP. Psychosocial variables and hypertension: A new look at an old controversy. *J Nerv Ment Dis* 1989;177:15–24.

Somogyi P, Minson JB, Morilak D, Llewellyn-Smith IJ, McIlhinney JRA, Chalmers JP. Evidence for an excitatory amino acid pathway in the brainstem and for its involvement in cardiovascular control. *Brain Res* 1989;496:401–407.

Sowers JR, Crane PD, Beck FWJ, McClanahan M, King ME, Mohanty PK. Relationship between urinary dopamine production and natriuresis after acute intravascular volume expansion with sodium chloride in dogs. *Endocrinology* 1984;115:2085–2090.

Sowers JR, Mohanty PK. Effect of advancing age on cardiopulmonary baroreceptor function in hypertensive men. *Hypertension* 1987;10:274–279.

Spann JF, Chidsey CA, Braunwald E. Reduction of cardiac stores of norepinephrine in experimental heart failure. *Science* 1964;145:1439–1441.

Spector S, Gordon R, Sjoerdsma A, Udenfriend S. End-product inhibition of tyrosine hydroxylase as a possible mechanism for regulation of norepinephrine synthesis. *Mol Pharmacol* 1967; 3:549–555.

Spector S, Sjoerdsma A, Udenfriend S. Blockade of endogenous norepinephrine synthesis by alpha-methyl-tyrosine, an inhibitor of tyrosine hydroxylase. *J Pharmacol Exp Ther* 1965; 147:86–95.

Spickler JW, Kezdi P, Geller E. Transfer characteristics of the carotid sinus pressure control system. In Kezdi P (Ed) *Baroreceptors and Hypertension*. Oxford, UK: Pergamon, 1967, pp 31–39.

Spilken AZ, Jacobs MA. Prediction of illness behavior from measures of life crisis, manifest distress and maladaptive coping. *J Psychosom Med* 1971;33:251–264.

Spokes EGS, Bannister R, Oppenheimer DR. Multiple system atrophy with autonomic failure: Clinical, histological and neurochemical observations on four cases. *J Neurol* 1979;43: 59–82.

Sreeharan N, Kappagoda CT, Linden RJ. The role of renal nerves in the diuresis and natriuresis caused by stimulation of atrial receptors. *Q J Exp Physiol* 1981;66:163–168.

Stanford SC, Nutt DJ, Cowen PJ. Comparison of the effects of chronic desmethylimipramine administration on α_2 and β adrenoceptors in different regions of rat brain. *Neuroscience* 1983;8:161–164.

Stanford SC, Nutt DJ. Comparison of the effects of repeated electroconvulsive shock on α_2 and β adrenoceptors in different regions of rat brain. *Neuroscience* 1982;7:1753–1757.

Starc TJ, Stalcup SA. Time course of changes in plasma renin activity and catecholamines during hemorrhange in conscious sheep. *Circ Shock* 1987;21:129–140.

Starke K, Montel H, Wagner J. Effect of phentolamine on noradrenaline uptake and release. *Naunyn-Schmiedeberg's Arch Pharmacol* 1971;271:181–192.

Starke K, Taube HD, Borowski E. Presynaptic receptor systems in catecholaminergic transmission. *Biochem Pharmacol* 1977;26:259–268.

Starke K. Alpha sympathomimetic inhibiton of adrenergic and cholinergic transmission in the rabbit heart. *Naunyn-Schmiedeberg's Arch Pharmacol* 1972;274:18–45.

Starkman MN, Cameron OG, Nesse RM, Zelnik T. Peripheral catecholamine levels and the symptoms of anxiety: Studies in patients with and without pheochromocytoma. *Psychosom Med* 1990;52:129–142.

Staszewska-Barczak J. The reflex stimulation of catecholamine secretion during the acute stage of myocardial infarction in the dog. *Clin Sci* 1971;41:419–439.

Staten MA, Matthews DE, Cryer PE, Bier DM. Physiological increments in epinephrine stimulate metabolic rate in humans. *Am J Physiol* 1987;253:E322–E330.

Steel CM, French EB. Aitchison WRC. Studies on adrenaline-induced leucocytosis in normal man. I. The role of the spleen and of the thoracic duct. *Br J Haematol* 1971;21:413–421.

Steele MK, Gardner DG, Xie P, Schultz HD. Interactions between ANP and ANG II in regulating blood pressure and sympathetic outflow. *Am J Physiol* 1991;260:R1145–R1151.

Steffens AB, Van der Gugten J, Godeke J, Luiten PG, Strubbe JH. Meal-induced increases in parasympathetic and sympathetic activity elicit simultaneous rises in plasma insulin and free fatty acids. *Physiol Behav* 1986;37:119–122.

Steiger JF, McCann DS. In vivo platelet aggregation and plasma catecholamines in acute myocardial infarction. *Am Heart J* 1982;104:1255–1261.

Steinberg SF, Kaplan LM, Inouye T, Zhang JF, Robinson RB. *Alpha*-1 adrenergic stimulation of 1,4,5-inositol triphosphate formation in ventricular myocytes. *J Pharmacol Exp Ther* 1989;250:1141–1148.

Stella A, Weaver L, Golin R, Genovesi S, Zanchetti A. Cardiovascular effects of afferent renal nerve stimulaiton. *Clin Exp Hyper* 1987;A9 (Suppl 1):97–111.

Stella A, Zanchetti A. Functional role of renal afferents. *Physiol Rev* 1991;71:659–682.

Stepanovic SR, Nikolic J, Varagic VM, Jozanov O. The effects of naloxone and atropine on the plasma catecholamine responses to eserine and to forced immobilization in rats. In Van Loon GR, Kvetnansky R, McCarty R, Axelrod J (Eds) *Stress. Neurochemical and Humoral Mechanisms*. New York: Gordon and Breach, 1989, pp 599–612.

Stephenson RB, Smith OA, Scher AM. Baroreceptor regulation of heart rate in baboons during different behavioral states. *Am J Physiol* 1981;241:R277–R285.

Stephenson RK, Sole MJ, Baines AD. Neural and extraneuronal catecholamine production by rat kidneys. *Am J Physiol* 1982;232:F261–F266.

Sternberg EM, Hill JM, Chrousos GP, Kamilaris T, Listwak SJ, Gold PW, Wilder RL. Inflammatory mediatory-induced hypothalamic-pituitary-adrenal axis activation is defective in streptococcal cell wall arthritis-susceptible Lewis rats. *Proc Nat Acad Sci USA* 1989;86:2374–2378.

Sternberg EM, Young WS III, Bernardini R, Calogero AE, Chrousos GP, Gold PW, Wilder RL. A central nervous system defect in biosynthesis of corticotropin-releasing hormone is associated with susceptibility to streptococcal cell wall-induced arthritis in Lewis rats. *Proc Nat Acad Sci USA* 1989;86:4771–4775.

Stewart JR, Burmeister WE, Burmeister J, Lucchesi BR. Electrophysiologic and antiarrhythmic effects of phentolamine in experimental coronary artery occlusion and reperfusion in the dog. *J Cardiovasc Pharmacol* 1980;2:77–91.

Stjarne L, Brundin J. β2 adrenoceptors facilitating noradrenaline secretion from human vasoconstrictor nerves. *Acta Physiol Scand* 1976;97:88–93.

Stjarne L, Lishajko F. Drug-induced inhibition of noradrenaline synthesis in vitro in bovine splenic nerve tissue. *Br J Pharmacol* 1966;27:398–404.

Stjarne L. New paradigm: A digital model of feedback regulation of sympathetic neurotransmitter secretion. In Vanhoutte PM (Ed) *Vasodilatation: Vascular Smooth Muscle, Peptides, Autonomic Nerves, and Endothelium*. New York: Raven Press, 1988, pp 145–160.

Stock G, Rupprecht U, Stumpf H, Schlor KH. Cardiovascular changes during arousal elicited by stimulation of amygdala, hypothalamus and locus coreuleus. *J Auton Nerv Sys* 1981;3:503–510.

Stoddard SL, Bergdall VK, Townsend DW, Levin BE. Plasma catecholamines associated with hypothalamically-elicited defense behavior. *Physiol Behav* 1986a;36:867–873.

Stoddard SL, Bergdall VK, Townsend DW, Levin BE. Plasma catecholamines associated with hypothalamically-elicited fight (escape) behavior in the freely moving cat. *Physiol Behav* 1986b;37:709–715.

Stoddard SL, Wilson PE, Bergdall VK. Sympathoadrenal activation related to feline aggression. *Aggress Behav* 1987;13:296 (Abstract).

Stoddard-Apter SL, Siegel A Levin BE. Plasma catecholamine and cardiovascular responses following hypothalamic stimulation in the awake cat. *J Auton Nerv Sys* 1983;8:343–360.

Stone EA, Slucky AV, Platt JE, Trullas R. Reduction of the cyclic adenosine 3'5' monophosphate response to catecholamines in rat brain slices after repeated restraint stress. *J Pharmacol Exp Ther* 1985;233:382–388.

Strack AM, Sawyer WB, Hughes JH, Platt KB, Loewy AD. A general pattern of CNS innervation of the sympathetic outflow demonstrated by transneuronal pseudorabies viral infections. *Brain Res* 1989a;491:156–162.

Strack AM, Sawyer WB, Platt KB, Loewy AD. CNS cell groups regulating the sympathetic outflow to adrenal gland as revealed by transneuronal cell body labeling with pseudorabies virus. *Brain Res* 1989b;491:274–296.

Stratton JR, Halter JB. Effect of a benzodiazepine (alprazolam) on plasma epinephrine and norepinephrine levels during exercise stress. *Am J Cardiol* 1985;56:136–139.

Strauss MB. *Familiar Medical Quotations.* Boston, MA: Little, Brown, 1968.

Strauss MB. The climate for the cultivation of clinical research. *New Engl J Med* 1960;262:805–810.

Streeten DHP, Anderson GH Jr, Lebowitz M, Speller PJ. Primary hyperepinephrinemia in patients without pheochromocytoma. *Arch Int Med* 1990;150:1528–1533.

Stricker EM, Zigmond MJ. Brain monoamines, homeostasis, and adaptive behavior. In Mountcastle VB (Ed) *The Nervous System.* Section 1. *Handbook of Physiology.* Bethesda, Md: American Physiological Society, 1986, pp 677–700.

Stromberg JS, Linares OA, Supiano MA, Smith MJ, Foster AH, Halter JB. Effect of desipramine on norepinephrine metabolism in humans: Interaction with aging. *Am J Physiol* 1991;261:R1484–R1490.

Struthers AD, Reid JL, Whitesmith R, Rodger JC. Effect of intravenous adrenaline on electrocardiogram, blood pressure, and serum potassium. *Br Heart J* 1983;49:90–93.

Struyker HAJ, van Rossum JM. Clonidine-induced cardiovascular effects after stereotaxic application in the hypothalamus of rats. *J Pharm Pharmacol* 1972;24:410–411.

Struyker-Boudier HAJ, Smeets GW, Brouwer GM, van Rossum JM. Hypothalamic alpha-adrenergic receptors in cardiovascular regulation. *Neuropharmacology* 1974;13:837–846.

Stute N, Trendelenburg U. The outward transport of axoplasmic noradrenaline induced by a rise of the sodium concentration in the adrenergic nerve endings of the rat vas deferens. *Naunyn-Schmiedeberg's Arch Pharmacol* 1984;327:124–132.

Suarez EC, Williams RB. Situational determinants of cardiovascular and emotional reactivity in high- and low-hostile men. *Psychosom Med* 1989;51:404–418.

Sudhir K, Jennings GL, Esler MD, Korner PI, Blombery PA, Lambert GW, Scoggins B, Whitworth JA. Hydrocortisone-induced hypertension in humans: Pressor responsiveness and sympathetic function. *Hypertension* 1989;13:416–421.

Sullivan PA, Procci WR, DeQuattro V, Schoentgen S, Levine D, van der Meulen J, Bornheimer JF. Anger, anxiety, guilt and increased basal and stress-induced neurogenic tone: Causes or effects in primary hypertension? *Clin Sci* 1981a;61 (Suppl 7):389s–392s.

Sullivan PA, Schoentgen S, DeQuattro V, Procci WR, Levine D, van der Meulen J, Bornheimer JF. Anxiety, anger, and neurogenic tone at rest and in stress in patients with primary hypertension. *Hypertension* 1981b;3:II119–II123.

Sun M-K, Guyenet PG. Arterial baroreceptor and vagal inputs to sympathoexcitatory neurons in rat medulla. *Am J Physiol* 1987;252:R699–R709.

Sun M-K, Guyenet PG. Excitation of rostral medullary pacemaker neurons with putative sympathoexcitatory function by cyclic AMP and beta-adrenoceptor agonists 'in vitro'. *Brain Res* 1990;511:30–40.

Sun M-K, Guyenet PG. GABA-mediated baroreceptor inhibition of reticulospinal neurons. *Am J Physiol* 1985;249:R672–R680.

Sun M-K, Reis DJ. Hypoxia selectively excites vasomotor neurons of rostral ventrolateral medulla in rats. *Am J Physiol* 1994;266:R245–R256.

Sun M-K, Young BS, Hackett JT, Guyenet PG. Rostral ventrolateral medullary neurons with intrinsic pacemaker properties are not catecholaminergic. *Brain Res* 1988;451:345–349.

Sundlof G, Wallin BG. Effect of lower body negative pressure on human muscle nerve sympathetic activity. *J Physiol (Lond)* 1978b;278:525–532.

Sundlof G, Wallin BG. Human muscle nerve sympathetic activity at rest. Relationship to blood pressure and age. *J Physiol (Lond)* 1978a;274:621–637.

Supiano MA, Linares OA, Smith MJ, Halter JB. Age-related differences in norepinephrine kinetics: Effect of posture and sodium-restricted diet. *Am J Physiol* 1990;259:E422–E431.

Supiano MA, Neubig RR, Linares OA, Halter JB, Rosen SG. Effects of low-sodium diet on regulation of platelet alpha 2-adrenergic receptors in young and elderly humans. *Am J Physiol* 1989;256:E339–E344.

Surawicz B. Ventricular fibrillation. *Am J Cardiol* 1971;28:268–287.

Suzuki H, Ferrario CM, Speth RC, Brosnihan KB, Smeby RR, DeSilva P. Alterations in plasma and cerebrospinal fluid norepinephrine and angiotensin II during the development of renal hypertension in conscious dogs. *Hypertension* 1983;5 (Suppl I):I139–I148.

Suzuki H, Nakane H, Kawamura Takeshita E, Saruta T. Excretion and metabolism of dopa and dopamine by isolated perfused rat kidney. *Am J Physiol* 1984;247:E285–E290.

Suzuki S, Takeshita A, Imaizumi T, Hirooka Y, Yoshida M, Ando S-I, Nakamura M. Central nervous system mechanisms involved in inhibition of renal sympathetic nerve activity induced by arginine vasopressin. *Circ Res* 1989;65:1390–1399.

Sved AF, Imaizumi T, Talman WT, Reis DJ. Vasopressin contributes to hypertension caused by nucleus tractus solitarius lesions. *Hypertension* 1985;7:262–267.

Sved AF, Reis DJ. Contributions of arginine vasopressin and the sympathetic nervous system to fulminating hypertension after destruction of caudal ventrolateral medulla in the rat. *J Hypertens* 1985;3:491–501.

Sved AF. Clonidine can lower blood pressure by inhibiting vasopressin release. *Eur J Pharmacol* 1985;19:111–116.

Swanson LW. Organization of mammalian neuroendocrine system. In Bloom FE (Ed) *Handbook of Physiology. The Nervous System.* Vol IV. Baltimore: Waverly Press, 1986, pp 317–363.

Swanson LW. The hypothalamus. In Bjorklund A, Hokfelt T, Swanson LW (Eds) *Handbook of Chemical Neuroanatomy.* Vol 5: *Integrated Systems of the CNS,* Part I. *Hypothalamus, Hippocampus, Amygdala, Retina.* New York: Elsevier Science, 1987, pp 1–124.

Swedberg K, Eneroth P, Kjekshus J, Wilhelmsen L. Hormones regulating cardiovascular function in patients with severe congestive heart failure and their relation to mortality. *Circulation* 1990;82:1730–1736.

Swedberg K, Waagstein F, Hjalmarson A, Wallentin I. Prolongation of survival in congestive cardiomyopathy by beta-receptor blockade. *Lancet* 1979;1:1374–1376.

Sylven C. Angina pectoris. Clinical characteristics, neurophysiological and molecular mechanisms. *Pain* 1989;36:145–167.

Syme SL. Socioenvironmental factors in heart disease. In Beamish RE, Singal PK, Dhalla NS (Eds) *Stress and Heart Disease*. Boston: Martinus Nijhoff, 1985, pp 60–70.

Szabadi E, Bradshaw CM. Alpha-1 adrenergic receptors in the central nervous system. In Ruffolo RR Jr (Ed) *The Alpha-1 Adrenergic Receptors*. Clifton, NJ: Humana Press, 1987, pp 405–453.

Szabo B, Hedler L, Ensinger H, Starke K. Opioid peptides decrease noradrenaline release and blood pressure in the rabbit at peripheral receptors. *Naunyn-Schmiedeberg's Arch Pharmacol* 1986;332:50–56.

Szabo B, Hedler L, Schurr C, Starke K. Peripheral presynaptic facilitatory effect of angiotensin II on noradrenaline release in anesthetized rabbits. *J Cardiovasc Pharmacol* 1990;15:968–975.

Szabo B, Hedler L, Starke K. Facilitation of the release of noradrenaline: An extra-adrenal effect of adrenocorticotropic hormone. *Resuscitation* 1989b;18:229–242.

Szabo B, Hedler L, Starke K. Peripheral presynaptic and central effects of clonidine, yohimbine and rauwolscine on the sympathetic nervous system in rabbits. *Naunyn-Schmiedeberg's Arch Pharmacol* 1989a;340:648–657.

Szabo B, Schultheiss A. Desipramine inhibits sympathetic nerve activity in the rabbit. *Naunyn-Schmiedeberg's Arch Pharmacol* 1990;342:469–476.

Szafarczyk A, Malaval F, Laurent A, Gibaud R, Assenmacher I. Further evidence for a central stimulatory action of catecholamines on adrenocorticotropin release in the rat. *Endocrinology* 1987;121:883–892.

Szemeredi K, Bagdy G, Kopin IJ, Goldstein DS. Neurocirculatory regulation in cortisol-induced hypertension. *Clin Exp Hyper* 1989 ϒ 1:1425–1439.

Szemeredi K, Bagdy G, Stull R, Calogero AE, Kopin IJ, Goldstein DS. Sympathoadrenomedullary inhibition by chronic glucocorticoid treatment in conscious rats. *Endocrinology* 1988a;123:2585–2590.

Szemeredi K, Bagdy G, Stull R, Kopin IJ, Goldstein DS. Cortisol and alpha-2 adrenergic regulation of sympathoneural activity. *Biogenic Amines* 1990;7:445–454.

Szemeredi K, Bagdy G, Stull R, Kopin IJ, Goldstein DS. Excessive sympathoadrenomedullary responsiveness to yohimbine in young spontaneously hypertensive rats. *Life Sci* 1988b;43:1063–1068.

Szemeredi K, Komoly S, Kopin IJ, Bagdy G, Keiser HR, Goldstein DS. Simultaneous measurement of plasma and extracellular fluid concentrations of catechols after yohimbine administration in rats. *Brain Res* 1991;542:8–14.

Szemeredi K, Pacak K, Kopin IJ, Goldstein DS. Sympathoneural and skeletal muscle contributions to plasma dopa responses in pithed rats. *J Auton Nerv Sys* 1991;35:169–174.

Tache Y, Pittman Q, Brown M. Bombesin-induced poikilothermy in rats. *Brain Res* 1980;188:525–530.

Taddei S, Pedrinelli R, Salvetti A. Sympathetic nervous system-dependent vasoconstriction in humans: Evidence for mechanistic role of endogenous purine compounds. *Circulation* 1990;82:2061–2067.

Taggart P, Carruthers M, Somerville W. Electrocardiogram, plasma catecholamines and lipids and their modification by oxprenolol when speaking before an audience. *Lancet* 1973;2:341–346.

Taggart P, Carruthers M, Somerville W. Emotions, catecholamines, and the electrocardiogram. *Cardiology* 1978;7:103–124.

Taggart P, Carruthers M. Endogenous hyperlipidemia induced by emotional stress of racing driving. *Lancet* 1971;1:363–366.

Takahashi Y, Satoh K, Sakumoto T, Tohyama M, Shimizu N. A major source of catecholamine terminals in the nucleus tractus solitarii. *Brain Res* 1979;172:372–377.

Takamine J. The isolation of the active principle of the suprarenal gland. *J Physiol (Lond)* 1901; 27:30P–39P.

Takeda K, Ikajima H, Nakata T, Kawasaki S, Hayashi J, Oguro M, Sasaki S, Nakagawa M. Clonidine abolishes exaggerated pressor responses to shaker stress in spontaneously hypertensive rats. *Am J Hypertens* 1990;3:39–44.

Takemoto Y. Decreases in catecholamine concentrations of cisternal cerebrospinal fluid and plasma in rats caused by pentobarbital anesthesia. *Jpn J Physiol* 1992;42:141–145.

Takeuchi T, Manning JW. Muscle cholinergic dilators in the sinus baroreceptor response in cats. *Circ Res* 1971;29:350–357.

Takiyyuddin MA, Cervenka JH, Pandian MR, Stuenkel CA, Neumann HP, O'Connor DT. Neuroendocrine sources of chromogranin-A in normal man: Clues from selective stimulation of endocrine glands. *J Clin Endocrinol Metab* 1990b;71:360–369.

Takiyyuddin MA, Cervenka JH, Sullivan PA, Parmer RJ, Barbosa JA, O'Connor DT. Is physiologic sympathoadrenal catecholamine release exocytotic in humans? *Circulation* 1990a; 81:185–191.

Tanabe S, Bunag RD. Aging escalates baroreceptor reflex suppression by the posterior hypothalamus in rats. *Hypertension* 1991;17:80–90.

Tanaka M. Electron microscopic study of cardiac lesions induced in rats by isoproterenol and by repeated stress. With suggestion that idiopathic cardiomyopathy may be a "disease of adaptation." *Jpn Circ J* 1981;45:1342–1354.

Tanaka T, Yokoo H, Mizoguchi K, Yoshida M, Tsuda A, Tanaka M. Noradrenaline release in the rat amygdala is increased by stress: Studies with intracerebral microdialysis. *Brain Res* 1991;544:174–176.

Tanner O. *Stress.* Alexandria, Va: Time-Life Books, 1976.

Tarizzo VI, Dahlof C. Adrenaline-induced enhancement of the blood pressure response to sympathetic nerve stimulation in adrenal demedullated pithed rats. *Naunyn-Schmiedeberg's Arch Pharmacol* 1989;340:144–150.

Tavares I, Lima D, Batten TFC, Coimbra A. Is the pathway connecting the caudal ventrolateral medulla with the dorsal horn of the spinal cord of the rat noradrenergic? *Regional Anesth* 1993; 18 (Suppl):1.

Taylor AA, Davies AO, Mares A, Raschko J, Pool JL, Nelson EB, Mitchell JR. Spectrum of dysautonomia in mitral valvular prolapse. *Am J Med* 1989;86:267–274.

Teitelman G, Ross RA, Joh TH, Reis DJ. Differences in utero in activities of catecholamine biosynthetic enzymes in adrenals of spontaneously hypertensive rats. *Clin Sci* 1981;61 (Suppl 7):227s-230s.

Tennant C. Psychological stress and ischaemic heart disease: An evaluation in the light of the diseases' attribution to war service. *Aust N Z J Psychiatry* 1982;16:31–36.

Terui N, Masuda N, Saeki Y, Kumada M. Activity of barosensitive neurons in the caudal ventrolateral medulla that send axonal projections to the rostral ventrolateral medulla in rabbits. *Neurosci Lett* 1990;118:211–214.

Teuber HL. Some effects of frontal lobotomy in man. In Warren JM, Akert K (Eds) *The Frontal Granular Cortex and Behavior.* San Francisco: McGraw-Hill, 1964, pp 332–333.

Thames MD, Ballon BJ. Occlusive summation of carotid and aortic baroreflexes in control of renal nerve activity. *Am J Physiol* 1984;246:H851–H857.

Thames MD, Schmid PG. Interaction between carotid and cardiopulmonary baroreflexes in control of plasma ADH. *Am J Physiol* 1981;241:H431–H434.

The Parkinson Study Group. Effects of tocopherol and deprenyl on the progression of disability in early Parkinson's disease. *N Engl J Med* 1993;328:176–183.

Thiagarajan AB, Gleiter CH, Mefford IN, Eskay RL, Nutt DJ. Effect of single and repeated electroconvulsive shock on the hypothalamic-pituitary-adrenal axis and plasma catecholamines in rats. *Psychopharmacology* 1989;97:548–552.

Thoenen H, Hurliman A, Haefely W. Dual site of action of phenoxybenzamine in the cat's spleen: blockade of a-adrenergic receptors and inhibition of reuptake of neurally released norepinephrine. *Experientia* 1964;20:272–273.

Thoenen H. Induction of tyrosine hydroxylase in peripheral and central adrenergic neurons by cold-exposure in rats. *Nature* 1970;228:861–862.

Thomaides TN, Chaudhuri KR, Maule S, Watson L, Marsden CD, Mathias CJ. Growth hormone responses to clonidine in central and peripheral primary autonomic failure. *Lancet* 1992; 340:263–266.

Thomas CB, Duszynski KR. Blood pressure levels in young adulthood as predictors of hypertension and the fate of the cold pressor test. *Johns Hopkins Med J* 1982;151:93–100.

Thomas CB, Murphy EA. Further studies on cholesterol levels in the Johns Hopkins medical students: Effect of stress at examinations. *J Chron Dis* 1958;8:661–669.

Thomas CB. Experimental hypertension from section of moderator nerves. *Bull Johns Hopkins Hosp* 1944;74:335–377.

Thomas DN, Holman RB. A microdialysis study of the regulation of endogenous noradrenaline release in the rat hippocampus. *J Neurochem* 1991;56:1741–1746.

Thomas DP. Effect of catecholamines on platelet aggregation caused by thrombin. *Nature* 1967; 215:298–299.

Thomas JA, Marks BH. Plasma norepinephrine in congestive heart failure. *Am J Cardiol* 1978; 41:233–243.

Thomas MR, Calaresu FR. Localization and function of medullary sites mediating vagal bradycardia in the cat. *Am J Physiol* 1974;226:1344–1349.

Thor KB, Helke CJ. Catecholamine-synthesizing neuronal projections to the nucleus tractus solitarii of the rat. *J Comp Neurol* 1988;268:264–280.

Thor KB, Helke CJ. Serotonin- and substance P-containing projections to the nucleus tractus solitarii of the rat. *J Comp Neurol* 1987;265:275–293.

Thoren O, Skarphedinsson JO, Carlsson S. Sympathetic inhibition from vagal afferents during severe hemorrhage in rats. *Acta Physiol Scand* 1988;133 (Suppl 571):97–105.

Thoren P, Mark AL, Morgan DA, O'Neil TP, Needleman P, Brody MJ. Activation of vagal depressor reflexes by atriopeptins inhibits renal sympathetic nerve activity. *Am J Physiol* 1986;251:H1252–H1259.

Thoren P, Skarphendinsson JO, Carlsson S. Sympathetic inhibition from vagal afferents during severe hemorrhage in rats. *Acta Physiol Scand* Suppl 1988;571:97–105.

Thornton EW, Van-Toller C. Operant conditioning of heart-rate changes in the functionally decorticate curarised rat. *Physiol Behav* 1973;10:983–988.

Thrivikraman KV, Plotsky PM. Absence of glucocorticoid negative feedback in moderate hemorrhage in conscious rats. *Am J Physiol* 1993;264:E497–E503.

Thureson-Klein A, Klein RL, Johansson O. Catecholamine-rich cells and varicosities in bovine splenic nerve, vesicle contents and evidence of exocytosis. *J Neurobiol* 1979;10:309–324.

Thureson-Klein A. Exocytosis from large and small dense cored vescicles in noradrenergic nerve terminals. *Neuroscience* 1983;10:245–252.

Tidgren B, Hjemdahl P, Theodorsson E, Nussberger J. Renal responses to lower body negative pressure in humans. *Am J Physiol* 1990;259:F573–F579.

Tidgren B, Hjemdahl P. Renal responses to mental stress and epinephrine in humans. *Am J Physiol* 1989;257:F682–F689.

Tidgren B, Theodorsson E, Hjemdahl P. Renal and systemic plasma immunoreactive neuropeptide Y and calcitonin gene-related peptide responses to mental stress and adrenaline in humans. *Clin Physiol* 1991;11:9–19.

Timms RJ. Cortical inhibiton and facilitation of the defense reaction. *J Physiol (Lond)* 1977;266: 98–99.

Tischler AS, Perlman RL, Morse GM, Sheard BE. Glucocorticoids increase catecholamine synthesis and storage in PC12 pheochromocytoma cell cultures. *J Neurochem* 1983;40:364–370.

Todd GL, Clayton FC, McKinney ME, Ruddel H, Buell JC, Eliot RS. Plasma catecholamine variations in physiologically reactive and nonreactive individuals to cold pressor test. In Beamish RE, Panagia, V, Dhalla NS (Eds) *Pathogenesis of Stress-Induced Heart Disease.* Boston: Martinus Nijhoff, 1984, pp 185–195.

Todd GL. Morphological correlates of catecholamine-induced heart cell damage. In Beamish RE, Panagia, V, Dhalla NS (Eds) *Pathogenesis of Stress-Induced Heart Disease.* Boston: Martinus Nijhoff, 1984, pp 237–250.

Tofler GH, Brezinski D, Schafer AI, Czeisler CA, Rutherford JD, Willich SN, Gleason RE, Williams GH, Muller JE. Concurrent morning increase in platelet aggregability and the risk of myocardial infarction and sudden cardiac death. *N Engl J Med* 1987;316:514–518.

Togashi H, Skuma I, Yoshioka M, Kobayashi T, Yasuda H, Kitabatake A, Saito H, Gross SS, Levi R. A central nervous system action of nitric oxide in blood pressure regulation. *J Pharmacol Exp Ther* 1992;262:343–347.

Togashi H, Yoshioka M, Tochihara M, Matsumoto M, Saito H. Differential effects of hemorrhage on adrenal and renal nerve activity in anesthetized rats. *Am J Physiol* 1990;259:H1134–H1141.

Topel DG, Bicknell EJ, Preston KS, Christian LL, Matsushima CY. Porcine stress syndrome. *Mod Vet Pract* 1968;49:40–60.

Trapani AJ, Undesser KP, Keeton TK, Bishop VS. Neurohumoral interactions in conscious dehydrated rabbit. *Am J Physiol* 1988;254:R338–R347.

Trautwein W, Cavalic A, Flockerzi V, Normann F, Pelzer D. Modulation of calcium channel function by phosphorylation in guinea pig ventrical cells and phospholipid bilayer membranes. *Circ Res* 1987;61:117–123.

Trendelenburg U. The extraneuronal uptake and metabolism of catecholamines. In Trendelenburg U, Weiner N (Eds) *Catecholamines* I. New York: Springer-Verlag, 1988, pp 279–319.

Trendelenburg U, Weiner N (Eds) *Catecholamines* I. New York: Springer-Verlag, 1988.

Trendelenburg U, Weiner N (Eds) *Catecholamines* II. New York: Springer-Verlag, 1989.

Trevisan M, Celentano E, Meucci C, Farinaro E, Jossa F, Krogh V, Giumetti D, Panico S, Scottoni A, Mancini M. Short-term effect of natural disasters on coronary heart disease risk factors. *Arteriosclerosis* 1986;6:491–494.

Trichopoulos D, Katsouyani K, Zavitsanos X, Tzonou A, Dalla-Vargia P. Psychological stress and fatal heart attack: The Athens (1981) earthquake natural experiment. *Lancet* 1983;1: 441–444.

Trimarco B, Ricciardelli B, De Luca N, De Simone A, Cuocolo A, Galva MD, Picotti GB, Condorelli M. Participation of endogenous catecholamines in the regulation of left ventricular mass in progeny of hypertensive parents. *Circulation* 1985;72:38–46.

Troullos ES, Hargreaves KM, Goldstein DS, Stull R, Dionne RA. Epinephrine suppresses stress-induced increases in plasma immunoreactive β-endorphin in humans. *J Clin Endocrinol Metab* 1989;69:546–551.

Tsai CF, Lin MT. Pain sensitivity, thermal capability, and brain monoamine turnover in hypertensive rats. *Am J Physiol* 1987;253:R910–R916.

Tsuda K, Kuchii M, Nishio I, Masyama Y. Presynaptic alpha 2-adrenoceptor mediated regulation of norepinephrine release in perfused mesenteric vasculatures in young and adult spontaneously hypertensive rats. *Jpn Circ J* 1987b;51:25–32.

Tsuda K, Kuchii M, Nishio I. Peripheral neural mechanism of hypertension in rat models—peripheral sympathetic neurotransmission in hypertension. *J Hypertens* 1986;4 (Suppl 3): S189–S192.

Tsuda K, Kusuyama Y, Hano T, Kuchii M, Nishio I, Masuyama Y. Neurotransmitter release and vascular reactivity in spontaneously hypertensive rats. *Jpn Circ J* 1984a;48:1263–1269.

Tsuda K, Nishio I, Masuyama Y. Diminished prostaglandin-mediated inhibition of norepinephrine release from the sympathetic nerve endings in spontaneously hypertensive rats. *Clin Exp Hypertens* 1987a;A9:1601–1614.

Tsuda, K., Kusuyama, Y., Hano, T., Kuchii, M., Nishio, I., and Masuyama, Y. Alteration of presynaptic alpha-2-mediated inhibition of norepinephrine release in perfused mesenteric arteries of young and adult spontaneously hypertensive rats. *J Hypertens* 1984b;2 (Suppl 3):95–97.

Tuck ML, Stern N, Sowers JR. Enhanced 24-hour norepinephrine and renin secretion in young patients with essential hypertension: Relation with the circadian pattern of arterial blood pressure. *Am J Cardiol* 1985;55:112–115.

Tuck ML, Williams GH, Dluhy RG, Greenfield M, Moore TJ. A delayed suppression of the renin-aldosterone axis following saline infusion in human hypertension. *Circ Res* 1976; 39:711–716.

Tucker DC, Saper CB, Ruggiero DA, Reis DJ. Organization of central adrenergic pathways: I. Relationships of ventrolateral medullary projections to the hypothalamus and spinal cord. *J Comp Neurol* 1987;259:591–603.

Tuckman J, Slater S, Mendlowitz M. The role of the carotid sinus reflexes in hemodynamic regulation in normotensive and hypertensive man. In Kezdi P (Ed) *Baroreceptors and Hypertension*. Oxford, UK: Pergamon, 1967, pp 333–347.

Turkkan JS, Goldstein DS. Chronic effects of high salt intake and conflict stress on blood pressure in primates. *Integ Physiol Behav Sci.* 1991b;26:269–281.

Turkkan JS, Goldstein DS. Production and reversal of DOCA-salt hypertension in baboons. *Clin Exp Hypertens* 1987;A9:125–140.

Turkkan JS, Goldstein, DS. Stress and sodium hypertension in baboons: Neuroendocrine and pharmacotherapeutic assessments. *J Hypertens* 1991a;9:969–975.

Turkkan JS, Harris AH, Goldstein DS. Do chronically repeated pressor episodes cause sustained elevations in blood pressure? In Weiss SM, Matthews KA, Detre T, Graef JA (Eds) *Stress, Reactivity, and Cardiovascular Disease*, 1984, p 237; NIH Publication No 84-2698.

Turkkan JS. Individual behavioral and neuroendocrine changes are correlated with blood-pressure elevations during conflict alone and combined with high-salt diet in baboons. *Psychobiology* 1991;19:161–167.

Tyce GM, Van Dyke RA, Rettke SR, Atchison SR, Wiesner RH, Dickson ER, Krom RA. Human liver and conjugation of catecholamines. *J Lab Clin Med* 1987;109:532–537.

Tyce GM. Demethylation of O-methyl metabolites of catecholamines in erythrocytes: A methanol-forming reaction. *Res Comm Chem Pathol Pharmacol* 1977;16:669–685.

U'Prichard DC, Reisine TD, Mason ST, Fibiger HC, Yamamura HI. Modulation of rat brain alpha- and beta-adrenergic receptor populations by lesion of the dorsal noradrenergic bundle. *Brain Res* 1980;187:143–154.

Udelsman R, Goldstein DS, Loriaux DL, Chrousos GP. Catecholamine-glucocorticoid interactions during surgical stress. *J Surg Res* 1987a;43:539–545.

Udelsman R, Harwood JP, Millan MA, Chrousos GP, Goldstein DS, Zimlichman R, Catt KL, Aguilera G. Functional corticotropin releasing factor receptors in the primate peripheral sympathetic nervous system. *Nature* 1986;319:147–150.

Udelsman R, Norton JA, Jelenich SE, Goldstein DS, Linehan WM, Loriaux DL, Chrousos GP. Responses of the hypothalamic-pituitary-adrenal and renin-angiotensin axes and the sympathetic system during controlled surgical and anesthetic stress. *J Clin Endocrinol Metab* 1987b;64:986–994.

Udenfriend S. Tyrosine hydroxylase. *Pharmacol Rev* 1966;18:43–51.

Ueyama T, Hamada M, Hano T, Nishio I, Masuyama Y, Furukawa S. Increased nerve growth factor levels in spontaneously hypertensive rats. *J Hypertens* 1992;10:215–219.

Unnerstall JR. Localizing the alpha-1 adrenergic receptor in the central nervous system. In Ruffolo RR Jr (Ed) *The Alpha-1 Adrenergic Receptors*. Clifton, NJ: Humana Press, 1987, pp 71–109.

Urabe M, Kawasaki H, Takasaki K. Effect of endothelium removal on the vasoconstrictor response to neuronally released 5-hydroxytryptamine and noradrenaline in the rat isolated mesenteric and femoral arteries. *Br J Pharmacol* 1991;102:85–90.

Usdin TB, Mezey E, Chen C, Brownstein MJ, Hoffman BJ. Cloning of the cocaine-sensitive bovine dopamine transporter. *Proc Natl Acad Sci USA* 1991;88:11168–11171.

Ushiyama K, Ogawa T, Ishii M, Ajisaka R, Sugishita Y, Ito I. Physiologic neuroendocrine arousal by mental arithmetic stress test in healthy subjects. *Am J Cardiol* 1991;67:101–103.

Vale W, Spiess J, Rivier C, Rivier J. Characterization of a 41-residue ovine hypothalamic peptide that stimulates the secretion of corticotropin and β-endorphin. *Science* 1981;213:1394–1397.

Valenta LJ, Elias ANB, Eisenberg H. ACTH stimulation of adrenal epinephrine and norepinephrine release. *Hormone Res* 1986;23:16–20.

Valentino RJ, Curtis AL, Parris DG, Wehby RG. Antidepressant actions on brain noradrenergic neurons. *J Pharmacol Exp Ther* 1990;253:833–840.

Valentino RJ, Foote SL. Corticotropin-releasing factor disrupts sensory responses of brain noradrenergic neurons. *Neuroendocrinology* 1987;45:28–36.

Valentino RJ, Foote SL. Corticotropin-releasing hormone increases tonic but not sensory-evoked activity of noradrenergic locus coeruleus neurons in unanesthetized rats. *J Neurosci* 1988; 8:1016–1025.

Van Bockstaele E, Pieribone V, Aston-Jones G. Diverse afferents converge on the nucleus paragigantocellularis in the rat ventrolateral medulla: Retrograde and anterograde tracing studies. *J Comp Neurol* 1989;290:561–584.

van den Berg DT, de Kloet ER, van Dijken HH, de Jong W. Differential central effects of mineralocorticoid and glucocorticoid agonists and antagonists on blood pressure. *Endocrinology* 1990;126:118–124.

van den Buuse M, De Kloet ER, Vesteeg DHG, de Jong, W. Regional brain catecholamine levels and the development of hypertension in the spontaneously hypertensive rat: The effect of 6-hydroxydopamine. *Brain Res* 1984;301:221–229.

van den Buuse M, Veldhuis HD, Versteeg DHG, de Jong W. Substantia nigra lesions attenuate the development of hypertension and behavioural hyperreactivity in spontaneously hypertensive rats. *Pharmacol Biochem Behav* 1986;25:317–324.

van den Buuse M, Versteeg DHG, de Jong, W. Role of dopamine in the development of spontaneous hypertension. *Hypertension* 1984;6:899–905.

van der Hoorn FAJ, Man in't Veld AJ, Schalekamp MADH. Determination of catecholamines in human plasma by high-performance liquid chromatography: Comparison between a new method with fluorescence detection and an established method with electrochemical detection. *J Chromatog* 1989;487:17–28.

van der Linden P-W G, Struyvenberg A, Kraaijenhagen RJ, Hack CE, van der Zwan JK. Anaphylactic shock after insect-sting challenge in 138 persons with a previous insect-sting reaction. *Ann Int Med* 1993;118:161–168.

van Huysse JW, Bealer SL. Central nervous system norepinephrine release during hypotension and hyperosmolality in conscious rats. *Am J Physiol* 1991;260:R1071–R1076.

van Lieshout JJ, Wieling W, Karemaker JM, Eckberg DL. The vasovagal response. *Clin Sci* 1991;81:575–586.

van Loon J, Shivalkar B, Plets C, Goffin J, Tjandra-Maga TB, Fleming W. Catecholamine response to a gradual increase of intracranial pressure. *J Neurosurg* 1993;79:705–709.

Vanoli E, Stramba-Badiale M, De Ferrari G, Cerati D, Billman G, Schwartz PJ. Baroreflex sensitivity and sudden death in conscious dogs before and after myocardial infarction. *J Am Coll Cardiol* 1987;9:80A (Abstract).

Varner KJ, Grosskreutz CL, Cox BF, Brody MJ. Differential regulation of sympathetic nerve activity by lateral and medial subregions of the rostral ventral medulla. *Prog Brain Res* 1989;81:99–103.

Vatner DE, Lavallee M, Amano J, Finizola A, Homcy CJ, Vatner SF. Mechanisms of supersensitivity to sympathomimetic amines in the chronically denervated heart of the conscious dog. *Circ Res* 1985;57:55–64.

Vatner SF, Manders WT, Knight DR. Vagally mediated regulation of renal function in conscious primates. *Am J Physiol* 1986;250:H546–H549.

Vatner SF, Pagani M, Manders WT, Pasipoularides AD. Alpha adrenergic vasoconstriction and nitroglycerin vasodilation of large coronary arteries in the conscious dog. *J Clin Invest* 1980;65:5–14.

Veith RC, Featherstone JA, Linares OA, Halter JB. Age differences in plasma norepinephrine kinetics in humans. *J Gerontol* 1986;41:319–324.

Velasquez MT, Menitove JE, Skelton MM, Cowley AW Jr. Hormonal responses and blood pressure maintenance in normal and hypertensive subjects during acute blood loss. *Hypertension* 1987;9:423–428.

Ventura HO, Messerli FH, Barron RE. Norepinephrine-induced hypertension in Guillain Barre syndrome. *J Hypertens* 1986;4:265–267.

Verrier RL, Dickerson LW. Autonomic nervous system and coronary blood flow changes related to emotional activation and sleep. *Circulation* 1991;83 (Suppl II):II81–II89.

Verrier RL, Hagestad EL, Lown B. Delayed myocardial ischemia induced by anger. *Circulation* 1987;75:249–254.

Verrier RL, Lown B. Autonomic nervous system and malignant cardiac arrhythmias. In Weiner H, Hofer MA, Stunkard AJ (Eds) *Brain, Behavior, and Bodily Disease*. New York: Raven Press, 1981, pp 273–291.

Victor RG, Leimbach WN Jr, Seals DR, Wallin BG, Mark AL. Effects of the cold pressor test on muscle sympathetic nerve activity in humans. *Hypertension* 1987;9:429–436.

Victor RG, Thoren P, Morgan DA, Mark AL. Differential control of adrenal and renal sympathetic nerve activity during hemorrhagic hypotension in rats. *Circ Res* 1989;64:686–694.

Vieira MA-Coelho MA, Soares-da-Silva P. Dopamine formation, from its immediate precursor 3,4-dihydroxyphenylalanine, along the rate digestive tract. *Fundam Clin Pharmacol* 1993; 7:235–243.

Villacres EC, Hollifield M, Katon WJ, Wilkinson CW, Veith RC. Sympathetic nervous system activity in panic disorder. *Psychiatry Res* 1987;21:313–321.

Vincent HH, Boomsma F, Man in 't Veld AJ, Schalekamp MADH. Stress levels of adrenaline amplify the blood pressure response to sympathetic stimulation. *J Hypertens* 1986;4:255–260.

Vincent HH, Boomsma F, Man in't Veld AJ, Derkx FH, Wenting GJ, Schalekamp MA. Effects of selective and non-selective β-agonists on plasma potassium and norepinephrine. *J Cardiovasc Pharmacol* 1984;6:107–114.

Vincent HH, Man in't Veld AJ, Boomsma F, Wenting GJ, Schalekamp MADH. Elevated plasma noradrenaline in response to beta-adrenoceptor stimulation in man. *Br J Clin Pharmacol* 1982;13:717–721.

Virtanen R. *Claude Bernard and His Place in the History of Ideas.* Lincoln, Neb: University of Nebraska Press, 1960.

Vissing SF, Scherrer U, Victor RG. Relation between sympathetic outflow and vascular resistance in the calf during perturbations in central venous pressure. Evidence for cardiopulmonary afferent regulation of calf vascular resistance in humans. *Circ Res* 1989;65:1710–1717.

Viveros OH, Abou-Donia MM, Lee C-L, Wilson SP, NIchol CA. Control of tissue tetrahydro-biopterin levels through GTP-cyclohydrolase: A factor in the regulation of monoamine synthesis. In Usdin E, Weiner N, Youdim MBH (Eds) *Function and Regulation of Monoamine Enzymes.* New York: Macmillan, 1981, pp 241–250.

Vizi ES, Labos E. Non-synaptic interactions at presynaptic level. *Prog Neurobiol* 1991;37:145–163.

Vlachakis ND, Alexander N. Plasma catecholamines and their major metabolites in spontaneously hypertensive rats. *Life Sci* 1981;29:467–472.

Vlachakis ND, Lampano C, Alexander N, Maronde RF. Catecholamines and their major metabolites in plasma and cerebrospinal fluid of man. *Brain Res* 1981;229:67–74.

Vogel JHK, Jacobowitz D, Chidsey CA. Distribution of norepinephrine in the failing bovine heart. *Circ Res* 1969;24:71–84.

Vogt M. The concentration of sympathin in different parts of the central nervous system under normal conditions and after the administration of drugs. *J Physiol (Lond)* 1954;123:451–481.

Voigt K, Ziegler M, Grunert-Fuchs M, Bickel U, Fehm-Wolfsdorf G. Hormonal responses to exhausting physical exercise: The role of predictability and controllability of the situation. *Psychoneuroendocrinology* 1990;15:173–184.

Vollmer RB, Baruchin A, Kolibal-Pegher SS, Corey SP, Stricker EM, Kaplan BB. Selective activation of norepinephrine- and epinephrine-secreting chromaffin cells in rat adrenal medulla. *Am J Physiol* 1992;263:R716–R721.

von Eiff AW, Czernik A. Der Effekt einer elektrischen Carotis-Sinus-Stimulation auf autonome Funktionen wahrend emotionaler Belastung. *Klin Wochenschr* 1970;48:60–62.

von Euler US, Franksson C, Hellstrom J. Adrenaline and noradrenaline output in urine after unilateral and bilateral adrenalectomy in man. *Acta Physiol Scand* 1954;31:1–5.

von Euler US, Hamberg U. Colorimetric determination of noradrenaline and adrenaline. *Acta Physiol Scand* 1949;19:74–84.

von Euler US, Ikkos D, Luft R. Adrenaline excretion during resting conditions and after insulin in adrenalectomized human subjects. *Acta Endocrinol* 1961;38:441–448.

von Euler US, Lishajko F. Reuptake and net uptake of noradrenaline in adrenergic nerve granules with a note on the affinity of l- and d-isomers. *Acta Physiol Scand* 1967;71:151–162.

von Euler US. A specific sympathomimetic ergone in adrenergic nerve fibres (sympathin) and its relations to adrenaline and nor-adrenaline. *Acta Physiol Scand* 1946;12:73–96.

von Euler US. Identification of the sympathomimetic ergone in adrenergic nerves of cattle (sympathin N) with laevo-noadrenaline. *Acta Physiol Scand* 1948;16:63–74.

von Euler US. Synthesis, uptake and storage of catecholamines in adrenergic nerves, the effect of drugs. In Eichler O, Farah A, Herken H, Welch AD (Eds) *Handbook of Experimental Pharmacology,* Vol XXXIII. New York: Springer-Verlag, 1972, pp 186–230.

von Euler US. The development and applications of the trihydroxyindole method for catechols. *Pharmacol Rev* 1959;11:262–268.

Waagstein F, Hjalmarson A, Varnauska E, Wallentin I. Effect of chronic beta-adrenergic receptor blockade in congestive cardiomyopathy. *Br Heart J* 1975;37:1022–1036.

Wade CE. Response, regulation, and actions of vasopressin during exercise: A review. *Med Sci Sports Exerc* 1984;16:506–511.

Wahi PL, Chakravartai RN, Anand IS, Kumar M, Khuller M, Bhattacharya SK. Noradrenaline induced myocardiopathy in normal and hypercholesterolaemic rhesus monkeys. In Beamish RE, Panagia, V, Dhalla NS (Eds) *Pathogenesis of Stress-Induced Heart Disease.* Boston: Martinus Nijhoff, 1984, pp 261–269.

Wakade TD, Blank MA, Malhotra RK, Pourcho R, Wakade AR. The peptide VIP is a neurotransmitter in rat adrenal medulla: Physiological role in controlling catecholamine secretion. *J Physiol (Lond)* 1991;444:349–362.

Wallach R, Karp RB, Reves JG, Oparil S, Smith LR, James TN. Pathogenesis of paroxysmal hypertension developing during and after coronary bypass surgery: A study of hemodynamic and humoral factors. *Am J Cardiol* 1980;46:559–565.

Wallick DW, Martin PJ, Masuda Y, Levy MN. Effects of autonomic activity and changes in heart rate on atrioventricular conduction. *Am J Physiol* 1982;243:H523–H527.

Wallin BG, Kunimoto MM, Sellgren J. Possible genetic influence on the strength of human muscle nerve sympathetic activity at rest. *Hypertension* 1993;22:282–284.

Wallin BG, Morlin C, Hjemdahl P. Muscle sympathetic activity and venous plasma noradrenaline concentrations during static exercise in normotensive and hypertensive subjects. *Acta Physiol Scand* 1987;129:489–497.

Wallin BG, Sundlof G, Eriksson B-M, Dominiak P, Grobecker H, Lindblad LE. Plasma noradrenaline correlates to sympathetic muscle nerve activity in normotensive man. *Acta Physiol Scand* 1981;111:69–73.

Wallin BG, Sundlof G. Sympathetic outflow to muscles during vasovagal syncope. *J Autonom Nerv Sys* 1982;6:287–291.

Wang P-C, Kuchel O, Buu NT, Genest J. Catecholamine glucuronidation: An important metabolic pathway for dopamine in the rat. *J Neurochem* 1983;40:1435–1440.

Wang PS, Gonzalez HA, Porter JC. Saline ingestion stimulates the in situ molar activity of tyrosine hydroxylase in the median eminence and superior cervical ganglion. *Brain Res* 1988;446:363–368.

Wang SC, Chai CY. Central control of baroreceptor reflex mechanism. In Kezdi P (Ed) *Baroreceptors and Hypertension.* Oxford, UK: Pergamon, 1967, pp 117–130.

Wang SC, Ranson SW. Autonomic responses to electrical stimulation of the lower brain stem. *J Comp Neurol* 1939;71:437–455.

Ward DG, Gunn CG. Locus coeruleus complex: Elicitation of a pressor response and a brain stem region necessary for its occurrence. *Brain Res* 1976;107;401–406.

Ward MM, Mefford IN, Parker SD, Chesney MA, Taylor CB, Keegan DL, Barchas JD. Epinephrine and norepinephrine responses in continuously collected human plasma to a series of stressors. *Psychosom Med* 1983;45:471–486.

Warheit GJ. Occupation: A key factor in stress at the manned space center. In Eliot RS (Ed) *Stress and the Heart*. Mount Kisco, NY: Futura, 1974, pp 51–65.

Warner MR, Sennayake PD, Ferrario CM, Levy MN. Sympathetic stimulation-evoked overflow of norepinephrine and neuropeptide Y from the heart. *Circ Res* 1991;69:455–465.

Warner MR, Wisler PL, Hodges TD, Watanabe AM, Zipes DP. Mechanisms of denervation supersensitivity in regionally denervated canine hearts. *Am J Physiol* 1993;264:H815–H820.

Watabe T, Tanaka K, Kumagae M, Itoh S, Takeda F, Morio K, Hasegawa M, Horiuchi T, Miyabe S, Shimizu N. Hormonal responses to insulin-induced hypoglycemia in man. *J Clin Endocrinol Metab* 1987;65:1187–1191.

Wearn J, Sturgis C. Studies on epinephrine. I: Effects of the injection of epinephrine in soldiers with ''irritable heart.'' *Arch Int Med* 1919;24:247–268.

Webb RL, Brody MJ. Functional identification of the central projections of afferent renal nerves. *Clin Exp Hypertens* 1987;A9 (Suppl 1):47–57.

Webb SA, Adgey AAJ, Pantridge JF. Autonomic disturbance at onset of acute myocardial infarction. *Br Med J* 1972;3:89–92.

Weber F, Brodde OE, Anlauf M, Bock KD. Subclassification of human beta-adrenergic receptors mediating renin release. *Clin Exp Hypertens* 1983;A5:225–238.

Wehrmacher WH, Randall WC. Regulation of the heart in health and disease. In Randall WC (Ed) *Nervous Control of Cardiovascular Function*. New York: Oxford University Press, 1984, pp 3–19.

Weidenfeld J, Feldman S. Effect of hypothalamic norepinephrine depletion on median eminence CRF-41 content and serum ACTH in control and adrenalectomized rats. *Brain Res* 1991; 532:201–204.

Weidmann P, Keusche G, Flammer J, Ziegler WH, Reubi FC. Increased ratio between changes in blood pressure and plasma norepinephrine in essential hypertension. *J Clin Endocrinol Metab* 1979;48:727–731.

Weil-Malherbe H, Axelrod J, Tomchick R. Blood-brain barrier for adrenaline. *Science* 1959;129: 1226–1227.

Weil-Malherbe H, Whitby LG, Axelrod J. The uptake of circulating [³H]norepinephrine by the pituitary gland and various areas of the brain. *J Neurochem* 1961;8:55–64.

Weil-Malherbe H. The fluorimetric estimation of adrenaline, noradrenaline and hydroxytyramine in urine. *Biochem J* 1956;63:4P (Abstract).

Weinberg SJ, Fuster JM. Electrocardiographic changes produced by localized hypothalamic stimulations. *Ann Int Med* 1960;53:332–341.

Weinberger MH, Luft FC, Henry DP. The role of the sympathetic nervous system in the modulation of sodium excretion. *Clin Exp Hypertens* 1982;A4:719–735.

Weiner H. Behavioral biology of stress and psychosomatic medicine. In Brown MR, Koob GF, Rivier C (Eds) *Stress. Neurobiology and Neuroendocrinology*. New York: Marcel Dekker, 1991a, pp 23–51.

Weiner H. Overview. In Weiner H, Florin I, Murison R, Hellhammer D (Eds) *Frontiers of Stress Research*. New York: Hans Huber, 1989, pp 405–418.

Weiner H. Stressful experience and cardiorespiratory disorders. *Circulation* 1991b;83 (Suppl II): II2–II8.

Weiner N, Lee FL, Dreyer E, Barnes E. The activation of tyrosine hydroxylase in noradrenergic neurons during acute nerve stimulation. *Life Sci* 1978;22:1197–1216.

Weinshilboum RM, Thoa NB, Johnson DG, Kopin IJ, Axelrod J. Proportional release of norepinephrine and dopamine-beta-hydroxylase from sympathetic nerves. *Science* 1971;174: 1349–1351.

Weinstock M, Schorer-Apelbaum D, Rosin AJ. Endogenous opiates mediate cardiac sympathetic inhibition in response to a pressor stimulus in rabbits. *J Hypertens* 1984;2:639–646.

Weise VK, Kopin IJ. Assay of catecholamines in human plasma. Studies of a single isotope radioenzymatic procedure. *Life Sci* 1976;19:1673–1685.

Weiss JM, Goodman PA, Losito BG, Corrigan S, Charry JM, Bailey WH. Behavioural depression produced by an uncontrollable stressor: Relationship to norepinephrine, dopamine and serotonin levels in various regions of rat brain. *Brain Res Rev* 1981;3:167–205.

Weiss JM. Effects of coping behaviour in different warning signal conditions on stress pathology in rats. *J Comp Physiol Psychol* 1971;77:1–13.

Weiss JM. Somatic effects of predictable and unpredictable shock. *Psychosom Med* 1970;32: 397–408.

Welsh JH, Catecholamines in the invertebrates. In Eichler O, Farah A, Herken H, Welch AD (Eds) *Handbook of Experimental Pharmacology,* Vol XXXIII. New York: Springer-Verlag, 1972, pp 79–109.

Wenger MA, Clemens T, Darsie MC, Engel BT, Estess FM, Sonnenschein RR. Autonomic response patterns during intravenous infusion of epinephrine and norepinephrine. *Psychosom Med* 1960;22:294–307.

Wertlake PT, Wilcox AA, Haley MI, Peterson JE. Relationship of mental and emotional stress to serum cholesterol levels. *Proc Soc Exp Biol Med* 1958;97:163–168.

Westfall TC, Badino L, Naes L, Meldrum MJ. Alterations in the field stimulation-induced release of endogenous norepinephrine from the coccygeal artery of spontaneously hypertensive and Wistar-Kyoto rats. *Eur J Pharmacol* 1987;135:433–437.

Westlund K, Denney R, Kochersberger L, Rose R, Abell C. Distinct monoamine oxidase A and B populations in primate brain. *Science* 1985;230:180–183.

Westlund KN, Bowker RM, Ziegler MG, Coulter JD. Organization of descending noradrenergic systems. In Ziegler MG, Lake CR (Eds) *Norepinephrine.* Baltimore: Williams & Wilkins, 1984, pp 55–73.

White TD. Role of adenine compounds in autonomic neurotransmission. *Pharmacol Ther* 1988; 38:129–168.

Wichter T, Hindricks G, Lerch H, Bartenstein P, Borggrefe M, Schober O, Breithardt G. Regional myocardial sympathetic dysinnervation in arrhythmogenic right ventricular cardiomyopathy. An analysis using ^{123}I-meta-iodobenzylguanidine scintigraphy. *Circulation* 1994; 89:667–683.

Widimsky J, Fejfarova MH, Fejfar Z. Changes of cardiac output in hypertensive disease. *Cardiologia* 1957;31:381–389.

Widmaier EP, Lim AT, Vale W. Secretion of corticotropin-releasing factor from culture rat hypothalamic cells: Effects of catecholamines. *Endocrinology* 1989;124:583–590.

Wieland DM, Rosenspire KC, Hutchins GD, Van Dort M, Rothley JM, Mislankar SG, Lee HT, Massin CC, Gildersleeve DL, Sherman PS, Schwaiger M. Neuronal mapping of the heart with 6-[^{18}F]fluorometaraminol. *J Med Chem* 1990;33:956–964.

Wikberg JES, Andersson JR, Lundholm L. Differentiation of adrenergic alpha-receptors in guinea pig intestine and rabbit aorta. *Blood Vessels* 1975;12:383–384.

Wikberg JES, Lefkowitz RJ. Adrenergic receptors in the heart: Pre- and postsynaptic mechanisms. In Randall WC (Ed) *Nervous Control of Cardiovascular Function*. New York: Oxford University Press, 1984, pp 95–129.

Wikberg JES. Pharmacological classification of adrenergic alpha receptors in the guinea pig. *Nature* 1978;273:164–166.

Wiley RG. Lesioning autonomic neurones using suicide transport and immunolesioning. *Clin Auton Res* 1993;3:215.

Wilffert B, Timmermans PBMWM, van Zwieten PA. Extrasynaptic location of *alpha*-2 and noninnervated *beta*-2 adrenoceptors in the vascular system of the pithed normotensive rat. *J Pharmacol Exp Ther* 1982;221:762–768.

Will-Shahab L, Schubert B. Functional status of sympathetic system in cardiovascular disease: Myocardial infarction. In Ganguly PK (Ed) *Catecholamines and Heart Disease*. Boca Raton, Fla: CRC Press, 1991, pp 123–143.

Willette RN, Barcas PP, Krieger AJ, Sapru HN. Vasopressor and depressor areas in the rat medulla. Identification by microinjection of L-glutamate. *Neuropharmacology* 1983;22:1071–1079.

Willette RN, Krieger AJ, Barcas PP, Sapru HN. Medullary aminobutyric acid (GABA) receptors and the regulation of blood pressure in the rat. *J Pharmacol Exp Ther* 1983;226:893–899.

Williams GH, Hollenberg NK. Are non-modulating patients with essential hypertension a distinct subgroup? Implications for therapy. *Am J Med* 1985;79 (Suppl 3C):3–9.

Williams LT, Lefkowitz RJ, Watanabe AM, Hathaway DR, Besch HR. Thyroid hormone regulation of beta adrenergic receptor number. *J Biol Chem* 1977;57:149–155.

Williams M, Young JB, Rosa RM, Gunn S, Epstein FH, Landsberg L. Effect of protein ingestion on urinary dopamine excretion. Evidence for the functional importance of renal decarboxylation of circulating 3,4-dihydroxyphenylalanine in man. *J Clin Invest* 1986;78:1687–1693.

Williams PD, Puddey IB, Beilin LJ, Vandongen R. Genetic influences on plasma catecholamines in human twins. *J Clin Endocrinol Metab* 1993;77:794–799.

Williams RB Jr, Haney TL, Lee KI, Kong YH, Blumenthal JA, Whalen RE. Type A behavior, hostility and coronary atherosclerosis. *Psychosom Med* 1980;42:539–549.

Williams RB Jr. *Neurocardiology*. Kalamazoo, Mich: The Upjohn Company, 1989.

Williams RB Jr. The role of the brain in physical disease. Folklore, normal science, or paradigm shift? *J Am Med Assoc* 1990;263:1971–1972.

Williams RB, Lane JD, Kuhn CM, Melosh W, White AD, Schanberg SM. Type A behavior and elevated physiological and neuroendocrine responses to cognitive tasks. *Science* 1982;218:483–485.

Willich SN, Linderer T, Wegscheider K, Leizorovicz A, Alamercery I, Schroder R. Increased morning incidence of myocardial infarction in the ISAM study: Absence with prior β-adrenergic blockade. *Circulation* 1989;80:853–858.

Willich SN, Maclure M, Mittleman M, Arntz H-R, Muller JE. Sudden cardiac death. Support for a role of triggering in causation. *Circulation* 1993;87:1442–1450.

Willius FA, Keys TE. *Classics of Cardiology*. New York: Dover Publications, 1961.

Winkler H. Occurrence and mechanism of exocytosis in adrenal medulla and sympathetic nerve. In Trendelenburg U, Weiner N (Eds) *Catecholamines*, Vol I. New York: Springer-Verlag, 1988, pp 43–118.

Winternitz SR, Wyss JM, Oparil S. The role of the posterior hypothalamic area in the pathogenesis of hypertension in the spontaneously hypertensive rat. *Brain Res* 1984;324:51–58.

Winters RW, Ironson GH, Schneiderman N. The neurobiology of anxiety. In Byrne DG, Rosenman RH (Eds) *Anxiety and the Heart.* New York: Hemisphere Publishing, 1990, pp 187–210.

Witze DJ, Kaye MP. Hypertrophic cardiomyopathy induced by administration of nerve growth factor. *Circulation* 1976; 53/54 (Suppl 2):II88 (Abstract).

Wolf S, Goodell H, Harold G. *Wolff's Stress and Disease,* 2nd ed. Springfield, Ill: CC Thomas, 1968.

Wolf S. Psychosocial forces in myocardial infarction and sudden death. *Circulation* 1969; (Suppl IV):39–40:74–81.

Wolf SG. History of the study of stress and heart disease. In Beamish RE, Singal PK, Dhalla NS (Eds) *Stress and Heart Disease.* Boston: Martinus Nijhoff, 1985, pp 3–16.

Wolf SG. Stress and heart disease. *Mod Concepts Cardiovasc Dis* 1960;29:599–603.

Wolf SG, Cardon PV, Shepard EM, Wolff HG. *Life Stress and Essential Hypertension.* Baltimore: Williams & Wilkins, 1955.

Wolf SG, McCabe WR, Yamamoto J, Adsett CA, Schottstaedt WW. Changes in serum lipids in relation to emotional stress during rigid control of diet and exercise. *Circulation* 1962; 26:379–387.

Wolfovitz E, Grossman E, Folio CJ, Keiser HR, Kopin IJ. Derivation of urinary dopamine from plasma dihydroxyphenylalanine (DOPA) in humans. *Clin Sci* 1993; 84:549–557.

Wollenberger A, Shahab L. Anoxia-induced release of noradrenaline from the isolated perfused heart. *Nature* 1965;207:88–89.

Woodward DJ, Moises HC, Waterhouse BD, Hoffer BJ, Freedman R. Modulatory actions of norepinephrine in the central nervous system. *Fed Proc* 1979;2109–2116.

Wortsman J, Frank S, Cryer PE. Adrenomedullary response to maximal stress in humans. *Am J Med* 1984;77:779–784.

Wortsman J, Nowak RM, Martin GB, Paradis NA, Cryer PE. Plasma epinephrine levels in resuscitation with cardiopulmonary bypass. *Crit Care Med* 1990;18:1134–1137.

Woulfe JM, Flumerfelt BA, Hrycyshyn AW. Efferent connections of the A1 noradrenergic cell group: A DBH immunohistochemical and PHA-L anterograde tracing study. *Exp Neurol* 1990;109:308–322.

Wurtman RJ, Axelrod J. Control of enzymatic synthesis of adrenaline in the adrenal medulla by adrenal cortical steroids. *J Biol Chem* 1966;241:2301–2305.

Wurtman RJ, Hefti F, Melamed E. Precursor control of neurotransmitter synthesis. *Pharmacol Rev* 1981;32:315–335.

Xie P, McDowell TS, Chapleua MW, Hajduczok G, Abboud FM. Rapid baroreceptor resetting in chronic hypertension. Implications for normalization of arterial pressure. *Hypertension* 1991;17:72–79.

Yadid G, Pacak K, Kopin IJ, Goldstein DS. Modified microdialysis probe for sampling extracellular fluid and administering drugs *in vivo. Am J Physiol* 1993; 265:R1205–R1211.

Yaksh TL. Pharmacology of spinal adrenergic systems which modulate spinal nociceptive processing. *Pharmacol Biochem Behav* 1985;22:845–858.

Yamada Y, Miyajima E, Tochikubo O, Matsukawa T, Ishii M. Age-related changes in muscle sympathetic nerve activity in essential hypertension. *Hypertension* 1989;13(6 Pt 2):870–877.

Yamaguchi I, Jose PA, Mouradian M, Canessa LM, Monsma FJ Jr, Sibley DR, Takeyasu K,

Felder RA. Expression of dopamine D_{1A} receptor gene in proximal tubule of rat kidneys. *Am J Physiol* 1993;264:F280–F285.

Yamaguchi I, Kopin IJ. Plasma catecholamines and blood pressure responses to sympathetic stimulation in pithed rats. *Am J Physiol* 1979;237:H305–H310.

Yamaguchi N, Brassard M. A differential effect of yohimbine on adrenal and neuronal catecholamine release during bilateral carotid occlusion in the dog. *J Auton Nerv Sys* 1988; 25:141–153.

Yamaguchi N, Briand R, Brassard M. Direct evidence that an increase in aortic norepinephrine level in response to insulin-induced hypoglycemia is due to increased adrenal norepinephrine output. *Can J Physiol Pharmacol* 1989;67:499–505.

Yamaguchi N, De Champlain J, Nadeau RA. Regulation of norepinephrine release form cardiac sympathetic fibers in the dog by presynaptic alpha- and beta-receptor. *Circ Rec* 1977;41: 108–117.

Yamamoto J, Akabane S, Yoshimi H, Nakai M, Ikeda M. Effects of taurine on stress-evoked hemodynamic and plasma catecholamine changes in spontaneously hypertensive rats. *Hypertension* 1985;7:913–922.

Yamamoto J, Nakai M, Natsume T. Cardiovascular responses to acute stress in young-to-old spontaneously hypertensive rats. *Hypertension* 1987;9:362–370.

Yamashita H, Kannan H, Ueta Y. Involvement of caudal ventrolateral medulla neurons in mediating visceroceptive information to the hypothalamic paraventricular nucleus. *Prog Brain Res* 1989;81:293–302.

Yamori Y, Iawawa T, Kanbe T, Kihara M, Nara Y, Horie R. Mechanisms of structural vascular changes in genetic hypertension: Analyses of cultured vascular smooth muscle cells from spontanouesly hypertensive rats. *Clin Sci* 1981;61:121s–123s.

Yamori Y, Tarazi RC, Ooshima A. Effect of beta-receptor-blocking agents on cardiovascular structural changes in spontaneous and noradrenaline-induced hypertension in rats. *Clin Sci* 1980;59:457s–460s.

Yao H, Fukiyama K, Takada Y, Fujishima M, Omae T. Neurogenic hypertension in the Guillain-Barre syndrome. *Jpn Heart J* 1985;26:593–596.

Yarbrough GG, Taylor DA, Antolik EK, Robinson EL. Spontaneously hypertensive rats exhibit an enhanced mydriatic response to clonidine. Evidence for enhanced sensitivity of central alpha 2-adrenoceptors. *Can J Physiol Pharmacol* 1983;61:764–766.

Yeh BK, McNay JL, Goldberg LI. Attenuation of dopamine renal and mesenteric vasodilation by haloperidol: Evidence for a specific dopamine receptor. *J Pharmacol Exp Ther* 1969; 168:303–309.

Yokoo H, Tanaka M, Yoshida M, Tsuda A, Tanaka T, Mizoguchi K. Direct evidence of conditioned fear-elicited enhancement of noradrenaline release in the rat hypothalamus assessed by intracranial microdialysis. *Brain Res* 1990;536:305–308.

Yoshimatsu H, Oomura Y, Katafuchi T, Niijima A. Effects of hypothalamic stimulation and lesion on adrenal nerve activity. *Am J Physiol* 1987;253:R418–R424.

Yoshimura M, Kambara S, Takahashi H, Okabayashi H, Ijichi H. Involvement of dopamine in development of hypertension in spontaneously hypertensive rat: Effect of carbidopa, inhibitor of peripheral DOPA decarboxylase. *Clin Exp Hypertens* 1987;A9:1585–1599.

Youdim MBH, Finberg JPM, Tipton KF. Monoamine oxidase. In Trendelenburg U, Weiner N (Eds) *Catecholamines I.* New York: Springer-Verlag, 1988, pp 119–192.

Youdim MBH, Finberg JPM. Monoamine oxidase inhibitor antidepressants. In Grahame-Smith DG, Cowen PJ (Eds) *Psychopharmacology I, Part 1: Preclinical Psychopharmacology.* Amersterdam: Excerpta Medica, 1982, pp 38–70.

Young IM. Some observations on the mechanism of adrenaline hyperpnoea. *J Physiol (Lond)* 1957;137:374–395.

Young JB, Landsberg L. Sympathoadrenal activity in fasting pregnant rats. Dissociation of adrenal medullary and sympathetic nervous system responses. *J Clin Invest* 1979;64:109–116.

Young JB, Rosa RM, Landsberg L. Dissociation of sympathetic nervous system and adrenal medullary responses. *Am J Physiol* 1984;247:E35–E40.

Zanchetti A, Mancia G. Cardiovascular reflexes and hypertension. *Hypertension* 1991;18 (Suppl III):III13–III21.

Zandberg P, De Jong W, De Wied D. Effect of catecholamine-receptor stimulating agents on blood pressure after local application in the nucleus tractus solitarii of the medulla oblongata. *Eur J Pharmacol* 1979;55:43–56.

Zavodskaya IS, Moreva EV, Novikova NA. *Neurogenic Heart Lesions.* Oxford, UK: Pergamon Press, 1980.

Zeiher AM, Drexler H, Wollschlaeger H, Saurbier B, Just H. Coronary vasomotion in response to sympathetic stimulation in humans: Importance of the functional integrity of the endothelium. *J Am Coll Cardiol* 1989;14:1181–1190.

Zerbe RL, Feuerstein G, Meyer DK, Kopin IJ. Cardiovascular, sympathetic, and renin-angiotensin system responses to hemorrhage in vasopressin-deficient rats. *Endocrinology* 1982;111:608–613.

Zhang T-X, Ciriello J. Lesions of paraventricular nucleus reverse the elevated arterial pressure after aortic baroreceptor denervation in the rat. *Neurosci Abstr* 1982;8:434.

Zhang T-X, Harper RM, Ni H. Cryogenic blockade of the central nucleus of the amygdala attenuates aversively conditioned blood pressure and respiratory responses. *Brain Res* 1986;386:136–145.

Ziegler MG, Echon C, Wilner KD, Specho P, Lake CR, McCutchen JA. Sympathetic nervous withdrawal in the vasodepressor (vasovagal) reaction. *J Auton Nerv Sys* 1986;17:273–278.

Ziegler MG, Kennedy B, Elayan H. Rat renal epinephrine synthesis. *J Clin Invest* 1989;84:1130–1133.

Ziegler MG, Lake CR, Ebert MH. Norepinephrine elevations in cerebrospinal fluid after *d-* and *l-*amphetamine. *Eur J Pharmacol* 1979a;57:127–133.

Ziegler MG, Lake CR, Kopin IJ. Plasma noradrenaline increases with age. *Nature* 1976;261:333–335.

Ziegler MG, Lake CR, Kopin IJ. The sympathetic-nervous-system defect in primary orthostatic hypotension. *N Engl J Med* 1977a;296:293–297.

Ziegler MG, Lake CR, Williams AC, Teychenne PF, Shoulson I, Steinsland O. Bromocriptine inhibits norepinephrine release. *Clin Pharmacol Ther* 1979b;25:137–142.

Ziegler MG, Lake CR, Wood JH, Brooks BR, Ebert MH. Relationship between norepinephrine in blood and cerebrospinal fluid in the presence of a blood-cerebrospinal fluid barrier for norepinephrine. *J Neurochem* 1977b;28:677–679.

Ziegler MG, Milano AJ, Lake CR. Increased cerebrospinal fluid norepinephrine in essential hypertension. *Clin Exp Hypertens* 1982;4:663–674.

Ziegler MG, Morrissey EC, Kennedy B, Elayan H. Sources of urinary catecholamines in renal denervated transplant recipients. *J Hypertens* 1990;8:927–931.

Zierhut W, Zimmer H-G. Significance of myocardial α- and β-adrenoceptors in catecholamine-induced cardiac hypertrophy. *Circ Res* 1989;65:1417–1425.

Zimanyi I, Folly G, Vizi ES. Inhibition of K^+ permeability diminishes alpha$_2$-adrenoceptor mediated effects on norepinephrine release. *J Neurosci Res* 1988;20:102–108.

Zimlichman R, Goldstein DS, Eisenhofer G, Stull R, Keiser HR. Comparison of norepinephrine and isoproterenol removal in the canine hindlimb and kidney. *Clin Exp Pharmacol Physiol* 1986;13:777–781.

Zimlichman R, Goldstein DS, Stull R, Folio CJ, Keiser HR. Dietary salt intake and the clonidine suppression test. *J Clin Pharmacol* 1987;27:199–205.

Zimlichman R, Goldstein DS, Zimlichman S, Keiser HR. Angiotensin II increases cytosolic calcium and stimulates catecholamine release in cultured bovine adrenomedullary cells. *Cell Calcium* 1987;8:315–325.

Zimlichman R, Levinson PD, Kelly G, Stull R, Keiser HR, Goldstein DS. Derivation of urinary dopamine from plasma dihydroxyphenylalanine. *Clin Sci* 1988;75:515–520.

Zimmerman BG. Actions of angiotensin on adrenergic nerve endings. *Fed Proc* 1978;37:199–202.

Zimmerman BG. Adrenergic facilitation by facilitation by angiotensin: does it serve a physiological function? *Clin Sci* 1981;60:343–348.

Zipes DP, Inoue H. Autonomic neural control of cardiac excitable properties. In Kulbertus HE, Franck G (Eds) *Neurocardiology*. Mount Kisco, NY: Futura, 1988, pp 59–84.

Zipes DP. Influence of myocardial ischemia and infarction on autonomic innervation of heart. *Circulation* 1990;82:1095–1105.

Zweifler A, Gross M, Sisson J. Effect of phenoxybenzamine on cardiovascular and plasma catecholamine responses to clonidine. *Clin Pharmacol Ther* 1983;33:156–162.

Index